RADIOLOGY
SECRETS PLUS

RADIOLOGY SECRETS PLUS

THIRD EDITION

E. SCOTT PRETORIUS, MD

Director of Magnetic Resonance Imaging
USTeleradiology
Palm Springs, California

JEFFREY A. SOLOMON, MD, MBA

Assistant Professor of Radiology and
Health Care Management
Hospital of the University of Pennsylvania
Philadelphia, Pennsylvania

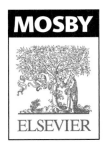

MOSBY

ELSEVIER

MOSBY
ELSEVIER

1600 John F. Kennedy Blvd.
Ste 1800
Philadelphia, PA 19103-2899

RADIOLOGY SECRETS PLUS   ISBN: 978-0-323-06794-2

Notice

Knowledge and best practice in this field are constantly changing. As new research and experience broaden our knowledge, changes in practice, treatment, and drug therapy may become necessary or appropriate. Readers are advised to check the most current information provided (i) on procedures featured or (ii) by the manufacturer of each product to be administered, to verify the recommended dose or formula, the method and duration of administration, and contraindications. It is the responsibility of the practitioner, relying on his or her own experience and knowledge of the patient, to make diagnoses, to determine dosages and the best treatment for each individual patient, and to take all appropriate safety precautions. To the fullest extent of the law, neither the Publisher nor the Editors assume any liability for any injury and/or damage to persons or property arising out of or related to any use of the material contained in this book.

The Publisher

Library of Congress Cataloging-in-Publication Data
Radiology secrets plus. – 3rd ed. / [edited by] E. Scott Pretorius, Jeffrey A. Solomon.
    p. ; cm. – (Secrets series)
  Rev. ed. of: Radiology secrets / E. Scott Pretorius, Jeffrey A. Solomon. c2006.
  Includes bibliographical references and index.
  ISBN 978-0-323-06794-2
  1. Diagnostic imaging–Examinations, questions, etc.   2. Diagnostic imaging–Miscellanea.   I. Pretorius, E. Scott.
II. Solomon, Jeffrey A.   IIII. Radiology secrets.   IV. Series: Secrets series.
  [DNLM: 1. Radiology–Examination Questions. WN 18.2 R1296 2011]
  RC78.7.D53R352 2011
  616.07'54076–dc22   2010011616

Acquisitions Editor: James Merritt
Developmental Editors: Andrea Vosburgh, Andrew Hall
Publishing Services Manager: Hemamalini Rajendrababu
Project Managers: Shereen Jameel/Srikumar Narayanan
Designer: Steven Stave
Marketing Manager: Jason Oberacker

Printed in Canada

Last digit is the print number: 9 8 7 6 5 4 3 2 1

To the memory of our dear departed colleagues,
Sridhar R. Charagundla, MD, PhD and
Saroja Adusumilli, MD

PREFACE

We both came to Penn Radiology in 1995 to be first-year residents at the University of Pennsylvania. Throughout our residencies and our preparation for our radiology board examinations, we yearned for a book that contained what we "really" needed to know, a book that neatly distilled the most important points from each subspecialty of radiology.

Sadly, we never found such a book. That, however, is exactly what we have sought to create: an eminently practical book that touches on all of the "high points" of each of radiology's subspecialties. To the extent that we have succeeded, we are indebted to our coauthors and to our many students, residents, and fellows. This book was written for you.

E. Scott Pretorius, MD
Jeffrey A. Solomon, MD, MBA

ACKNOWLEDGMENT

The authors thank Charles T. Lau, MD, for his considerable assistance in the preparation of this third edition.

CONTRIBUTORS

Linda J. Bagley, MD
Associate Professor of Radiology, Neuroradiology Section, Hospital of the University of Pennsylvania, Philadelphia, Pennsylvania

Jonathan N. Balcombe, MBBS
Fellow, Cardiovascular Imaging, Hospital of the University of Pennsylvania, Philadelphia, Pennsylvania

Richard D. Bellah, MD
Associate Professor of Radiology, Children's Hospital of Philadelphia, Philadelphia, Pennsylvania

Judy S. Blebea, MD
Professor of Radiology, Musculoskeletal Section, Hospital of the University of Pennsylvania, Philadelphia, Pennsylvania

William W. Boonn, MD
Associate Clinical Director of Imaging Informatics, Hospital of the University of Pennsylvania, Philadelphia, Pennsylvania

Kerry Bron, MD
Radiologist, Philadelphia, Pennsylvania

Lucas Buchanan, MBA
Wharton School of Business, Philadelphia, Pennsylvania

Sridhar R. Charagundla, MD, PhD
Assistant Professor of Radiology, Magnetic Resonance Imaging and Cardiovascular Sections, Department of Radiology, Hospital of the University of Pennsylvania, Philadelphia, Pennsylvania

Beverly G. Coleman, MD, FACR
Professor of Radiology, Associate Chair for Abdominal Imaging, Ultrasound Section Chief, Hospital of the University of Pennsylvania, Philadelphia, Pennsylvania

Keith A. Ferguson, MD
Radiologist, Radiology Associates of West Florida, Brandon, Florida

Denise Fog, DO
Radiologist, Booth Radiology Associates, Woodbury, New Jersey

Jeffrey Scott Friedenberg, MD
Radiologist, Manalapan, New Jersey

Sara Chen Gavenonis, MD
Breast Imaging Section, Hospital of the University of Pennsylvania, Philadelphia, Pennsylvania

Gregory Goodworth, MD
Radiologist, Cherry Hill, New Jersey

Andrew Gordon, MD
Radiologist, Upland, Pennsylvania

Susan Hilton, MD
Clinical Professor of Radiology, CT Section Co-Chief, Hospital of the University of Pennsylvania, Philadelphia, Pennsylvania

Wendy C. Hsu, MD
Associate Program Director, Radiology Residency, Virginia Mason Medical Center, Seattle, Washington

Maxim Itkin, MD
Adjunct Assistant Professor, Interventional Radiology Section, Hospital of the University of Pennsylvania, Philadelphia, Pennsylvania

Saurabh Jha, MBBS
Assistant Professor of Radiology, Cardiovascular Section, Hospital of the University of Pennsylvania, Philadelphia, Pennsylvania

Lisa Jones, MD, PhD
Assistant Professor of Radiology, Hospital of the University of Pennsylvania, Philadelphia, Pennsylvania

Andrew J. Kapustin, MD
Radiologist, Mecklenburg Radiology Associates, Charlotte, North Carolina

Ann K. Kim, MD
Assistant Professor of Neurology, Neuroradiology Section, Hospital of the University of Pennsylvania, Philadelphia, Pennsylvania

Woojin Kim, MD
Assistant Professor of Radiology, Musculoskeletal Section, Hospital of the University of Pennsylvania, Philadelphia, Pennsylvania

Charles T. Lau, MD
Fellow, Thoracic Imaging Section, Hospital of the University of Pennsylvania, Philadelphia, Pennsylvania

Harold I. Litt, MD, PhD
Assistant Professor of Radiology, Cardiovascular Imaging, and Section Chief, Hospital of the University of Pennsylvania, Philadelphia, Pennsylvania

Laurie A. Loevner, MD
Professor of Radiology, Otorhinolaryngology, Head and Neck Surgery, and Neurosurgery, Hospital of the University of Pennsylvania, Philadelphia, Pennsylvania

Gautham Mallampati, MD
Radiologist, Atlanta, Georgia

Wallace T. Miller, Jr., MD
Associate Professor of Radiology, Thoracic Imaging Section, Hospital of the University of Pennsylvania, Philadelphia, Pennsylvania

Jeffrey I. Mondschein, MD
Assistant Professor of Radiology, Interventional Section, Hospital of the University of Pennsylvania, Philadelphia, Pennsylvania

D. Andrew Mong, MD
Pediatric Radiologist, Nighthawk Radiology Services, San Francisco, California

Gul Moonis, MD
Assistant Professor of Radiology, Beth Israel Deaconess Medical Center, Harvard Medical School, Boston, Massachusetts

Andrew Newberg, MD
Associate Professor of Radiology, Nuclear Medicine Section, Hospital of the University of Pennsylvania, Philadelphia, Pennsylvania

Joseph R. Perno, MD, PhD
Radiologist, VA Medical Center of Philadelphia; Clinical Assistant Professor of Radiology, University of Pennsylvania School of Medicine, Philadelphia, Pennsylvania

Linda K. Petrovich, MD
Radiologist, Lutz, Florida

Avrum N. Pollock, MD, FRCPC
Assistant Professor of Radiology, Children's Hospital of Philadelphia, Philadelphia, Pennsylvania

E. Scott Pretorius, MD
Director of Magnetic Resonance Imaging, USTeleradiology, Palm Springs, California

Parvati Ramchandani, MD
Professor of Radiology, Genitourinary Section, Hospital of the University of Pennsylvania, Philadelphia, Pennsylvania

Neil Roach, MD
Radiologist, Diagnostic Imaging, Inc., Philadelphia, Pennsylvania

Mark Rosen, MD, PhD
Magnetic Resonance Imaging Section, Hospital of the University of Pennsylvania, Philadelphia, Pennsylvania

Susan E. Rowling, MD
Clinical Assistant Professor of Radiology, Hospital of the University of Pennsylvania, Philadelphia, Pennsylvania

Stephen E. Rubesin, MD
Professor of Radiology, Gastrointestinal Section, Hospital of the University of Pennsylvania, Philadelphia, Pennsylvania

Mary Scanlon, MD
Clinical Associate Professor, Neuroradiology Section, Hospital of the University of Pennsylvania, Philadelphia, Pennsylvania

Milan Sheth, MD
Chief of Chest Radiology, Morristown Memorial Hospital, Morristown, New Jersey

Richard Shlansky-Goldberg, MD
Associate Professor of Radiology, Magnetic Resonance Imaging Section Chief, Hospital of the University of Pennsylvania, Philadelphia, Pennsylvania

Conor P. Shortt, MBBCh, MSc, FFR, RCSI
Fellow, Abdominal Imaging, Hospital of the University of Pennsylvania, Philadelphia, Pennsylvania

Evan S. Siegelman, MD
Section Chief Body MRI, Hospital of the University of Pennsylvania, Philadelphia, Pennsylvania

Ross I. Silver, MD
Radiologist, St. Luke's Hospital, Bethlehem, Pennsylvania

Jeffrey A. Solomon, MD, MBA
Assistant Professor of Radiology and Health Care Management, Hospital of the University of Pennsylvania, Philadelphia, Pennsylvania

S. William Stavropoulos, MD
Assistant Professor of Radiology, Interventional Section, Associate Chair of Clinical Operations, Hospital of the University of Pennsylvania, Philadelphia, Pennsylvania

Drew A. Torigian, MD, MA
Assistant Professor of Radiology, Thoracic, and Magnetic Resonance Imaging Sections, Hospital of the University of Pennsylvania, Philadelphia, Pennsylvania

Susan P. Weinstein, MD
Abdominal Imaging, Hospital of the University of Pennsylvania, Philadelphia, Pennsylvania

Courtney Woodfield, MD
Assistant Professor, Department of Diagnostic Imaging, The Warren Alpert Medical School of Brown University; Women and Infants Hospital; Rhode Island Hospital, Providence, Rhode Island

Christopher J. Yoo, MD
Radiologist, San Francisco, California

Hanna M. Zafar, MD, MHS
Assistant Professor of Radiology, Abdominal Imaging, Hospital of the University of Pennsylvania, Philadelphia, Pennsylvania

CONTENTS

TOP 100 SECRETS

These secrets are 100 of the top board alerts. They summarize the concepts, principles, and most salient details of radiology.

1. Increasing voltage (kV) decreases contrast and increases exposure, making the film darker. Increasing milliampere-seconds (mAs) increases exposure, making the film darker.

2. A scout film should always be obtained before performing a fluoroscopy study with a contrast agent. The scout film allows the radiologist to determine whether an object that appears "white" on a radiograph is bone or metal versus contrast (the latter would not be on the scout film).

3. Structures in the body that are very dense (such as structures that contain calcium) attenuate a large amount of the x-ray beam; the x-ray beam is unable to reach the film and darken it, and such structures appear white on a radiograph. Conversely, structures that are not very dense (such as air) allow the x-ray beam to penetrate and darken the film; such structures appear black.

4. Regions with many acoustic interfaces reflect a lot of sound back to the transducer. These are termed *echogenic* or *hyperechoic,* and by convention are viewed as bright areas on ultrasound (US). Regions with few acoustic interfaces do not reflect many sound waves; they are termed *hypoechoic* and are viewed as dark areas.

5. Electron-dense structures, such as metal and bone, stop a large number of x-rays and are bright on computed tomography (CT). Regions with lower electron density, such as air or fat, stop very few x-rays and are rendered as dark. Because CT images are created with x-rays, the same things that are bright and dark on plain films are bright and dark on CT.

6. T1-weighted images have a short "time to repetition" (TR) (<1000 ms) and a short "time to echo" (TE) (<20 ms). T2-weighted images have a long TR (>2000 ms) and a long TE (>40 ms).

7. To differentiate between T1-weighted and T2-weighted images, look for simple fluid. Fluid tends to be hyperintense to virtually everything else on T2-weighted images. On T1-weighted images, fluid is of low intermediate signal. Good places to look for fluid include the urinary bladder and the cerebrospinal fluid.

8. Nuclear medicine is unique in that its strength lies in portraying the functional status of an organ, rather than producing images that are predominantly anatomic in content.

9. In nuclear medicine studies, the radiologist administers a radioactive atom, either alone or coupled to a molecule, that is known to target a certain organ or organs. Its distribution is examined to determine any pathologic condition in that particular organ.

10. PACS stands for *picture archiving and communication systems.* These are the systems used by digital radiology departments to store, network, and view imaging studies.

11. RIS stands for *radiology information system*. RIS manages patient scheduling and tracking, examination billing, and receipt/display of radiology reports.

12. The American College of Radiology recommends that women begin getting mammograms at age 40 and annually thereafter.

13. The BIRADS (Breast Imaging Reporting and Dictation System) lexicon was developed by the American College of Radiology to provide a clear and concise way to report mammographic results: 1 = normal; 2 = benign finding; 3 = probably benign finding (6-month follow-up mammogram recommended); 4 = suspicious finding (biopsy recommended); 5 = high likelihood of malignancy (biopsy recommended); and 6 = confirmed malignancy. Category 0 indicates that further imaging is required.

14. Breast US is useful in characterizing palpable masses or mammographically detected masses as cystic or solid. Findings in a solid lesion that are suspicious for malignancy include a hypoechoic appearance with posterior acoustic shadowing, angular margins, spiculations, microlobulations, lesion morphology "taller" than "wide," and ductal extension of the mass.

15. Findings on breast magnetic resonance imaging (MRI) suspicious for malignancy in an enhancing lesion include avid arterial phase enhancement, washout of contrast agent in a delayed phase, spiculated or microlobulated margins, greater enhancement peripherally than centrally, and architectural distortion.

16. Anomalous origin of the coronary arteries occurs rarely (about 1% of cardiac catheterizations). Sudden death is associated with a left main coronary artery that arises from the right sinus (particularly when the artery courses between the aorta and pulmonary artery), a right coronary artery that arises from the left sinus, and a single coronary artery. The left main coronary artery may also arise from the pulmonary trunk; this anomaly tends to manifest earlier, with congestive heart failure or sudden death.

17. Aortic dissections that involve the ascending aorta are surgical emergencies because the mortality rate is significantly greater in medically managed patients (approximately 90% in the first 3 months) compared with surgically treated patients. This high mortality rate is mostly due to hemopericardium, causing tamponade; acute aortic regurgitation; or involvement of coronary artery origins, causing myocardial infarction. Descending aortic dissections are usually treated medically with antihypertensive agents.

18. The most specific finding of a pulmonary embolus is a partial or complete intraluminal filling defect in a pulmonary artery. On CT angiography, the filling defect should be present on at least two contiguous sections. Abrupt cutoff of the artery also indicates a pulmonary embolus.

19. A stenosis is generally considered significant if the luminal diameter is reduced by 50%, and the systolic pressure gradient is greater than 10 mm Hg across the lesion. A vessel lumen that is diminished by 50% would have a corresponding 75% reduction in a cross-sectional area, which would likely reduce flow to a clinically significant level.

20. Contraindications to barium studies of the upper gastrointestinal tract include known or suspected perforation (use water-soluble agent) and the inability of the patient to swallow (use nasogastric tube).

21. Focal hepatic lesions with T1 components that are isointense to mildly hyperintense to the surrounding liver are almost always hepatocellular in origin.

22. Almost all hepatic cysts and hemangiomas can be differentiated from malignant liver disease by the use of heavily T2-weighted (>180 ms) MR images.

23. On postcontrast images, the normal spleen displays alternating bands of high and low attenuation (CT) or signal (MRI) in the arterial phase. The spleen appears more homogeneous in a more delayed phase.

24. Splenic laceration can be differentiated from developmental splenic cleft. Patients with laceration have a trauma history, display a low attenuation defect with sharp edges, and have perisplenic hemoperitoneum.

25. MRI and CT are less specific in the characterization of splenic lesions than they are in characterization of liver, adrenal, or renal lesions.

26. A pseudocyst is the most common cystic lesion of the pancreas, accounting for about 90% of all cystic lesions in the pancreas.

27. The pancreatic neck and body are the most common portions of the pancreas to be injured in blunt trauma because they are compressed against the spine in blunt traumatic injuries to the abdomen.

28. The most specific CT imaging finding of acute appendicitis is an abnormal appendix that is typically dilated 6 mm or greater and fluid-filled. A calcified appendicolith with periappendiceal fat stranding is another highly specific CT finding.

29. If bowel ischemia is suspected on CT, one should assess the patency of the celiac artery, superior mesenteric artery, inferior mesenteric artery, portal vein, superior mesenteric vein, and inferior mesenteric vein. When the central superior mesenteric vessels are affected, the entire small bowel and the large bowel proximal to the distal third of the transverse colon tend to be affected. When the central inferior mesenteric vessels are affected, the distal third of the transverse colon, the descending colon, and the sigmoid colon are generally involved.

30. A fixed filling defect in the urinary collecting system is highly suggestive of transitional cell carcinoma and should be evaluated further with brush biopsy.

31. In a male patient with pelvic trauma, the urethra should be evaluated with a retrograde urethrogram before placement of a bladder drainage catheter.

32. An enhancing renal mass that does not contain macroscopic fat is a renal cell carcinoma until proven otherwise.

33. An enhancing renal lesion with macroscopic fat is a benign angiomyolipoma.

34. Cystic renal lesions that contain thick internal septations, thick mural calcification, or enhancing mural nodules are suggestive of cystic renal cell carcinomas and should be excised.

35. Patients with limited renal function (creatinine ≥1.5 mg/dL) generally should not receive an iodinated intravenous contrast agent for CT. Gadolinium chelate contrast agents used for MRI are generally safe for these patients.

36. There are three ways to show that an adrenal lesion is a benign adenoma: attenuation of less than 10 HU on unenhanced CT, washout of greater than 50% on delayed CT, or signal loss of 10% to 15% on chemical shift MRI.

37. Most pheochromocytomas occur in the adrenal glands and enhance avidly on CT and MRI.

38. In premenopausal women, because normal dominant follicles can be 3 cm (or sometimes larger), simple ovarian cysts smaller than 3 cm need no follow-up and typically resolve spontaneously.

39. MRI can generally distinguish between a septate and bicornuate uterus. A septate uterus has a smooth outer contour and a fibrous septum. A bicornuate uterus displays a depression 1 cm or greater of the outer contour of the fundus, and a thicker, more muscular septum.

40. Most intratesticular masses are malignant. Most extratesticular masses are benign.

41. The following equipment should be present when administering conscious sedations: pharmacologic antagonists, appropriate equipment to establish airway and provide positive-pressure ventilation, supplemental oxygen, and defibrillator.

42. Inferior vena cava filters should be placed below the lowest renal vein when possible.

43. Embolization on both sides of a pseudoaneurysm, aneurysm, or arteriovenous fistula is necessary to prevent reconstitution of flow via collaterals, which causes recurrence of the lesion.

44. The two most common indications for placement of a transjugular intrahepatic portosystemic shunt (TIPS) are variceal bleeding related to portal hypertension that is refractory to endoscopic therapy and ascites refractory to medical management. TIPS placement may act as an effective bridge to liver transplantation for patients with end-stage liver disease and the manifestations of portal hypertension.

45. There is a high association between Segond fracture and anterior cruciate ligament tear and meniscal injury.

46. When you see a fracture of the medial malleolus, do not forget to look at the proximal fibula for Maisonneuve fracture.

47. On a cervical spine radiograph, if you cannot visualize the lower cervical spine, obtain either a swimmer's view or a CT scan. You must visualize C7-T1 to "clear" the cervical spine.

48. Osteoporosis has many secondary causes. Medical evaluation for multiple myeloma and endocrine diseases should be done before one assumes primary osteoporosis.

49. If you see multiple lytic bone lesions in an adult, think of metastatic disease versus multiple myeloma. Primary tumors to consider in a patient with metastatic bone lesions are lung, prostate, breast, kidney, thyroid, and colorectal.

50. Patients with an osteoid osteoma classically present with pain at night relieved by aspirin.

51. Primary bone tumors that are known to occur in the epiphyseal region include giant cell tumor, chondroblastoma, and clear cell chondrosarcoma.

52. Rotator cuff tears are rare in individuals younger than 40 years except in athletes or in the setting of trauma.

53. MRI is the most sensitive modality for detection of early osteonecrosis, before femoral head cortical collapse. Early detection allows for possible joint-sparing therapies such as steroid reduction, supportive therapies such as non–weight bearing, and core decompression.

54. A meniscal tear is diagnosed on MRI by identifying increased internal meniscal signal intensity that extends to the articular surface.

55. After the Achilles tendon, the next most likely ankle tendon to tear is the posterior tibial tendon.

56. The anterior talofibular ligament, part of the lateral ligamentous complex, is the most commonly sprained and torn ankle ligament.

57. Early plain film findings of osteomyelitis include soft tissue swelling and blurred fascial planes. After 7 to 10 days, bone lucencies and periosteal reaction may be seen. On MRI, bone infection generally is depicted as a region of abnormal marrow signal, which is T1 hypointense and short-tau inversion recovery (STIR) hyperintense to normal marrow.

58. Epidural hematoma is a surgical emergency. It is usually caused by an arterial injury (most commonly middle meningeal artery), often associated with temporal bone fracture, confined by the lateral sutures, and usually lenticular in shape. Subdural hematoma is usually caused by injury to the bridging cortical veins, is not confined by the lateral sutures, and is usually crescentic in shape.

59. The differential diagnosis of an intracranial mass in a patient with human immunodeficiency virus includes toxoplasmosis, other brain abscess, and lymphoma. Progressive multifocal leukoencephalopathy, a demyelinating disease, can sometimes appear masslike.

60. Head CT is often normal in acute stroke. The earliest sign (within 6 hours) of an acute infarct on CT is loss of the gray-white differentiation with obscuration of the lateral lentiform nucleus. Acute ischemic changes can be seen within minutes of onset of the ictus on diffusion-weighted MRI.

61. C8 is a nerve root without a body. It exits between C7 and T1. Cervical nerve roots exit above the pedicles of the same-numbered body; thoracic and lumbar nerve roots exit below the pedicles of the same-numbered body.

62. One should be consistent in describing spinal degenerative disc disease. A disc bulge is a diffuse, symmetric extension of the disc beyond the end plate. A disc protrusion is a more focal extension of the disc in which the "neck" is wider than the more distal portion. A disc herniation is an extrusion of a portion of the disc in which the "neck" is the narrowest part. A disc sequestrum is a free disc fragment in the epidural space that has lost connection to the disc.

63. Inflammatory and vascular disorders of the spinal cord may mimic neoplasms.

64. Low density in a lymph node in an adult with head and neck cancer is characteristic of metastatic disease until proven otherwise.

65. The parotid glands are the only salivary glands that contain lymph nodes.

66. Neck lesions above the hyoid bone should be studied first with MRI. Pathologic findings of the neck below the hyoid bone should be primarily imaged with CT.

67. CT is the imaging modality of choice for conductive hearing loss. MRI is the imaging modality of choice in adult-onset sensorineural hearing loss.

68. Tumors and other lesions within the spinal canal may be classified as extradural (outside the thecal sac), intradural-extramedullary (inside the thecal sac, but outside the cord), or intramedullary (inside the cord). Making this determination is the first step to selecting the correct differential diagnosis for a lesion.

69. Positron emission tomography (PET) with fluorodeoxyglucose may change the surgical management of patients in 40% of cases. In some cases, distant metastases or restaging indicates that the cancer is inoperable, preventing surgery that would have not been useful. In 20% of patients, PET shows that enlarged nodes that may have prevented surgery from being considered were actually benign, so that surgery can be performed.

70. A "superscan" on bone scan implies that so much of the methylene diphosphate is taken up by the bones that there is no significant excretion in the kidneys and bladder or uptake in the soft tissues. In a patient with cancer, a "superscan" implies widespread osseous metastases that cannot be individually distinguished, but rather occupy almost the entire skeleton.

71. To classify a ventilation-perfusion ($\dot{V}/\dot{Q}$) scan as a "high probability" for pulmonary embolism (PE), the scan must have the equivalent of two or more large segmental perfusion defects (75% to 100% involvement of the segment) that are not matched by ventilatory abnormalities. Four or more moderately sized perfusion defects (25% to 75% involvement of the segment) would also represent a high probability for PE. The implication of a high-probability scan suggests a greater than 80% chance of having a PE.

72. Younger male patients with "cold" thyroid nodules are more likely to have cancer than are older female patients with similar findings. Exposure of the neck to radiation is also an important risk factor for cancer in a cold nodule. US findings of mixed cystic and solid components within a cold nodule are also more suggestive of thyroid cancer. Cold nodules in the setting of a multinodular goiter are substantially less likely to be cancer than other cold nodules.

73. After renal transplantation, acute tubular necrosis (ATN) occurs almost immediately, whereas chronic rejection occurs over several days to weeks or longer. Patients with ATN have normal or only slightly diminished perfusion of the kidney with a delayed cortical transit time (how long it takes for urine to appear in the collecting system). Rejection usually is associated with diminished flow with mildly impaired cortical function.

74. An exercise stress test should be stopped when (1) the patient cannot continue because of dyspnea, chest pain, fatigue, or musculoskeletal problems; (2) the patient has a hypertensive response; (3) the patient develops ST segment depressions of greater than 3 mm; (4) the patient has ST segment elevation, heralding a possible myocardial infarction; or (5) the patient experiences the onset of a potentially dangerous arrhythmia, such as ventricular tachycardia, ventricular fibrillation, very rapid supraventricular tachycardia, or heart block.

75. A right-sided arch is associated with tetralogy of Fallot (TOF) and truncus arteriosus (TA), but is more closely associated with TA. Because TOF is more common, however, you are more likely to see a right-sided arch with TOF.

76. Thickened aryepiglottic folds with a thickened epiglottis are indicative of epiglottitis and warrant emergent intubation.

77. If you suspect an aspirated foreign body, you should order bilateral lateral decubitus films. A normal lung would lose volume, whereas an obstructed lung would remain lucent and inflated.

78. The double-bubble sign on plain films represents an air-filled or fluid-filled distended stomach and duodenal bulb. It is seen in malrotation, duodenal atresia, and jejunal atresia.

79. A fleck of calcium in a normal-sized globe of a child younger than 6 years is characteristic of retinoblastoma until proven otherwise.

80. In a child's elbow, the medial epicondyle ossification center appears before the trochlear ossification center. If you see an ossific density in the region of the trochlea in the absence of a medial epicondylar ossification center, this is an avulsed fragment.

81. Metaphyseal corner fractures are highly sensitive and specific for child abuse.

82. The most common cause of death of an abused child is injury to the central nervous system.

83. If a pulmonary infiltrate does not resolve over time despite treatment with antimicrobial agents, a potential bronchoalveolar cell subtype of lung carcinoma should be suspected.

84. Interstitial pulmonary edema, usually caused by congestive heart failure, is the most common interstitial abnormality encountered in daily practice.

85. Most patients with asymptomatic mediastinal tumors have benign tumors, whereas most patients with symptomatic mediastinal tumors have malignant tumors.

86. If you see a pneumothorax on chest radiography that is associated with contralateral mediastinal shift and inferior displacement of the ipsilateral hemidiaphragm, immediately notify the physician caring for the patient because a tension pneumothorax may be present. Emergent treatment is required to prevent rapid death.

87. If you see focal ovoid lucency surrounding an endotracheal tube or a tracheostomy tube with an associated bulge in the adjacent tracheal walls, suspect overinflation of the cuff, and notify the clinical staff immediately.

88. If a nasogastric, orogastric, or feeding tube is seen to extend into a distal bronchus, lung, or pleural space, notify the clinical staff immediately; suggest that tube removal be performed only after a thoracostomy tube set is at the bedside in case a significant pneumothorax develops.

89. When air embolism is suspected during line placement or use, the patient should be placed in the left lateral position immediately to keep the air trapped in the right heart chambers, supplemental oxygen should be administered, and vital signs should be monitored.

90. In a normal early pregnancy, the yolk sac should be visible on US by a mean gestational sac diameter of 8 mm transvaginally and 20 mm transabdominally. Similarly, an embryo should be visible on US by a mean gestational sac diameter of 16 mm transvaginally and 25 mm transabdominally.

91. If a pregnant patient presents with vaginal bleeding, pelvic pain, and uterine tenderness, placental abruption must be excluded.

92. The most dreaded complication of oligohydramnios is pulmonary hypoplasia.

93. Omphalocele has a worse prognosis than gastroschisis because the former is associated with an increased incidence of chromosomal abnormalities leading to other structural abnormalities.

94. Most strokes are due to emboli rather than carotid stenosis. It is important to identify irregular atherosclerotic surfaces when examining the carotid circulation.

95. US findings in early or uncomplicated acute cholecystitis may include gallstones (which may be impacted in the gallbladder neck or cystic duct), gallbladder wall thickening, and gallbladder distention. Murphy sign (focal tenderness over the gallbladder when compressed by the US transducer) may also be elicited.

96. The combination of gallstones and Murphy sign on US has a positive predictive value of 92% and a negative predictive value of 95% for acute cholecystitis.

97. For a physician to be found liable for malpractice, the following four things must be shown: establishment of a duty of care (i.e., physician-patient relationship); breach of the duty of care, or negligence; adverse outcome with injury or harm; and direct causality between negligence and outcome.

98. The three most common reasons radiologists are sued are failure of diagnosis, failure to communicate findings in an appropriate and timely manner, and failure to suggest the next appropriate procedure.

99. To become board-certified in diagnostic radiology, you must pass the written and oral examinations of the American Board of Radiology (www.theabr.org). The written examination consists of a physics portion and a clinical portion. You may take the physics portion in your second, third, or fourth year of radiology training. The clinical written portion is taken in the fall of the fourth year, and the oral examination is taken in Louisville, Kentucky, in June of the fourth year of residency.

100. The only thing more stressful than going to Louisville is going back to Louisville.

INTRODUCTION TO IMAGING MODALITIES

I

INTRODUCTION TO PLAIN FILM RADIOGRAPHY AND FLUOROSCOPY

Linda K. Petrovich, MD, and
E. Scott Pretorius, MD

CHAPTER 1

PLAIN FILM RADIOGRAPHY

1. How do diagnostic x-rays differ from other kinds of electromagnetic radiation?

X-rays have higher frequencies and shorter wavelengths than visible light, microwaves, and radio waves. Diagnostic x-rays typically have energies between 20 keV and 150 keV. Gamma rays, which are emitted by many agents used in nuclear medicine, have even higher frequencies and shorter wavelengths than x-rays.

2. What are the components of an x-ray tube?

An x-ray tube contains a negatively charged cathode and a positively charged anode. The cathode contains a filament (usually made of coiled tungsten wire) that is the source of electrons. The electrons are accelerated toward the anode. The anode contains the target (most commonly made of tungsten), where x-rays are produced.

3. How are diagnostic x-rays produced?

In an x-ray tube, x-rays are produced when an energetic electron passes close to an atomic nucleus in the anode of the x-ray tube. The attractive force of the positively charged nucleus causes the electron to change direction and lose energy. The energy difference between the initial energy of the electron and the energy of the electron after it changes direction is released as an x-ray photon. This process is called *bremsstrahlung,* which means "braking radiation" in German.

4. What happens to most of the energy entering the x-ray tube?

Most (99%) of the electrical energy entering the tube is converted to heat, and tube heating is often the limiting factor in how much the x-ray tube can be used. About 1% of the electrical energy entering the tube is converted to x-rays.

5. What are the key parameters that can be manipulated on an x-ray generator?

The voltage across the x-ray tube (measured in kilovolts [kV]), the current flowing through the x-ray tube (measured in milliamperes [mA]), and the exposure time (measured in milliseconds [ms]) can be manipulated. Current and exposure time can be combined and expressed in milliampere-seconds (mAs).

6. What happens if kV is increased?

X-ray penetration increases, exposure increases (darker film), and contrast decreases. The maximal energy of the x-rays produced is increased. Film contrast primarily depends on kV.

7. What happens if mAs is increased?

Increasing mAs means increased film exposure (more x-rays produced), which darkens the film. The maximal energy of the x-rays produced is not changed.

8. How are plain film radiographs generated?

The patient is placed between an x-ray tube and a film cassette. The x-ray tube produces x-rays that pass through the human body and are attenuated by interaction with body tissues. The film cassette contains film that is adjacent to fluorescent screens. When the x-rays reach the film cassette, a photochemical interaction occurs between the x-rays and the screen coated with fluorescent particles. The x-rays activate the fluorescent particles to emit light rays. The light rays expose the photographic film, and an image is produced.

9. What are collimators, grids, and screens? Where are they?

From the x-ray tube, x-rays pass through a collimator, which consists of lead sheets (Fig. 1-1). Collimators narrow the x-ray beam. X-rays travel through air to the patient and then through a grid, which consists of narrow lead strips separated by plastic. The grid allows passage of x-rays that have passed directly through the patient (and contain useful information) and stops scattered x-rays, which would contribute to noise and decreased contrast. After passing through the grid, x-rays penetrate the film cassette, which in standard dual-screen systems includes an intensifying screen, the film, and a second intensifying screen. The screens absorb the x-ray photons and emit visible light. The light exposes the film.

10. What is the inverse square law?
The intensity of the x-ray beam decreases with the square of the distance from the x-ray tube. In other words, if one doubles the distance between oneself and the x-ray tube, x-ray exposure decreases by a factor of 4. This concept is important in determining x-ray exposure and absorbed dose.

11. What are the advantages and disadvantages of a small focal spot?
The focal spot is the source of x-rays in the tube. Smaller focal spots produce sharper images, but larger focal spots can tolerate greater amounts of heat. Small focal spots are used for mammography (which has few exposures, but very sharp images are required). Large focal spots are used in fluoroscopy (for continuous exposure, but lesser resolution). Regular diagnostic x-rays use focal spot sizes between the sizes used for mammography and fluoroscopy.

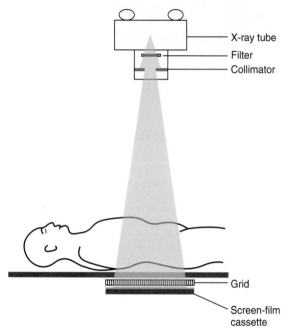

Figure 1-1. Apparatus for film screen radiography.

Key Points: Radiographic Exposures

1. Increasing voltage (kV) increases the maximal energy of the x-rays produced, decreases the film contrast, and increases exposure, making the film darker.
2. Increasing mAs increases the amount of x-rays produced, does not change the maximal energy of the x-rays produced, and increases exposure, making the film darker.
3. The focal spot is the source of x-rays in the tube.
4. A small focal spot produces sharper images and is used in mammography.
5. A large focal spot can tolerate more heat and is used in fluoroscopy.

12. What are the five basic densities seen on an x-ray? How do they appear?
The five basic densities are air, fat, soft tissue, bone, and metal. Air attenuates very little of the x-ray beam, allowing nearly the full force of the beam to darken the film, so air appears black. Bone and metals attenuate a large proportion of the x-ray beam, allowing very little radiation through to blacken the film. Bone and metallic objects appear white on radiographs. Fat and soft tissues attenuate intermediate amounts of the x-ray beam. They appear somewhere between white and black as a spectrum of shades of gray.

13. How does computed radiography differ from film screen radiography?
In computed radiography, a phosphor plate is used to capture x-ray exposure information. Electrons are trapped in the phosphor layer by the x-ray exposure, and the plate is "read" by a device that uses lasers to compel the electrons to emit light. This pattern is electronically stored as a digital image. The ability of the observer to manipulate the brightness and contrast of the digital image is a great advantage of this technique.

14. How do mammography film screen combinations differ from combinations used for chest and abdominal examinations?
Mammography film screen combinations are slower than combinations used for chest and abdominal imaging. This means that mammography film screen combinations are thinner and have higher spatial resolution.

15. What is the difference between a posteroanterior (PA) and an anteroposterior (AP) film?
The names of these views describe the path of the x-ray beam through the patient. In a standing PA chest radiograph, the beam enters the patient from the back, and the image is acquired in front of the patient. For acquiring portable chest radiographs, a cassette is placed behind the patient, and the x-ray beam is transmitted from the front, creating an AP film. A similar naming convention is followed for all radiographic and mammographic images.

MAMMOGRAPHY

16. How does mammographic technique (kV and mA) selection differ from that selected for chest and abdominal examinations?

Mammography uses lower kV (for higher image contrast) and higher mA (for shorter exposure times) compared with the technique for chest and abdominal examinations.

17. What are the two standard views obtained in mammography?

The two standard views are medio-lateral oblique (MLO) and craniocaudal (CC). The direction of the x-ray beam is defined by the name of the view. In CC views, the x-ray beam enters the cranial portion of the breast, traverses the breast, and exits on the caudal side of the breast onto the film. By convention, metallic markers indicating view type are placed closest to the axilla—laterally on the CC view and superiorly on the MLO view.

18. Can any other views be obtained?

Yes. If an abnormality is seen on only one of the previously described views, or if it is seen on both views but needs further characterization, or if it is unclear whether an apparent mass is real or just superimposed tissue, additional views are often obtained. If a lesion is seen on only one of the two standard views (MLO, CC), a 90-degree medio-lateral (ML) view may be helpful to localize the lesion. Rolled views may be performed in any projection, and tissue can be rolled in any direction desired. This is done to position the area of a potential lesion away from adjacent tissue that may obscure it.

19. How are spot compression and magnification views used in diagnostic mammography?

Spot compression views are often obtained to determine whether a density "presses out"—meaning that on a compression view it is found to have represented a superimposition of normal breast tissue rather than an actual mass. Magnification views are obtained to visualize calcifications better or to characterize a mass better.

20. How are women with breast implants imaged with mammography?

Four views of each breast are done:
- Two CC views—one with the implant in the field of view and one with the implant displaced as much out of the field as possible.
- Two MLO views—one with the implant in the field of view and one with the implant displaced as much out of the field as possible.

21. What are the two main tissue types in the breast? How do they appear on a mammogram?

The two main tissues are fibroglandular tissue, which appears bright, and fat, which appears darker.

22. Why are single screens (rather than dual screens) usually used in mammography?

Dual-screen systems are more efficient in detecting x-rays and are used for most purposes. The two screens produce more scatter than a single screen, however, and decrease image sharpness. Because sharpness is so important in mammography to characterize calcifications, single-screen systems are used.

FLUOROSCOPY

23. What is fluoroscopy? How are fluoroscopic images obtained?

Fluoroscopy uses continuously emitted x-rays and allows real-time visualization of anatomic structures. An x-ray tube located beneath the table emits a continuous x-ray beam that passes through the patient and falls onto a continuously fluorescing screen and image intensifier located above the patient (Fig. 1-2). The fluorescing screen emits a faint light. The emitted light is amplified electronically by an image intensifier, and the image is displayed on a television screen. When an image of interest is identified, a radiograph may be obtained by placing a film between the patient and image intensifier and exposing the film with a pulse of radiation.

24. Why are image intensifiers used?

Image intensifiers substantially decrease the amount of radiation needed to produce clinically useful images.

25. How do fluoroscopic conventions differ from radiographic conventions?

On fluoroscopy, things that are white on x-rays (e.g., bones or oral contrast agent) are presented as dark. Things that are dark on x-ray (e.g., air) are presented as white on fluoroscopy.

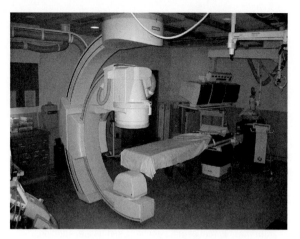

Figure 1-2. Typical C-arm unit for fluoroscopically guided procedures.

26. Discuss the contrast agents used in fluoroscopic studies of the upper and lower gastrointestinal (GI) tract.
Barium sulfate is the standard contrast agent for routine fluoroscopic contrast studies of the upper and lower GI tract. "Thin," more fluid suspensions are used for single-contrast studies. "Thick," more viscous suspensions are used for double-contrast (air and oral contrast agent) studies. If perforation of the GI tract is suspected, a water-soluble, iodinated contrast agent such as diatrizoate (Gastrografin) is used instead of barium because of the high mortality rate from barium peritonitis. Water-soluble agents are quickly resorbed through the peritoneal surface. Aspiration of water-soluble agents may result in chemical pneumonitis and should not be used in patients with an increased risk of aspiration.

27. Why is it important to obtain a scout film before administering a contrast agent in a fluoroscopic study?
Objects that appear "white" on a radiograph include contrast agents and calcium. If a white object is seen after contrast administration, it may be either the contrast agent or calcium. The way to differentiate is to see whether it was present on the scout (precontrast) image. If it was present, it is calcium; if it was not present, it is the contrast agent. Before administration of a barium enema examination, the scout film may help determine the adequacy of the bowel preparation before the procedure. This scout film helps avoid nondiagnostic examinations because of retained stool.

28. Name four types of fluoroscopic studies and a possible clinical indication for each.
- Esophagogram: dysphagia (to rule out stricture or mass)
- Upper GI study: abdominal pain (to rule out gastric or duodenal ulcer disease)
- Small bowel follow-through: diarrhea or constipation (to rule out Crohn disease or other small bowel pathologic conditions)
- Barium enema: rectal bleeding (to rule out a polyp or mass)

29. What is digital subtraction angiography?
Digital subtraction angiography is a technique in which a precontrast image is electronically subtracted from an image obtained after intravascular contrast injection. This technique results in a greater contrast-to-background image because background structures such as bone and soft tissues have been removed.

CHAPTER 2

INTRODUCTION TO ULTRASOUND, CT, AND MRI

E. Scott Pretorius, MD

ULTRASOUND

1. How is an ultrasound (US) image created?

US is an imaging technique that uses sound waves, generally in the range of 2 million to 20 million cycles per second (2 to 20 MHz), much greater than the frequencies audible to humans or animals. A hand-held transducer is applied to the body. This transducer sends US waves into the body and receives reflected sound waves. The transducer's information is communicated via cable to the US scanner, and the data are rendered on a monitor (Fig. 2-1).

2. Why is the gel used?

US coupling gel (Fig. 2-2) is used to help transmit US waves to and from the transducer. Reflection of sound waves occurs at interfaces where there is a difference in the speed of propagation of sound waves, and because sound/US waves travel relatively slowly through air, the air-skin interface has potential to reflect a great deal of the waves we would like to use for imaging. Placing US coupling gel between the transducer and skin greatly reduces this effect, and the system is designed so that the transducer face and the coupling gel have acoustic impedances similar to that of skin.

3. What makes something bright or dark on US?

Sound waves encountering a tissue can be attenuated, reflected, or transmitted by the tissue. Reflected sound waves returning to the transducer are used by the computer to make an image. Sound is generally reflected when waves traveling in one kind of tissue encounter a different kind of tissue, which has different properties of US wave propagation. These are called *acoustic interfaces*.

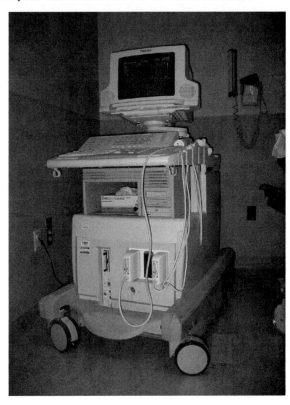

Figure 2-1. US scanner.

Regions with many acoustic interfaces reflect a lot of sound returning to the transducer. These are termed *echogenic* or *hyperechoic* and by convention are viewed as bright areas. Regions with few acoustic interfaces do not reflect many sound waves. These are termed *hypoechoic* and are viewed as dark areas.

4. What are some things that are hyperechoic?

Hyperechoic and *hypoechoic* are terms that refer to the brightness of an object relative to other things in the image. Air-tissue interfaces reflect a great deal of sound, and such interfaces are markedly hyperechoic. US is not useful for identifying an aerated lung and air-filled bowel. Gel is applied to the patient's skin to minimize this effect at the air-skin interface. Bone–soft tissue interfaces also reflect a great deal of sound. Imaging inside bone is generally impossible with US.

5. What are some things that are hypoechoic?

Fluid is usually homogeneous, and fluid-filled objects, such as the urinary bladder, cysts, and large blood vessels, are generally very hypoechoic.

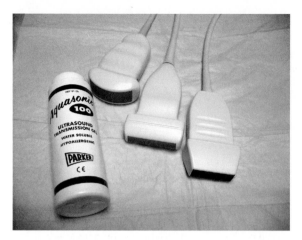

Figure 2-2. US transducers, with a bottle of coupling gel. Gel is placed on the skin to facilitate transmission of US waves to and from the transducer.

6. What transducer should I choose for the examination?

It depends largely on what you are examining. Lower US frequencies penetrate to greater depths, whereas higher US frequencies generally provide higher resolution. For a general examination of the abdomen, which requires large depths to see the liver, pancreas, and spleen, a 3- or 5-MHz transducer is a good choice. For a superficial examination, such as the scrotum or thyroid, a 10-MHz transducer is often used.

7. What kinds of specialized transducers exist?

Endovaginal probes are commonly used for gynecologic examinations and for evaluation of early pregnancies. They are usually 7.5-MHz probes. Endorectal probes are available for prostate imaging. They are generally in the range of 9 MHz.

8. Why are patients asked to come with a full bladder for a pelvic US?

Fluid in the urinary bladder facilitates transmission of sound waves so that the uterus and ovaries can be seen better using a transabdominal probe. If the bladder is not full, endovaginal examination is more often necessary.

9. What is the difference between posterior acoustic enhancement and posterior acoustic shadowing?

Posterior acoustic enhancement refers to the increased brightness seen beyond objects that transmit a lot of sound waves. Because fluid-filled cysts transmit a great deal of sound, the area beyond cysts often displays posterior acoustic enhancement.

Posterior acoustic shadowing has the opposite effect—decreased brightness seen beyond objects that reflect a great deal of sound. Gallstones, which are echogenic, reflect a lot of sound, and shadowing is often seen in the tissue beyond the gallstones.

10. What is Doppler US?

Doppler US is used primarily to evaluate flowing blood in blood vessels. It is based on the principle that sound waves originating from a moving source appear to have a different frequency/wavelength than sound waves originating from a stationary source. Echoes returning from blood flowing away from the transducer appear to have a lower frequency and longer wavelength than the original wave. Similarly, blood flowing toward the transducer appears to have a higher frequency and shorter wavelength than the original wave.

COMPUTED TOMOGRAPHY

11. How is a computed tomography (CT) image created?

The patient lies on a mechanical table that slowly moves through a doughnut-shaped scanner (Fig. 2-3). Inside the scanner, an x-ray emitter rotates around the patient in the axial plane. On the opposite side of the patient, 180 degrees from the emitter, electronic x-ray detectors receive the x-ray beam and calculate how much of the beam was transmitted and how much was absorbed by the patient. The computer calculates the x-ray absorption of each voxel within the slice and assigns it a numeric value.

12. What makes something bright or dark on CT?

Because CT images are created with x-rays, the same things that are bright and dark on plain films are bright and dark on CT. Electron-dense structures, such as metal and bone, stop a large number of x-rays and are bright on CT. Regions with lower electron density, such as air or fat, stop very few x-rays and are rendered as dark.

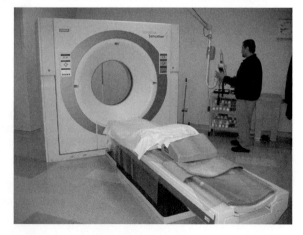

Figure 2-3. Multidetector row CT scanner.

13. What is the difference between serial CT and helical (or spiral) CT?
In *serial CT scanning,* the emitter/detector whirls 360 degrees around the patient to acquire a slice; the table then moves the patient, and the emitter/detector whirls 360 degrees the other way to acquire the next slice.

In *helical (spiral) scanning,* the emitter/detector array moves around the patient continuously in the same direction, and the table moves continuously through the scanner while the patient is being imaged. This technologic advance was made possible by the development of the slip-ring gantry, which eliminated the cables that brought power to the emitter/detector and allows it to move continuously in one direction. Helical scanning is generally much faster than serial scanning. All multidetector row scanners are also, by definition, helical.

14. In helical CT, what is pitch?
Pitch is the longitudinal distance (in millimeters) that the table moves during one revolution of the x-ray tube.

15. What is the difference between single detector row and multidetector row scanners?
Multidetector row scanners have more than one row of x-ray detectors, which allow them to acquire more than one image slice at the same time. Multidetector row scanners are much faster than single detector row scanners. Radiologists have used this technology to acquire ever greater numbers of increasingly thinner slices, which has led to the emergence of many new CT applications, including CT angiography and CT urography.

16. What is the Hounsfield scale?
The Hounsfield scale is a scale that is used to assign voxel values in CT. It extends from −1000 to +1000. The center value, 0 Hounsfield units (HU), is the attenuation of water. Things that absorb more x-rays have greater HU values. Cortical bone is approximately 1000 HU; muscle, about 40 HU; gray matter, 40 HU; white matter, 30 HU; cerebrospinal fluid, 10 HU; fat, −60; and air, −1000.

17. What are *window* and *level*?
After the CT data are acquired, and an HU value is assigned to each voxel in a slice, the data can be viewed in different ways. The *window* is a range of HU values that are chosen to be viewed as shades of gray; assigned HU values greater than this range are depicted as white, and values less than this range are depicted as black. The *level* is the HU value that is the center value of the window. Commonly used window/level combinations include those for viewing lung, bone, liver, and brain.

18. What is the difference between a pixel and a voxel?
A pixel is a single "dot" within a two-dimensional image and has unique coordinates along the *x* and *y* axes of the image. A voxel is a pixel with three dimensions. A voxel that is the same length in all three dimensions is an isotropic voxel.

19. What is field of view?
The field of view is the width of the image in CT or magnetic resonance imaging (MRI). It is most commonly reported in centimeters.

20. What is the matrix?
In diagnostic imaging, *matrix* size refers to the number of pixels contained on each axis of a CT or MRI slice, such as a square matrix of 512 × 512 pixels (typical in CT) or a rectangular matrix of 256 × 192 pixels (common in MRI).

21. What is the difference between spatial resolution and contrast resolution?
Spatial resolution is a measure of the ability of an imaging technique to show that two nearby objects are separate objects. It is measured in "line pairs per millimeter," referring to the ability of a modality to show that very small pairs of lines are separate lines and not a single line. CT has the highest spatial resolution of the digital cross-sectional modalities.

Contrast resolution refers to the ability of an imaging modality to render different objects or tissues as different shades of gray. MRI has the highest contrast resolution of the digital cross-sectional modalities.

MAGNETIC RESONANCE IMAGING

22. How is the MR image created?
The patient is placed in a scanner that generates a very strong magnetic field (Fig. 2-4). Hydrogen nuclei have a net magnetic moment and behave like little magnets, aligning themselves either parallel (spin up) or antiparallel (spin down) with the magnetic field. Radiofrequency waves are pulsed in, which scatter the hydrogen nuclei in all directions. When the radiofrequency pulse is stopped, the hydrogen nuclei tend to realign themselves along the magnetic field, but this occurs at different rates in different tissues. These differential relaxation rates are used to create the MR image.

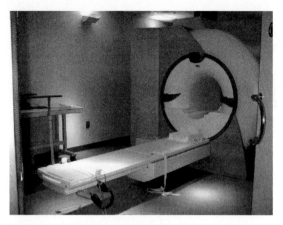

Figure 2-4. A 1.5-T MRI scanner. The central bore of the scanner is narrower than that of a CT scanner.

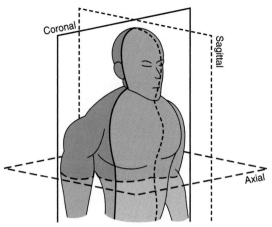

Figure 2-5. Planes used for cross-sectional imaging: axial, sagittal, and coronal.

23. What are the three basic planes used in imaging?

The three basic planes are axial, sagittal, and coronal (Fig. 2-5). An advantage of MRI over CT is that MRI data can be obtained in any plane. CT data are acquired axially, but can be reformatted to generate other planes.

24. What is the difference between T1 and T2?

T1 is a measure of relaxation time in the longitudinal plane, and T2 is a measure of relaxation time in the transverse plane.

25. What are T1-weighted and T2-weighted images?

- *T1-weighted images* are created primarily by using data from differential proton relaxation rates in the plane longitudinal to the main magnetic field.
- *T2-weighted images* primarily make use of data from differential proton relaxation rates in the plane transverse to the main magnetic field.

26. What is a pulse sequence?

A pulse sequence is a series of instructions that is repeated many times to build up the data to create the MR image.

27. What are TR and TE?

TR is the "time to repetition," or the time it takes to complete one full iteration of a pulse sequence. *TE* is the "time to echo," or the time between the start of a pulse sequence and the acquisition of data from the excited protons. TR and TE are, by convention, reported in milliseconds (ms).

28. What is a spin-echo (SE) pulse sequence?

The SE pulse sequence begins with a 90-degree pulse, followed by a 180-degree pulse. After the 180-degree pulse, MRI signal is acquired from the protons. SE pulse sequences may be used to create T1-weighted or T2-weighted images.

29. What is the difference between SE imaging and fast spin-echo (FSE) imaging?

FSE is a technique that takes advantage of the fact that, after the 90-degree and 180-degree pulses have been applied, there are multiple "echoes"—bits of MRI signal—that can be acquired. FSE is much faster than conventional SE, especially for T2-weighted imaging, because it requires going through many fewer iterations of the pulse sequence (fewer TRs) to create the image. In practice, FSE is almost always used instead of SE.

30. How can I tell the difference between T1 and T2 by looking at the TR and TE?

- T1-weighted images have a short TR (<1000 ms) and a short TE (<20 ms).
- T2-weighted images have a long TR (>2000 ms) and a long TE (>40 ms).

Key Points: Methods of Generating Contrast between Different Tissues

1. US uses US waves. *Acoustic interfaces,* regions in tissues where the speed of the US wave changes, are rendered as bright. Areas that are more internally homogeneous (e.g., fluid), without acoustic interfaces, are rendered as dark.
2. CT uses x-rays. Tissues of higher electron density (e.g., bone) stop more x-rays and are rendered as bright.
3. MRI uses magnets and radio waves. Different sequences of radio waves (pulse sequences) generate different types of images. MRI has greater contrast than US and CT, and, with different pulse sequences, has multiple different ways of generating contrast between tissues.

31. How can I tell the difference between T1 and T2 by looking at an image?

The best way is to look for fluid, which tends to be hyperintense to virtually everything else on T2-weighted images. On T1-weighted images, fluid is of low intermediate signal. Good places to look for fluid include the urinary bladder and the cerebrospinal fluid.

Fat is an unreliable predictor of image weighting. Although fat is brighter than most other tissues on T1, its appearance on T2-weighted images is often manipulated. Fat tends to be relatively hypointense to other tissues on SE T2-weighted images and hyperintense on FSE T2-weighted images. Also, a technique known as *fat saturation* is often used to decrease the signal from fat on T1-weighted images and FSE T2-weighted images. Because of these complexities, fat is an unreliable marker of image weighting.

32. What kinds of things tend to be bright on T1-weighted images?

Fat, hemorrhage, proteinaceous substances, melanin, and paramagnetic agents such as gadolinium chelates tend to be bright on T1-weighted images.

33. I see something dark on T1-weighted and T2-weighted images. What kinds of things do that?

Air, flowing blood (on SE or FSE images), and cortical bone can appear dark on T1-weighted and T2-weighted images. Ligaments, tendons, and other dense fibrous tissues are also usually of low T1, low T2 signal.

34. How strong is 1.5 Tesla (T)?

The earth's magnetic field is about 0.5 gauss. Because 1.5 T is equal to 15,000 gauss, the magnetic field of such a scanner is 30,000 times the strength of the earth's magnetic field.

35. Are low-magnetic-field open scanners as good as high-field scanners?

No. Generally, low-field (≤0.5 T) scanners require longer imaging times to produce poorer images. With good surface coils and a lot of imaging time, open scanners can often produce good images of stationary body parts, such as joints, spine, and brain. For imaging applications requiring high resolution (breast imaging) or rapid imaging, such as abdominal MRI, magnetic resonance angiography (MRA), and dynamic gadolinium-enhanced MRI, low-field scanners are markedly inferior to high-field systems.

36. What is the difference between SE images and gradient-echo (GE) images?

SE images start with a 90-degree pulse, followed by a 180-degree refocusing pulse. GE sequences use pulses of less than 90 degrees and do not have 180-degree refocusing pulses. TR and TE are often very short, and GE sequences usually are used for acquiring T1-weighted images. Because these images can be obtained very rapidly, they are the most common type of image to be acquired after rapid gadolinium injection and are used for performing contrast-enhanced MRA.

37. What kinds of images are acquired before and after gadolinium chelate administration?

Gadolinium chelates that are used as contrast agents for MRI primarily shorten T1 relaxation times, making things appear more hyperintense on T1-weighted images. Precontrast and postcontrast images are T1-weighted images. T1-weighted SE imaging is often performed in regions where longer imaging times are acceptable, such as brain. For the abdomen and pelvis, however, where imaging must be completed in a breath-hold, T1-weighted GE images are almost exclusively used.

38. Why is it important that the precontrast image and the postcontrast image have the same imaging parameters?

Nothing can be changed on the scanner between the acquisition of the precontrast image and the postcontrast image. The reason is that, in contrast to CT, there is no absolute scale of "brightness" and "darkness" on MRI. The only way to know whether something enhances on MRI is to compare its signal on the postcontrast image with its signal on the identical precontrast image. One cannot compare signal intensities between two images acquired with different TRs or different TEs.

39. What are contraindications to MRI?

Patients with implanted electronic devices, such as pacemakers, defibrillators, neurostimulators, and cochlear implants, should not be placed in the magnetic field. A patient who is dependent on a pacemaker for cardiac pacing may die in the scanner if the device malfunctions. Even if the patient is not dependent on the device for survival, the battery life would be shortened by exposure to the field.

Extreme claustrophobia is a relative contraindication to MRI. Such patients may need to be sedated for examination. In some cases, low-field imaging on an open scanner may be able to be used instead.

40. Who should not receive gadolinium chelates?

Patients with a prior true allergic response to gadolinium chelates, including hives, bronchospasm, and anaphylaxis, should not be injected. True allergic response is very rare, on the order of 1 in 200,000 injections. The most common side effects of these agents are mild headache and a metallic taste.

Pregnant patients should not receive gadolinium chelates. Many of the agents are known to be able to cross the blood-placental barrier, and their effect on the fetus is unknown.

CHAPTER 3

INTRODUCTION TO NUCLEAR MEDICINE

Linda K. Petrovich, MD, and
E. Scott Pretorius, MD

1. How is a nuclear medicine test performed?

A radiopharmaceutical agent, which is a radioactively tagged compound, is administered to a patient. Many radiopharmaceutical agents act like analogues of natural biologic compounds and localize to specific organs. Photons are emitted from the radiopharmaceutical agent in the patient, and a gamma camera is used to detect the tracer distribution. An image is created by a computer system (Fig. 3-1).

2. What is the difference between the x-rays used in plain films and computed tomography (CT) and the gamma rays used in nuclear medicine?

X-rays are produced from the interaction of bombarding photons or electrons within an atom. Gamma rays are produced when an unstable nucleus transitions to a more stable state. Diagnostic x-ray imaging is referred to as *transmission imaging*. This term is used because images are formed as x-ray photons from an external source traverse tissue and emerge to form the image. Nuclear medicine is referred to as *emission imaging* because photons are emitted from inside the patient and subsequently detected by the gamma camera imaging system.

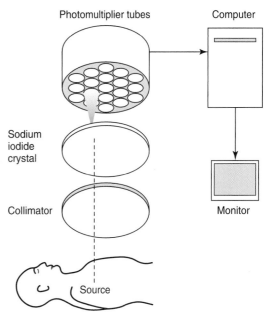

Figure 3-1. Line drawing showing the flow of information of a typical nuclear medicine study, such as a bone scan, obtained with a gamma camera.

3. How does nuclear medicine differ from other imaging modalities used in radiology, such as plain film, ultrasound (US), CT, and magnetic resonance imaging (MRI)?

Plain films, US, CT, and MRI produce anatomic images with very high spatial resolution. A viewer can see anatomy very well, but function generally is not assessed. Nuclear medicine studies sacrifice spatial resolution, but in return offer information about organ function.

Key Points: How Nuclear Medicine Differs from Other Imaging Modalities

1. Radiopharmaceutical agents are administered to the patient before imaging.
2. Images are indicative of the functional status of an organ.
3. The spatial resolution in nuclear medicine is less than that of x-rays, US, CT, and MRI.
4. Photons are emitted from the patient and detected by a gamma camera.
5. The total time for a nuclear medicine test may range from minutes to days, depending on the half-life and distribution of the radiopharmaceutical agent.

---

4. List some common clinical indications for performing nuclear medicine imaging.

- To rule out pulmonary embolism, a ventilation-perfusion (V̇/Q̇) scan may be performed.
- To evaluate for acute cholecystitis, a hepato-iminodiacetic acid (HIDA) scan may be performed.
- To detect a potential gastrointestinal (GI) bleed, a bleeding scan may be performed.
- To evaluate for osteomyelitis, a three-phase bone scan may be performed.

5. What radiopharmaceutical agents are used in a V̇/Q̇ scan?

A V̇/Q̇ scan attempts to identify regions of lung that are aerated lung but not perfused (such regions are suspicious for pulmonary embolism). The scan consists of two parts: a ventilation phase where the aerated lung is imaged, and a perfusion phase that maps blood flow to the lungs. The two sets of images are compared for discrepancies. For the ventilation portion of the study, xenon-133 and technetium (Tc)-99m diethylenetriaminepentaacetic acid (DTPA) are the most commonly used agents. For the perfusion portion of the study, Tc-99m macroaggregated albumin (MAA) is used.

6. How is a V̇/Q̇ scan performed?

The ventilation portion is performed using either radioactive gas (xenon) or radioactive aerosol (Tc-99m DTPA). When radioactive gas is used, the study is accomplished in three phases: single-breath/wash-in phase, equilibrium phase, and washout phase. For studies that use radioaerosols, the radiopharmaceutical agent is placed in a special nebulizer system, and the patient breathes through the mouthpiece until sufficient radioaerosol is delivered to the lungs. Tc-99m remains in the lung long enough to obtain multiple views with a gamma camera. Tc-99m MAA is injected into a peripheral vein to assess perfusion. The particles travel to the right side of the heart and then to the lungs, where they are filtered or trapped in the pulmonary vascular bed. The emissions from the trapped particles are imaged with a gamma camera.

7. How are the results of a V̇/Q̇ scan interpreted?

If an acute pulmonary embolism is present, the thrombus in the blood vessel prevents radiotracer from reaching the portion of lung supplied by the vessel, and a perfusion defect results. An acute thrombus does not prevent air from being distributed to the lung via bronchi, however, and the results of the ventilation scan are normal. This combination of a perfusion defect without a corresponding ventilation defect is called a *mismatch*. The results of a V̇/Q̇ scan are classified as low, intermediate, or high probability for a pulmonary embolism. The classification is based on the number and size of defects, with higher numbers and sizes resulting in greater probability that an embolus is present.

8. What radiopharmaceutical agent is used in HIDA scan?

Tc-99m–labeled iminodiacetic acid (IDA) compounds are used. They share biologic activity with bilirubin and are also taken up, transported, and excreted by hepatocytes.

9. How is HIDA scan performed?

The patient is required to fast for at least 4 hours, but not longer than 24 hours. If the test is performed after a recent meal, the gallbladder may still be contracted, and this could lead to false-positive test results. After a prolonged fast, the gallbladder may be filled with concentrated bile, and this may also lead to false-positive test results by preventing tracer accumulation in the gallbladder. Tc-99m IDA is injected into a peripheral vein, followed by immediate imaging of the right upper quadrant.

10. How are the results of HIDA scan interpreted?

Because the tracer behaves similar to bilirubin, it should be taken up by hepatocytes and excreted into the bile ducts. The liver should be visualized first, followed by visualization of the bowel and gallbladder. The appearance of tracer in the bowel and gallbladder by 60 minutes after administration is defined as normal. Nonvisualization of the gallbladder by 60 minutes is diagnostic of acute cholecystitis because this implies a functional obstruction of the cystic duct. False-positive results can be caused by chronic cholecystitis, hepatic insufficiency, and fasting for less than 4 hours or more than 24 hours as previously described.

Key Points: Common Clinical Indications for a Nuclear Medicine Study

1. To rule out pulmonary embolism (ventilation-perfusion scan)
2. To rule out acute cholecystitis, bile duct obstruction, or biliary leak (HIDA scan)
3. To rule out lower GI bleed (Tc-99m sulfur colloid or Tc-99m–labeled red blood cells)
4. To rule out infection (bone scan, indium-111–labeled white blood cells, gallium 67)
5. To evaluate for metastatic disease (bone scan, positron emission tomography (PET) scan)
6. To evaluate for thyroid pathologic conditions (iodine-123)
7. To evaluate for renal pathologic conditions, such as obstruction, hypertension, reflux, and transplant (Tc-99m–labeled compounds)

---

11. What radiopharmaceutical agents are used for GI bleeding scan?

Tc-99m sulfur colloid or Tc-99m–labeled red blood cells (RBCs) are used. Tc-99m–labeled RBCs are more difficult to prepare, but have a longer plasma half-life and are able to detect a GI bleed over a longer period.

12. How do you tell whether the results of the bleeding scan are positive?

An abnormal radiotracer hot spot appears and conforms to bowel anatomy. The activity should increase over time and move through the GI tract. Because blood acts as an intestinal irritant, movement can be rapid and bidirectional.

13. What are some indications for performing a renal scan?

Renal scans have various clinical applications, including evaluating renal transplants, differentiating between obstructed and dilated collecting systems, and diagnosing reflux and renovascular hypertension.

14. What are the four major renal functions that can be evaluated with radionuclide imaging?

Renal scans are helpful in evaluating blood flow to the kidney, glomerular filtration, tubular function (resorption and secretion), and drainage of the collecting systems.

15. What are the main radiopharmaceutical agents used in renal scans? How do they differ?

Tc-99m DTPA is a glomerular agent, meaning that it is cleared primarily by glomerular filtration and is neither reabsorbed nor secreted by the renal tubules. It can be used to measure the glomerular filtration rate. Tc-99m mertiatide (MAG3) is a tubular agent, meaning that its mechanism of renal clearance is solely tubular secretion. Tc-99m dimercaptosuccinic acid (DMSA) is a cortical agent, meaning that it binds to tubular cells in the renal cortex, making possible static imaging of the renal parenchymal cortex.

16. What three main factors should be examined when interpreting a renal scan?

Blood flow, radiotracer uptake, and radiotracer excretion should be examined.

17. What radiopharmaceutical agents are used in thyroid imaging?

Iodine-123 is the diagnostic agent of choice for imaging the thyroid. Iodine is administered orally. It is absorbed from the GI tract and trapped and organified (incorporated into thyroglobulin molecules) in the thyroid. Tc-99m pertechnetate is used if imaging has to be performed within 1 hour or if the patient is unable to ingest orally. Iodine-131 is used for whole-body scans after thyroidectomy for thyroid cancer and for therapeutic purposes.

18. Describe the appearance of Graves disease, thyroiditis, and tumor on a nuclear imaging study.

Graves disease is manifested by an enlarged gland that shows diffusely increased uptake. *Thyroiditis* appears as diffusely decreased uptake. *Thyroid cancer* tends to appear as a focal area of decreased activity (a solitary cold nodule) rather than showing increased activity on a nuclear medicine study.

19. What radiopharmaceutical agents are used in bone scanning?

Tc-99m–labeled diphosphonates are injected intravenously to perform a bone scan. The radiotracer distribution is representative of osteoblastic activity and regional blood flow to bone. Dynamic blood flow imaging is performed immediately after the injection of radiotracer. Static imaging is performed 2 to 4 hours after injection and is indicative of osteoblastic activity.

20. What are the two types of bone scans that can be performed, and what are the indications for each?

Focal three-phase imaging and whole-body imaging are the two types of bone scans. Focal three-phase imaging is used to differentiate cellulitis from osteomyelitis. The three phases are the flow phase (1 minute after injection), the blood pool (5 minutes after injection), and the skeletal phase (2 to 4 hours after injection). Cellulitis and osteomyelitis have increased uptake in the first two phases of the bone scan; however, only osteomyelitis shows increased activity in the third phase.

Whole-body imaging consists of static images obtained 2 to 4 hours after injection. It is used for detection of metastatic and metabolic diseases and bone dysplasia.

21. If you are concerned about an infection outside the skeletal system, what nuclear imaging studies can you perform?

Indium (In)-111–labeled white blood cells (WBCs) and gallium-67 citrate can be used to detect occult infection. To label WBCs with In-111, the cells must be removed from plasma. Blood is taken from the patient, labeled, and reinjected. Imaging is performed 24 hours after the injection. The normal distribution of WBCs is spleen, liver, and bone marrow. Activity seen outside the normal expected distribution is evidence of a focus of infection. Gallium, the other agent useful in locating sources of infection, binds to iron-binding molecules. Its normal distribution is liver and bone marrow. It is excreted by the kidneys for the first 24 hours and through the large bowel after 24 hours. As with an In-111 WBC scan, activity seen outside the expected normal organs of uptake is evidence of infection.

22. What is a PET scan?

PET stands for *positron emission tomography*. A tracer that emits positrons is injected into the patient. After the positrons are emitted from the nucleus of an atom, they travel through surrounding tissue and collide with electrons. This collision between positrons and electrons is called *annihilation* and produces gamma rays. The gamma rays are detected by a PET scanner and analyzed by a computer to form an image. Because positronic decay produces two 511-keV photons that travel in exactly opposite directions, acquisition of PET data is sometimes called *coincidence detection*—only photons of the correct energy that are detected simultaneously by detectors 180 degrees from each other are registered as true events, and the rest are assumed to be noise.

23. What radiopharmaceutical agent is used in PET? What type of pathologic conditions can it detect?

Fluorodeoxyglucose (FDG) is used in PET. This is a radionuclide combined with glucose, which is the currency of metabolism for malignant and benign cells. Because malignant cells tend to grow and metabolize glucose faster than healthy tissue, however, malignant cells use more of the tracer. PET uses the difference in metabolism to differentiate normal from abnormal tissue.

Key Points: Main Radionuclides Used in Nuclear Medicine
1. Tc-99m (most common)
2. Iodine-123
3. Gallium-67
4. Thallium-201
5. In-111
6. FDG (for PET imaging)

24. What is SUV?

SUV is *standardized uptake value*. It is a very important concept in interpretation of PET and PET/CT scans, and is a measurement of the activity seen in a region of interest relative to the body as a whole. By definition, if the activity of an injected dose were normalized over the entire body, the SUV everywhere would be 1.

25. What types of cancer are best detected on PET?

PET scans can be used to detect malignant tumors, determine cancer stage, and judge the effectiveness of cancer treatment. They are most often used in patients with head and neck tumors, colorectal cancer, lymphoma, melanoma, and lung cancer.

26. Should PET/CT be done with or without an intravenous contrast agent?

There is increasing evidence that the use of an intravenous contrast agent for the CT portion of PET/CT increases detection of liver lesions and allows for more accurate characterization of the lesions detected.

BIBLIOGRAPHY

[1] S. Badiee, B.L. Franc, E.M. Webb, et al., Role of IV iodinated contrast material in ^{18}F-FDG PET/CT of liver metastases, AJR Am. J. Roentgeol. 191 (2008) 1436–1439.
[2] J.H. Thrall, Nuclear Medicine: The Requisites, second ed., Mosby, St. Louis, 2001.

CHAPTER 4

COMPUTERS IN RADIOLOGY

William W. Boonn, MD

1. What is PACS?

PACS stands for *picture archiving and communication system*. On the most basic level, PACS integrates image acquisition modalities, workstation displays, the image archiving system, and the underlying network.

2. How are PACS images stored?

The PACS archive traditionally has been composed of short-term and long-term storage. Short-term storage usually is composed of a redundant array of inexpensive (or identical) discs (RAID) arrays (see question 3) that provide quick access to image data. After a certain amount of time (which depends on the size of the short-term archive, but can be 3 to 30 days), images from the short-term archive are moved to the long-term archive, which is usually composed of magnetic tape or magneto-optical media. Images cannot be viewed directly from the long-term archive. Instead, images need to be "fetched" from the long-term archive and copied back to the short-term archive before being viewed on a workstation. This compromise was made because of the high cost of RAID storage. The cost of RAID storage has decreased enough more recently so that several PACS archives are now being designed as "always online" systems. These new systems are composed only of RAID arrays, which essentially place all images in the short-term archive and eliminate the need for fetching.

3. What is a RAID?

A RAID is a group of hard discs and a system that sorts and stores data in various forms to improve data-acquisition speed and provide improved data protection. To accomplish this, a system of levels (from 1 to 5) "mirrors," "stripes," and "duplexes" data onto a group of hard discs.

4. What is image compression?

Image compression is the process of reducing image file size using various mathematical algorithms. Compression is usually expressed as a ratio (e.g., 10:1). A 10-megabyte (MB) file that is compressed at a ratio of 10:1 would have a final size of 1 MB. Generally, as compression ratios increase, file sizes decrease; however, a price is inevitably paid in decreased image fidelity.

5. What is the difference between "lossy" and "lossless" compression?

Encoding an image is a process that converts a raw image (e.g., the original radiograph) into a more compact coded file. Decoding converts the coded file to a decoded image. If the raw image and the decoded image are the same, the compression method is considered lossless. If there is a difference between the raw image and the decoded image, the method of encoding and decoding is considered lossy. Lossless compression can usually achieve ratios of 2:1 or 3:1. Lossy compression can achieve much higher compression ratios; however, overcompression may destroy fine detail, making the image unacceptable for diagnostic purposes.

6. What is RIS?

RIS stands for *radiology information system*. RIS is a system responsible for the workflow within a radiology department. These tasks include patient scheduling and tracking, billing, and handling of radiology reports.

7. What is HIS?

HIS stands for *hospital information system*. HIS manages patient demographics; insurance and billing; and often other clinical information systems, including laboratory results, physician orders, and electronic medical records.

8. What is DICOM?

DICOM stands for *Digital Imaging and Communications in Medicine*. DICOM is a standard that establishes rules that allow medical images and associated information to be exchanged between imaging equipment from different vendors, computers, and hospitals. A computed tomography (CT) scanner produced by vendor A and a magnetic resonance imaging (MRI) scanner produced by vendor B can send images to a PACS from vendor C using DICOM as a common language. In addition to storing image information, other DICOM standard services include query/retrieve, print management, scheduling of acquisition and notification of completion, and security profiles.

9. What determines image storage size?

Image size, generally expressed in megabytes, is determined by spatial resolution and bit depth. Spatial resolution for a two-dimensional (2D) image is defined by a matrix of horizontal and vertical pixels. A single image in a typical CT scan is composed of a matrix of 512 vertical pixels × 512 horizontal pixels, whereas a chest radiograph image might have a matrix size of 2500 vertical pixels × 2000 horizontal pixels. For a given anatomic area of interest, images with a larger matrix size have greater spatial resolution.

Bit depth is defined by the number of shades of gray within the image, where $2n$ equals shades of gray and n equals bit depth. An image with a bit depth of 1 has 2 shades of gray (pure black and pure white). A 6-bit image contains 64 shades of gray; 7-bit, 128 shades; 8-bit, 256 shades; and 12-bit, 4096 shades. Most diagnostic-quality digital images in MRI, CT, and computed radiography/digital radiography are displayed in 10 or 12 bits.

The file size of an imaging study also depends on the number of images in that study. A chest radiograph may have 2 images (posteroanterior and lateral), whereas a CT scan of the abdomen may have 50 images. With the advent of multidetector row CT scanners, it is now possible to acquire thinner slices in much less time, often resulting in much larger studies. This capability also allows images to be reconstructed in different planes. All of this contributes to an increased number of images and, overall, larger study sizes for storage. A CT angiogram may contain 500 to 1000 images or more.

10. How large are these studies?

Table 4-1 shows approximate matrix and file sizes for various imaging modalities. These values vary depending on bit depth, number of images acquired, and compression technique.

11. What is teleradiology?

Teleradiology is the process of sending digital radiology images over a computer network to a remote location (this can be across town or across the globe) for viewing and interpretation. The American College of Radiology publishes a set of guidelines and standards for teleradiology that include minimal display requirements, security and privacy provisions, and documentation standards.

12. What is IHE?

Integrating the Healthcare Enterprise (IHE) is an initiative undertaken by medical specialists and other care providers, administrators, information technology professionals, and industry professionals to improve the way computer systems in health care share information. IHE promotes coordinated use of established communications standards such as DICOM and HL7 (see question 13) to address specific clinical needs that support optimal patient care. Systems developed in accordance with IHE communicate with one another better, are easier to implement, and enable care providers to use information more effectively.

Table 4-1. Approximate Matrix and File Sizes for Various Imaging Modalities

| MODALITY | Image Matrix | | Per Study Basis | | | |
| | | | Images | | Size (MB) | |
	X	Y	AVERAGE	RANGE	AVERAGE	RANGE
Computed radiography (CR)	2000	2500	3	2-5	30	20-50
Digital radiography (DR)	3000	3000	3	2-5	54	40-90
Film digitizer	2000	2500	3	2-5	30	20-50
CT	512	512	60	40-300	32	20-150
Multidetector row CT	512	512	500	200-1000	250	100-600
MRI	256	256	200	80-1000	25	10-150
Digital mammography	3000	3000	6	4-8	100	75-150
US	640	480	30	20-60	20	10-40
Nuclear medicine	256	256	10	4-30	1	0.5-4
Digital fluoroscopy (without digital subtraction angiography [DSA])	1024	1024	20	10-50	20	10-50
Digital fluoroscopy (with DSA)	1024	1024	150	120-240	450	360-720

13. What is HL7?

Health Level 7 (HL7) is the standard used by most RIS and HIS to exchange information between systems. It was designed for sending notifications about events in a health system (e.g., a patient is admitted) and transmitting information (e.g., laboratory data and radiology reports). It was not designed to handle image information; that role is primarily served by DICOM.

14. How are conventional radiographs integrated into an all-digital PACS?

There are three methods. The first method is to obtain a conventional radiograph on film and digitize the image using a scanner. In fully digital environments, this method is usually reserved for digitizing "outside" films or films from settings where digital acquisition has not yet been implemented, such as in the operating room. The second and third methods for acquiring digital radiographs are computed radiography and digital radiography.

Key Points: Computers in Radiology

1. The storage size for a given image is determined by the spatial resolution and bit depth of the image.
2. Digital radiology (DR) systems eliminate the plate and cassette completely and acquire digital images directly, using flat-panel detectors.
3. RIS and PACS are essential elements of DR.

---

15. What is three-dimensional (3D) reconstruction?

3D reconstruction is the process of analyzing a 2D data set and displaying it in three dimensions using various postprocessing techniques and algorithms. The most common 3D reconstructions are multiplanar reformat (MPR), maximum intensity projection (MIP), surface shaded display (SSD), volume rendering (VR), and virtual intraluminal endoscopy (also called "virtual fly-through").

MPR processes images acquired in one plane (e.g., axial CT) and reconstructs the image in other planes (sagittal, coronal, or oblique) so that one may view and scroll through images from multiple perspectives. Curved MPR is another algorithm that is more commonly used in angiographic studies in which curved structures (e.g., the aorta or other blood vessels) are viewed in a single plane. This algorithm is helpful for studying vascular stenosis and aneurysms.

MIP processes a volume of data and assigns a value to each voxel along a line to the viewer's eye. Only the maximum voxel value along that line is displayed. This technique is commonly used in CT angiography and magnetic resonance angiography (MRA), where vascular structures (usually containing contrast agent and having high voxel values) can be separated from background structures and be better visualized.

VR displays all of the 3D data at once, using voxel intensities to determine the transparency of each structure. High-voxel-intensity structures are more opaque, whereas low-voxel-intensity structures are more translucent. The user can assign colors to particular voxel intensities (e.g., red for soft tissues, white for bone density, and yellow for fat density) to create more realistic 3D images.

16. What is voice recognition (or speech recognition)?

Voice recognition is the process by which a computer system recognizes spoken words and converts them to text. Comprehending human languages falls under a different field of computer science called *natural language processing*. Early systems required that the speaker speak slowly and distinctly and separate each word with a short pause. These systems were called *discrete speech systems*. More recently, *continuous speech systems* have become available that allow the user to speak more naturally.

17. What are the advantages and disadvantages of voice or speech recognition relative to conventional dictation/transcription?

There are several *advantages* to voice recognition over conventional dictations for radiology reporting. Report turnaround time is vastly reduced, overall cost is decreased (because transcriptionists are no longer required), and users who take advantage of text macros can dictate standard reports in less time.

The *disadvantages* include erroneous reports because of poor recognition of the speech of certain individuals (sometimes because of lack of training) and difficulty in recognizing similar sounding words (e.g., "hypodense" vs. "hyperdense"). Poor recognition and inefficient use of macros often result in increased dictation time and frustration on the part of the radiologist, which is usually remedied with better training and support.

18. What is structured reporting?

Structured reporting enables the capture of radiology report information so that it can be retrieved later and reused. A key feature of a structured report is consistent organization. A report of an abdominal CT study might follow subheadings that describe each of the anatomic areas described in the report, such as the liver, spleen, pancreas, and kidneys. This feature of structured reporting is sometimes called "itemized reporting" or "standardized reporting," and is preferred by referring physicians, presumably because specific information can be found more easily than in a narrative report. There are no reliable data on the frequency with which reports of this type are currently used. Structured reports also use standard language.

When defined terms from a standard lexicon are associated with imaging reports, the information in the report becomes more accessible and reusable. For many years, mammography has fostered the use of structured reporting as strictly defined—choosing from a limited set of options, such as the six Breast Imaging Reporting and Data System (BI-RADS) categories, to express the likelihood of cancer on a mammogram. BI-RADS reduces the variability and improves the clarity of communication among physicians. Correlation of the recorded structured data items to histopathologic findings (which can often be performed automatically) provides regular feedback to radiologists on their strengths and weaknesses, improving the overall quality of mammographic interpretation.

19. What is RadLex?

RadLex is a comprehensive lexicon for the indexing and retrieval of online radiology resources developed by the Radiological Society of North America and other radiology organizations, including the American College of Radiology (ACR). It has been designed to satisfy the needs of software developers, system vendors, and radiology users by adopting the best features of existing terminology systems, while producing new terms to fill critical gaps. RadLex also provides a comprehensive and technology-friendly replacement for the ACR Index for Radiological Diagnoses. Rather than "reinventing the wheel," RadLex unifies and supplements other lexicons and standards, such as SNOMED-CT and DICOM.

BIBLIOGRAPHY

[1] K. Dreyer, D. Hirschorn, J. Thrall, A. Mehta, PACS: A Guide to the Digital Revolution, Springer-Verlag, New York, 2005.
[2] S.C. Horii, Primer on computers and information technology, part four: a nontechnical introduction to DICOM, RadioGraphics 17 (1997) 1297–1309.
[3] C.P. Langlotz, RadLex: a new method for indexing online educational materials, RadioGraphics 26 (2006) 1595–1597.
[4] B. Liu, F. Cao, M. Zhou, et al., Trends in PACS image storage and archive, Comput. Med. Imaging Graph 27 (2003) 165–174.
[5] O. Ratib, Y. Ligier, D. Bandon, D. Valentino, Update on digital image management and PACS, Abdom. Imaging 25 (2000) 333–340.
[6] E.L. Siegel, R.M. Kolodner, Filmless Radiology, Springer-Verlag, New York, 1999.
[7] D.L. Weiss, C.P. Langlotz, Structured reporting: patient care enhancement or productivity nightmare? Radiology 249 (2008) 739–747.

SCREENING MAMMOGRAPHY

Susan P. Weinstein, MD

CHAPTER 5

1. What is a screening mammogram?

A screening mammogram is a radiographic examination of the breasts performed for early detection of breast cancer in asymptomatic women.

2. When should an average woman start getting mammograms?

The American College of Radiology recommends that a woman get a first mammogram at age 40 and annual mammograms thereafter.

3. Are there instances when screening should start earlier than 40?

Patients with a history of Hodgkin disease treated with radiation or women with a strong family history of breast cancer may be candidates for earlier screening. In women treated for Hodgkin disease, surveillance may begin 10 years after chest wall/mediastinal radiation exposure. Patients who received radiation therapy during puberty are at greatest risk for breast cancer. Patients who received radiation therapy after age 30 have a minimally increased risk over the general population. For patients with a history of a first-degree relative with breast cancer, screening should begin 10 years before the age at which the relative was diagnosed. If the relative was diagnosed after age 50, there would be no impact on the screening recommendation. If the relative was diagnosed before age 50, the woman should begin screening before the age of 40.

4. How many views are obtained for a routine mammogram?

Four views are obtained for a routine mammogram. Craniocaudal (CC) and medio-lateral oblique (MLO) views of each breast are obtained. In some patients, more than four images may be needed to visualize all of the breast parenchyma adequately.

5. Which view visualizes the most breast tissue?

MLO view visualizes the most breast tissue.

6. Which portion of the breast is better visualized on CC view than on MLO view?

The medial breast is better visualized on CC view.

7. How should a film screen mammogram be hung?

CC views are hung next to one another, and MLO views are hung adjacent to each other (Fig. 5-1). The films are hung with the labels in the upper corner. On CC views, the labels are placed adjacent to the lateral breast. On MLO views, the labels are placed adjacent to the superior breast. The comparison films are hung in the same manner above the current study.

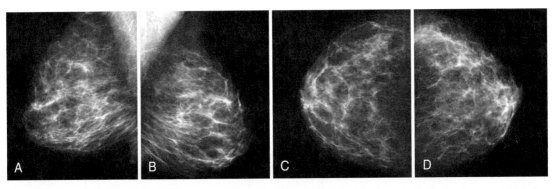

Figure 5-1. Screening mammogram hung for viewing. **A-D,** From the viewer's left, the images are the left MLO view (**A**), the right MLO view (**B**), the left CC view (**C**), and the right CC view (**D**). The comparison films are typically hung above the current study.

8. How old should the comparison films be?

If the patient has multiple sets of prior films, we like to compare with the studies that are 2 years old. Early changes from breast cancer can be subtle, and the changes are easier to detect over the 2-year interval.

9. What if there are comparison films elsewhere? Do we need to get them?

If the mammogram results are considered to be negative, no. Studies have shown that it is not cost-effective and does not improve patient care to obtain comparison films for studies with normal results. If there is an abnormal finding, an attempt should be made to get the prior studies from the outside institution. If the prior films cannot be obtained, the patient should be recalled for additional evaluation.

10. What is the incidence of screening-detected breast cancer?

In a population that has never been screened, the incidence is about 6 to 10/1000. In a population that is routinely screened, the incidence decreases to about 2 to 4/1000.

11. What is the reported sensitivity of screening mammography?

False-negative interpretation (mammograms that are interpreted as negative, but a cancer is present) is usually 15% to 20%. The sensitivity decreases as the glandularity of the breast tissue increases. The sensitivity of mammography in women with dense breast tissue is about 50%. In fatty breast tissue, the sensitivity of mammography is quite high, in the high 90s.

12. What is the difference between a screening mammogram and a diagnostic mammogram?

A screening mammogram is performed on asymptomatic patients as part of routine annual surveillance. A diagnostic mammogram is performed when the patient has a history of breast cancer or presents with a breast-related complaint or symptom.

13. Are there other types of breast cancer screening modalities? Which modalities are used in everyday clinical practice?

Digital mammography is similar to film screen mammography, but the images are acquired in a digital form. After acquisition, image processing is possible with the digitized images. The images can be printed and viewed as hard copies similar to film screen mammography or reviewed on a computer monitor. The soft copy images can be manipulated to enhance the image interpretation. The contrast can be changed, and the images can be magnified. Although film screen mammography has better spatial resolution than digital mammography, digital mammography has better contrast resolution than film screen images.

Screening breast ultrasound (US) consists of US examination of both breasts in asymptomatic women. The largest prospective study to date was sponsored by American College of Radiology Imaging Network (ACRIN) 6666. The goal of the prospective, multicenter trial was to compare the diagnostic yield of screening breast mammography plus US versus mammography alone in high-risk women. Although the added screening US examinations found additional breast cancers, there was a high false-positive rate. That is, many biopsies were recommended for benign findings, resulting in a low positive predictive value.

Screening magnetic resonance imaging (MRI) is not likely to be used in everyday clinical practice because of the lack of availability, high cost, and variable specificity leading to many false-positive interpretations. MRI screening has shown to be promising in very high-risk patients, however. The American Cancer Society guidelines recommend MRI screening in women with a greater than 20% to 25% lifetime risk for breast cancer. The screening groups include women who are carriers of the *BRCA* mutations or untested women with a first-degree relative who is a known carrier; women with a history of mantle radiation before age 30; and women with Li-Fraumeni, Cowden, and Bannayan-Riley-Ruvalcaba syndromes. MRI screening cancer yield in high-risk patients has consistently been 2% to 3%.

Key Points: Screening Mammography

1. Annual screening mammography should begin at age 40.
2. Mammography is still the best screening test to detect subclinical breast cancer.
3. The sensitivity of mammography is in the range of 85%.
4. Most breast cancers occur in women with no family history of the disease.

14. Is digital mammography better than film screen mammography in detecting breast cancer?

The largest prospective multicenter trial comparing digital mammography with film screen mammography is the Digital Mammographic Imaging Screening Trial (DMIST) sponsored by ACRIN. The study recruited more than 49,000 women. Overall, in the general population, the accuracy of digital mammography was similar to film screen mammography. The accuracy of digital mammography was higher than film screen mammography, however, in certain subpopulations, including women younger than age 50 years, women with heterogeneously or extremely dense breasts, and premenopausal or perimenopausal women.

15. Is there an age at which breast cancer screening should stop?

In the United States, there are no guidelines for when screening should stop. In other countries, the recommended age at which screening should stop ranges from 59 to 74 years.

16. What is batch reading of screening mammograms?

Batch reading is the most efficient way to read screening mammograms. The women are imaged. The films are hung on a multiviewer or loaded onto a workstation, and all the studies are batch read by the radiologist, typically the following day. This approach increases efficiency. The results are mailed to the patients.

17. What are some risk factors for developing breast cancer?

Perhaps the greatest risk factor is being a female. Men get breast cancer, but male breast cancer accounts for less than 1% of all breast cancers diagnosed annually. Other risk factors include being genetic mutation carrier (*BRCA1* and *BRCA2*) status, history of mantle radiation, first-degree relative with breast cancer, personal history of breast cancer, history of atypia such as atypical ductal hyperplasia and lobular carcinoma in situ on biopsy, early menarche, late menopause, nulliparous status, late first-term pregnancy (>30 years old), and advancing age.

18. *True or false*: Most breast cancers occur in women with a family history of breast cancer.

False. About 20% of breast cancers occur in patients with a positive family history. About 75% to 80% of breast cancers are sporadic.

19. *True or false*: With increased use of breast cancer screening, the incidence of breast cancer has been declining

False. The incidence of breast cancer has been steadily increasing since the 1980s. This increase has been partly attributed to early detection owing to increased breast cancer screening with mammography during this time period. The incidence leveled off in the 1990s and began to decline starting about 1999 according to the National Cancer Institute Surveillance Epidemiology and End Results (SEER) data. The reason for this decreased incidence is unclear. According to the SEER data, it was estimated that 182,460 women would be diagnosed with breast cancer in 2008 and 40,480 women would die of cancer from breast cancer (National Cancer Institute Surveillance Epidemiology and End Results [SEER], Table I-1. Available at: http://seer.cancer.gov/csr/1975_2005/results_single/sect_01_table.01.pdf).

20. It has been said that one in eight women has a risk of developing breast cancer. Does a 40-year-old woman have the same risk as an 80-year-old woman?

No. The one-in-eight risk of developing breast cancer refers to an overall lifetime risk if the woman lives to age 85. Given identical circumstances, a 40-year-old woman does not have the same risk as an 80-year-old woman. The National Cancer Institute gives an overall risk based on the age of the patient (Tables 5-1 and 5-2). The incidence peaks between ages 45 and 74, then decreases.

21. What are *BRCA1* and *BRCA2*? What is the risk of getting breast cancer by age 70 in a patient who is a *BRCA1* gene carrier?

BRCA1 and *BRCA2* are genetic mutations. Both genes have autosomal dominant expression and may be inherited from the maternal or the paternal side. Women who carry a *BRCA1* or *BRCA2* gene have increased risk of developing cancers, with breast and ovarian cancers being the two most common types. In regards to breast cancer, the women who have the genetic mutation tend to develop breast cancer at an earlier age than the general population and are more likely to develop bilateral breast cancer. Men with *BRCA1* and *BRCA2* mutations are at increased risk of developing prostate cancer. Men who carry the *BRCA1* mutation are also at increased risk for breast cancer. Genetic testing for *BRCA1* and *BRCA2* is available. In a woman who is a *BRCA1* carrier, the risk of developing breast cancer can be 85%.

Table 5-1. Age-Related Incidence of Breast Cancer

AGE	INCIDENCE (%)
<20	0
20-34	1.9
35-44	10.6
45-54	22.4
55-64	23.3
65-74	19.8
75-84	16.5
>85	5.5

Data from National Cancer Institute Surveillance, Epidemiology, and End Results Program 2008 website. Most of the data can be found in Ries LAG, Melbert D, Krapcho M, et al (eds): SEER Cancer Statistics Review, 1975-2005. Bethesda, MD, National Cancer Institute, 2007. Available at: http://seer.cancer.gov/csr/1975_2005/.

22. How much radiation does a woman receive from a routine screening mammogram?

The amount of radiation is 0.2 rad (2 mGy) for two views of one breast. Although there is radiation exposure, the amount is considered small and is believed to be outweighed by the benefits of early detection from screening.

23. How is a patient who has undergone screening informed of her test results?

Usually, a letter is sent in the mail. There are two potential results. The patient may be informed that her mammogram was normal. Alternatively, the patient may be informed of the need for additional evaluation, which may be in the form of additional imaging or obtaining the patient's prior mammograms for comparison.

Table 5-2. Definitions

Annual percent change (APC)	Average annual percent change over several years. APC is used to measure trends or the change in rates over time. For information on how this is calculated, go to "Trend Algorithms" in the SEER*Stat Help system. The calculation involves fitting a straight line to the natural logarithm of the data when it is displayed by calendar year
Joinpoint analyses	Statistical model for characterizing cancer trends that uses statistical criteria to determine how many times and when the trends in incidence or mortality rates have changed. The results of joinpoint are given as calendar-year ranges and APC in the rates over each period
Survival rate	Survival rate examines how long after diagnosis people live. Cancer survival is measured in many different ways depending on the intended purpose
Relative survival rate	Measure of net survival that is calculated by comparing observed (overall) survival with expected survival from a comparable set of individuals who do not have cancer to measure the excess mortality that is associated with a cancer diagnosis
Stage distribution	Stage provides a measure of disease progression, detailing the degree to which the cancer has advanced. Two methods commonly used to determine stage are AJCC and SEER historic. The AJCC method (see Collaborative Staging Method) is more commonly used in clinical settings, whereas SEER has standardized and simplified staging to ensure consistent definitions over time
Lifetime risk	Probability of developing cancer in the course of one's life span. Lifetime risk may also be discussed in terms of the probability of developing or dying from cancer. Based on cancer rates from 2003-2005, it was estimated that men had about a 44% chance of developing cancer in their lifetimes, whereas women had about a 37% chance
Probability of developing cancer	Chance that an individual will develop cancer in his or her lifetime
Prevalence	Number of people who have received a diagnosis of cancer during a defined time period, and who are alive on the last day of that period. Most prevalence data in SEER are for limited duration because information on cases diagnosed before 1973 is not generally available

AJCC, American Joint Committee on Cancer; SEER, Surveillance, Epidemiology, and End Results.

24. What happens if additional imaging evaluation is needed based on findings on the screening mammogram?

The patient is sent a letter advising her that additional evaluation is needed. In addition, at our institution, a coordinator calls the patient to schedule the necessary appointment.

25. What is the call-back rate? What should the call-back rate be for a radiologist?

The call-back rate is the percentage of the screening cases that the radiologist recommends for additional imaging evaluations. The rate should be 10% or less.

26. Is the breast a modified skin gland, fatty tissue, muscle, or lymphatic structure?

The breast tissue is derived from ectodermal origin and is a modified skin gland.

27. How does accessory breast tissue form? Where is it most commonly located?

Breast tissue development begins at about 6 weeks of gestation and originates from ectodermal elements. The "milk line" extends from the groin region to the axillary region. Most of the potential breast tissue atrophies except in the fourth intercostal region, where "normal" mammary tissue eventually develops. The lack of appropriate regression results in accessory breasts anywhere along the "milk line."

BIBLIOGRAPHY

[1] W.A. Berg, J.D. Blume, J.B. Cormack, et al., ACRIN 6666 Investigators: Combined screening with ultrasound and mammography vs mammography alone in women at elevated risk of breast cancer, JAMA 299 (2008) 2151–2163.

[2] D.B. Kopans, Breast Imaging, third ed., Lippincott Williams & Wilkins, Philadelphia, 2007.

[3] C.D. Lehman, C. Isaacs, M.D. Schnall, et al., Cancer yield of mammography, MR, and US in high-risk women: prospective multi-institution breast cancer screening study, Radiology 244 (2007) 381–388.

[4] E.D. Pisano, C. Gatsonis, E. Hendrick, et al., Diagnostic performance of digital versus film mammography for breast-cancer screening, N. Engl. J. Med. 353 (2005) 1773–1783.

[5] D. Saslow, C. Boetes, W. Burke, et al., American Cancer Society guidelines for breast screening with MRI as an adjunct to mammography, CA Cancer J. Clin. 57 (2007) 75–89.

[6] S. Shapiro, E.A. Coleman, M. Broeders, et al., Breast cancer screening programs in 22 countries: current policies, administration and guidelines, Int. J. Epidemiol. 27 (1998) 735–742.

6 CHAPTER

DIAGNOSTIC MAMMOGRAPHY

Susan P. Weinstein, MD

1. What are the indications for a diagnostic mammogram?

Some indications for a diagnostic mammogram include a history of breast cancer, breast lump, nipple discharge, focal breast pain, breast implants, history of breast biopsy, and follow-up for a previously evaluated mammographic finding (BI-RADS category 3 lesion [see question 3]).

2. What views are performed for diagnostic mammography? How are patients who have undergone diagnostic mammography informed of results?

Routine views are performed with additional views as needed. These additional views may include spot compression views, magnification views, exaggerated views, and rolled views. Ultrasound (US) may also be performed if indicated. The imaging evaluation is completed while the patient is present, and the patient is informed of the results before she leaves. At our institution, the physician discusses the results with the patient.

3. What is BI-RADS?

The Breast Imaging Reporting and Data System (BI-RADS) lexicon was developed by the American College of Radiology to provide a clear, concise way to report the mammographic results. A BI-RADS category is reported at the end of every mammogram report and summarizes the findings of the mammogram (Table 6-1).

4. What types of mammographic changes may be seen after breast conservation?

There may be persistent distortion and edema. Other findings include skin thickening and trabecular thickening. The first mammogram after completion of therapy serves as a baseline study for the patient. The post-therapy changes should remain stable or improve over time.

5. Does mammography have a very high sensitivity in detecting recurrent breast cancer after breast conservation?

The sensitivity of mammography in detecting recurrent tumor is limited by the post-therapy changes present on the mammogram. Overall, mammography does not detect recurrence about one third of the time. Mammography detects

Table 6-1. BI-RADS Lexicon

BI-RADS CATEGORY	DEFINITION
1	Normal mammogram. The patient should return in 1 yr for her annual mammogram
2	Benign finding on the mammogram. The patient should return in 1 yr for her annual mammogram
3	A finding is present, but there is a high likelihood of benignity (>98%). A short-term follow-up is recommended in 6 mo. Normally, the follow-up is performed over a total of 2 yr
4	A finding is present, and a biopsy is warranted
4a	Low likelihood of malignancy
4b	Intermediate likelihood of malignancy
4c	Moderate likelihood of malignancy
5	A finding is present, and a biopsy is recommended. There is a high likelihood of malignancy (>95%)
6	Confirmed malignancy
0	Indicates that the imaging evaluation is incomplete. Additional evaluation or prior films are needed for comparison

recurrent disease manifested by calcifications, although early fat necrosis may be difficult to differentiate from intraductal carcinoma. The sensitivity of mammography is lower in detecting masses. Physical examination plays a complementary role in evaluating the patient after breast conservation.

6. What is the incidence of recurrent breast cancer in a patient after breast conservation?
The risk of recurrence is about 1% to 2% per year. At 5 years, the risk of recurrence is about 5% to 10%.

7. *True or false*: In patients who develop recurrence after breast conservation, survival rates are about the same as for patients who had a mastectomy as the initial treatment.
True. Recurrence after breast conservation does not seem to affect the overall survival rate for patients with breast cancer. Survival depends on the size of the recurrence, however.

8. What are contraindications to breast conservation?
- Multicentric cancer. The presence of breast cancer in different quadrants is a contraindication. If there is multifocal tumor or more than one foci of cancer localized to the same quadrant, breast conservation therapy is feasible.
- Size of the cancer relative to the breast size. This is a relative contraindication. Some clinicians use 5 cm as a cutoff, but others use a relative measurement as a size cutoff. A 6-cm cancer in a large breast may result in acceptable cosmesis, whereas in a small breast it would result in unacceptable cosmetic results.
- First-trimester or second-trimester pregnancy.
- History of prior radiation therapy to the chest or mediastinum.
- Active collagen vascular disease.

9. In a patient who is planning to have breast conservation, when is it necessary to obtain a postbiopsy mammogram shortly after a successful excisional biopsy?
If the malignancy was associated with calcifications on the mammogram, a postbiopsy mammogram should be obtained to ensure that all the suspicious microcalcifications have been removed. If there are residual calcifications, the likelihood that there is residual disease is quite high. The inverse is not true. If there are no residual calcifications, this does not indicate that there is no residual disease. There may be portions of the cancer that are not calcified. The decision to re-excise is based on pathologic margin status.

For breast cancers that manifest as a mass on the mammogram, a postbiopsy mammogram is not needed. The decision to re-excise should be based on the histologic margins. Because of the postbiopsy changes in the surgical bed, it would be difficult to differentiate between postbiopsy changes and residual tumor.

10. *True or false*: In a patient with a history of breast cancer, it is beneficial to get a mammogram more frequently than once a year.
False. No studies have shown the benefit of increased frequency of screening. Our institution recommends mammography once a year.

11. How do you hang a mammogram of a patient who has had a mastectomy?
The craniocaudal (CC) and medio-lateral oblique (MLO) views should be hung on the appropriate side on the light box. The old films should be hung in mirror image.

12. What is a 6-month follow-up? How long is the follow-up performed for BI-RADS category 3 lesions?
Six-month follow-up is performed for BI-RADS category 3 lesions (after an appropriate imaging evaluation). The follow-up is performed for a total of 2 years at 6-month intervals. For lesions that fit the "probably benign" category, less than 2% of the lesions are malignant. That is, greater than 98% of the lesions are benign.

13. How is the mastectomy bed evaluated?
We do not recommend routine imaging evaluation of the mastectomy bed. No studies have shown the benefit of routine imaging evaluation of the surgical bed. Instead, clinical evaluation is recommended. If there is a palpable area of concern on the physical examination, US should be performed as the next step in the evaluation.

14. What types of surgical reconstruction are available after a mastectomy?
There are various types of tissue flaps, such as transverse rectus abdominis musculocutaneous flaps and latissimus dorsi flaps. Alternatively, silicone or saline implants may be used for reconstruction.

15. *True or false*: **After a benign breast biopsy, significant residual changes are usually visible on a mammogram.**
False. After a benign breast biopsy, the breast tissue usually heals with few residual changes. Infrequently, distortion and postbiopsy changes may persist.

16. **For all breast biopsies, approximately what percentage of the pathology results should be malignant?**
The positive predictive value for all breast biopsies should be approximately 25% to 40%. This rate is considered acceptable.

17. **A 47-year-old woman presents with a newly palpable breast mass and has a negative mammogram. What should be done next?**
The next step in the evaluation should be a directed US evaluation of the area of palpable concern. If a solid mass is present, a biopsy should be recommended.

18. **If US results are negative, what should be done next? What percentage of the time can a cancer be missed on US and mammography?**
If US and mammography results are negative, clinical management is advised. This may include clinically following the patient or doing a biopsy if the palpable area is clinically suspicious. Depending on the literature, the negative predictive value of combined mammography and US is 95% to 100%. That is, if both studies are negative, a cancer may be missed 5% of the time or less.

Key Points: Diagnostic Mammography

1. The BI-RADS categories (see Table 6-1) are essential for reporting results of diagnostic mammography.
2. Diagnostic mammography is indicated for women with a specific breast-related problem that needs to be evaluated. Screening mammography is indicated for asymptomatic patients.
3. In patients who have had breast conservation, the postbiopsy changes may limit the sensitivity of mammography.
4. In a patient presenting with a palpable breast mass, if the mammogram results are negative, the imaging evaluation should not stop at that point. Directed US evaluation is necessary to complete the evaluation.

---

19. **What types of nipple discharge are considered suspicious and warrant additional imaging evaluation? What imaging work-up is recommended for suspicious nipple discharge?**
Nipple discharge that is spontaneous, bloody, clear, or serosanguineous is considered suspicious. The first step in the evaluation should be a mammogram. The mammogram results may be normal or show a finding. At our institution, we also perform US looking for any suspicious lesions that may be causing the discharge. Typically, we look in the subareolar and periareolar regions.

If the mammogram and US are normal, the next step may be a galactogram. The involved ductal orifice is cannulated, and a catheter is inserted. A small amount of contrast agent is injected into the ductal system until resistance is felt. A mammogram is obtained to look for filling defects that may be the cause of the discharge (Fig. 6-1). If there is a filling defect, the defect may be due to various causes, such as debris, a papilloma, or a malignancy.

Magnetic resonance imaging (MRI) may also have a role in the evaluation of nipple discharge. Ultimately, if there is clinically suspicious discharge with no clear explanation, surgical duct exploration may be performed.

20. **What types of nipple discharge are associated with benign etiologies?**
The typical benign discharge may be greenish, brownish, or milky in color. Bilaterality and discharge arising from multiple ductal orifices are also benign characteristics.

21. **In a patient with a suspicious type of nipple discharge, what is the likelihood that the discharge is due to cancer?**
The likelihood is about 10%.

22. **What is the most common etiology for bloody nipple discharge?**
Benign papillomas are the most common etiology.

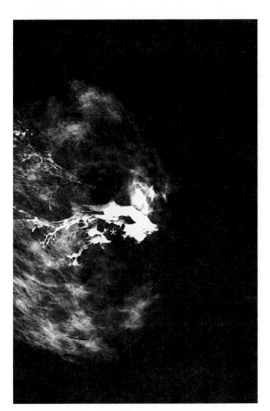

Figure 6-1. Image from a galactogram in a patient presenting with bloody nipple discharge. Contrast agent is seen filling a ductal system. Lobulated filling defect is marked with an *asterisk*. Biopsy revealed a papilloma.

23. What are the most common histologic types of breast cancer?

The most common histologic types of breast cancer are invasive ductal carcinoma, intraductal (ductal carcinoma in situ) carcinoma, and invasive lobular carcinoma. Subtypes of invasive ductal carcinoma include medullary, mucinous, papillary, cribriform, papillary, metaplastic, micropapillary, and tubular. Less common histologic types of breast cancer include sarcoma and lymphoma. Secondary neoplasms of the breast are rare, but may occur.

24. Is lobular carcinoma in situ (LCIS) a form of cancer? What is the significance of LCIS?

LCIS has no clinical or mammographic correlate. It is a histologic diagnosis. LCIS is not a cancer, but is considered a risk lesion. In a woman previously diagnosed with LCIS, the risk of developing breast cancer in either breast is about 33%.

25. What is the differential diagnosis for a red swollen breast?

The differential diagnosis includes infection, inflammatory breast cancer, history of prior radiation, and lymphatic or vascular obstruction. The history of prior radiation should be easy to corroborate with the patient. Patients with infection and inflammatory breast cancer can present with similar histories: red, swollen, tender breast. Imaging should be performed to exclude a mass or an abscess. If the patient's symptoms do not improve with treatment (antibiotics), inflammatory breast cancer should be excluded. The skin appears red and swollen in inflammatory carcinoma because the dermal lymphatics are infiltrated with tumor cells. Typically, punch biopsy of the skin confirms the diagnosis. Occasionally, punch biopsy findings are negative.

26. Is there such a thing as a mammographic emergency?

Probably the only breast imaging–related emergency is an abscess that needs to be drained, but this problem can usually be managed clinically. If a fluctuant mass is present, it can be drained by palpation. Otherwise, if there is clinical concern of an abscess, the patient can be treated symptomatically. Patients are usually in too much pain to get a mammogram anyway; if they undergo imaging, US is usually performed to look for a collection.

27. How many views are obtained in a patient with breast augmentation?

At our institution, four routine views (CC and MLO views) and four implant-displaced views are obtained. (At some institutions, an implant-displaced medio-lateral view may also be obtained.) On the four routine views, the breast implant is imaged. The glandular tissue is not well compressed. The implant-displaced views are obtained with the implant pushed back so that the breast tissue can be compressed. Usually the presence of the breast implants limits the visualization of the posterior breast tissue.

28. Where can the implants be placed in the breast?

They can be placed retropectorally, behind the pectoralis muscle. Alternatively, they can be placed in the retroglandular position, or in front of the muscle.

29. What types of implants are available?

Currently, saline and silicone implants are available. In the past, silicone implants were available only for reconstruction in patients with a history of breast cancer. Silicone implants are available now for cosmetic augmentation as well. In 2006, the U.S. Food and Drug Administration approved silicone implants for cosmetic surgery after taking them off the market in 1992 because of a controversy regarding silicon implants and possible association with connective tissue disease. No studies to date have definitively associated silicone implants with connective tissue disease.

30. What is the most sensitive imaging evaluation for implant rupture?

MRI is the gold standard. US may be used to evaluate for rupture as well, but the examination is operator dependent. Rupture may be contained within the fibrous capsule surrounding the implant (intracapsular) or may extend outside the fibrous capsule (extracapsular). Although mammography detects extracapsular rupture, it is limited in the evaluation of intracapsular rupture, the more common form of rupture. MRI findings of implant rupture are the linguine sign (most reliable), the keyhole sign, and the noose sign.

31. A man presents with a breast lump. How should the patient be imaged? What is the most common etiology for a breast lump in a man?

For a man presenting with a breast lump, we usually recommend a bilateral mammogram. Sometimes US may be needed if there is dense tissue in the area of the breast lump on the mammogram. The most common etiology for a breast lump in a man is gynecomastia. Usually this is bilateral, although it commonly can be asymmetric (Fig. 6-2). Clinical work-up should be recommended to evaluate for the etiology of the gynecomastia.

32. What is the etiology of gynecomastia?

There is a long differential diagnosis for gynecomastia. In infants and in teenagers, it is most commonly due to hormonal influences. Transplacental maternal hormones are responsible in infants. In teenagers, the hormonal fluctuations of adolescence are thought to be responsible. Other pathologic processes should be excluded, however. A few common etiologies for gynecomastia are marijuana use, certain types of medications, liver dysfunction, androgen deficiency, or any condition that causes an imbalance of estrogen to testosterone. Finally, hormone-secreting tumors should be excluded.

33. Do men get breast cancer? What is the frequency?

Yes, but male breast cancers are rare, accounting for less than 1% of all breast cancers (Fig. 6-3). Male breast cancer is most commonly diagnosed between 60 and 70 years of age. The most common symptom is a painless mass. Other

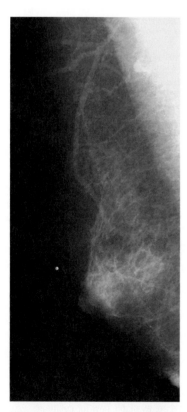

Figure 6-2. MLO view of a male patient who presented with breast pain. Glandular tissue is seen in subareolar region consistent with gynecomastia.

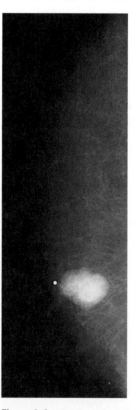

Figure 6-3. MLO view of a male patient who presented with a breast lump. A lobulated, circumscribed mass is seen in the subareolar region. The mass is definitely masslike, in contrast to the changes of gynecomastia seen in Figure 6-2. Biopsy showed invasive carcinoma.

symptoms include mass, skin dimpling or retraction, and occasionally discharge. Men are treated with mastectomy. Breast conservation therapy is not a standard of care in men. In addition, male patients may get radiation therapy or chemotherapy or both depending on stage, lymph node status, and final surgical margins. Some also get hormonal therapy because most male breast cancers are estrogen receptor positive. Overall, stage for stage, the prognosis for male breast cancer is similar to that for female breast cancer. In the past, it was thought that male breast cancer had a worse prognosis than female breast cancer; however, this was due to the late stage at which the disease was diagnosed.

34. **_True or false_: Breast cancer can manifest in the following ways: calcifications, masses, architectural distortion, and density.**
True for all of the above. Benign lesions may also manifest in the same ways.

35. **The following terms are commonly used to describe calcifications. Classify the terms as describing _benign, indeterminate,_ or _malignant_ calcifications.**
a. Popcorn
b. Centrally lucent
c. Amorphous
d. Heterogeneous
e. Indistinct
f. Round
g. Milk of calcium
h. Linear, branching
i. Rodlike
j. Eggshell
k. Dystrophic
l. Pleomorphic
Benign: a, b, f, g, i, j, k; _indeterminate:_ c, e; _malignant:_ d, h, l.

36. **Figs. 6-4 through 6-9 show images of calcifications. Classify them as benign or malignant calcifications**
Figs. 6-4 and 6-5 display malignant calcifications. Figs. 6-6, 6-7, 6-8, and 6-9 show different types of benign calcifications: Fig. 6-6 shows milk of calcium, Fig. 6-7 shows round calcifications, Fig. 6-8 shows popcorn calcifications, and Fig. 6-9 shows secretory calcifications.

37. **What is a triple-negative breast cancer? What is the significance of a triple-negative cancer?**
A cancer is termed _triple-negative_ when it does not express receptors for estrogen, progesterone, and human epidermal growth factor receptor-2. Depending on the tumor receptor expression, different types of therapies may be used to treat breast cancer. Triple-negative cancers do not express any of the three receptors; drugs such as tamoxifen and trastuzumab (Herceptin) are not effective against these cancers. Triple-negative cancers tend to be more aggressive with a higher rate of recurrence than other subtypes. Studies have shown triple-negative cancers also disproportionately affect premenopausal African-American women and are more common in carriers of _BRCA1_ mutation.

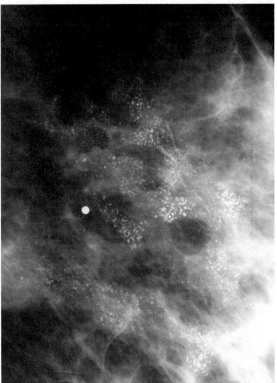

Figure 6-4. Malignant calcifications.

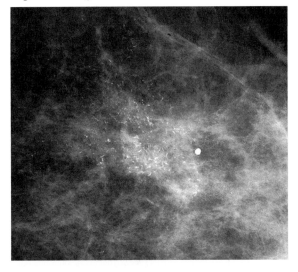

Figure 6-5. Malignant calcifications.

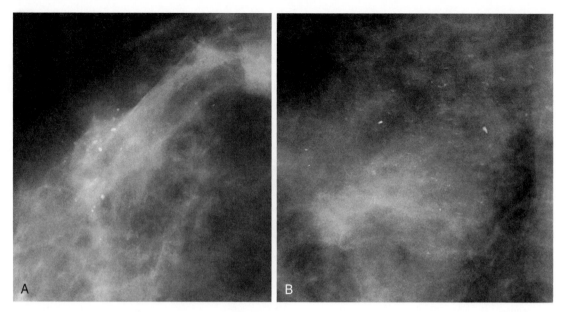

Figure 6-6. Benign calcifications, milk of calcium. **A,** CC view. **B,** MLO view.

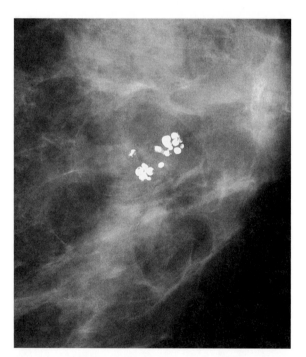

Figure 6-7. Benign round calcifications.

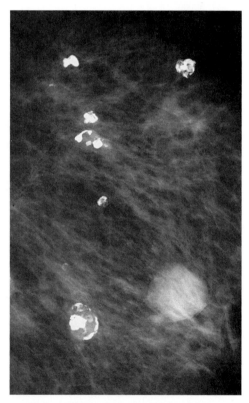

Figure 6-8. Benign popcorn calcifications.

38. A patient presents with a palpable breast mass and a stable mammogram. The mass in Fig. 6-10 is seen on US. What should be the radiologist's recommendation?
Although the mammogram was considered stable, the next step in the evaluation of the patient should include a targeted US examination. The mass is very hypoechoic, but does not have any features that would suggest that this is a cyst. The indistinct margins also makes the mass suspicious. In this case, core needle biopsy was performed under US with subsequent diagnosis of invasive ductal carcinoma.

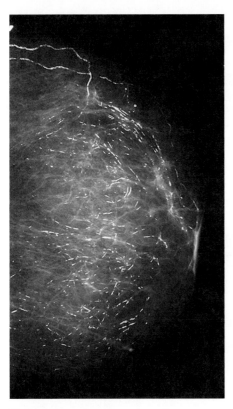

Figure 6-9. Benign secretory calcifications.

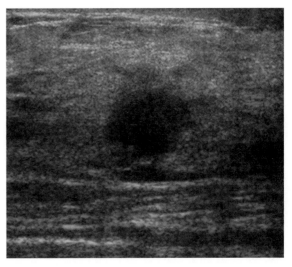

Figure 6-10. Ultrasound of hypoechoic breast mass, without posterior through-transmission.

BIBLIOGRAPHY

[1] L.W. Bassett, Imaging of breast masses, Radiol. Clin. North Am. 38 (2000) 669–692.
[2] M.A. Dennis, S.H. Parker, A.J. Klaus, et al., Breast biopsy avoidance: the value of normal mammograms and normal sonograms in the setting of a palpable lump, Radiology 219 (2001) 186–191.
[3] D.D. Dershaw, Breast imaging and the conservative treatment of breast cancer, Radiol. Clin. North Am. 40 (2002) 501–516.
[4] J.S. Kaiser, M.A. Helvie, R.L. Blacklaw, M.A. Roubidoux, Palpable breast thickening: role of mammography and US in cancer detection, Radiology 223 (2002) 839–844.
[5] H. Nakahara, K. Namba, R. Watanabe, et al., A comparison of MR imaging, galactography and ultrasonography in patients with nipple discharge, Breast Cancer 10 (2003) 320–329.
[6] S.G. Orel, C.S. Dougherty, C. Reynolds, et al., MR imaging in patients with nipple discharge: initial experience, Radiology 216 (2000) 248–254.
[7] M.S. Soo, E.L. Rosen, J.A. Baker, et al., Negative predictive value of sonography with mammography in patients with palpable breast lesions, AJR Am. J. Roentgenol. 177 (2001) 1167–1170.

BREAST ULTRASOUND AND BREAST PROCEDURES

Susan P. Weinstein, MD

1. What are the labeled structures on the ultrasound (US) image in Fig. 7-1?
The structures are skin (*A*), subcutaneous fat (*B*), glandular tissue (*C*), fat (*D*), muscle (*E*), and rib (*F*).

2. What type of transducer should be used to perform breast US?
A linear array transducer should be used. It should be at least 7 MHz, ideally 10 MHz or greater.

3. List the indications for breast US after a mammographic evaluation.
- To evaluate a palpable abnormality further.
- To characterize a mammographic finding or abnormality.

4. In what situations would you not perform a mammogram but go directly to breast US in evaluating patients with palpable breast masses?
In patients who are younger than 30 and in pregnant patients, it is recommended to go directly to breast US. For all other patients, mammography should be obtained first. At our institution, a mammogram is obtained first in women who are older than 30. To evaluate the palpable abnormality further, US follows the mammogram. If the patient is younger than 30, US is obtained first. Age 30 is an arbitrary number; different institutions may have a different cutoff age.

5. What are some suspicious lesion features on US?
Suspicious features on US include a markedly hypoechoic appearance, posterior acoustic shadowing, angular margins, spiculations, microlobulations, a mass that is taller than wide, and ductal extension. Although these features are usually seen in malignant lesions, there is an overlap, and benign masses may also exhibit some of these findings (Fig. 7-2).

6. What are some benign lesion features on US?
Benign features on US include absence of malignant features, well-circumscribed mass, ellipsoid shape, macrolobulations, and hyperechogenicity. Although these features are typically seen in benign lesions, some malignant masses may exhibit some of these features. Well-circumscribed cancers include invasive ductal carcinoma (not otherwise specified) and medullary and colloid subtypes of ductal carcinoma (Fig. 7-3).

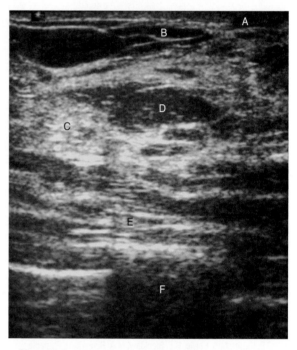

Figure 7-1. US image of normal breast tissue.

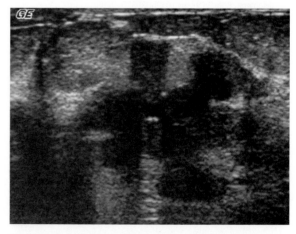

Figure 7-2. Highly suspicious hypoechoic lobulated solid mass with irregular margins in a woman who presented with a palpable breast mass. Biopsy revealed invasive carcinoma.

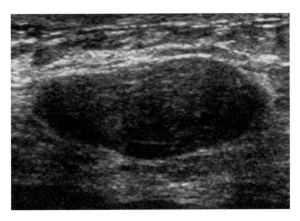

Figure 7-3. A 26-year-old woman presented with a palpable mass. US shows a benign-appearing, well-circumscribed oval mass. US findings are consistent with a benign mass such as a fibroadenoma.

7. What types of biopsy procedures may be performed to evaluate breast lesions?

Fine needle aspiration (FNA) is readily available and needs no special equipment. Overall, it is less traumatic than core biopsy or excisional biopsy.

Core needle biopsy is a minimally invasive percutaneous procedure that can be performed under US guidance or stereotactic mammographic guidance. A wide range of needles is available on the market in terms of needle gauge and vacuum versus nonvacuum assistance. The type of needle that is used tends to be based on personal preferences, although stereotactic biopsies are almost always done with vacuum assistance to maximize the retrieval of calcifications. Biopsies performed under US tend to be easier and faster to perform than stereotactic biopsies, partly because of the real-time imaging available with US guidance. At our institution, we reserve the stereotactic method to obtain biopsy samples of calcifications, although biopsy samples of solid masses may also be obtained using this method. Percutaneous core biopsies are less expensive, are faster to perform, and are less traumatic than surgical biopsies. The false-negative rates are similar to open biopsies.

Needle localization followed by excisional biopsy in the operating room is the gold standard. To confirm removal of the lesion, a specimen radiograph is obtained. At our institution, we image the specimen while the patient is still in the operating room. The findings are called to the surgeon.

8. What are the relative disadvantages of FNA, core needle biopsy, and needle localization/excision?

- *FNA*: The results depend on the skill of the individual performing the procedure and the cytopathologist. There can be a high percentage of unsatisfactory aspirates (20% to 30% of cases). Invasive versus in situ cancer cannot be differentiated on FNA. The false-negative rate for image-guided FNA is unknown.
- *Core needle biopsy*: Tissue displacement may occur during the biopsy procedure, resulting in misinterpretation of intraductal carcinoma as invasive carcinoma. Inversely, cancer can occasionally be understaged.
- *Needle localization with excisional biopsy*: This is the most expensive and most traumatic of all the biopsy procedures.

9. After core biopsy, how can one be certain that the lesion of interest was actually what was sampled?

After a stereotactic biopsy, a specimen radiograph is used to confirm that representative amounts of the targeted calcifications are in the specimen. Real-time visualization during the US-guided biopsy confirms that samples of the appropriate area of concern were obtained.

10. What is stereotaxis?

Stereotaxis is a technique used to localize breast lesions for biopsy. A digital image of the lesion, the scout image, is taken on the stereotactic machine. This image is obtained at 0 degrees. Two views are taken at ±15 degrees from the original 0-degree scout image. From the three views, the machine calculates the z axis, which is the depth the needle needs to be placed to obtain a biopsy sample of the lesion.

Key Points: Ultrasound/Interventional Procedures

1. For optimal imaging evaluation, at least a 7-MHz transducer (ideally ≥10 MHz) should be used to perform breast US.
2. In addition to doing the percutaneous breast biopsy, the radiologist's role includes evaluating the pathology results for concordance with the imaging findings.
3. If atypical ductal hyperplasia is present on pathologic evaluation of a percutaneous biopsy specimen, excisional biopsy should be recommended.

11. In what circumstances would stereotactic biopsy be difficult to perform?
- Lesions in the subareolar location.
- If the breast tissue is thin. Compression thickness of less than 2.5 cm may make biopsy sampling difficult.
- Lesions that are very posterior in location.
- If the calcifications are indistinct and difficult to see. The calcifications need to be easily visible to target them appropriately for biopsy sampling. A loosely grouped cluster would also make targeting difficult. A tight cluster would be easier to target for biopsy sampling.

12. In what circumstances would a US-guided biopsy be difficult to perform?
- Lesions that are very small and close to the skin surface.
- Lesions behind the nipple.
- Lesions close to the chest wall.

13. What is discordance in relation to percutaneous biopsies?
When a percutaneous breast biopsy is performed, one of the radiologist's roles is to ensure the histologic diagnosis is concordant, or makes sense with the imaging appearance. If the imaging appearance is highly suspicious, and the pathologic results are benign, this may suggest a discordance. If there is discordance, the radiologist may suggest excisional biopsy for further evaluation.

14. In what situations or histologic diagnosis should an excisional biopsy be recommended after a percutaneous breast biopsy?
When there is pathologic-imaging discordance, excisional biopsy should be recommended. When atypical ductal hyperplasia is present on pathologic evaluation, excisional biopsy should also be recommended. When atypical ductal hyperplasia is present, cancer is present on excisional biopsy 20% to 56% (14G needle) and 0% to 38% (11G needle) of the time. Other controversial pathologic diagnoses include papillary lesions, radial scars, atypical lobular hyperplasia, and lobular carcinoma in situ. The literature would advocate excisional biopsy for these lesions as well.

BIBLIOGRAPHY

[1] G. Gardenosa, Breast Imaging Companion, third ed., Lippincott Williams & Wilkins, Philadelphia, 2007.
[2] D.B. Kopans, Breast Imaging, third ed., Lippincott Williams & Wilkins, Philadelphia, 2007.
[3] L. Liberman, Percutaneous image-guided core breast biopsy, Radiol. Clin. North Am. 40 (2002) 483–500.

CHAPTER 8

BREAST MRI

Sara Chen Gavenonis, MD, and
Mark Rosen, MD, PhD

BREAST MRI TECHNIQUE

1. How is breast magnetic resonance imaging (MRI) performed?

The patient is required to lie on her stomach in the prone position. A breast-specific coil is used, with the breasts placed into openings or wells that house the receiver coils (devices that detect emitted MRI signal from the body). Prone positioning helps minimize the motion of the breast during respiration. Dependent positioning of the breast also helps to extend the breast away from the chest wall and allows for mild compression of the breast, further minimizing unwanted motion during the MRI examination.

2. What pulse sequences are required for breast MRI?

The pulse sequences used to create the different MRI images in a breast MRI examination depend on several factors, including the capabilities and performance of the MRI system used and the type of information (e.g., implant evaluation or cancer identification) sought by the referring physician. In addition, the imaging techniques used by a particular MRI center reflect the experience and preferences of the local radiologists at that center. At our institution, breast MRI is performed in the sagittal plane and includes T1-weighted spin-echo, fat-saturated T2-weighted fast spin-echo (FSE), and fat-saturated three-dimensional T1-weighted spoiled gradient-recalled-echo. Dynamic postcontrast images are obtained resulting in three postcontrast series. Delayed axial T1-weighted fat-saturated images are also obtained for multiplanar imaging correlation and improved visualization of the axillary regions.

Computer-generated subtraction images using the precontrast series as a mask are also routinely used to assess for areas of enhancement. It is important to assess for artifacts from possible motion between the precontrast and postcontrast series to avoid pitfalls when interpreting subtraction images.

3. Is 3-Tesla (T) imaging superior to 1.5-T imaging for breast cancer detection?

Compared with imaging at 1.5-T, imaging at 3-T improves the signal-to-noise ratio (S/N) by approximately a factor of 2. This added S/N can be translated into higher spatial resolution and faster imaging (with parallel imaging techniques) without sacrificing image quality. Preliminary results suggest that higher resolution breast MRI at 3-T is feasible. In addition, tissue T1 relaxation rates are longer at 3-T, theoretically improving the image contrast and sensitivity of breast MRI to gadolinium enhancement. The quality of magnetic resonance spectroscopy (MRS) can also be improved at 3-T through improved spectral resolution and the potential for spectroscopy of smaller lesions. No studies have yet shown, however, that 3-T imaging results in superior diagnostic accuracy than imaging at 1.5-T.

4. Can MRS complement MRI for identifying malignant breast lesions?

MRS provides information on the relative concentrations of small molecular metabolites in tissue. In clinical breast MRS, the detection of elevated choline levels is associated with malignancy. Preliminary studies have shown that MRS can independently predict malignancy in solid breast lesions. Currently, MRS can be used only in lesions approximately 1 cm or larger in diameter, however, limiting the potential usefulness in routine clinical practice. Nevertheless, several investigators have shown the feasibility of incorporating MRS into breast MRI protocols as an adjunctive method for identifying malignant lesions.

NORMAL ANATOMY ON BREAST MRI

5. What are the components of the female breast?

The mature female breast is divided into the following components: glandular elements (ducts and lobules), fibrous supporting structure (Cooper ligaments), and surrounding adipose tissue. Blood vessels and, occasionally, lymph nodes are also found within the breast. Anatomically, the breast is bounded anteriorly, inferiorly, and medially by skin. Posteriorly, it is bounded by the chest wall (pectoralis major and minor muscles, ribs, and intercostal muscles). Superolaterally, the glandular breast tissue variably extends into the axilla, where adipose tissue, major blood vessels, and lymph nodes reside.

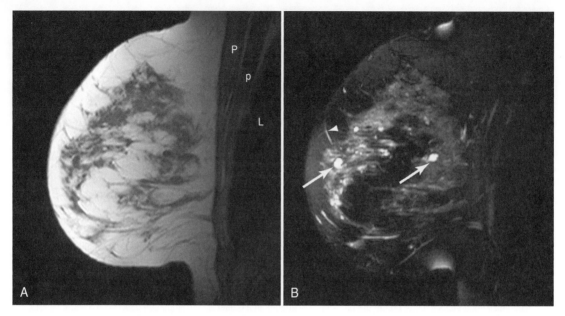

Figure 8-1. A, Sagittal T1-weighted image of normal breast. The fat within the breast is bright, and the fibroglandular elements are intermediate to dark. P = pectoralis major, p = pectoralis minor, L = lung. **B,** Sagittal FSE T2-weighted image with fat saturation, at same location as **A**. The suppressed fat is now dark on this image, and the fibroglandular elements are variably intermediate to bright. Higher signal intensity is seen in small cysts (*arrows*) and in peripheral veins (*arrowhead*).

The breast is divided into 8 to 20 segments, each of which is supplied by a major lactiferous duct. The ducts extend from the nipple, each communicating with a separate nipple orifice. The lactiferous duct subdivides into numerous ductules, each of which ramifies into several lobules. A terminal ductule and its associated lobules are classified together as a terminal ductule-lobular unit (TDLU). Most breast cancers develop within the TDLU.

6. What is the normal appearance of the breast on MRI?

On MRI, one can distinguish between the fatty adipose tissue and the fibroglandular elements, or parenchyma, on the basis of signal intensity. On T1-weighted imaging, the fat is bright, whereas the parenchyma is intermediate to dark (Fig. 8-1A). The appearance of the breast on T2-weighted imaging depends on whether fat suppression is used. Most radiologists use fat suppression on T2-weighted imaging. On fat-suppressed T2-weighted imaging, breast tissue is intermediate to bright (Fig. 8-1B). This fat suppression eliminates or reduces the high signal intensity of fat to highlight the bright signal of fluid in ducts or cysts or the bright signal intensity of certain masses, such as lymph nodes or fibroadenomas.

INDICATIONS FOR BREAST MRI

7. What are the indications for diagnostic breast MRI?

Two general categories of use of a breast imaging modality are screening and diagnostic. The use of breast MRI as a diagnostic study has been well established. In patients with a known breast cancer, breast MRI is useful in defining the extent of disease in the ipsilateral breast for surgical planning purposes and useful in screening for a synchronous cancer in the contralateral breast. Breast MRI can also be used for monitoring local tumor response to neoadjuvant chemotherapy. Breast MRI can be used to look for an index breast lesion when there is metastatic axillary lymphadenopathy with no suspicious mammographic findings in the ipsilateral breast. In addition, breast MRI can sometimes be helpful in the work-up of indeterminate mammographic and ultrasound (US) findings, or in cases of an area of clinical concern with no suspicious mammographic or US findings. Breast MRI can also be performed for evaluation of the integrity of breast prostheses (implants) (see subsequent section on implant evaluation).

8. What are the indications for screening breast MRI?

In March 2007, the American Cancer Society published guidelines for the use of breast MRI as a screening modality. Based on evidence, annual screening breast MRI is now recommended for patients with a deleterious *BRCA* mutation, for untested first-degree relatives of *BRCA* carriers, and for patients with a lifetime risk approximately 20% to 25% or greater, as defined by BRCAPRO or other models that are largely dependent on family history. Also, annual screening breast MRI is recommended for specific subgroups, such as patients who received radiation to the chest between age 10 and 30 years and patients (and their first-degree relatives) with syndromes known to predispose to malignancy (Li-Fraumeni, Cowden, and Bannayan-Riley-Ruvalcaba syndromes).

Beyond these specific groups of patients, annual screening breast MRI is not currently recommended, especially given the relatively low specificity of breast MRI and the propensity for false-positive findings. Investigation continues into the use of breast MRI as a screening modality in patients with a prior personal history of breast cancer, patients with heterogeneously dense or extremely dense breasts on mammography, and in patients with a prior history of a breast biopsy with pathology results of atypia or lobular carcinoma in situ.

9. **What is the appearance of (invasive) breast cancer on MRI? Do all breast cancers appear as focal enhancing masses?**
   Breast cancer can appear as an enhancing mass or an enhancing region of the breast after contrast agent administration (Fig. 8-2). Certain malignancies, such as invasive lobular cancer or ductal carcinoma in situ (DCIS), may manifest as focal or segmental areas or regions of enhancement (also termed *nonmass enhancement*) (Fig. 8-3).

10. **Do all enhancing abnormalities in the breast represent cancer?**
    No. Although MRI is very sensitive for detecting breast cancer, it is less specific because many other breast entities can be enhancing. Many benign masses, such as fibroadenomas and intramammary lymph nodes, also enhance after gadolinium administration. Proliferative breast changes, such as fibrocystic disease or ductal hyperplasia, may also enhance after gadolinium administration. Even normal breast parenchyma may enhance after contrast administration, especially in premenopausal women or women receiving hormone replacement therapy.

11. **Does an irregular or spiculated margin in an enhancing lesion always represent breast cancer?**
    Generally, an enhancing mass with irregular or spiculated margins is more suspicious for malignancy than a mass with smooth or lobulated margins. Some enhancing masses with irregular margins are ultimately benign (e.g., radial scars), however, and some cancers may manifest with smooth margins. Internal morphology is also an important indicator of malignancy on MRI. Masses that are centrally necrotic (often seen in larger cancers) may show heterogeneous internal enhancement or irregular peripheral rim enhancement (Fig. 8-4), or both.

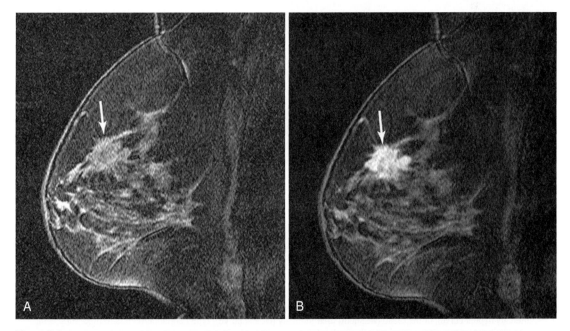

Figure 8-2. A, Breast cancer on T1-weighted spoiled gradient-recalled-echo image (TR = 7.7 ms, TE = 1.8 ms). The cancer (*arrow*) is isointense to the background glandular tissue. **B,** After gadolinium administration, the cancer is seen as an avidly enhancing mass. The contrast-enhanced images also help depict the irregular and spiculated borders of the mass.

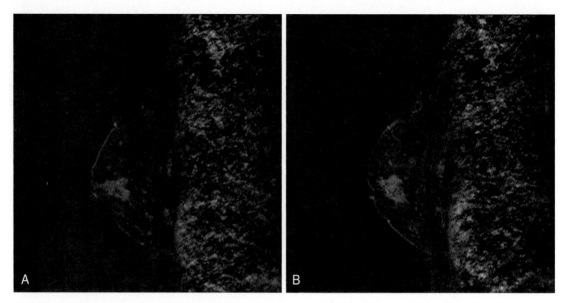

Figure 8-3. **A** and **B,** DCIS on MRI (sagittal subtraction images, first postcontrast series). In the lower inner left breast, avid segmental enhancement extends from the nipple posteriorly toward the chest wall.

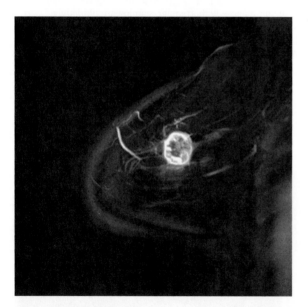

Figure 8-4. Invasive ductal carcinoma on MRI (T1-weighted spoiled gradient-recalled-echo image, first postcontrast series). Note the index mass has smooth margins compared with Figure 8-2. There is also heterogeneous enhancement of the lesion, with irregular peripheral enhancement.

12. Do malignant lesions enhance more strongly and more rapidly than benign lesions?

Although breast cancers do tend to enhance more rapidly and more intensely than benign lesions, some cancers may enhance less prominently; invasive lobular cancer can be a subtle area of enhancement on MRI (Fig. 8-5). In such cases, identification of the cancer may require close comparison between the unenhanced and enhanced T1-weighted images or the use of computer-generated subtraction images. Occasionally, noninvasive cancers (e.g., DCIS) enhance minimally or not at all.

Kinetic patterns of enhancement are crucial when evaluating suspicious enhancing lesions. Lesions that enhance minimally during the "first-pass" of a contrast agent (generally within 1 to 2 minutes after the intravenous bolus of gadolinium) but then steadily increase in intensity over time are typically benign, whereas lesions that enhance markedly in the first pass, but then decrease in their intensity are usually malignant. Exceptions exist in both cases, however, and a combination of morphologic and vascular enhancement information should be analyzed in the interpretation of breast MRI.

13. How are breast lesion kinetic patterns categorized?

The rate of initial enhancement (between the precontrast and first postcontrast series) can be described as rapid, intermediate, or slow. Generally, more vascular lesions have a more rapid rate of enhancement during this initial time period. Malignant breast lesions tend to be more vascular and often enhance markedly during the first pass of contrast agent. After the initial phase of enhancement, lesions continue to enhance gradually (type I curve), stabilize (plateau) their intensity (type II curve), or decrease (washout) their intensity (type III curve). Type I enhancement is termed *persistent*; type II enhancement, *plateau;* and type III, *washout.* Type III enhancement generally is the most suspicious pattern for malignancy.

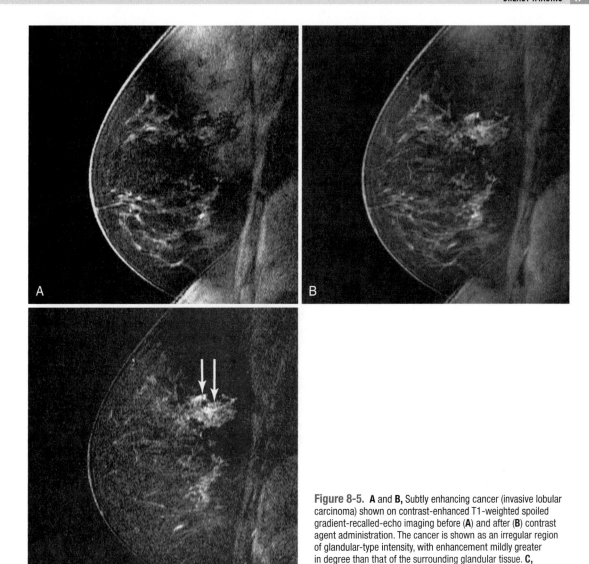

Figure 8-5. A and **B,** Subtly enhancing cancer (invasive lobular carcinoma) shown on contrast-enhanced T1-weighted spoiled gradient-recalled-echo imaging before (**A**) and after (**B**) contrast agent administration. The cancer is shown as an irregular region of glandular-type intensity, with enhancement mildly greater in degree than that of the surrounding glandular tissue. **C,** Enhancement (*arrows*) is much more apparent in the computer-generated subtraction (postcontrast minus precontrast) image.

14. Do all breast cancers show early rapid enhancement, followed by washout (type III enhancement)?

Although this pattern is not always seen in breast cancer, many invasive cancers show at least some areas of this pattern of enhancement (termed *washout pattern*). Malignant breast lesions often have higher degrees of angiogenesis, which has been shown to be essential for tumor growth and metastasis. New vessels in this microenvironment are abnormally leaky to gadolinium. As a result, malignant lesions tend to enhance markedly after gadolinium contrast administration, and washout more rapidly as the arterial contrast concentration declines.

15. How can biopsy specimens of suspicious lesions that are identified only on breast MRI be obtained?

When a suspicious breast lesion is identified by MRI, it is imperative to correlate the findings with findings on mammography and US. Often, an MRI abnormality has a corresponding mammographic or US finding. If there are no suspicious intermodality correlates for a suspicious breast MRI finding, an MRI-guided tissue sampling procedure is required. MRI-guided needle localization and core biopsy can be performed with specialized MRI-compatible equipment. If MRI-guided core biopsy is performed, MRI-compatible tissue markers are often also placed to mark the site of biopsy.

> **Key Points: MRI Breast Cancer Detection**
>
> 1. Intravenous contrast agent (gadolinium) is required to evaluate the breast parenchyma for malignancy on MRI.
> 2. MRI is nearly 100% sensitive for invasive breast cancer, but is less sensitive for DCIS. MRI can detect foci of cancer that are occult on mammography and physical examination.
> 3. Cancer detection requires identification of foci or regions of abnormal enhancement.
> 4. Differentiation between benign and malignant on breast MRI requires evaluation of lesion morphology (e.g., borders) and enhancement kinetics.
> 5. The use of breast MRI for diagnostic purposes has been established. It is useful in defining extent of disease in a patient with known cancer, for monitoring local tumor response to neoadjuvant chemotherapy, and for implant evaluation.
> 6. In 2007, the American Cancer Society published guidelines for use of screening MRI, with annual screening breast MRI recommended in specific patient groups at high risk for breast cancer. Investigation continues into the use of breast MRI as a screening modality in many other patient groups.

IMPLANT EVALUATION BY MRI

16. What are the components of a breast prosthesis?

There are two broad categories of breast implants: saline-only implants and silicone-containing implants. All implants (including saline-only implants) have a thin elastomer shell, generally derived from a silicone polymer. Saline implants often contain an access port that allows for injection of additional saline into the lumen because these implants are also used as tissue expanders. Silicone implants may be single-lumen or dual-lumen, usually with a silicone-containing inner lumen surrounded by a saline-containing outer lumen.

17. How does one distinguish between silicone and saline implants on MRI?

Because silicone and saline are hypointense on T1-weighted imaging and hyperintense on T2-weighted imaging, differentiation between the two requires more sophisticated MRI. More heavily T2-weighted sequences (with echo times on the order of 200 ms) accentuate slight differences in the T2 relaxation times of these substances (Fig. 8-6A). Frequency-selective water saturation can effectively eliminate the signal intensity of saline, while preserving the bright silicone signal on T2-weighted images (Fig. 8-6B). More advanced imaging methods can be used to create images with signal contribution from only one moiety or the other.

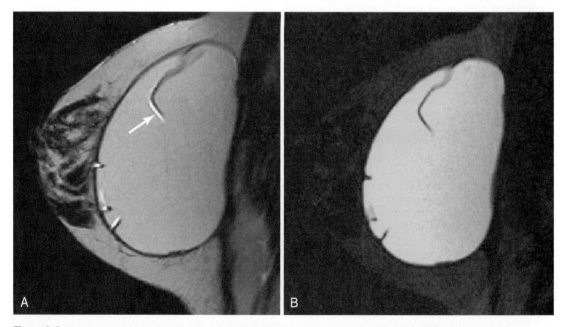

Figure 8-6. A, Normal appearance of a silicone implant on MRI. Sagittal heavily T2-weighted FSE (TR = 5016 ms, TE = 202 ms) image shows an intact single-lumen silicone implant. Dark lines extending into the center of the implant are normal radial folds of the outer elastomer shell. The silicone is intermediately high in signal intensity, and fluid condensation within the radial folds (*arrow*) is brighter than silicone. **B,** Silicone-only imaging on MRI. Sagittal short-tau inversion recovery image (TR = 4600 ms, TE = 105 ms) with frequency-selective water suppression yields an image in which only silicone contributes bright signal intensity. This sequence is useful for showing extracapsular ruptures with extravasation of free silicone into the breast or chest wall.

18. What is the normal MRI appearance of a breast implant?

A normal breast implant is oval or ellipsoid in shape. An outer fibrous capsule forms as part of the normal tissue response to the implant. On T2-weighted MRI, the lumen of the implant should be uniformly bright with no internal debris. Infolding of the outer implant shell is common and manifests as radially oriented protrusions ("radial folds") into the lumen of the implant. This is a common appearance of the normal implant and is not a sign of implant rupture. Condensation of fluid outside the implant shell but within the fibrous capsule is also a common phenomenon and should not be viewed as a sign of rupture.

19. What are the different types of implant rupture?

The different types of implant rupture include gel bleed, contained (intracapsular) rupture, and extracapsular rupture. These categories refer to the degree of disruption of the elastomer shell of the implant and the external fibrous capsule that develops around it.

20. What is gel bleed?

Gel bleed refers to transudation of small amounts of silicone gel through tiny perforations, or microtears, of the outer elastomer shell. Gel bleed is diagnosed by visualization of a small amount of silicone gel external to an otherwise intact elastomer shell, but contained within the external fibrous capsule. The term *gel bleed* is reserved for MRI evaluation of silicone implants. It is impossible on MRI to distinguish between saline extrusion through a microtear of the elastomer shell and normal fluid condensation between the elastomer shell and the fibrous capsule.

21. Describe the appearance of a contained implant rupture.

A contained rupture can occur in either saline or silicone implants. In a contained rupture, there is complete or near-complete separation of the elastomer shell from the fibrous capsule and fragmentation of the elastomer shell. The contents of the implant lumen (saline or silicone) remain contained, however, within the external fibrous capsule. The hallmark of contained rupture on MRI is the "linguine sign" (Fig. 8-7), in which strands of the remnant elastomer shell float freely in the contents of the implant lumen. These are identified as dark linear strands on T2-weighted images.

22. What are the MRI findings of extracapsular rupture?

Extracapsular rupture refers to rupture of the external fibrous capsule. For either silicone or saline implants, an extracapsular rupture can be diagnosed when there is gross deformity or collapse of the fibrous capsule. For silicone-containing implants, an extracapsular rupture is diagnosed whenever free silicone is identified within the extracapsular soft tissues of the breast or within axillary lymph nodes. When one seeks to identify the presence of free silicone within

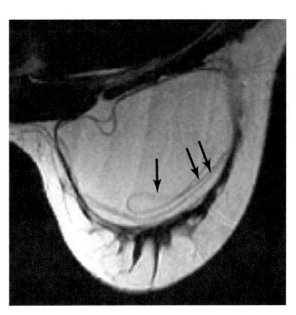

Figure 8-7. Axial T2-weighted FSE image of a silicone implant with contained (intracapsular) rupture. The silicone is contained by the outer fibrous capsule that develops within the breast after implant placement. The fragmented strands of the outer elastomer shell of the implant can be seen floating freely within the contained silicone, resembling strands of linguine (*arrows*).

breast tissue, one must separate not only silicone and saline signals, but also signals of breast parenchyma and fat. Silicone-only imaging sequences are essential for detecting free silicone in the breast or axilla.

Key Points: Implant Evaluation

1. Breast implants can be saline-only, silicone-only, or a combination of saline and silicone (dual-lumen).
2. MRI is the most accurate imaging modality for evaluating implant integrity.
3. Implant rupture can be intracapsular or extracapsular.
4. Depiction of free silicone in the breast tissue is the hallmark of extracapsular rupture.

BIBLIOGRAPHY

[1]   W.A. Berg, C.I. Caskey, U.M. Hamper, et al., Single- and double-lumen silicone breast implant integrity: prospective evaluation of MR and US criteria, Radiology 197 (1995) 45–52.

[2]   R. Gilles, J.M. Guinebretiere, O. Lucidarme, et al., Nonpalpable breast tumors: diagnosis with contrast-enhanced subtraction dynamic MR imaging, Radiology 191 (1994) 625–631.

[3]   K. Kinkel, N.M. Hylton, Challenges to interpretation of breast MRI, J. Magn. Reson. Imaging 13 (2001) 821–829.

[4]   C.K. Kuhl, S. Klaschik, P. Mielcarek, et al., Do T2-weighted pulse sequences help with the differential diagnosis of enhancing lesions in dynamic breast MRI? J. Magn. Reson. Imaging 9 (1999) 187–196.

[5]   C.K. Kuhl, R.K. Schmutzler, C.C. Leutner, et al., Breast MR imaging screening in 192 women proved or suspected to be carriers of a breast cancer susceptibility gene: preliminary results, Radiology 215 (2000) 267–279.

[6]   S.G. Lee, S.G. Orel, I.J. Woo, et al., MR imaging screening of the contralateral breast in patients with newly diagnosed breast cancer: preliminary results, Radiology 226 (2003) 773–778.

[7]   L. Liberman, E.A. Morris, D.D. Dershaw, et al., MR imaging of the ipsilateral breast in women with percutaneously proven breast cancer, AJR Am. J. Roentgenol. 180 (2003) 901–910.

[8]   S.G. Orel, M.D. Schnall, V.A. LiVolsi, R.H. Troupin, Suspicious breast lesions: MR imaging with radiologic-pathologic correlation, Radiology 190 (1994) 485–493.

[9]   R. Rakow-Penner, B. Daniel, H. Yu, et al., Relaxation times of breast tissue at 1.5T and 3T measured using IDEAL, J. Magn. Reson. Imaging 23 (2006) 87–91.

[10] D. Saslow, C. Boetes, W. Burke, et al., American Cancer Society guidelines for breast screening with MRI as an adjunct to mammography, CA Cancer J. Clin. 57 (2007) 75–89.

III

CARDIAC AND NONINVASIVE VASCULAR IMAGING

CARDIAC IMAGING: X-RAY AND MRI

Sridhar R. Charagundla, MD, PhD, and
Harold I. Litt, MD, PhD

CHAPTER 9

1. What forms the borders of the heart on the frontal posteroanterior (PA) or anteroposterior (AP) chest radiograph?

The chest radiograph represents an important first step in the imaging work-up of cardiovascular disease. Analysis of the cardiac silhouette can yield valuable information about chamber enlargement. The right atrium comprises the right heart border. This border becomes bulbous when the right atrium is enlarged. Superiorly, three convexities (called the "three moguls") comprise the left heart border, which, from superior to inferior, are the aortic knob, main pulmonary artery, and left atrial appendage. Inferiorly, the left ventricle (lateral wall and apex) comprises the left heart border.

2. What forms the borders of the heart on the lateral chest radiograph?

Superiorly, the left atrium comprises the posterior heart border. Inferiorly, the left ventricle comprises the posterior heart border. The right ventricle comprises the anterior heart border; inferiorly, this abuts the posterior aspect of the sternum (Fig. 9-1).

3. What are signs of left atrial enlargement on the chest radiograph?

Chamber enlargement can be identified generally by increased prominence of convexity of the corresponding heart border. In particular, left atrial enlargement causes a posterior bulging of the superoposterior heart border. On the frontal chest radiograph, signs of left atrial enlargement include enlargement of the left atrial appendage, "splaying" of the carina and elevation of the left main stem bronchus, and a "double density" projecting over the central portions of the heart, sometimes extending over toward the right (Fig. 9-2).

Key Points: Chest X-Ray Evaluation of Cardiac Chamber Size

1. Right atrium: right heart border on frontal view.
2. Right ventricle: anterior heart border on lateral view.
3. Left atrium: posterior-superior heart border on lateral view.
4. Left ventricle: left inferior heart border on frontal view.

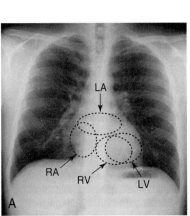 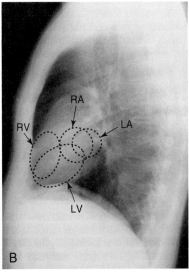

Figure 9-1. A and **B,** Normal PA (**A**) and lateral (**B**) chest radiographs with location of cardiac chambers outlined. LA = left atrium, RA = right atrium, RV = right ventricle, LV = left ventricle.

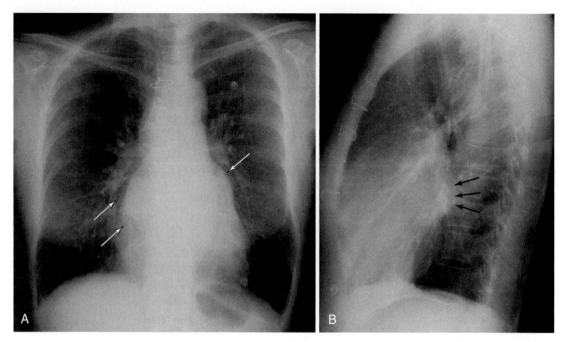

Figure 9-2. **A** and **B,** Left atrial enlargement (*arrows*) on PA (**A**) and lateral (**B**) chest radiographs. Note "double density" projecting over the right heart, enlarged left atrial appendage ("third mogul"), and convexity of the superoposterior heart border.

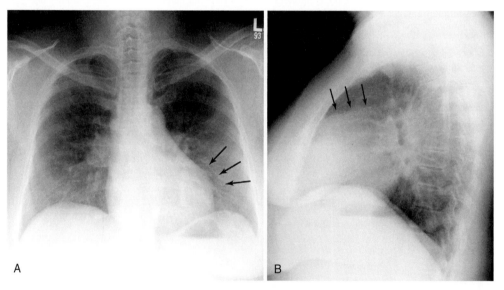

Figure 9-3. **A** and **B,** Right ventricular enlargement (*arrows*) on PA (**A**) and lateral (**B**) chest radiographs. Note rounded, uplifted left heart border and extra density in retrosternal clear space.

4. What are signs of right ventricular enlargement on the chest radiograph?

On the frontal radiograph, right ventricular enlargement can cause rounding of the left heart border (obscuring the normal shadow created by the left ventricle) and uplifting of the cardiac apex. On the lateral radiograph, right ventricular enlargement can displace normal retrosternal aerated lung (fill in the "anterior clear space"), although this is an unreliable finding (Fig. 9-3).

5. What are common causes of an intra-atrial mass?

The most common cause is thrombus. Patients with indwelling central venous catheters are at risk for developing right atrial thrombus, and patients with atrial fibrillation are at increased risk for developing left atrial thrombus. Deep venous thrombi of the extremities can migrate to the right atrium before causing a pulmonary embolism (see Figs. 12-1 and 12-2). Other causes of clot in the atria include hypercoagulable states and tumors that invade the inferior vena cava and propagate as "tumor thrombus" into the right atrium (e.g., renal cell carcinoma, adrenal carcinoma, and hepatocellular carcinoma). The most common primary atrial neoplasm is a myxoma (Fig. 9-4).

6. What are the types of atrial septal defect (ASD)? Which chambers and vessels become enlarged with an ASD?
ASDs are classified as ostium primum, ostium secundum, or sinus venosus defects, depending on their position in the septum. Secundum defects are the most common, and sinus venosus defects are often associated with partial anomalous pulmonary venous return. A defect in the interatrial septum creates a communication between the left and right atria. Usually, because the left atrium has slightly higher pressures, the direction of flow through the septal defect is left to right. This results in increased flow through the right atrium, right ventricle, and pulmonary arteries and can ultimately cause enlargement of any or all of these structures. The left atrium should be normal in size.

7. What are the types of ventricular septal defects (VSDs)? Which chambers and vessels become enlarged with a VSD?
The most common VSDs are classified as muscular, membranous, or supracristal, depending on their location in the muscular or membranous septum or in the outflow tract. A defect in the interventricular septum creates a communication between the ventricles, resulting in blood flowing from the left ventricle into the right ventricle. This results in right ventricular, pulmonary arterial, and left atrial enlargement.

8. What is a patent ductus arteriosus (PDA)? Which chambers and vessels become enlarged with a PDA?
A PDA is a persistent communication between the aorta and main pulmonary artery just beyond the origin of the left subclavian artery. Flow is directed from the aorta into the pulmonary artery, causing enlargement of the pulmonary arteries, left atrium, and left ventricle.

9. What is the most sensitive imaging technique for the detection of myocardial infarction?
Cardiac magnetic resonance imaging (MRI) with delayed postgadolinium imaging ("viability study") is the most sensitive imaging technique. Echocardiography can detect areas of myocardial wall thinning or abnormal myocardial contraction. Cardiac single photon emission computed tomography (SPECT) can detect areas of nonviable myocardium. MRI has greater specificity than echocardiography, however, and far greater spatial resolution and sensitivity than SPECT. Acute or chronic myocardial infarction shows accumulation of gadolinium in a delayed fashion (10 to 15 minutes after administration), probably owing to a combination of increased vascular permeability and enlargement of the extracellular space. The percentage of the myocardial thickness showing delayed enhancement correlates inversely with the likelihood of return of function of that segment of myocardium after a revascularization procedure.

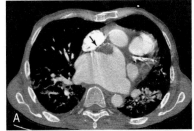

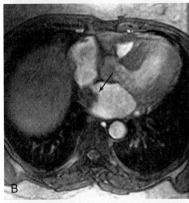

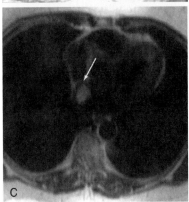

Figure 9-4. A-C, Intra-atrial thrombus (*arrow* in **A**) and intra-atrial myxoma (*arrows* in **B** and **C**). **A,** Contrast-enhanced CT image shows a filling defect in anterior aspect of the left atrium, representing thrombus. This patient had undergone heart transplant. **B** and **C,** Gradient-echo (**B**) and T2-weighted spin-echo (**C**) MR images show a mass in the left atrium that is hyperintense on T2-weighted images and represents a myxoma.

10. How long after myocardial infarction does a ventricular aneurysm develop?
A ventricular aneurysm develops in the setting of remote prior myocardial infarction. Areas of the heart muscle that have undergone infarction ultimately become thin and fibrotic; these weak areas of myocardium can balloon out over time because of chronic exposure to systemic blood pressure. Ventricular aneurysms usually have a wide mouth and may undergo mural calcification, resulting in a characteristic curvilinear density on chest radiographs (Fig. 9-5).

11. How long after myocardial infarction does a ventricular pseudoaneurysm develop?
Infarcted myocardial tissue undergoes a predictable sequence of histologic changes. As the tissue undergoes necrosis, it becomes mechanically weak and is prone to rupture. This most commonly occurs approximately 3 to 7 days after the infarction. Myocardial rupture most often occurs in the ventricular free wall, but can also occur in the interventricular septum (causing a left-to-right shunt) or in a papillary muscle (causing mitral regurgitation). If the myocardial rupture

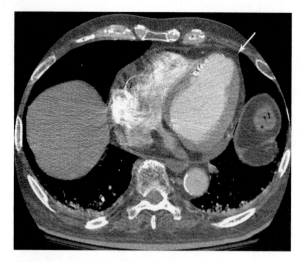

Figure 9-5. True ventricular aneurysm. Contrast-enhanced CT image shows marked thinning (*arrow*) of myocardium at the left ventricular apex, a characteristic location for a true ventricular aneurysm.

is contained, a ventricular pseudoaneurysm forms. These pseudoaneurysms characteristically have a narrow mouth because they essentially represent rupture through a small hole in the myocardium. Myocardial pseudoaneurysms are generally considered to be unstable because they themselves may rupture (Fig. 9-6).

12. What are some imaging findings of chronic (constrictive) pericarditis?
Chronic (constrictive) pericarditis can be caused by cardiac surgery, radiation, or tuberculosis; however, most cases are idiopathic. Patients commonly present with right heart failure. Imaging findings include pericardial thickening (>3 mm), pericardial calcification, and abnormal motion of the interventricular septum. None of these findings is pathognomonic. In the appropriate clinical setting, and with invasive or noninvasive hemodynamic findings suggesting constriction or restriction, thickened pericardium on MRI or computed tomography (CT) is sufficient to make the diagnosis of constrictive pericarditis.

13. In a patient with an abnormal electrocardiogram (ECG) finding and a family history of sudden death, cardiac MRI shows a dilated right ventricle with abnormal wall motion and a normal left ventricle. What is the most likely diagnosis?
Arrhythmogenic right ventricular dysplasia or cardiomyopathy is the most likely diagnosis; this is a disease of unknown etiology, characterized by fatty or fibrous infiltration of the myocardium. It is a common cause of sudden death and may be familial. Diagnosis is made through a combination of clinical, imaging, ECG, and pathologic findings. MRI is a useful test for evaluating right ventricular morphology, composition, and function. Suggestive findings on MRI include dysfunction, dilation, or thinning of the right ventricular wall; aneurysms of the right ventricle; and fatty infiltration of the right ventricular wall. Treatment consists of placement of an implantable cardioverter defibrillator. The diagnosis of arrhythmogenic right ventricular dysplasia should not be made on the basis of imaging findings alone.

14. How is bright blood MRI accomplished? Why is it used?
As its name implies, *bright blood* imaging is an MRI technique whereby flowing blood has high signal compared with tissue. This technique is accomplished through the use of gradient-echo imaging. Bright blood imaging techniques are useful because they are fast and have high spatial resolution; they are commonly used for depicting blood vessels, cardiac chambers, and valve leaflets. Turbulent blood flow causes dark "jets" in bright blood images, allowing the detection of valvular stenosis or incompetence.

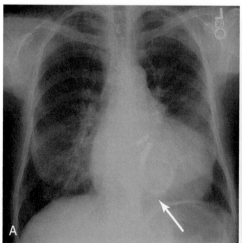
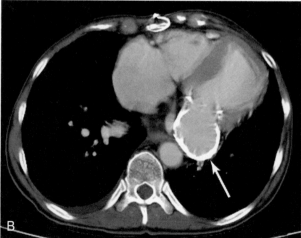

Figure 9-6. Ventricular pseudoaneurysm. **A** and **B,** PA chest radiograph (**A**) and contrast-enhanced CT image (**B**) show a pseudoaneurysm (*arrows*) arising from posteroinferior portion of the left ventricle. In this case, there is extensive mural calcification, indicating that the pseudoaneurysm is old.

15. How is dark blood MRI accomplished? Why is it used?

Dark blood imaging is an MRI technique whereby the blood signal is suppressed; this can be done with spin-echo or inversion recovery imaging. By reducing the signal from blood, myocardial tissue and vessel walls stand out from the background and can be seen in great detail. Dark blood imaging techniques are useful for detailed analysis of myocardial morphology and composition, cardiac anatomy, and vascular anatomy.

16. How is cine imaging accomplished?

Cine imaging portrays the heart in motion. Images are acquired during all phases of the cardiac cycle and require synchronization with the ECG signal. In MRI, this is accomplished with gradient-echo imaging (these images are bright blood).

17. Why is cine imaging used?

Cine imaging is necessary to evaluate cardiac function and can be used to detect wall motion abnormalities, calculate ejection fraction, and study the motion of valve leaflets.

18. Which congenital coronary artery anomalies can cause sudden death?

Normally, the right and left main coronary arteries arise from the aorta at the right and left sinuses of Valsalva. Anomalous origin of the coronary arteries occurs rarely (about 1% of cardiac catheterizations). Sudden death is associated with the left main coronary artery arising from the right sinus (particularly when the artery courses between the aorta and the pulmonary artery), the right coronary artery arising from the left sinus, or a single coronary artery. The left main coronary artery may also arise from the pulmonary trunk; this anomaly tends to manifest earlier, with congestive heart failure or sudden death (Fig. 9-7).

19. What are the standard planes for cross-sectional cine cardiac imaging?

The oblique orientation of the heart with respect to the body axis requires special planes of imaging. The four-chamber view of the heart captures all four cardiac chambers in a single image and includes the tricuspid and mitral valves. The short-axis view of the heart is perpendicular to the four-chamber view and allows accurate measurement of septal thickness and ventricular free wall thickness. In the short-axis view, the left ventricle is depicted in cross section and appears almost circular. Standard axial images also are commonly used. Coronal images are sometimes used to evaluate the diaphragmatic surface of the heart (Fig. 9-8).

20. What is the most common malignancy of the heart and pericardium?

Metastatic disease is most common. Lung cancer, lymphoma, breast cancer, and melanoma all can involve the heart or pericardium. Lung cancer is the most common primary tumor of patients with cardiac metastases; however, melanoma is the most likely tumor to spread to the heart. Primary tumors of the heart are rare, and primary malignant tumors of the heart are exceedingly rare.

21. What are some causes of dilated cardiomyopathy and restrictive cardiomyopathy?

Cardiomyopathies are diseases that involve primary dysfunction of the heart muscle. This broad collection of diseases can be divided on a pathophysiologic basis into dilated, hypertrophic, and restrictive subtypes, with some overlap occurring between these categories. A few causes of dilated cardiomyopathy include previous myocarditis related to viral infection (especially coxsackievirus B and cytomegalovirus), and toxic exposure (e.g., cocaine, alcohol, and doxorubicin). Causes of restrictive cardiomyopathy include infiltrative systemic disorders such as sarcoidosis, amyloidosis, eosinophilic cardiomyopathy (Löffler syndrome), and Fabry disease.

22. How can cardiac MRI distinguish between ischemic heart disease and nonischemic diseases such as cardiomyopathies?

Delayed postgadolinium imaging in patients with ischemic heart disease shows subendocardial or transmural late enhancement in a coronary territory distribution (see question 26). In patients with cardiomyopathy, areas of late enhancement may be mid-myocardial or epicardial and are distributed in a noncoronary territory distribution (Fig. 9-9).

23. What is Eisenmenger syndrome?

Small left-to-right shunts, such as ASDs and VSDs, are commonly asymptomatic early in life and may go undetected. Over time, the right side of the cardiopulmonary circulation responds to the increased volume with pulmonary arterial hyperplasia. This hyperplasia ultimately leads to elevated pulmonary vascular resistance and an increase in right-sided pressures (pulmonary hypertension). When right-sided pressures exceed left-sided pressures, the left-to-right shunt switches and becomes a right-to-left shunt. Dyspnea, fatigue, and cyanosis develop. This syndrome usually manifests in young adulthood.

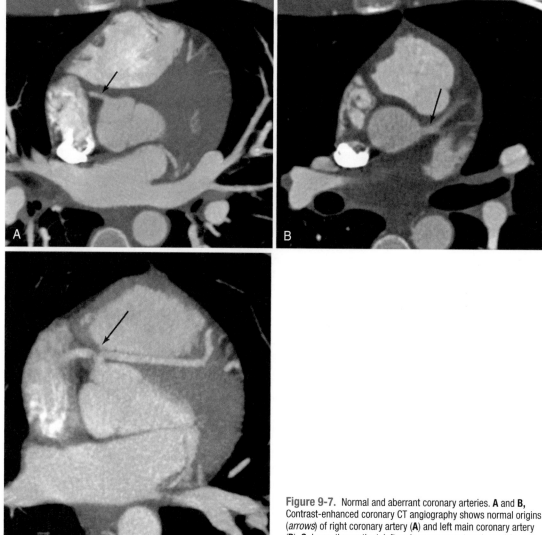

Figure 9-7. Normal and aberrant coronary arteries. **A** and **B,** Contrast-enhanced coronary CT angiography shows normal origins (*arrows*) of right coronary artery (**A**) and left main coronary artery (**B**). **C,** In another patient, left main coronary artery (*arrow*) is seen arising from the right coronary artery.

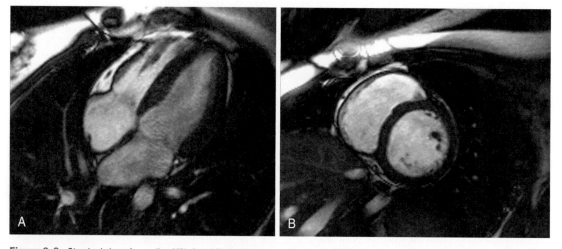

Figure 9-8.   Standard views for cardiac MRI. **A** and **B,** Bright blood gradient-echo MR images, four-chamber (**A**) and short-axis (**B**) views.

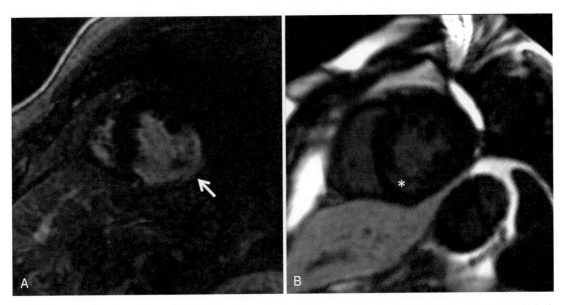

Figure 9-9. Ischemic versus nonischemic heart disease shown by delayed enhancement cardiac MRI. **A** and **B,** Short-axis images obtained 12 minutes after gadolinium DTPA administration show subendocardial and transmural late enhancement in inferior and lateral walls (*arrow*) reflecting prior myocardial infarction (**A**), and area of mid-myocardial late enhancement in a noncoronary distribution (*asterisk*) typical of nonischemic cardiomyopathy, in this case secondary to sarcoidosis (**B**).

24. What are some noninvasive methods of coronary artery imaging?

Imaging the coronary arteries is a major part of evaluating ischemic heart disease. Traditionally, this imaging has been performed through cardiac catheterization, a procedure that requires arterial puncture. Newer technologies promise noninvasive, cross-sectional imaging of coronary artery patency and can offer the potential to characterize coronary artery plaque. MRI, using bright blood, dark blood, and gadolinium-enhanced techniques, can image vessel patency, and determine lipid content in coronary plaques. Coronary CT angiography can image vessel patency, potentially with a higher spatial resolution than MRI, and measure coronary calcification (see Chapter 11).

25. What are some diseases that affect valvular function? How can they be diagnosed with imaging?

The aortic, pulmonic, mitral, and tricuspid valves can become stenotic, incompetent, or both. A chamber draining through a stenotic valve experiences a pressure load; if this chamber is a ventricle, it responds with muscular hypertrophy. If this chamber is an atrium, however, it responds with enlargement. A chamber draining through an incompetent (regurgitant) valve experiences a volume load and responds with enlargement (whether it is an atrium or a ventricle). Echocardiography and MRI can measure chamber size and velocity and direction of blood flow across a valve orifice, detecting and quantifying valvular disease.

26. What is the differential diagnosis of a regional wall motion abnormality?

A wall motion abnormality indicates a portion of myocardium that has abnormally reduced contractility. This reduced contractility usually occurs on the basis of previous or ongoing ischemia and suggests heart muscle that is acutely ischemic, dead, stunned, or hibernating. Acutely ischemic myocardium cannot contract properly because of inadequate blood flow and poor energy supply. Infarcted myocardium does not contract and may eventually exhibit "paradoxic" motion—ballooning out during systole instead of thickening. When a portion of heart muscle remains viable after a temporary episode of ischemia, it can become "stunned," where wall motion abnormality persists because of chemical changes in the myocardium that resolve over time. Finally, ischemic myocardium can downregulate its own contractility to match its energy demands with energy supply; this is termed *hibernating* and may signify tissue at risk for becoming infarcted.

27. What portions of the heart are supplied by the right coronary, left anterior descending, and circumflex arteries?

The left anterior descending artery supplies the left ventricular apex and the anterior portion of the interventricular septum. The right coronary artery supplies the posteroinferior wall of the left ventricle and the posterior portion of the interventricular septum. The left circumflex artery supplies the lateral wall of the left ventricle (Fig. 9-10).

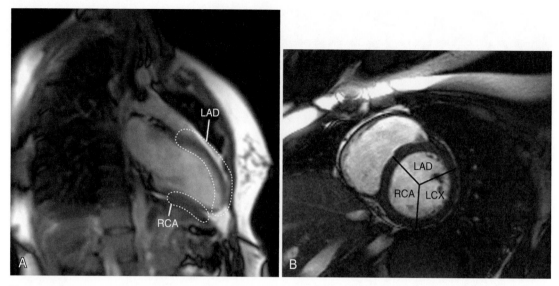

Figure 9-10. Coronary vascular territories. **A** and **B,** Bright blood gradient-echo MR images with coronary vascular territories delineated on vertical long-axis (**A**) and short-axis (**B**) views. LAD = left anterior descending (artery), RCA = right coronary artery, LCX = left circumflex (artery).

BIBLIOGRAPHY

[1] C. Bomma, J. Rutberg, H. Tandri, et al., Misdiagnosis of arrhythmogenic right ventricular dysplasia/cardiomyopathy, J. Cardiovasc. Electrophysiol. 15 (2004) 300–306.
[2] F. Kimura, F. Sakai, Y. Sakomura, et al., Helical CT features of arrhythmogenic right ventricular cardiomyopathy, RadioGraphics 22 (2002) 1111–1124.
[3] W.J. Manning, D.J. Pennell (Eds.), Cardiovascular Magnetic Resonance, Churchill Livingstone, New York, 2002.
[4] G.C. Mueller, A. Attili, Cardiomyopathy: magnetic resonance imaging evaluation, Semin. Roentgenol. 43 (2008) 204–222.
[5] R.W. Troughton, C.R. Asher, A.L. Klein, Pericarditis, Lancet 363 (2004) 717–727.

CT ANGIOGRAPHY AND MRA OF THE AORTA

CHAPTER 10

Andrew J. Kapustin, MD, and
Harold I. Litt, MD, PhD

1. How do aneurysms and pseudoaneurysms differ?

An *aneurysm* (also known as a *true aneurysm*) is dilation of a vessel in which all three layers of the vessel wall remain intact. A *pseudoaneurysm* (also known as a *false aneurysm*) is a contained rupture and implies disruption of at least part of the aortic wall (i.e., the intima or media or both), with intact adventitia. Pseudoaneurysms are potentially highly unstable lesions. They are often post-traumatic or iatrogenic (Fig. 10-1).

2. What is a mycotic aneurysm? Which imaging findings help suggest the diagnosis?

One might think *mycotic* means "related to fungus," but *mycotic aneurysm* refers to an aneurysm caused by any type of infection, usually bacterial. Imaging features that may suggest the diagnosis are rapid change in size, adjacent inflammation, perivascular gas, eccentric (see Fig. 10-1) or saccular configuration, or lack of atherosclerotic calcification.

3. What is an inflammatory aneurysm?

Inflammatory aneurysms are a form of retroperitoneal fibrosis associated with aortic aneurysms. These aneurysms are surrounded by extensive inflammation and fibrosis that often lead to complications such as ureteral obstruction. Some authorities believe that the surrounding fibrosis is a result of microscopic leakage of the aneurysm causing a severe secondary inflammatory response, whereas others espouse a viral or immune reaction–related etiology. Inflammatory aneurysms are much less common than atherosclerotic aneurysms.

4. How is aortic dissection different from aortic transection?

Aortic dissection is caused by a tear of the intima, creating a false channel or lumen within the wall of the artery. Flowing blood dissects along the course of the aorta, extending the false lumen longitudinally and into branch vessels. The classic presentation is "ripping" back or chest pain.

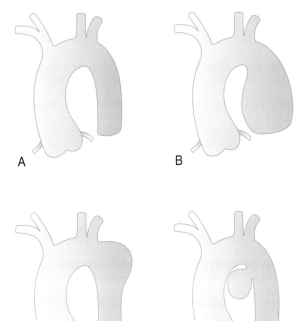

Figure 10-1. Types of aortic aneurysm. **A,** Normal configuration of thoracic aorta. **B,** Fusiform aneurysmal dilation of descending thoracic aorta. Fusiform aneurysms are common in atherosclerosis. **C,** Eccentric, or saccular, aneurysm of descending thoracic aorta, perhaps caused by infection. **D,** Pseudoaneurysm, a contained rupture. In true aneurysms, all three layers of the vessel wall are intact. In pseudoaneurysms, the intima or media or both have been disrupted, leaving intact adventitia.

Aortic transection (perhaps better referred to as *traumatic aortic injury*) occurs in trauma patients. The entire aortic wall is injured or transected, leading to hemorrhage or pseudoaneurysm formation. Transection is usually a focal injury, and imaging should focus on the region of interest, usually in the chest. Dissections extend for some distance and require more extensive imaging of the entire aorta and its branch vessels.

5. **In the setting of blunt trauma, where do aortic injuries most commonly occur?**
Most injuries seen by radiologists occur at the aortic isthmus, which is just distal to the takeoff of the left subclavian artery. Most authorities believe this is due to asymmetric aortic fixation at this location, leading to shear stress. Radiologists less commonly see injuries to the ascending aorta because many patients with this type of injury die before reaching the hospital.

6. **How are traumatic aortic injuries diagnosed?**
Clinical suspicion or chest x-ray findings should be enough to send a patient with an unstable condition to surgery. If the patient's condition is relatively stable, most authorities now recommend CT angiography, preferably with a multidetector computed tomography (CT) scanner. Catheter angiography, previously the mainstay of diagnosis, is now most useful for problem solving when CT angiography is nondiagnostic or equivocal.

7. **Name the chest x-ray findings of a thoracic aortic pathologic condition.**
Primary signs include an enlarged or enlarging aorta, an indistinct aortic contour, and displacement of intimal atherosclerotic calcifications (in aortic dissection). Secondary signs, indicating mass effect from an aneurysm or hematoma, include mediastinal widening; displacement of adjacent structures such as the trachea, the left main stem bronchus, or a nasogastric tube in the esophagus; an "apical cap," or mediastinal hematoma extending above the lung apex; or pleural or pericardial effusion (can be hemorrhagic, but is more commonly exudative fluid secondary to the adjacent acute aortic process). Many of these findings are not specific for aortic pathologic conditions. Even mediastinal hematoma in the setting of trauma is not specific because it may be secondary to venous rather than arterial injury.

8. **What are the two classification schemes for aortic dissection?**
The *Stanford classification* categorizes dissections into dissections involving the ascending aorta regardless of involvement of the descending aorta, and dissections involving the descending aorta only:

- Type A: Ascending aorta involved with or without descending aorta
- Type B: Descending aorta only

The *DeBakey classification* denotes three categories of aortic dissection: singular involvement of the ascending or the descending aorta or involvement of both ascending and descending aortas. The mnemonic for this system is *BAD*:

- Type 1: Both ascending and descending
- Type 2: Ascending only
- Type 3: Descending only

The descending aorta is defined as distal to the takeoff of the left subclavian artery.

9. **How are dissections that involve the ascending aorta managed differently from dissections that involve the descending aorta only?**
Dissections involving the ascending aorta (Stanford type A and DeBakey types 1 and 2) are surgical emergencies because mortality is significantly greater in medically managed patients (approximately 90% in the first 3 months) compared with surgically treated patients. This high mortality rate is mostly due to hemopericardium causing tamponade, acute aortic regurgitation, or involvement of coronary artery origins causing myocardial infarction. Descending aortic dissections are usually treated medically (antihypertensive agents) because morbidity and mortality are greater with surgery than with medical management. Complicated descending aortic dissections may require surgical or endovascular intervention, however.

10. **Which lumen is usually larger in aortic dissection—the true or false lumen?**
Approximately 90% of the time, the false lumen is larger than the true lumen.

11. Describe other acute aortic syndromes that are often called variants of aortic dissection.

Penetrating atherosclerotic ulcer is a focal tear of the intima caused by ruptured plaque, leading to ulceration into the aortic wall. It is different from a dissection because a dissection is not focal, but rather propagates along the length of the vessel. *Intramural hematoma* is a term that describes hemorrhage into the wall of the vessel, generally between the inner and outer layers of the media. Intramural hematoma may occur without an intimal tear, such as secondary to rupture of the vasa vasorum (small blood vessels in the wall of the aorta); this is usually secondary to hypertension, but can be caused by trauma. Alternatively, intramural hematoma may be associated with an intimal tear, such as secondary to a penetrating atherosclerotic ulcer (Fig. 10-2).

Warning: These terms can become extremely confusing because one form of an aortic pathologic condition can lead to another. In part because of this confusion in terminology, there are numerous controversies in the surgical literature regarding prognosis and management of the "dissection variants."

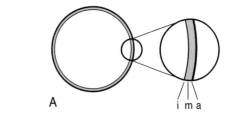
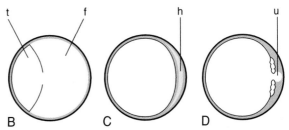

Figure 10-2. Aortic wall anatomy and pathologic conditions. **A,** Layers of the aortic wall. i = intima, m = media, a = adventitia. **B,** Aortic dissection, between the intima and media. t = true lumen, f = false lumen. **C,** h = intramural hematoma. **D,** u = penetrating atherosclerotic ulcer.

12. What is the best imaging modality for diagnosing each of these conditions?

CT and magnetic resonance imaging (MRI) are the two best modalities for evaluating these conditions. CT (particularly multidetector CT) is generally preferred because it is faster (important in patients with an unstable condition) and has better spatial resolution. MRI is often used for problem solving in patients with a stable condition or in patients with a contrast agent allergy. For patients with renal disease on permanent dialysis, CT should be performed because of the risk of nephrogenic systemic fibrosis related to gadolinium-based MRI contrast agents. For patients with renal disease who are not on permanent dialysis, noncontrast magnetic resonance angiography (MRA) techniques can be used; although these techniques generally have lower spatial resolution and take longer to acquire than contrast-enhanced MRA, they are usually sufficient to exclude an acute aortic syndrome. Ultrasound also has been used, but it cannot visualize the entire aorta and misses the extent of disease or associated complications. At this time, the main indication for use of catheter angiography for these conditions is treatment of complications.

13. How can these conditions be distinguished on axial MR or CT images?

A dissection flap most often appears as a line across the vessel, separating the true lumen from the false lumen (Fig. 10-3). Intramural hematomas usually appear as a crescentic region of high attenuation or signal intensity with smooth borders. The presence of an irregular luminal border with peripheral low attenuation may reflect ulcerated atherosclerotic plaque or thrombus.

14. What is the utility of precontrast imaging when performing CT angiography or MRA of the aorta?

Subacute hemorrhage has higher attenuation than flowing blood on noncontrast CT and high signal intensity on precontrast T1-weighted MRI. These findings can be easily obscured in the presence of an intravenous contrast agent; precontrast imaging is mandatory to detect the presence of intramural hematoma.

15. How large must the thoracic and abdominal aortas be to be called aneurysmal?

Any artery dilated by more than 50% of its normal size is called aneurysmal. Most authorities define aortic aneurysm as 4 cm in the thoracic aorta and 3 cm in the abdomen. The aorta should normally decrease in size as it extends distally, and any focal dilation should be considered abnormal.

16. When is an abdominal aortic aneurysm usually repaired?

Surgical repair of an abdominal aortic aneurysm is generally considered for aortas larger than 5 cm or for aortas that are symptomatic or display rapid growth.

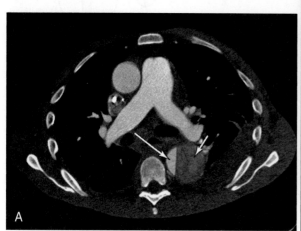
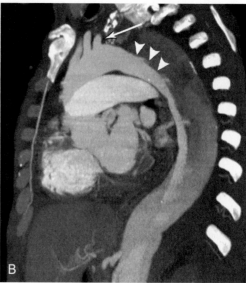

Figure 10-3. A, Axial CT angiography image shows aortic dissection, with differential flow in the true lumen (*long arrow*) and false lumen (*short arrow*). **B,** Oblique sagittal maximum intensity projection reformatted image shows this to be a type B dissection, beginning just distal to the takeoff of the left subclavian artery (*arrow*). The dissection flap is indicated by *arrowheads*.

17. What is Laplace's law? How is it relevant to aortic aneurysms?

Laplace's law states that the larger the radius of a sphere, the greater the wall stress. In regard to aneurysms, this means that as an aneurysm increases in size, the stress on the aortic wall also increases. The aneurysm becomes more prone to rupture with increasing size.

18. Can the overall size of an aortic aneurysm be determined by catheter angiography?

No. Often there is an extensive mural thrombus in an aneurysm, and a large aneurysm can have a normal-sized lumen. Only the lumen is opacified by catheter angiography, and the outer size of the aneurysm cannot be determined by this method.

19. How is the size of the aorta most accurately measured on CT or MRI?

Drawing a line perpendicular to the course of the aorta is required for accurate measurement of the aortic diameter. This is often different than the cross section of the aorta commonly seen on axial CT and MR images because these images are axial to the patient's body, not axial relative to the aorta. Accurate measuring, especially of a tortuous vessel, often requires multiplanar or three-dimensional reformatting (Fig. 10-4).

20. Name two methods of repairing aneurysms, and compare their advantages and disadvantages.

Surgical repair and endovascular stent-graft are two methods of repairing aneurysms. Surgical repair is a more definitive treatment, requiring no imaging follow-up, and has known long-term durability. Endovascular repair is newer, and long-term data are unavailable. Because of potential complications of endovascular repair, follow-up imaging and reintervention often are required. Many patients with aortic aneurysm are not surgical candidates, however, because of comorbidities such as cardiopulmonary disease; endovascular repair is preferred for these patients. More recent large studies have shown lower operative mortality and short-term morbidity, but an increase in repeat procedures for endovascular repair compared with open surgical repair of abdominal aortic aneurysms. Thoracic aortic endovascular repair is a newer procedure, with fewer outcomes studies at present.

21. What criteria are used to determine whether an aortic aneurysm can be treated by endovascular technique?

- *The relationship of the aneurysm to the origins of other vessels:* In the abdomen, the relationship of the aneurysm to the renal arteries is paramount because the angiographer would not want to occlude the origin of these arteries with a stent graft. In the chest, it is preferable not to cover the origin of the left subclavian artery with the stent, but this can be done if needed, with placement of a carotid-subclavian bypass graft.
- *The luminal size of the common and external iliac arteries:* Because the stent-graft is delivered to the aorta via a femoral artery approach, the angiographer needs a vessel large enough to accommodate the size of the delivery system (currently 6 to 8 mm).
- *The length of the aneurysm and whether it extends into the iliac arteries:* This determines the size and type of stent-graft used.

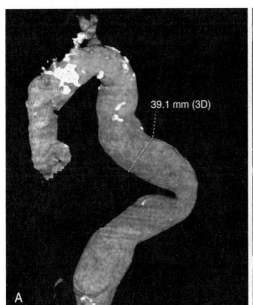
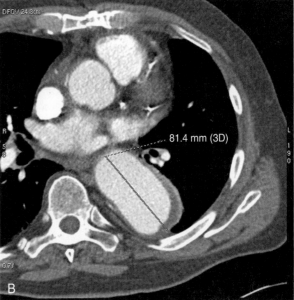

Figure 10-4. **A,** Oblique sagittal volume-rendered CT angiography image of a tortuous aorta shows the proper way to measure a tortuous aorta. An imaginary line is drawn down the center of the long axis of the vessel, and the transverse diameter is measured perpendicular to that line. Measurements such as this must be made using multiplanar or three-dimensional reformatting to compensate for vessel tortuosity. **B,** Axial CT image from same study shows how reliance on axial images can result in overestimation of aortic size. At this level, the tortuous aorta is flowing roughly in the axial plane and appears much more dilated than it actually is.

22. Why is follow-up imaging of stent-grafts needed?

Follow-up imaging is performed to look for complications and re-evaluate the size of the aneurysm after endovascular repair. Ideally, the aneurysm sac gradually decreases in size after repair. Complications include migration of the stent-graft, hemorrhage, infection, and endoleak.

23. What are endoleaks? What imaging technique is used to find them?

An *endoleak* is defined as residual blood flow in the "aneurysm sac" (in other words, between the native aortic wall and the wall of the stent-graft). This complication is subcategorized based on the origin of the blood flow to the aneurysm sac. Type II endoleaks are the most common and are related to reversed flow into the aneurysm sac from collateral vessels such as the inferior mesenteric artery or lumbar arteries (Fig. 10-5). Screening for endoleaks is usually performed with CT angiography or MRA. An appropriate protocol requires precontrast images and postcontrast arterial phase and delayed phase images because endoleaks may be identified only on delayed imaging. CT and MRI cannot always delineate the type of endoleak. Catheter angiography can be used to define an endoleak better. Many endoleaks can be repaired percutaneously.

24. What other types of aortic procedures can be performed through an endovascular approach?

Newer endovascular procedures involving the aorta include treatment of aortic coarctation (see next question) using stents, and placement of percutaneous aortic valves for patients with severe aortic stenosis who are not surgical candidates. Both of these procedures require appropriate iliac artery access vessels, similar to endovascular aneurysm repair.

25. How do aortic coarctation and pseudocoarctation differ?

Aortic coarctation is a hemodynamically significant stenosis of the aorta, most commonly seen just distal to the takeoff of the left subclavian artery. Pseudocoarctation mimics coarctation because there is an apparent focal narrowing of the proximal descending aorta. This narrowing is due to buckling of a tortuous aorta, however, and does not result in a hemodynamically significant pressure gradient across the area of narrowing. Rib notching, owing to collateral intercostal arteries, is seen in true coarctation, not in pseudocoarctation.

26. What is a bovine aortic arch?

Most people have three large arteries originating from the aortic arch: the innominate artery (brachiocephalic artery), the left common carotid artery, and the left subclavian artery. The most common variant of aortic arch anatomy is termed a *bovine arch,* in which there are two vessels that arise from the aorta. The more proximal of these is a common trunk of the innominate artery and left common carotid artery. The more distal vessel is the left subclavian artery. This anatomic variant is of no clinical significance except when planning aortic surgery.

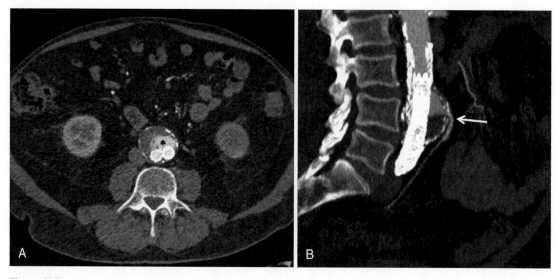

Figure 10-5. Images from CT angiography showing type II endoleak. **A,** Axial image showing contrast material outside the stent lumen indicating endoleak (*asterisk*). **B,** Oblique sagittal maximum intensity projection showing endoleak communicating with the inferior mesenteric artery (*arrow*).

BIBLIOGRAPHY

[1] M.A. Coady, J.A. Rizzo, J.L. Goldstein, J.A. Elefteriades, Natural history, pathogenesis, and etiology of thoracic aortic aneurysms and dissections, Cardiol. Clin. North Am. 17 (1999) 615–635.

[2] J.D. Creasy, C. Chiles, W.D. Routh, R.B. Dyer, Overview of traumatic injury of the thoracic aorta, RadioGraphics 17 (1997) 27–45.

[3] M.E. Debakey, C.H. McCollum, E.S. Crawford, et al., Dissection and dissecting aneurysms of the aorta: twenty-year follow up of 527 patients treated surgically, Surgery 92 (1982) 1118–1134.

[4] D.S. Dyer, E.E. Moore, M.F. Mestek, et al., Can chest CT be used to exclude aortic injury? Radiology 213 (1999) 195–202.

[5] M.A. LePage, L.E. Quint, S.S. Sonnad, et al., Aortic dissection: CT features that distinguish true lumen from false lumen, AJR Am. J. Roentgenol. 177 (2001) 207–211.

[6] T.A. Macedo, A.W. Stanson, G.S. Oderich, et al., Infected aortic aneurysms: imaging findings, Radiology 231 (2004) 250–257.

[7] K.J. Macura, F.M. Corl, E.K. Fishman, D.A. Bluemke, Pathogenesis in acute aortic syndromes: aortic dissection, intramural hematoma, and penetrating atherosclerotic aortic ulcer, AJR Am. J. Roentgenol. 181 (2003) 309–316.

[8] W.J. Manning, D.J. Pennell (Eds.), Cardiovascular Magnetic Resonance, Churchill Livingstone, New York, 2002.

[9] S.W. Stavropoulos, S.R. Charagundla, Imaging techniques for detection and management of endoleaks after endovascular aortic aneurysm repair, Radiology 243 (2007) 641–655.

CHAPTER 11

CORONARY CT ANGIOGRAPHY

Jonathan N. Balcombe, MBBS, and
Harold I. Litt, MD, PhD

1. What is coronary CT angiography, and how does it differ from regular chest computed tomography (CT)?

Coronary CT angiography is a CT angiogram of the coronary arteries (Fig. 11-1). On a regular CT scan of the chest, the heart appears blurred because of its motion, so coronary CT requires synchronization of image acquisition to the electrocardiogram (ECG) signal. The challenge of imaging the coronary arteries is compounded by the fact that these vessels are very small and move a large amount in every cardiac cycle. The left main coronary artery measures a maximum of 5 mm in diameter, and for much of their course the other arteries are only about 2 mm in diameter. The resolution of the CT scanner must be submillimeter. The right coronary artery can move 5 cm in each cardiac cycle, as the heart contracts and expands. Imaging a 2-mm structure that moves 5 cm in each direction every second is demanding. To acquire high-quality images, the following techniques are employed: ECG-gating, multidetector image acquisition, fast gantry rotation, and, in some scanners, dual x-ray tubes.

2. What is multidetector image acquisition? Are more slices always better?

Coronary arteries do not respect simple axial, coronal, or sagittal planes. They curve and twist in all dimensions, in a variable manner, as they supply the heart. Optimal coronary artery evaluation requires that the physician is able to evaluate the arteries in any plane. To allow this, the image data must be isotropic (i.e., of equal spatial resolution in all three planes). Modern CT scanners enable this evaluation by having multiple rows of detectors, each of which are very thin. A common detector array has 64 rows of detectors, each 0.6 mm wide. Because of the helical nature of scanning, the images can be reconstructed at an even smaller pixel size of 0.3 mm if necessary. The large number of detector rows speeds imaging. The above-mentioned array would be able to acquire a 4-cm slab of data in one acquisition. Newer scanners with 256 or 320 slices are able to acquire 16 cm—the whole heart—in a single acquisition. This capability avoids many of the technical issues involved in scanning different portions of the heart during multiple different heartbeats and "stitching" the data together.

3. How long does a cardiac CT acquisition take?

To acquire an image, the gantry of the CT scanner must rotate 180 degrees around the patient. With a rotation speed of 330 ms, a modern scanner acquires the image in 165 ms, which is the *temporal resolution*. Some scanners have two x-ray tubes, which allows image acquisition after only 90 degrees of gantry rotation, reducing the temporal resolution to 83 ms. This 83-ms shutter speed is still long, however, compared with digital subtraction angiography catheter angiography, with its temporal resolution of 7 to 10 ms, and so gating is also required.

4. What is gating?

ECG leads are placed on the patient and connected to the scanner. Images can be acquired with either *prospective* or *retrospective gating*. The aim is to leverage the temporal resolution of the scanner to maximal advantage by acquiring data during phases in the cardiac cycle when cardiac motion is least; this is usually in late diastole.

In *prospective gating,* the x-ray tube is turned on only during a specific phase of the cardiac cycle, usually in late diastole when cardiac motion is at a minimum. During the remainder of the cycle, the table moves, and the patient is repositioned for the next set of images, which are taken during the same phase of the next heartbeat. Prospective gating exposes the patient to a lower radiation dose than retrospective gating. Strict heart rate control is required for a prospective scan, however, because if there is motion blur on an image, there are no data available from other points in the cardiac cycle to attempt a reconstruction at a different phase.

In *retrospective gating,* the patient is scanned in a continuous helical fashion. The x-ray tube is on throughout the cardiac cycle, although *tube current modulation* may be used to decrease the radiation dose during phases of the cardiac cycle where motion is most prominent (e.g., systole). Images are reconstructed from data acquired during specific portions of the cardiac cycle. Advantages include the ability to reconstruct images from any phase of the cardiac cycle, which may help in evaluation of a coronary artery segment that is blurred during the preferred late diastolic phase. In addition, if images are generated from all phases of the cardiac cycle, functional information is available regarding ejection fraction, valve motion, and wall motion. Retrospective gating is accompanied by a relative radiation dose penalty, however, compared with prospective gating of about 2 to 3:1.

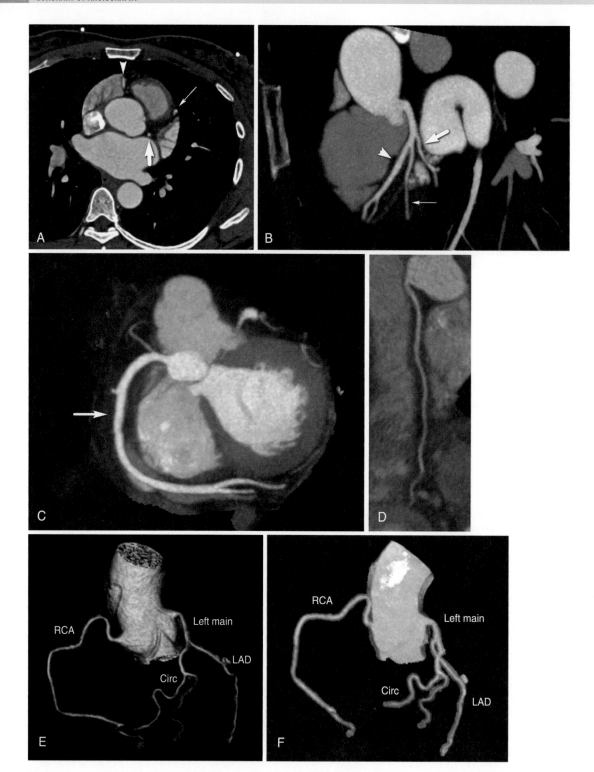

Figure 11-1. Normal coronary arteries. **A,** Axial image shows right coronary (*arrowhead*), left anterior descending (*thin arrow*), and circumflex (*thick arrow*) arteries. **B,** Maximum intensity projection (MIP) image shows left main artery branching into left anterior descending (*arrowhead*), first diagonal (*thin arrow*) and circumflex (*thick arrow*) arteries. **C,** Additional MIP image shows right coronary artery (*thin arrow*). **D,** Curved planar reformat image of right coronary artery allows evaluation of entire vessel on a single image. **E,** Volume-rendered three-dimensional image with subtraction of the heart permits evaluation of entire arterial tree with perspective. **F,** Wide-slab MIP with heart subtraction shows vessels with less three-dimensional perspective. RCA = right coronary artery; Circ = circumflex (artery); LAD, left anterior descending (artery).

5. Can coronary CT be performed at any heart rate?

To minimize motion and acquire images of diagnostic quality, a slow rate and regular cardiac rhythm are highly desirable. A rate of 60 beats/min or less is ideal because it allows effective use of prospective gating, minimizing radiation dose. Administration of oral β-blockers is a safe method of achieving this heart rate in most patients. Contraindications include severe asthma or congestive obstructive pulmonary disease, heart failure, and heart block. In the setting of acute chest pain, cocaine use is also a contraindication. Scanning at higher heart rates is sometimes unavoidable, and rates in the 60s almost always yield diagnostic images with retrospective gating.

6. Can I use nitroglycerin to dilate the coronary arteries and get better images?

Yes, an oral spray of nitroglycerin at the beginning of the scan is effective in dilating the coronary arteries and improving visualization. Nitroglycerin is contraindicated in patients with hypotension and patients with phosphodiesterase inhibitor use.

7. How much radiation exposure is there for a patient undergoing coronary CT angiography?

Radiation exposure is a perennial issue for all CT studies. Opponents of coronary CT angiography have touted high radiation dose from the study as a reason to choose the more established catheter angiography or nuclear stress test. Prospective gating results in an average of 4 mSv or less of exposure, however. Newer techniques with lower tube voltage and higher current can reduce the dose to 1 to 2 mSv in some cases. In comparison, diagnostic catheterization results in an average of 7 mSv, with considerable operator-dependent variation. A nuclear study using sestamibi with stress and rest phases measures about 15 mSv. Regardless, all efforts should be made to reduce dose and to consider which organs are exposed. It would be prudent to be especially conscious of radiation dose in young women because of the relatively high breast dose from coronary CT angiography.

8. What are the advantages and disadvantages of coronary CT angiography versus catheter angiography?

Coronary CT angiography is less invasive than catheter angiography and avoids the potential complications of groin hematoma, pseudoaneurysm, retroperitoneal hematoma, and dissection, and sedation-related complications. In addition to showing the lumen of the vessel, coronary CT angiography depicts the vessel wall and plaque or other pathology within it (Fig. 11-2), which can be inferred only from catheter angiography. Analysis of plaque composition is also possible. Coronary CT angiography easily shows anatomic abnormalities such as aberrant course or origin of the arteries (Fig. 11-3; see Fig. 9-7) and coronary artery fistulas, both of which are difficult to evaluate at catheterization. Coronary CT angiography depicts bypass grafts easily (Fig. 11-4)—another challenge for catheter angiography. Coronary CT angiography also depicts other causes of chest pain, such as pulmonary embolus, aortic dissection, or pneumonia. In the presence of a coronary artery stent (Fig. 11-5), stent patency versus obstruction is usually determinable by CT angiography, although evaluation of the degree of patency or extent of in-stent stenosis is limited by beam hardening artifact from the stent. The presence of a very large amount of coronary calcium also complicates the evaluation of the degree of stenosis. Intervention is possible only in catheter angiography, and in a patient for whom intervention is considered a likely outcome of the diagnostic procedure, catheter angiography should be used (Table 11-1).

9. Which patients can benefit from coronary CT angiography?

The largest group of referrals for coronary CT angiography comprises patients with atypical or low-risk chest pain. In these patients, a negative study prevents a chain of cardiac investigations such as stress tests. These patients may present to the emergency department or may be scanned on an outpatient basis. Chest pain patients with a high risk of acute coronary syndrome are not typically evaluated by coronary CT angiography because the probability of requiring intervention is high enough to justify catheterization in many cases. Evaluation for aberrant coronary artery origin and course is also a good indication for coronary CT angiography, as is further evaluation of a patient with an equivocal stress test.

10. Can I use coronary CT angiography as a single study for a patient with chest pain to rule out cardiac ischemia, aortic dissection, and pulmonary embolus?

Extending the range of coronary CT angiography to include the entire chest for additional indications is possible. It involves increasing the radiation dose, however, and the dose of intravenous contrast agent required for simultaneous opacification of pulmonary arteries, coronary arteries, and the aorta. The application of clinical acumen to focus the work-up more narrowly whenever possible is preferable. If this "triple-rule-out" is to be attempted, prospective gating would be advantageous in minimizing the radiation dose.

11. Are there uses for cardiac CT other than coronary artery evaluation?

Cardiac CT can be used for multiple purposes in addition to coronary artery evaluation. Common requests include evaluation of pulmonary vein ostia and anatomy in candidates for electrophysiologic studies and potential ablation therapy in the setting of atrial fibrillation. Cardiac masses and valvular pathology may also be evaluated by CT, although echocardiography and MRI may be more definitive. One advantage of CT in these scenarios is its ability to depict calcium accurately, which may be helpful for characterizing masses, and may affect treatment strategies in valvular disease.

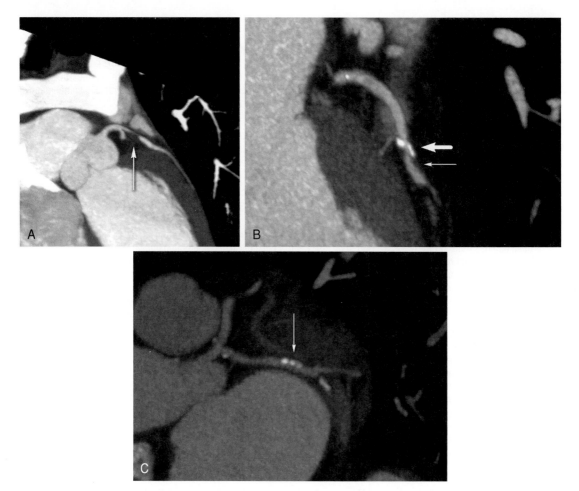

Figure 11-2. Atherosclerotic plaque in coronary arteries. **A,** Noncalcified plaque in proximal left anterior descending artery (*arrow*) causes 90% stenosis. **B,** Mixed plaque in left anterior descending artery composed of calcified (*thick arrow*) and noncalcified (*thin arrow*) components causes 70% stenosis. **C,** Calcified plaque (*thin arrow*) in circumflex artery causes mild stenosis.

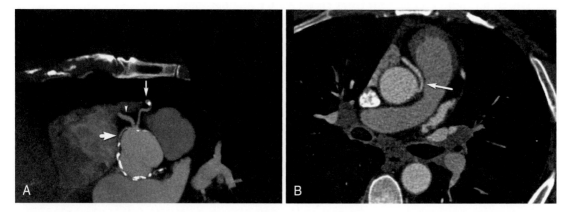

Figure 11-3. Anomalous origin of the coronary arteries. **A,** Left anterior descending (*thin arrow*), right coronary (*arrowhead*), and circumflex (*thick arrow*) arteries all arise from the right cusp. The left anterior descending artery and circumflex artery courses are anterior to the pulmonary artery and retroaortic. **B,** Right coronary artery (*arrow*) arises from the left cusp and passes between the aorta and pulmonary artery (interarterial course), a route that leaves the right coronary artery susceptible to compression between the two great arteries.

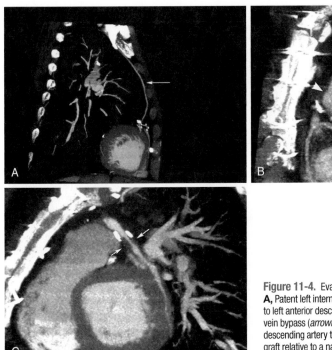

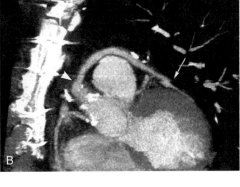

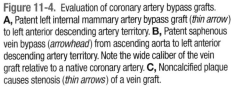

Figure 11-4. Evaluation of coronary artery bypass grafts. **A,** Patent left internal mammary artery bypass graft (*thin arrow*) to left anterior descending artery territory. **B,** Patent saphenous vein bypass (*arrowhead*) from ascending aorta to left anterior descending artery territory. Note the wide caliber of the vein graft relative to a native coronary artery. **C,** Noncalcified plaque causes stenosis (*thin arrows*) of a vein graft.

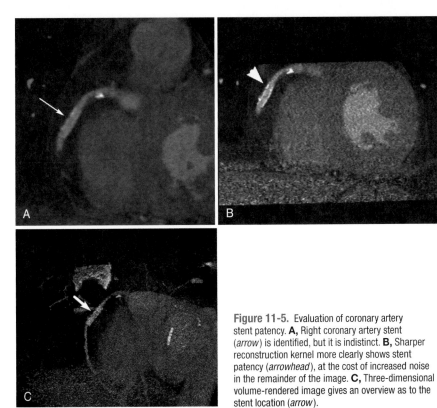

Figure 11-5. Evaluation of coronary artery stent patency. **A,** Right coronary artery stent (*arrow*) is identified, but it is indistinct. **B,** Sharper reconstruction kernel more clearly shows stent patency (*arrowhead*), at the cost of increased noise in the remainder of the image. **C,** Three-dimensional volume-rendered image gives an overview as to the stent location (*arrow*).

Table 11-1. Coronary CT Angiography versus Catheter Angiography

	CORONARY CT ANGIOGRAPHY	CATHETER ANGIOGRAPHY
Vessel stenosis	+	++
Plaque composition	+	−
Aberrant course	+	+/−
Graft evaluation	+	+/−
Stent evaluation	+/−	+
Extracardiac findings	+	−
Ability to intervene	−	+
Risk of complication	Very low	Intermediate

12. Is coronary CT the same as coronary artery calcium (CAC) scoring?

No, CAC scoring is an older technique. It involves use of an unenhanced scan, which accurately depicts the amount of calcific plaque in the coronary arteries. The calcified lesions are easily identified by their high attenuation. The plaque can measured by computerized methods to generate a "calcium score" based on the product of calcium volume and attenuation. The calcium score places the patient in a risk category for future cardiovascular events, according to population-based data. These data are an excellent risk predictor for cardiovascular events, and a positive test result may be used as a stimulus for aggressive medical therapy and risk factor reduction and behavior modification. The technique has limitations, however. It does not depict the coronary artery lumen, and it gives no information regarding actual stenoses in a specific patient. It is also unable to detect noncalcified plaque. Patients with noncalcified severe stenoses and a complete absence of any calcified plaque are uncommon, but they do appear. Such patients could receive false assurance from their negative CAC score reports. Although CAC scoring may have a role in screening, it cannot be the sole test in a patient with chest pain.

13. Does CAC scoring have a role in chest pain evaluation?

As noted previously, CAC scoring can miss noncalcified plaque and does not give information on luminal narrowing. It is useful, however, as the first step of a coronary CT angiography evaluation. The CAC score gives a useful indication as to the overall extent of atherosclerosis. A high score (>400 in the acute setting) is often used to abort the planned coronary CT angiography and progress directly to catheterization, given the high-risk category in which the patient is now found. In the outpatient setting, scores greater than 2000 make vessel analysis difficult on coronary CT angiography, and other diagnostic tests may be preferable. The unenhanced calcium scoring scan involves a much smaller radiation dose than the main coronary CT angiography examination and can be modified to cover the entire chest, aiding evaluation of the lungs and mediastinum to search for other causes of chest pain.

14. How is a coronary CT angiography examination reviewed?

Initially, the calcium scoring sequence is reviewed for lung and mediastinal pathology. Calcium score is calculated. Then the main coronary CT angiography sequence is reviewed. From the raw data of this scan, multiple reconstructions may be generated in various phases of the cardiac cycle (if retrospective gating was used). The reconstructed images are typically reviewed at a dedicated workstation axially and using multiplanar reformatted images generated by the interpreting physician to depict the arteries best. The myocardium, valves, pericardium, and extracardiac structures should also be thoroughly evaluated. More advanced workstation functions, such as curved planar reformat of coronary arteries, may be used as an aid to interpretation, but they must not be used to replace analysis of the entire data set by the radiologist. Finally, if retrospective gating is employed, a cine sequence of the heart should be reconstructed to evaluate wall motion and calculate ejection fraction.

15. How are coronary artery stenoses reported?

Coronary artery plaques are described by:

- The vessel and the vessel segment
- Plaque composition (i.e., calcified, mixed, or uncalcified)
- Plaque length
- Degree of stenosis caused

Degree of stenosis is best characterized by percentage values (e.g., "50%" stenosis). A percentage is more specific than "moderate" stenosis.

16. What is "myocardial bridging"? Is it important?

The coronary arteries are located in the epicardial fat, which is a fat layer deep to the pericardium, but superficial to the myocardium. Myocardial bridging is present if the artery courses into the myocardium and is surrounded by muscle for part of its course (Fig. 11-6). The significance of myocardial bridging is that, theoretically, an artery surrounded

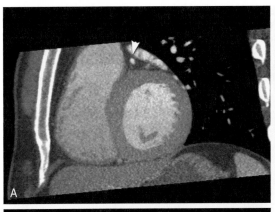

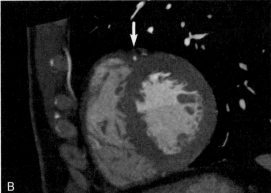

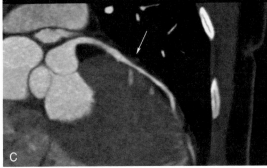

Figure 11-6. Myocardial bridging. **A,** Normal proximal left anterior descending artery (*arrowhead*) is located in and surrounded by epicardial fat. **B** and **C,** Bridged left anterior descending artery (*arrows*) is surrounded by myocardium for a short segment.

by myocardium may be compressed when the myocardium contracts during systole (systolic compression), limiting blood supply and causing ischemia. Catheter angiography has difficulty identifying bridging unless it causes systolic compression because the myocardium is not depicted. Until more recently, myocardial bridging has rarely been diagnosed. Coronary CT angiography shows bridging in 25% to 40% of patients, however, most commonly in the left anterior descending artery. If multiphase data are available, the vessel should be viewed in systole to ensure that there is no systolic compression. Myocardial bridging is almost always an incidental finding without systolic compression or any other clinical significance. Systolic compression may be more likely in cases in which the bridged arterial segment is relatively long and is located deep within the myocardium.

17. Have trials shown an advantage to using coronary CT angiography in place of catheter angiograms or nuclear stress tests?

Early coronary CT angiography studies performed on 4- and 16-slice scanners raised doubt as to the accuracy of coronary CT angiography. Newer studies performed on 40- and 64-slice scanners, using catheter angiography as the gold standard, show coronary CT angiography sensitivity of 96% to 99% for stenoses of greater than 50% on a per patient level, with specificity of 88% to 93%. Other studies have compared the use of coronary CT angiography in low-risk chest pain patients in the emergency department in place of serial cardiac enzymes and nuclear stress test. These studies show quicker discharge, lower cost, and no missed cardiac events (for follow-up periods of 1 year) for the coronary CT angiography group. These trials support the use of coronary CT angiography as accurate and cost-effective in low-risk chest pain patients. In addition, coronary CT angiography provides a large amount of data that are mostly unobtainable by catheter angiography and nuclear stress test, such as plaque composition, extent of vessel remodeling, extracardiac findings, aberrant coronary artery course, and numerous other pathologies.

18. Will the patient's insurance pay for coronary CT angiography? What do NCD, LCD, and CED mean?

When new medical technologies or procedures are introduced, the Center for Medicare & Medicaid Services (CMS) must decide whether to cover their cost for Medicare patients, and most private insurers generally follow Medicare reimbursement policies. These new technologies are usually examined during an initial evaluation period before a final decision is rendered. During this period, local Medicare offices around the United States may decide to cover or not cover a particular service under a *local coverage determination (LCD)*. When the evaluation period has passed, a *national coverage determination (NCD)* is made; if a procedure is covered by an NCD, all Medicare patients generally would be able to have the procedure with insurance coverage. In the case of coronary CT, CMS initially decided to allow *coverage with evidence development,* in which coronary CT studies would be covered only if they were performed as part of research studies designed to show the usefulness of coronary CT in specific clinical situations. After considerable negative feedback from physicians, patients, and members of Congress, in March 2008 CMS decided to leave things the way they were (i.e., with each local Medicare office deciding on its own LCD) for another 2 years before deciding on an NCD. The answer to "will the patient's insurance pay for coronary CT angiography" is that it depends on where the patient lives and what insurance coverage he or she has.

CHAPTER 12

CT ANGIOGRAPHY OF THE PULMONARY VASCULATURE

Milan Sheth, MD, and
Harold I. Litt, MD, PhD

1. What are the primary methods for imaging for pulmonary embolus (PE)?

There are three main methods of pulmonary arterial imaging. One is pulmonary arteriography, which is accomplished by inserting a catheter under fluoroscopic guidance into the pulmonary artery and injecting contrast agent to visualize the pulmonary arteries directly. Nuclear ventilation/perfusion ($\dot{V}/\dot{Q}$) examinations compare the location of radiolabeled ventilated particles with radiolabeled injected particles to help infer the presence of PE. The third method is computed tomography (CT) pulmonary angiography, which involves injecting contrast agent into a vein and using CT to evaluate the pulmonary arteries.

2. What plain film findings may suggest PE?

A chest radiograph is usually the first imaging modality used for a patient with suspected PE. The results of the chest film may be negative or have nonspecific findings, such as pleural effusions and atelectasis, but occasionally the film can have a wedge-shaped peripheral opacity, referred to as a *Hampton hump*. An area of lucency resulting from decreased perfusion that is termed *Westermark sign* also may be seen.

3. What are the advantages of CT angiography over other methods in the evaluation of PE?

One important advantage over catheter pulmonary arteriography and $\dot{V}/\dot{Q}$ nuclear medicine scans is that CT angiography may be used to diagnose other causes of the patient's symptoms, such as a pleural effusion or atelectasis. In contrast to arteriography, CT angiography is noninvasive and safer. CT angiography also takes less time to perform. CT angiography has several advantages over nuclear $\dot{V}/\dot{Q}$ imaging. It is less dependent on patient cooperation. In addition, nuclear $\dot{V}/\dot{Q}$ examinations may have a 60% to 70% indeterminate rate, especially in patients with underlying lung disease or other comorbidities, which limit specificity.

4. How do you perform a CT angiography examination for PE?

The technique for performing CT angiography optimally involves the use of a multidetector row CT scanner. Contrast agent is injected at a high rate into a peripheral vein. Scanning is timed to obtain optimal contrast opacification of the pulmonary arteries. Thin-section axial CT images of 1- to 2-mm thickness are obtained throughout the chest. With CT scanners containing 16, 64, or more slices, a CT scan for PE requires only a 5- to 10-second acquisition, and provides high-quality images, even in very dyspneic patients.

Key Points: CT Angiography

1. Multidetector row CT angiography has become the first-line imaging examination for evaluation of suspected PE.
2. CT angiography has greater specificity than a $\dot{V}/\dot{Q}$ scan.
3. CT angiography has greater availability and safety than pulmonary angiography.

---

5. What are the direct CT angiography findings of PE?

The most specific finding of a PE is a partial or complete intraluminal filling defect in a pulmonary artery (Fig. 12-1). It should be present on at least two contiguous sections. Abrupt cutoff of the artery also indicates a PE.

6. What are the indirect findings of PE?

A pulmonary artery with an embolus may be slightly enlarged. Parenchymal findings, such as wedge-shaped opacities denoting areas of infarction and atelectasis, sometimes can be seen as well. Areas of decreased perfusion can manifest as wedge-shaped hyperlucency.

7. How can acute PE be distinguished from chronic PE on CT angiography?

It may be difficult to differentiate acute from chronic PE. Chronic PE may be complicated by superimposed acute PE. Acute PE are often seen as central filling defects, in contrast to chronic emboli, which are more peripheral. This is easy to remember because the peripheral appearance of chronic PE is due to an acute clot in a vessel that recanalizes over time. Chronic emboli can also calcify, whereas acute emboli do not. Long-standing PE are more likely than acute emboli to cause pulmonary hypertension, leading to right heart enlargement and enlargement of the main and central pulmonary arteries (Fig. 12-2). Lastly, increased mediastinal collateral vessels can be seen in some cases of chronic PE.

8. What are other uses for CT in PE?

CT also can be used to evaluate the lower extremity venous system for thrombosis, using the same contrast bolus, by imaging several minutes after the PE study. Lower extremity ultrasound (US) is generally used to evaluate lower extremity veins, but CT has several advantages. One is that it is not operator dependent, in contrast to US. CT can be used to evaluate for clot in areas that are inaccessible to US or difficult to evaluate. This includes the deep pelvic veins (a common source of thrombus that may embolize to the lungs) and the region around the adductor canal. US can be of limited value in patients who are obese or have had recent surgery. Within certain limitations, CT may be a better choice than US in these situations.

9. What is a pulmonary arteriovenous malformation (AVM), and what symptoms can it cause?

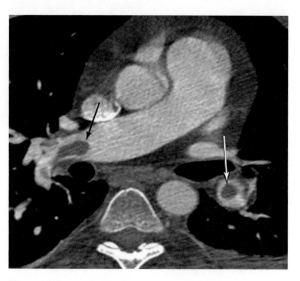

Figure 12-1. Axial image from pulmonary CT angiography examination shows bilateral PE, which are visualized as intraluminal filling defects in the pulmonary arterial system (*arrows*).

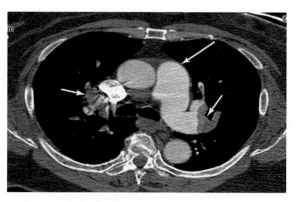

Figure 12-2. Axial CT angiography image shows bilateral chronic PE (*short arrows*). Although these emboli have not calcified, the main pulmonary artery (*long arrow*) is enlarged, indicating pulmonary hypertension.

A pulmonary AVM is an abnormal communication between the pulmonary artery and a draining vein, causing blood to bypass the pulmonary capillary bed before returning to the left heart. AVMs may be asymptomatic, but they can manifest with a wide range of clinical symptoms. Symptoms result from the loss of two essential physiologic functions of the lungs. Hypoxia may occur because of shunting, and paradoxic emboli, stroke, or brain abscess may occur because of the loss of the "filter" effect of the lung. Pulmonary AVMs may cause vague symptoms, such as chest pain and dyspnea on exertion, because of shunting of deoxygenated blood. With severe shunting, high-output cardiac failure can result from right-to-left shunting.

10. What is orthodeoxia?

The term *orthodeoxia* is used to describe position-dependent oxygen desaturation. Most pulmonary AVMs occur in the lower lobes. Shunting of blood and desaturation are maximum when blood flow to the lung bases is greatest. Patients with large pulmonary AVMs in the lower lobes have larger shunts and lower oxygen saturation when standing. When lying down, blood is redirected toward the lung apices, and the shunt fraction and desaturation may decrease.

11. What pulmonary AVMs are associated with what hereditary disorder?

Although pulmonary AVMs are often isolated, they can be associated with hereditary hemorrhagic telangiectasia, also known as Osler-Weber-Rendu disease. Hereditary hemorrhagic telangiectasia is a genetic disorder that causes vascular malformations that can lead to multiple pulmonary AVMs. It is characterized by telangiectasias of the skin and mucosal linings, epistaxis, and AVMs in various internal organs such as the brain and liver. It is wise to screen family members of patients who present with pulmonary AVMs so that they can receive treatment.

12. You are asked to start a peripheral intravenous line in a patient with a known pulmonary AVM. What special precautions should you take?

Patients with pulmonary AVMs lack the "filter" function performed by the pulmonary capillary bed. This situation predisposes patients to paradoxic emboli from endogenous and exogenous sources. Air or other material accidentally introduced into the venous system could pass through the shunt and cause a stroke. Care must be taken that all venous lines are free of air, and that filters are used to prevent paradoxic emboli.

13. What are the imaging characteristics of a pulmonary AVM on plain film and CT?

On plain film, pulmonary AVMs appear as serpiginous or nodular densities that can connect to the hilum. On CT, they appear as a homogeneous noncalcified nodule that has a vascular connection with an enlarged feeding artery and draining vein (Fig. 12-3). On dynamic images, the malformation enhances in a sequential manner from the feeding artery to the malformation to the vein.

14. What is partial anomalous pulmonary venous return (PAPVR)?

PAPVR occurs when part of the pulmonary venous system drains directly into the systemic circulation. It can occur in isolation or be associated with either atrial septal defect or a hypogenetic lung. When PAPVR is associated with atrial septal defect (usually a sinus venosus defect), the right upper lobe drains into the superior vena cava. When PAPVR occurs with a hypogenetic lung, it is a component of congenital pulmonary venolobar syndrome, also known as scimitar syndrome.

15. What is scimitar syndrome, and what are its associated imaging findings?

Scimitar syndrome is a hypogenetic lung (almost exclusively on the right) that is drained by an anomalous vein. This anomalous vein can drain into many structures, including the infradiaphragmatic inferior vena cava (IVC), suprahepatic IVC, portal vein, or right atrium. The chest x-ray shows a small right lung with a tubular opacity paralleling the right heart border (called the *scimitar*). Magnetic resonance imaging (MRI) and CT show the course and nature of the abnormal vascular anatomy better (Fig. 12-4).

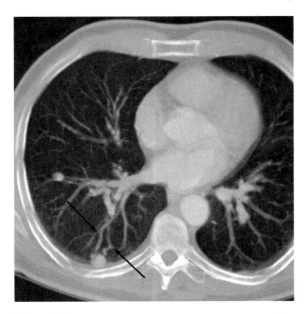

Figure 12-3. Axial CT angiography image shows a pulmonary AVM, with feeding artery and draining vein (*arrows*) associated with the lesion.

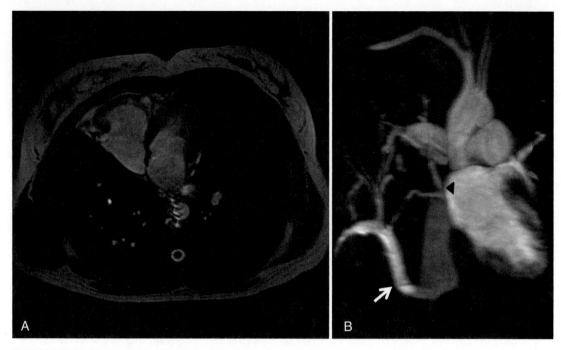

Figure 12-4. Findings of scimitar syndrome. **A,** Axial MR image shows small right lung and shift of the mediastinum to the right. **B,** Oblique maximum intensity projection of magnetic resonance angiography (MRA) of the chest showing anomalous pulmonary venous drainage of the right lower lobe to the IVC (*arrow*), the so-called scimitar vein. The upper lobe drains into the left atrium (*arrowhead*).

16. What is the most common primary tumor of the pulmonary artery?
Tumors associated with the pulmonary vascular system are exceedingly rare. Angiosarcomas are most common. These are rare tumors and sometimes can be difficult to distinguish from occlusive PE because both fill the lumen of the pulmonary artery.

CHAPTER 13

CT ANGIOGRAPHY AND MRA OF THE PERIPHERAL AND VISCERAL VASCULATURE

Maxim Itkin, MD, and
Harold I. Litt, MD, PhD

1. What are computed tomography (CT) angiography and magnetic resonance angiography (MRA)?

CT angiography and MRA are methods to image blood vessels noninvasively using CT or MRI. To make vessels visible, iodine-based contrast material (for CT angiography) or gadolinium chelate contrast material (for MRA) is injected through a peripheral intravenous line, and images are acquired at peak vascular enhancement.

2. When is peak contrast enhancement?

Contrast agent is injected intravenously as a bolus at a rate 2 to 4 mL/sec. The concentration of the contrast agent at a specific location changes with time, according to an enhancement curve. The maximum concentration in proximal systemic arteries usually occurs 20 to 30 seconds after beginning the injection. Peak opacification occurs at different time points in different parts of the body. To scan vessels at optimal enhancement, the scanning table moves to image the appropriate body part. This is a technique referred to as *bolus chase*.

3. How do we know the time of peak contrast enhancement?

The time of peak enhancement varies from patient to patient and is influenced by factors such as patient size, cardiac output, and contrast injection site. Although timing may be estimated, the peak opacification time is usually determined for each patient to obtain consistent results. This determination can be performed by injecting a "test bolus," a small amount of contrast agent (20 mL for iodine-based CT contrast material), and measuring the opacification curve at the most proximal point upstream to the area of interest (usually somewhere in the aorta) by scanning at the same location every 1 or 2 seconds. The time between start of the injection and peak enhancement determines the scan delay. Another method, called *bolus* tracking, measures the enhancement (or MRI signal intensity) at a given point every 1 or 2 seconds during the main contrast agent injection until a threshold enhancement is reached, and then scanning begins.

4. What images are obtained during a CT angiography or MRA study?

CT angiography images are acquired in the axial plane. Although experienced radiologists can interpret these images, it is easier to diagnose vessel pathology by creating an image in a plane that allows the long axis of the vessel to be viewed. To view vessels in this perspective, axial images are transferred to a three-dimensional (3D) workstation where the physician or a specially trained technologist performs reconstructions. There are several principal modes of 3D image presentation. Multiplanar reformatting allows reconstruction of the image along any oblique plane or a curve (curved planar reformatting). Maximum intensity projection (MIP) (Fig. 13-1) is a method in which only the brightest pixel at a given location in a slab of tissue is displayed. Images obtained with this method appear similar to a conventional angiogram. Shaded surface display (SSD) (Fig. 13-2) shows data in a 3D representation using only pixels that are on the surface of objects.

Volume-rendering techniques use the advantages of MIP and SSD methods, preserving all image data and displaying them as a 3D representation. This display is achieved by assigning different transparencies to tissues with different densities (Fig. 13-3).

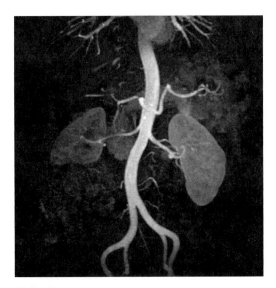

Figure 13-1. Coronal MIP image of dynamic, gadolinium-enhanced 3D MRA shows normal aorta and normal bilateral renal arteries. The patient has had right lower pole partial nephrectomy.

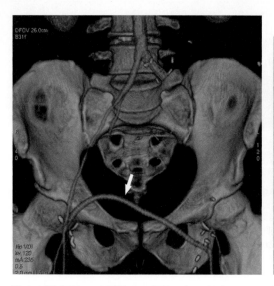

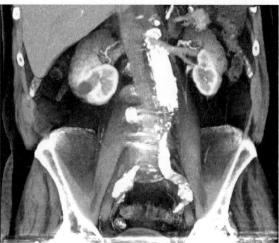

Figure 13-2. Coronal SSD image of CT angiography data set shows patent femoral-femoral bypass (*arrow*). The left common iliac and external iliac arteries are occluded.

Figure 13-3. Coronal volume-rendering image of CT angiography data set showing the kidneys, renal veins, and inferior vena cava.

An important advantage of MRA is the ability to acquire images in any plane. MRA acquisitions can be performed in the plane along the course of vessels (usually coronal for the legs), which may decrease the volume of tissue that needs to be covered by the examination. The data can be reformatted and displayed similarly to CT angiography data.

5. **When should one choose MRA versus CT angiography for a runoff examination?**
   Both methods have advantages and disadvantages, and sometimes they are complementary. CT angiography has a shorter acquisition time and higher spatial resolution, especially when machines with 16, 64, or more slices are used. An arterial scan from the diaphragm to the toes can take 10 to 20 seconds, and the whole study, including preparation and positioning, lasts only about 10 minutes. MRA is a much longer study and requires the patient to lie still in the magnet for the entire examination. This requirement may be problematic for patients who are claustrophobic or unstable. MRA is the study of choice for patients with an allergy to iodinated contrast agents. Although gadolinium-based contrast agents used for MRA were previously thought to be safe for use in patients with renal failure, the recently reported incidence of nephrogenic systemic fibrosis in these patients has removed this possibility (see question 22 for a full discussion). CT angiography can be performed when MRA is contraindicated, as in patients with pacemakers. One advantage of CT angiography over MRA is the ability to obtain images with fewer artifacts when the patient has metal intravascular stents, although MRA may be better for patients with heavily calcified vessels. Generally, both methods are acceptable substitutes for catheter angiography, and each institution has to tailor its own policy according to available resources and expertise.

6. **What do intravascular stents look like on MRA and CT angiography?**
   There are two main types of intravascular stents: balloon expandable, made from stainless steel, and self-expandable, made from a special alloy called *nitinol*. The first type of stent is paramagnetic and creates strong MRI artifacts that prevent imaging of the underlying vessel. Nitinol stents are made from a diamagnetic material that creates fewer artifacts. Stainless steel and nitinol stents cause minimal artifacts in CT angiography and usually do not obscure the underlying vessel.

7. **What is the definition of a hemodynamically significant artery stenosis?**
   Different arterial distributions can tolerate different degrees of stenosis, depending on the metabolic activity of the target organ and the availability of collateral blood supply. On CT angiography or MRA or both, most authors define "significant stenosis" as a diameter reduction of greater than 75%, although a more conservative definition is greater than 50%. Pressure gradients cannot be measured on CT angiography and MRA. Although quantitative measurements of the degree of stenosis are important, the presence of clinical symptoms should be the major determinant in the decision to treat an arterial lesion. Sequential subcritical stenoses result in a pressure decrease that approximates the sum of each stenosis. Additional signs of hemodynamically significant stenosis are poststenotic dilation of a vessel and delayed enhancement of the target organ.

8. **What is the best way to measure the degree of a stenosis?**
The most accepted way is to measure the ratio of the diameter of the stenosis to a "normal-appearing" vessel segment. This method was adopted from the technique used to measure stenoses during conventional angiography. Although well established, this method may lack precision because it uses a two-dimensional representation of a 3D object to estimate a stenosis. It also relies on the ability to select a "normal" segment of vessel to use as a reference. This may be problematic because even normal vessels taper distally, and it may be difficult to find an area adjacent to a stenosis that is not aneurysmal or affected by poststenotic dilation. CT angiography and MRA offer the unique opportunity to evaluate the stenosis precisely, by measuring the decrease in cross-sectional area. With the development of more automated vessel analysis tools, measurements of cross-sectional area are expected to become the gold standard.

> **Key Points: Measuring Degree of Vessel Stenosis**
>
> 1. *Most accurate method:* Compare cross-sectional area of stenotic lesion segment with that of a normal segment of the vessel.
> 2. *Most commonly used method:* Compare linear diameter of stenotic lesion segment with that of a normal segment of the vessel.

9. **What is the distribution of peripheral vascular disease in different age groups?**
Generally, young smokers have more proximal disease involving the iliac vessels. Older patients, especially patients with diabetes, have more distal disease involving the infrapopliteal vessels. This difference is important because patency rates after treatment of proximal disease using endovascular and surgical methods are significantly greater.

10. **What is meant by "single-, two-, or three-vessel" runoff?**
Normally, there are three infrapopliteal vessels: the anterior tibial, posterior tibial, and peroneal arteries. The number of these calf vessels that are continuously patent from the origin to the ankle defines the number of runoff vessels.
A higher number usually corresponds to a better prognosis after surgery or endovascular procedures.

11. **What structures separate the superficial femoral from the popliteal artery and the external iliac from the common femoral artery?**
The superficial femoral artery becomes the popliteal artery after entering the adductor (Hunter) canal. The external iliac artery becomes the femoral artery immediately after the takeoff of the deep circumflex iliac artery.

12. **On an anterior projection, which thigh vessel takes a more medial course—the superficial femoral artery or the deep femoral artery?**
The normal course of the superficial femoral artery is medial to that of the deep femoral artery (Fig. 13-4).

13. **Why are angiographic studies performed on potential renal donors?**
Donor kidney harvesting is often performed using a minimally invasive laparoscopic approach. The surgeon's field of view is limited, so precise information concerning the location, size, and

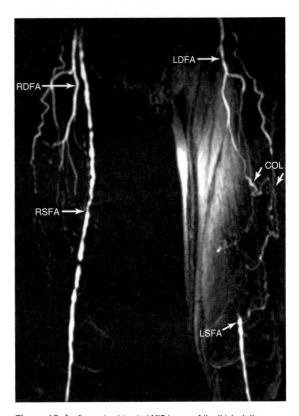

Figure 13-4. Coronal subtracted MIP image of the thigh station from a gadolinium-enhanced bolus chase runoff examination shows occlusion of the left superficial femoral artery. The left deep femoral artery (LDFA) is patent and gives rise to tortuous collateral (COL) vessels that reconstitute the distal left superficial femoral artery (LSFA) just above the knee joint. The right superficial femoral artery (RSFA) and right deep femoral artery (RDFA) are patent.

number of renal arteries and veins is required before surgery. This is extremely important because of the variability of the renal vasculature in humans.

14. What is the prevalence of accessory renal arteries in the general population?

Approximately 30% of people have accessory renal arteries (Fig. 13-5). Identification of the number, location, and size of the renal arteries is vital. Significant post-transplant complications may result if even a small vessel that supplies the ureter is accidentally sacrificed. Larger arteries that supply the renal pelvis or significant portions of renal parenchyma must be preserved, sometimes necessitating complicated reconstructive surgery.

15. What is the most common left renal vein anatomic variant?

Generally, renal veins have more consistent anatomy than renal arteries. Knowledge of the venous anatomy before laparoscopic surgery is important to prevent vascular injury and bleeding. The left vein is longer than the right vein, which is one reason why the left kidney is preferred for transplantation. The most common left renal vein anatomic variant is a circumaortic renal vein, which occurs in 5% to 7% of the population. With this anatomic variant, the left renal vein forms a ring around the aorta. The anterior segment of the ring connects with the inferior vena cava at the expected level of the left renal vein, and the posterior segment connects with the inferior vena cava below the insertion of the anterior segment. A retroaortic left renal vein is less common and occurs in 2% to 3% of people.

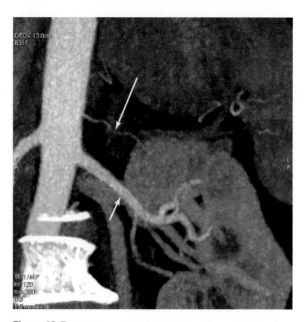

Figure 13-5. Multiplanar reformat MIP image of the renal arteries in a potential kidney donor, showing left upper pole accessory artery (*long arrow*) and main left renal artery (*short arrow*).

16. What are the secondary imaging signs of renal artery stenosis?

Secondary imaging signs are delayed parenchymal enhancement and an overall reduced kidney size. A difference of more than 1 to 2 cm in renal length is considered significant.

17. Can fibromuscular dysplasia (FMD) be diagnosed using MRA or CT angiography?

Currently, the gold standard for the diagnosis of FMD is still conventional arteriography. The main findings of FMD are subtle intimal changes, resulting in a beaded appearance to affected vessels. The resolution of MRA is insufficient for diagnosis. CT angiography, using 16- and 64-channel scanners, shows promise for detecting FMD, but it is not considered reliable enough at this time to diagnose FMD accurately.

18. What are the collateral pathways between the superior mesenteric artery (SMA) and inferior mesenteric artery (IMA) and the celiac artery and the SMA?

There are two collateral pathways that connect the SMA and IMA: the arc of Riolan proximally and the marginal artery of Drummond distally. The main collateral pathways between the celiac artery and the SMA are through the common hepatic artery, gastroduodenal artery, and pancreaticoduodenal arteries. The arc of Bühler is a direct connection between the SMA and celiac artery.

19. Can ostial SMA or celiac artery occlusion result in mesenteric ischemia?

Because of the extensive collaterals between the three main mesenteric vessels, occlusion of just one of these three vessels usually does not cause symptoms. Severe stenosis of at least two of the vessels is necessary for symptomatic mesenteric ischemia (Fig. 13-6).

20. Identify each of the vessels shown in Fig. 13-7.

Answers are given in figure legend.

21. What is the median arcuate ligament? What is its significance?

The median arcuate ligament is formed from fibers derived from the medial edge of left and right diaphragmatic crus during their ascent anterosuperiorly. The median arcuate ligament may occasionally cause a stenosis of the proximal celiac axis because of extrinsic compression. The clinical significance of the resulting narrowing is

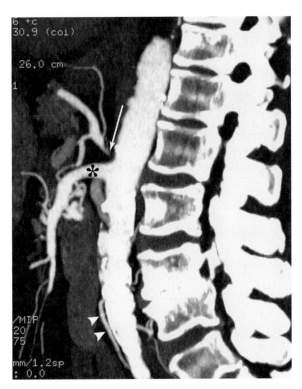

Figure 13-6. Sagittal multiplanar reformat image of CT angiography data set shows complete occlusion of the celiac artery at its origin (*arrow*) and patent superior mesenteric (*asterisk*) and inferior mesenteric (*arrowheads*) arteries.

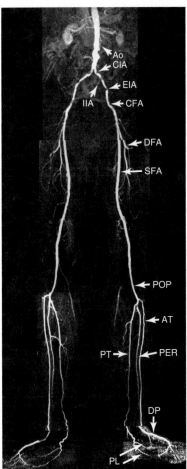

Figure 13-7. Coronal subtracted MIP image from a multistation, gadolinium-enhanced bolus chase runoff examination. The patient had claudication, and there are bilateral stenoses of the common iliac and external iliac arteries (*arrows*). Ao = aorta, CIA = common iliac artery, EIA = external iliac artery, IIA = internal iliac artery (not shown on right in this patient), CFA = common femoral artery, DFA = deep femoral artery, SFA = superficial femoral artery, POP = popliteal artery, AT = anterior tibial (artery), PT = posterior tibial (artery), PER = peroneal artery, DP = dorsalis pedis, PL = medial and lateral plantar arches.

uncertain. The finding is often made incidentally in asymptomatic patients. Severe celiac stenosis and even celiac occlusions are often well tolerated. The diagnosis of celiac compression can be made by imaging during inspiration and expiration. The degree of stenosis depends on the phase of the respiratory cycle, often becoming less pronounced during inspiration.

22. What is nephrogenic systemic fibrosis?

Nephrogenic systemic fibrosis is a more recently described disorder characterized by multiorgan proliferation of fibrous tissue. It was first described in the skin—hence the previous designation of *nephrogenic fibrosing dermopathy*. The first cases were reported in 2000, with a few thousand cases reported since then. All reported cases have been in patients with acute or chronic renal insufficiency, and almost all have been associated with administration of gadolinium-containing contrast agents for MRI. The largest number of cases have been reported in patients who received a specific MRI contrast agent, gadodiamide (Omniscan; GE Healthcare), but cases have been reported with other agents, and none are believed to be completely safe for administration to patients with poor renal function. At our institution, contrast-enhanced MRI is not performed in patients with a glomerular filtration rate of less than 30 mL/min/1.73 m^2, and is performed with caution in patients with glomerular filtration rate 30 to 60 mL/min/1.73 m^2.

23. How does this nephrogenic systemic fibrosis affect which patients should receive MRA versus CT angiography?

The emergence of nephrogenic systemic fibrosis has had a dramatic impact on MRA because many patients with suspicion of vascular disease also have impaired renal function and had previously received MRA as a "safe" alternative to CT angiography, which uses nephrotoxic iodinated contrast material. In patients with renal insufficiency who are on permanent dialysis, CT angiography is now the test of choice. Patients who are not yet on permanent dialysis pose a particular conundrum because neither CT angiography nor MRA with contrast enhancement is indicated; in these situations, noncontrast MRA techniques such as time-of-flight and steady state free procession can be used, although their performance is limited in small vessels.

WEBSITE

⊕

http://www.ctisus.org

BIBLIOGRAPHY

[1] W.J. Manning, D.J. Pennell (Eds.), Cardiovascular Magnetic Resonance, Churchill Livingstone, New York, 2002.
[2] F.G. Shellock, A. Spinazzi, MRI safety update 2008, part 1: MRI contrast agents and nephrogenic systemic fibrosis, AJR Am. J. Roentgenol. 191 (2008) 1129–1139.

IV
GASTROINTESTINAL TRACT

CHAPTER 14

PLAIN RADIOGRAPHS OF THE ABDOMEN

Stephen E. Rubesin, MD

1. What is a flat plate of the abdomen?

Flat plate is a historical term that refers to a past method of radiography when radiographs were recorded on flat plates of glass coated with an emulsion sensitive to x-rays. This examination also has been termed a *plain abdominal radiograph, plain film of the abdomen, abdominal plain film,* and *KUB. KUB* refers to the kidney, ureters, and bladder; this term is not preferred because the ureters are not visible on the plain radiograph, and other organs are visible. The term *plain film of the abdomen* is not accurate if the image is recorded either on a phosphor plate or directly by electronic means, stored electronically, and displayed on a monitor or plasma screen. No "film" is involved. The preferred terms are *plain radiograph of the abdomen* or *plain abdominal radiograph.*

2. What structures are visible on a plain radiograph?

Structures are visible on a plain radiograph as a result of differential attenuation of the x-ray beam by air, fat, soft tissue, calcium, and various metals. The edge of an organ composed of soft tissue is visible only where it interfaces with fat of the retroperitoneum or mesenteries, gas within the lumen of the adjacent bowel, or gas within the intraperitoneal or retroperitoneal spaces. Interfaces are best shown when the x-ray beam is tangential to the interface. Calcium density is detected in bones or abnormal calcifications, such as gallstones or kidney stones, or within vessel lumens or vascular walls.

The inferior edge of the liver may be visible. The soft tissue of the spleen may be outlined by air in the stomach and gas in the splenic flexure of the colon. The kidneys and lateral border of the psoas muscles are outlined by retroperitoneal fat. A moderately distended urinary bladder may be outlined by pelvic fat. Portions of the uterus may also be outlined by pelvic fat.

The stomach is defined by its rugal folds. Air and fluid in a nondistended stomach is a normal finding. The duodenal bulb may be shown by air. Small intestine is identified by its thin, transverse folds (valvulae conniventes). The colon is defined by its haustral sacculations (Fig. 14-1). A small amount of gas may be present in nondistended small intestine. Gas may outline the nondependent portions of the colon, in particular, the transverse colon. Although the lung bases and posterior sulcus are usually underexposed during chest radiography, they are well shown on plain abdominal radiographs.

3. What is an anteroposterior radiograph?

The standard plain abdominal radiograph is obtained with the patient in a recumbent position, lying on his or her back, and is termed a *supine radiograph.* The x-ray tube is anterior (superior) to the patient, and the radiographic image capture device is posterior (inferior) to the patient. The x-ray beam travels from anterior to the patient to be captured posterior to the patient. By convention, this is termed an *anteroposterior radiograph.*

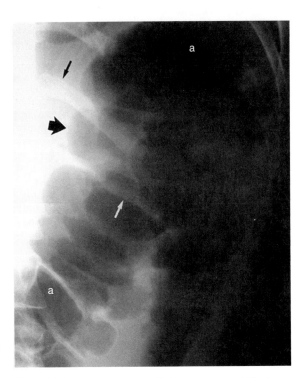

Figure 14-1. Coned-down image of left upper quadrant obtained with the patient standing. Air density (*a*) varies from black to gray. Bone density is shown in the lower left ribs (*small black arrow on left 11th rib*). The colon is identified by its air-filled haustral sacculations (*large black arrow*), interfaced with adjacent soft tissue density. The interhaustral folds of the descending colon are thick (*white arrow*) in this patient diagnosed with fulminant colitis ("toxic megacolon"). The interhaustral fold density is representative of soft tissue density.

4. What is a lateral decubitus radiograph?

The term *decubitus* means lying down. Without qualification, the term *decubitus radiograph* is meaningless. A "decub" is obtained with the patient lying with his or her left or right side down. A right lateral decubitus radiograph is an image obtained with the patient lying with his or her right side down, the x-ray tube oriented in a horizontal position on one side of the patient, and the image capture device (usually a "cassette") oriented perpendicular (upright) to the tube on the other side of the patient. To prevent any confusion, the best terms are *right-side-down decubitus* and *left-side-down decubitus* views, referring to the position of the patient.

5. What is the purpose of an image obtained with the patient in a lateral decubitus or erect position?

Images obtained with the patient in an erect position (chest x-ray or abdominal image) or images obtained with the patient in a lateral decubitus position are used to show air-fluid levels in the gastrointestinal (GI) tract or free intraperitoneal gas (Fig. 14-2). These views are important in patients with suspected perforation or bowel obstruction. An erect view is used in patients who can stand; decubitus views are performed in patients who are unable to stand.

6. List indications for a plain radiograph of the abdomen.

- Acute or subacute abdominal pain
- Suspected calculus in any viscus
- Suspected obstruction or adynamic ileus
- Suspected perforation of a viscus
- Abdominal trauma
- Abdominal distention

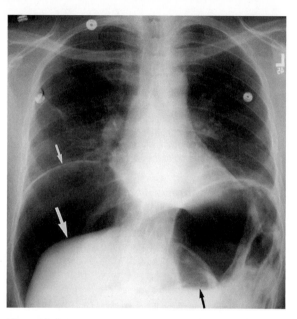

Figure 14-2. Radiograph of the chest obtained with the patient standing. A large amount of free intraperitoneal gas separates the right hemidiaphragm (*small white arrow*) from the superior edge of the liver (*large white arrow*). An air-fluid level (*black arrow*) in a small intestinal loop identifies this as an "erect chest x-ray."

7. What are the advantages and disadvantages of a plain abdominal radiograph versus a computed tomography (CT) scan?

A *plain abdominal radiograph* is a low-cost procedure that is easy to perform with inexpensive radiographic equipment. A radiograph requires little cooperation from the patient. The radiation dose is small. A *CT scan* is a high-cost procedure that also requires little cooperation from the patient. CT equipment is expensive and delivers a higher radiation dose to the patient. Given the rapid speed of new CT scanners, the time that a patient is lying on the radiographic tabletop is nearly equal for a plain film of the abdomen and CT scan. An abdominal film requires no patient preparation. There is about a 1-hour preparation time for a CT scan that uses intravenous (IV) and oral contrast agents.

CT has far greater contrast resolution than a plain film and is far superior in showing abnormal calcifications or fluid/gas patterns in the viscera or peritoneal space. CT is tremendously superior at showing the solid organs. A plain radiograph has better spatial resolution than CT, in particular, the overview scout image of a CT scan (variously termed *scanogram, topogram*). A plain film provides an overall "big picture" for bowel obstruction superior to a CT scan. This advantage is greatly surpassed, however, by individual bowel loops, fluid-filled bowel loops, and bowel wall thickness and intravenous contrast enhancement patterns shown on CT.

8. In the era of fast CT scanners, what is the role of a plain radiograph?

Plain radiographs are helpful when patients require serial studies, such as patients undergoing decompression for small bowel obstruction or follow-up for resolution of postoperative adynamic ileus. Plain radiographs are also helpful in determining positions of various tubes placed in the abdomen. If there is any question, however, that a tube tip is not within its expected location, a contrast study must be performed.

Plain radiographs may be valuable in patients in the intensive care unit (ICU) who are too seriously ill to move. The physicians have to balance the risk of patient transport from the intensive care unit to the CT scanner and the greater information obtained by a CT scan with the mediocre diagnostic capability but safety of an abdominal film obtained with portable radiographic equipment. In situations that require extreme speed, a CT scan without the use of either oral or intravenous contrast agent still provides much more information than a plain abdominal radiograph.

9. **Why is the term *free air* a misnomer?**

Gas in the stomach is initially similar in composition to atmospheric air swallowed by the patient. When various digestive processes occur, the gas in the luminal organs no longer has the same composition as atmospheric air. Carbon dioxide is generated when acid secreted by the stomach combines with bicarbonate secreted by the pancreas. Oxygen and carbon dioxide are resorbed in the small bowel. Only nitrogen is not absorbed. Colonic gas is also composed of gases such as methane and hydrogen sulfide, produced by bacterial fermentation.

Gas in the peritoneal cavity ascends to a nondependent position under the anterior abdominal wall with the patient in a supine position and underneath the diaphragm with the patient in an erect position. Intraperitoneal gas is also trapped in various crevices of the organs and mesenteries. A patient should be positioned in an erect or decubitus position for about 10 minutes before a radiograph is obtained to look for "free intraperitoneal gas."

10. **What are the best patient positions to detect free intraperitoneal gas on a plain radiograph?**

Free intraperitoneal gas is best shown on an erect chest x-ray centered over the diaphragm (see Fig. 14-2); 1 mL of gas may be detected under the curve of a hemidiaphragm. A left-side-down lateral decubitus view to show air above or under the liver edge is the second best choice.

11. **What percentage of supine radiographs shows free intraperitoneal gas?**

In some patients, an erect chest, erect abdominal, or lateral decubitus radiograph is impossible, and an image can be obtained only with the patient in a supine position. A supine abdominal radiograph shows free intraperitoneal gas in about 60% of patients with free intraperitoneal gas.

12. **What is the Rigler sign?**

Rigler sign is named after the radiologist Leo Rigler, MD, who described a sign of pneumoperitoneum in 1941. Normally, gas outlines only the luminal side of a bowel loop. The soft tissue side of the bowel is not visible as a sharp edge because there is no difference in density between the soft tissue of bowel wall and the remainder of the abdomen. When free intraperitoneal gas abuts a gas-filled loop of bowel, gas surrounds both sides of the bowel wall. If the interfaces of gas and bowel wall are perpendicular to the x-ray beam, the bowel wall is visible and appears as a thin stripe of soft tissue (Fig. 14-3).

13. **In what quadrant is free intraperitoneal gas best detected?**

Signs of free intraperitoneal gas are most commonly seen in the right upper quadrant, as lucency over the liver; curvilinear, triangular, or linear streaks of gas outlining the edge of liver near the porta hepatitis; or gas outlining the falciform ligament (Fig. 14-4). Other signs of free intraperitoneal gas include a curved lucency under the mid-diaphragm resembling a "cupola," gas trapped in the interhaustral folds (the triangle sign), and air in the pelvis outlining the lateral umbilical folds (Fig. 14-5).

14. **A coned-down image of the right upper quadrant is presented in Fig. 14-6. What structure is outlined by gas? Where is the gas located?**

Gas in the retroperitoneal space usually results from iatrogenic causes or gas-forming infections. Gas originates in the following retroperitoneal structures: the second through fourth portions of the duodenum; pancreas and distal common bile duct; ascending and descending colon and rectum; kidneys, ureters, and urinary bladder; and abdominal aorta and its branches. Gas rarely arises in the retroperitoneal adrenal glands.

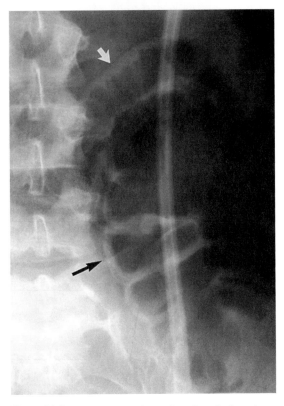

Figure 14-3. Rigler sign of free intraperitoneal gas. Radiograph of abdomen obtained with the patient supine. The outer walls of small and large bowel are normally invisible. Free intraperitoneal gas outlines the outer wall of a loop of small intestine (*white arrow*) and the proximal sigmoid colon (*black arrow*). The colon is identified by its sacculated outer contour structure. The small bowel is identified by a smooth outer contour.

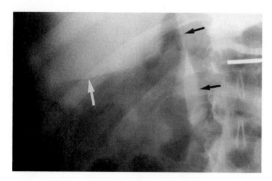

Figure 14-4. Falciform ligament sign of free intraperitoneal gas. The falciform ligament (*black arrows*) and inferior edge of the liver (*white arrow*) are outlined by free intraperitoneal gas.

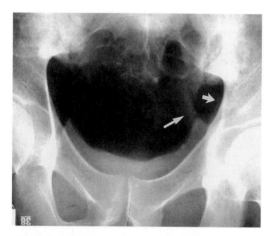

Figure 14-5. Free intraperitoneal gas in the pelvis in coned-down image of the pelvis obtained with the patient supine. Radiolucent free intraperitoneal gas outlines the lateral umbilical folds (*left fold identified by long arrow*) and inferior left (*short arrow*) and right paracolic gutters.

15. What is the most common noniatrogenic cause of pneumobilia?

Gas in the biliary tree, or pneumobilia, usually results from communication of bowel with the biliary tree, not a gas-forming infection. The most common cause of pneumobilia is probably endoscopically or surgically performed sphincterotomy or a choledochoenteric anastomosis. In patients who have not undergone iatrogenic interventions, the most common cause of pneumobilia is a penetrating duodenal ulcer. Other etiologic factors include choledochoduodenal or cholecystoduodenal fistula owing to gallstones eroding into the duodenum.

16. What is Rigler triad?

The combination of gas in the biliary tree; small bowel dilation; and a calcified, ectopic gallstone is a triad of findings described by Rigler; it also has been termed *gallstone ileus*. This triad is seen in less than half of patients in whom a gallstone erodes into the bowel and causes an obstruction in either the distal ileum or the sigmoid colon, the narrowest areas of the small and large bowel. The triad is uncommon in patients in whom a gallstone erodes into bowel because only a few gallstones are calcified; obstruction is not always present; and the fistula may close, resulting in lack of biliary air.

17. What does the linear form of pneumatosis imply?

Pneumatosis is gas in the intestinal wall. Linear streaks of gas (Fig. 14-7) within the small or large intestinal wall (Fig. 14-8) suggest ischemia, but not irreversible necrosis. In patients with ischemia, bowel does not contract normally and dilates. Ischemia is one of the most common causes of severe small bowel dilation. Edema or blood in the bowel wall associated with ischemia may appear as nodular soft tissue densities resembling "thumbprints."

Rounded air collections in bowel wall may be due to benign causes of rents in the mucosa, termed *pneumatosis cystoides intestinalis* or *benign pneumatosis coli*. The gas-filled blebs are most commonly detected in the colon and are associated with various clinical conditions, such as scleroderma, steroid use, and celiac disease.

18. In what portions of the GI tract is normal gas located when the patient is radiographed in a supine position?

Gas collects in nondependent portions of the GI tract. When the patient is lying in a supine position, the gastric antrum and transverse colon are the most anterior portions of the GI tract. When the patient lies in a prone position, the gastric fundus, ascending and descending colon, and mid-rectum are the most nondependent portions of the GI tract. An air-filled transverse colon less than 5 to 7 cm in diameter is a normal finding on a supine radiograph.

19. What does the term *ileus* mean?

Ileus is Greek, meaning "to wrap" or "to roll." The term initially was used to describe patients "doubled-over" with abdominal pain. The term later was used to describe bowel dilation. The term *ileus,* meaning dilation, needs a qualifier to imply either atony or obstruction. *Mechanical ileus* means bowel obstruction. The terms *adynamic ileus, paralytic ileus,* or *functional ileus* describe diminished bowel contraction or peristalsis, not obstruction, with accumulation of air and fluid in the intestinal lumen.

20. Which study is superior in diagnosing small bowel obstruction: plain radiograph or CT?

Before the advent of CT, plain abdominal radiographs (Fig. 14-9) and barium studies were used to diagnose small bowel obstruction. CT has become the imaging modality of choice, however, in patients with suspected small bowel obstruction. CT is superior in diagnosing the presence, location, and etiologic factors of small bowel obstruction. The value of plain radiographs is in follow-up of the resolution or progression of small bowel obstruction in patients who do not undergo surgery.

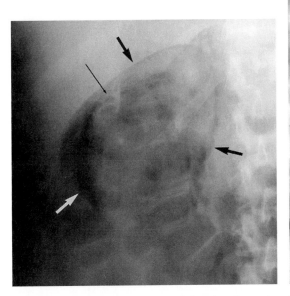

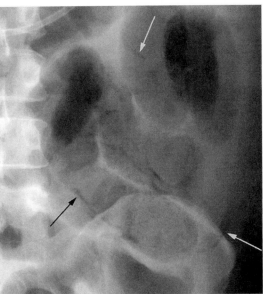

Figure 14-6. The kidney is outlined by gas in the retroperitoneum in coned-down image of the right upper quadrant.
An ovoid lucency outlines the kidney (*thick arrows*). Lobules of perirenal fat appear as 0.5- to 1-cm lucencies surrounded by rings of soft tissue (*thin arrow*). This retroperitoneal gas was the result of perforation of the rectum at endoscopy.

Figure 14-7. Linear form of pneumatosis. Coned-down image obtained from a radiograph with the patient supine shows linear streaks of gas (*arrows*) within the smooth-surfaced walls of small intestine. Soft tissue within the lumen of the bowel represents fluid and debris composed of blood and sloughed cells ("the small bowel feces sign"). The patient was hypotensive. Ischemia with transmural necrosis was found at surgery.

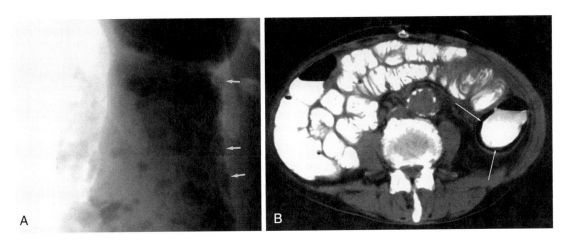

Figure 14-8. Pneumatosis coli. **A,** Coned-down image from an x-ray obtained with the patient supine shows small (1 to 2 mm), irregularly shaped bubbles of gas overlying the descending colon. Where the colonic wall is shown in profile, the bubbles of gas (*arrows*) are shown to be located in the colonic wall. This hypotensive patient had infarction in the portion of colon that is at the transition of arterial supply between the superior mesenteric artery and inferior mesenteric artery ("watershed zone"). **B,** Axial image from a CT scan of the abdomen shows curvilinear air density between the contrast-filled lumen of the descending colon and the soft tissue of the colonic wall (*arrows*).

21. What are the pitfalls of plain radiograph diagnosis of small bowel obstruction?
A small bowel loop is identified on plain abdominal radiography by intraluminal air outlining valvulae conniventes. If a small bowel loop is completely filled with fluid, it cannot be identified on a plain abdominal radiograph. Plain abdominal radiography misses fluid-filled loops, underdiagnoses small bowel obstruction, and is unable to estimate the level of obstruction accurately. In contrast, CT can identify fluid-filled bowel loops just proximal to the obstruction that plain radiography cannot identify.

The clue to an obstruction is a transition between dilated small bowel proximal to an obstructing lesion and collapsed small bowel distal to the obstruction (see Fig. 14-9). False-negative diagnoses may be made with CT and plain abdominal radiography when bowel is not dilated owing to vomiting or nasogastric tube/long tube decompression, or when an examination is performed before fluid can accumulate proximal to the obstruction. False-positive diagnosis of obstruction is frequent with CT and plain abdominal radiography. False-positive diagnoses may be made in patients with an adynamic ileus predominantly involving the small intestine (Fig. 14-10). Plain film radiography detects about 80% of small bowel obstructions.

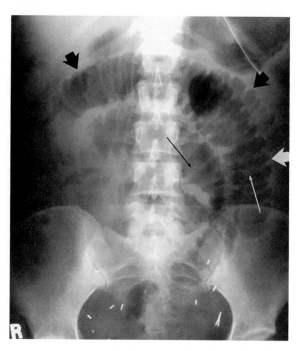

Figure 14-9. Closed-loop small bowel obstruction with ischemia. Plain abdominal radiograph obtained with the patient supine shows that the mid-small intestine is disproportionately dilated. The loops are "radially arranged" (*thick arrows*), with their mesenteric origin in the right lower quadrant. Normal valvulae conniventes are 1 to 2 mm thick. The small bowel folds are markedly thickened, about 4 to 5 mm (*thin arrows*).

22. What modality is able to diagnose an obstruction complicated by ischemia?

Ischemia may occur when the mesentery is twisted during a closed loop obstruction, compromising venous return and arterial inflow. Ischemia may also occur during any obstruction in which luminal dilation results in venous congestion. CT is the best radiologic modality to identify ischemia. CT diagnosis depends on identification of a thick-walled bowel that either does not enhance or has a mural stratification pattern because of marked submucosal edema (Fig. 14-11). In some patients, there is increased attenuation of bowel wall on unenhanced scans because of intramural hemorrhage. Enlargement of veins in the mesentery may be present in patients with venous obstruction. The mesentery may be of increased attenuation because of edema.

Key Points: Radiology of the Gastrointestinal Tract

1. Plain radiographs of the abdomen have been replaced by CT, ultrasound (US), and magnetic resonance imaging (MRI) in patients with acute clinical problems.
2. Plain radiographs are helpful to show the location of various tubes and for evaluation of ICU patients or patients who require serial studies.
3. The first examination the radiologist should obtain for a patient with suspected small bowel obstruction is a CT scan.
4. Free intraperitoneal gas is detected in a supine plain radiograph in 60% of patients with perforation.
5. Linear pneumatosis is highly suggestive of ischemia.

---

23. Can CT show adhesions?

CT diagnosis of small bowel obstruction relies on identification of the transition zone between dilated and nondilated bowel. CT can identify causes of obstruction that have bulk, such as a primary carcinoma or a metastasis, and CT can show an external hernia. CT identifies extrinsic inflammatory processes, such as appendicitis or diverticulitis, that may secondarily obstruct small bowel. CT diagnosis of adhesions as a cause of obstruction is a presumptive diagnosis only, however, made when no identifiable cause of obstruction is seen at the transition zone.

24. In what situations are barium studies most helpful for the diagnosis of small bowel obstruction?

Barium studies are superior to CT in diagnosing low-grade or intermittent small bowel obstructions. The site of obstruction is identified more reliably by a barium study than with CT. Barium studies are superior in determining whether a stricture in a patient with Crohn disease is functionally obstructive. Barium studies also are superior to CT in showing intraluminal tumors as a cause of intussusception/obstruction.

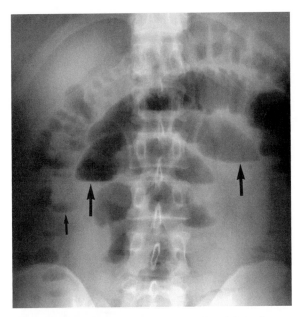

Figure 14-10. Adynamic ileus mimicking small bowel obstruction. Plain abdominal radiograph obtained with the patient erect shows that the mid-small intestine is disproportionately dilated. Air-fluid levels (*large arrows*) are seen in the small intestinal lumen. The nondistended colon is identified by its haustral sacculations. Air-fluid levels are also present in the colon (*small arrow*) and are a clue that this patient had (bacterial) enteritis with a hypersecretory state.

25. What is the most common form of colonic volvulus?

Sigmoid volvulus accounts for about three fourths of cases of colonic volvulus (Fig. 14-12). Radiographically, an inverted U-shaped loop of dilated colon extends far out of the pelvis into the upper abdomen. If the inner walls of the ascending and descending portions of the sigmoid loop are apposed to each other, a thick soft tissue stripe is seen radiating toward the pelvis. This has been described as resembling a coffee bean. The colon and even the small intestine proximal to the twist also are dilated.

26. What patient groups have a greater incidence of sigmoid volvulus?

Patients with elongated, dilated sigmoid colons are predisposed to sigmoid volvulus. Sigmoid volvulus is common in parts of the world (e.g., Africa) where people have high-fiber diets, bulky stools, and large colons. In the United States, sigmoid volvulus is common in patients who are either bedridden or taking medications that cause colonic hypomotility; patients in nursing homes and mental institutions are at the most risk for sigmoid volvulus.

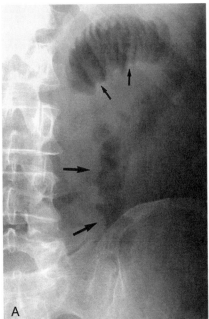
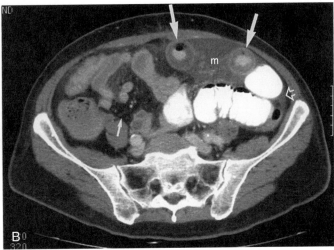

Figure 14-11. Small bowel ischemia shown by comparison of plain radiograph and CT scan. **A,** Coned-down image of the left upper quadrant from plain radiograph of the abdomen obtained with the patient supine shows a mildly dilated loop of small intestine with thick valvulae conniventes (*small arrows*). Smooth, 1-cm nodules (*large arrows*) seen on the mesenteric border of a second left upper quadrant loop are examples of "thumbprinting" owing to severe submucosal edema (in this case) or hemorrhage. **B,** Axial image from CT scan of the abdomen at the level of the upper sacrum shows two loops of ileum with a mural stratification pattern ("target sign") (*large arrows*). High-attenuation contrast material and bubbles of gas are seen within the ileal lumen surrounded by a thick band of fluid attenuation in the submucosa surrounded by high attenuation in the muscularis propria. Ascites is present in the paracolic gutters (left paracolic gutter identified by *open arrow*). The mesentery supplying these abnormal loops is engorged and of fluid attenuation (*m*) compared with the normal fat attenuation of normal small bowel mesentery (*small arrow*) of nonischemic loops.

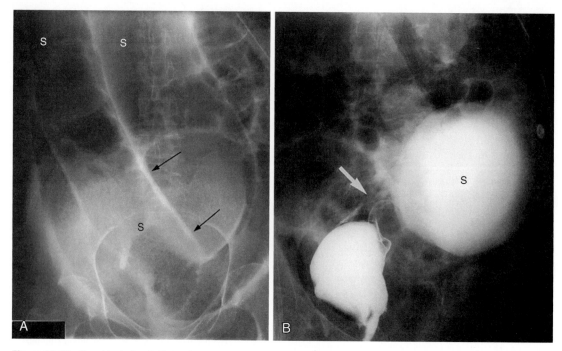

Figure 14-12. Sigmoid volvulus. **A,** Plain radiograph of abdomen shows a markedly dilated sigmoid colon (*S*). A thick soft tissue stripe (*arrows*) is seen between adjacent limbs of the dilated sigmoid colon, representing the walls of two adjacent loops coapted together. This overall appearance is said to resemble a coffee bean (radiologists are very imaginative individuals). **B,** Overhead image from a subsequent single-contrast barium enema shows a smooth narrowing (*arrow*) distal to a massively dilated sigmoid colon (*S*). When the obstruction has been shown, the radiologist does not fill the colon with barium because barium can form concretions in the colon behind a colonic obstruction. (Barium would not form concretions in an obstructed small intestine.)

27. In what quadrant of the abdomen does the cecum lie in a patient with cecal volvulus?
The ascending colon is fused to the retroperitoneum in most people. In patients in whom the right colon has incompletely fused to the retroperitoneum, the ascending colon can twist on its mesentery and become obstructed. The colon proximal to the twist, in particular the cecum, becomes dilated and is located in the mid-left abdomen or in the left upper quadrant. This condition is poorly termed a *cecal volvulus,* when, in reality, it is an *ascending colon volvulus.*

28. What percentage of gallstones are calcified?
About 15% of gallstones are radiopaque on plain abdominal radiography (Fig. 14-13). Calcification is detected in about 30% to 40% of gallstones on CT. CT detects about 80% of calcified or noncalcified gallstones (Fig. 14-14). Cholesterol calculi appear as low-attenuation filling defects, often floating in bile. US detects about 95% of gallstones.

Gallstones are an example of concretions formed in the abdomen. The calcification usually occurs around a central nidus of organic or inorganic foreign matter, thrombus, focal pus, or cellular debris. The calcification occurs within the lumen of tubular structures, such as blood vessels, biliary tree, or ureters, or within a hollow viscus, such as the gallbladder or urinary bladder. Concretions may have a round, ovoid, branched, or spiculated shape.

29. A plain radiograph of the abdomen is obtained in a patient who has a palpable abdominal mass (Fig. 14-15). What is your diagnosis?
There is a curvilinear calcification in the mid-abdomen centered at the L2 vertebral body level. A diagnosis of a calcified abdominal aortic aneurysm is made.

Linear or curvilinear calcifications are seen in tubular or cystic structures. In the walls of tubes, such as blood vessels, the bile duct, the ureter, and the vasa differentia, the calcifications are usually discontinuous and of varying thickness. If a tubular structure is seen en face, a thick, discontinuous ring of calcification may be detected. This type of calcification is typical of arterial calcifications, in particular, atherosclerotic calcification.

Calcifications in the walls of cysts appear as a curvilinear rim of calcification. This rim is often incomplete. Various lesions give this appearance, including renal cysts and renal cell carcinoma, aneurysms of the aorta and other major vessels, echinococcus cysts in the liver or spleen, pancreatic pseudocysts, adrenal cysts, mesenteric cysts, mucinous

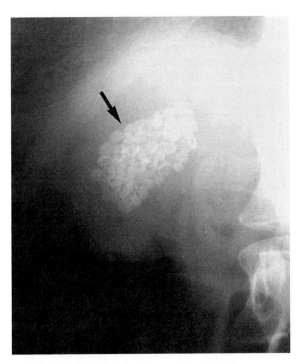

Figure 14-13. Calcified gallstones. Coned-down image from abdominal radiograph performed with the patient supine shows numerous 2- to 3-mm, polygonally shaped, calcified, "faceted" gallstones (*arrow*).

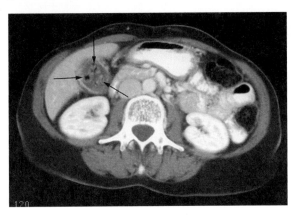

Figure 14-14. Noncalcified gallstones. Axial image at the level of the gallbladder from abdominal CT scan shows three noncalcified gallstones (*arrows*). The periphery of the stones has a higher attenuation than that of the surrounding bile. Tiny bubbles of air attenuation are seen in two of the stones, representing trapped nitrogen gas.

tumors of the appendix, and cystic tumors of the ovaries. Calcification of the gallbladder wall in chronic cholecystitis (porcelain gallbladder) has a similar appearance. The location of an abnormality is a clue to the location of a calcification in the abdomen detected on plain film radiography. CT shows the organ of origin and the cause of a calcified mass in most cases.

30. A coned-down view of the upper abdomen (Fig. 14-16) is obtained in a man with chronic abdominal pain. What is your diagnosis?
Dense, sharply angulated clumps of calcium are confined to a 4-cm area just to the right of the L2 vertebral body. A diagnosis of calcific pancreatitis is made.

Calcifications in abdominal masses and inflammatory processes have various shapes and sizes. Calcifications in mucin-producing tumors appear amorphous or punctate. Intraductal calcifications in patients with alcoholic pancreatitis appear as small clumps overlying the pancreas (see Fig. 14-16). Mottled, slightly irregular, ovoid masses of calcification are typically seen in calcified lymph nodes. Uterine leiomyomas are the most common pelvic tumor to calcify. These tumors may have a peripheral rim, central whorled, or clumplike calcification (Fig. 14-17).

31. A patient has a palpable abdominal mass (Fig. 14-18). What organ is enlarged?
Answer is provided in the figure legend. CT, MRI, and US are now the modalities of choice in the work-up of a palpable abdominal mass. If gynecologic disease is suspected, US of the pelvis or MRI is the preferred examination. For upper abdominal masses, CT or MRI is indicated.

32. A 45-year-old man has recently received a liver transplant. Identify the type and location of the two tubular structures below the diaphragm in Fig. 14-19A. What has the radiologist done in Fig. 14-19B and C?
Answers are provided in the figure legend.
A wide variety of man-made devices are placed in the abdomen at surgery or through various orifices. Clinically placed foreign objects are better seen on plain radiographs when a radiodense substance has been incorporated into the device by the manufacturer. Injection of various tubes with water-soluble contrast agent can confirm the location of the tubes (see Fig. 14-19C). Radiopaque wires and tubes outside of the patient make radiographic interpretation more difficult, unless the radiologist knows exactly what is supposed lie within or outside of the patient. The location of a tube in the GI tract is suggested by its configuration.

33. A 38-year-old man complains of nausea and vomiting. What type of tube has been placed in Fig. 14-20A?
Tubes used for decompression are typically of larger caliber than tubes used for feeding. The nasogastric tube used for decompression seen in Fig. 14-20A is wider than the feeding tube seen in Fig. 14-19A.

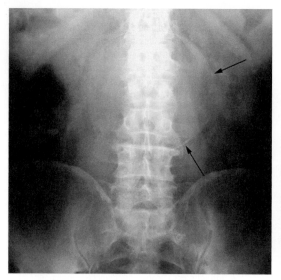

Figure 14-15. Plain radiograph of the abdomen obtained with the patient in supine shows a discontinuous ring of curvilinear calcification (*arrows*) surrounding a soft tissue mass (11 cm in diameter) in the mid-abdomen. This proved to be a saccular abdominal aortic aneurysm. This is an example of vascular calcification owing to atherosclerosis.

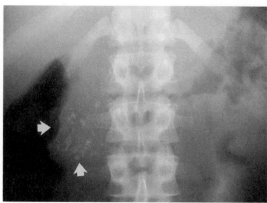

Figure 14-16. Calcific pancreatitis resulting from chronic alcohol abuse. Coned-down view of the upper abdomen shows dense clumps of calcification (*arrows*) to the right of the L2 vertebral body. These calcifications are not in the pancreatic parenchyma, but are within dilated pancreatic ducts.

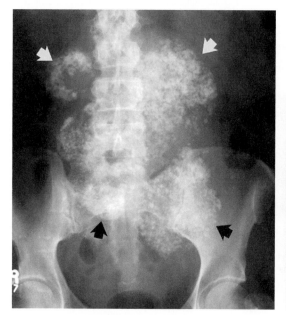

Figure 14-17. Calcified uterine leiomyomas. Plain radiograph of the abdomen shows a large calcified mass (*arrows*). Four round calcified masses are confluent in the midline. The calcifications are dense and punctate, but some are said to resemble "popcorn." This is the type of calcification typically seen in uterine leiomyomas.

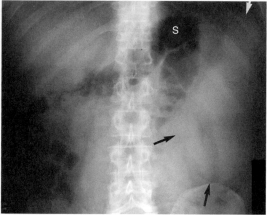

Figure 14-18. Plain abdominal radiograph obtained with the patient in supine shows a large (25-cm) mass (*arrows*) in the left upper quadrant that deviates the splenic flexure of the colon (*S*) medially. This mass is an enlarged spleen in a patient with leukemia.

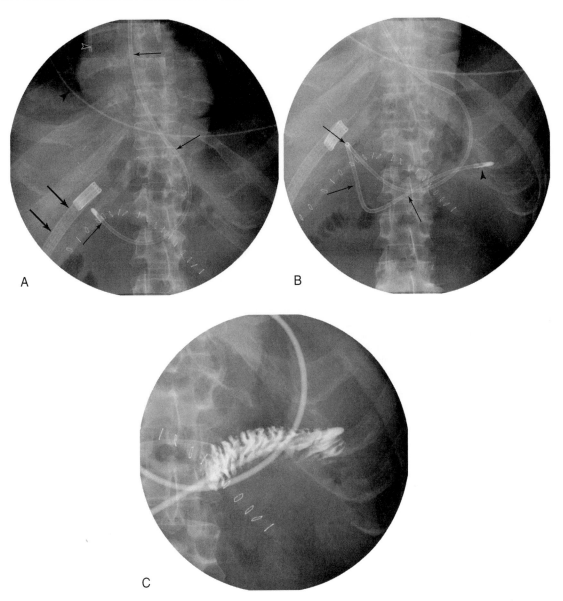

Figure 14-19. A, Spot radiograph of the upper abdomen shows a thin (5-mm) radiopaque tubular structure (*small arrows*) coursing parallel to the lower thoracic spine, entering the mid-upper abdomen, then curving gently to the right. This is a feeding tube, coursing along the greater curvature of the stomach, with its tip in the distal gastric antrum. A second tube (*large arrows*) is folded over itself in the right upper quadrant. This tube has four lumens and multiple small holes. This is a Jackson-Pratt drainage tube that was placed in the subhepatic space. The tip of a right venous catheter (*small arrowhead*) is in the distal superior vena cava. A metallic wire (an electrocardiogram lead) (*large arrowheads*) crosses the lower chest. This wire is outside of the patient because it does not conform to any anatomic structure. Multiple metallic skin staples are present in a curvilinear configuration. **B,** Under fluoroscopic guidance, a radiologist has advanced the feeding tube tip from the gastric antrum to the duodenal-jejunal junction. The configuration of the feeding tube (*arrows*) mimics the "C" shape of the duodenum. **C,** Injection of the feeding tube with water-soluble contrast agent confirms that the tip of the feeding tube is at the duodenal-jejunal junction.

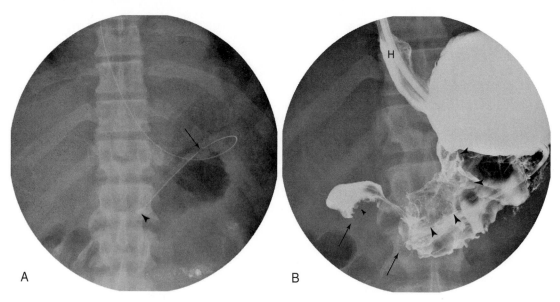

A B

Figure 14-20. A, Spot radiograph shows radiopaque tube of a caliber much wider than the feeding tube in Figure 14-19A. The tube is looped in the gastric fundus, and its tip (*arrowhead*) is in the distal gastric body. The side-hole of the tube (*arrow*) is identified. This is a nasogastric tube, typically used to decompress the stomach or small intestine. The stomach is not dilated. **B,** Spot radiograph obtained 30 minutes after the nasogastric tube has been injected with high-density barium. Complete gastric outlet obstruction is shown because no barium has left the stomach. There is a 4-cm-long annular constriction of the proximal gastric antrum (*between long arrows*), with nodular mucosa (*small arrowhead*). Plaquelike flattening and mucosal nodularity extend up the lesser curvature (*large arrowheads*). Thick rugal folds are seen along the distal greater curvature. Also note reflux of barium into a small hiatal hernia (*H*) and the distal esophagus. This gastric mass was an adenocarcinoma of the stomach infiltrating the lower gastric body and proximal gastric antrum causing complete gastric outlet obstruction. These images show how a plain radiograph reveals only the tip of the iceberg in some cases. Nasogastric decompression has removed fluid and made the stomach of normal size on the plain radiograph, without any indication of complete gastric outlet obstruction. Vomiting can also decompress an obstructed stomach.

BIBLIOGRAPHY

[1] S.R. Baker, Abdominal calcifications, in: R.M. Gore, M.S. Levine (Eds.), Textbook of Gastrointestinal Radiology, third ed., Saunders, Philadelphia, 2008, pp. 225–231.
[2] S.R. Baker, K.C. Cho (Eds.), The Abdominal Plain Film with Correlative Imaging, second ed., Appleton & Lange, Stamford, CT, 1998.
[3] J.M. Messmer, Gas and soft tissue abnormalities, in: R.M. Gore, M.S. Levine (Eds.), Textbook of Gastrointestinal Radiology, third ed., Saunders, Philadelphia, 2008, pp. 205–223.
[4] R.E. Miller, S.W. Nelson, The roentgenologic demonstration of tiny amounts of free intraperitoneal gas: experimental and clinical studies, AJR Am J Roentgenol 112 (1971) 574–585.
[5] W.M. Thompson, Abdomen: normal anatomy and examination techniques, in: R.M. Gore, M.S. Levine (Eds.), Textbook of Gastrointestinal Radiology, third ed., Saunders, Philadelphia, 2008, pp. 189–203.

UPPER GASTROINTESTINAL TRACT

Stephen E. Rubesin, MD

CHAPTER 15

1. What organs are studied during an upper gastrointestinal (GI) series?
The esophagus, stomach, and duodenum are studied. The radiologist evaluates the morphology and motility of these organs.

2. What organs are studied during a pharyngoesophagogram?
The radiologist evaluates the motility of the oral cavity, pharynx, and esophagus, and the morphology of the pharynx, esophagus, and gastric cardia. The radiologist records oral, pharyngeal, and esophageal motility via a VCR (video), via a DVD recorder, or on film ("cine"). Film has been almost completely replaced as the recording medium for motility because of increased radiation exposure, cost, and difficulty of film processing. The term *cine-esophagram* is outdated.

3. What organ is shown in Fig. 15-1?
Fig. 15-1 shows a normal lower thoracic esophagus. The esophagus is a muscular tube within the mediastinum. The esophagus is usually collapsed unless distended by liquid or solid food; swallowed air; or, in this image, swallowed air and barium. In this patient, swallowed high-density barium coats the mucosa. The swallowed carbon dioxide (effervescent agent) and swallowed air distend the lumen of the esophagus. The mucosa of the esophageal tube seen in profile appears as a white line (*arrows*). The mucosal surface of the normal esophagus seen en face is smooth and varies from white to gray (representative mucosa identified by *S*). Normal structures in the mediastinum push on the distended esophagus, manifested as alterations of the normal straight tubular contour of the esophagus. These indentations are identified as the bottom of the aortic arch (*a*), the left main stem bronchus (*b*), and the left atrium (*l*).

4. What organs are shown in Fig. 15-2? Identify the numbered parts of the organs as labeled.
This image is a double-contrast image of the stomach and duodenum. See the figure legend for the answers.

5. What curvatures do the *black* and *open arrows* in Fig. 15-2 identify?
The *black arrows* identify the lesser curvature of the stomach; the *open arrows* identify the greater curvature.

6. Why does the gastric fundus appear white in Fig. 15-2, whereas the antrum appears gray?
Barium sulfate absorbs and scatters x-rays, but air does not. X-rays passing through barium are blocked and do not reach the film. X-rays easily pass through GI structures filled with air and expose the film. The relatively exposed areas of the film appear as shades of black; the relatively unexposed areas of the film appear as shades of white. The heavy barium falls to the lowest or most "dependent" portion of the stomach. This image was obtained with the patient recumbent, back against the fluoroscopic tabletop (a supine radiograph). The gastric fundus is posterior to the gastric antrum; barium falls into the gastric fundus when the patient lies in a supine position. Because barium absorbs more x-rays than air, the gastric fundus appears "white." In this radiograph, the anteriorly located gastric antrum is filled with air and is also "etched in white" by a thin layer of barium. Most of the x-rays, but not all, pass through the antrum, partially exposing the film. The gastric antrum appears "gray," not black as a purely air-filled structure would appear.

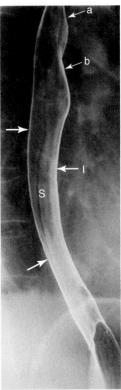

Figure 15-1. Normal esophagus (see question 3 for description).

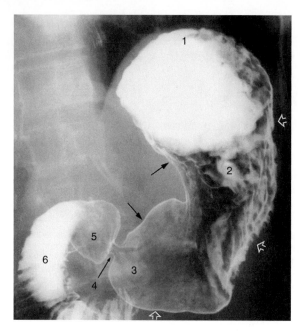

Figure 15-2. Normal stomach. *1* = gastric fundus, *2* = gastric body, *3* = gastric antrum, *4* = pylorus [pyloric channel], *5* = duodenal bulb, and *6* = second portion of duodenum.

Today, most radiographs are not obtained using real film as the recording medium, but they use some type of image capture device. The relative exposures on the image capture device are digitized and are assigned gray-scale values, from white to black. The images are displayed on a monitor or flat panel. Depending on the radiologist, large exposures are assigned either "white" or "black" values. In the United States, barium is usually assigned a "white" value; in Japan, barium often is assigned a "black" value.

7. **Two images of the esophagus are presented in Fig. 15-3. What is your diagnosis?**
This is a semiannular carcinoma of the esophagus. The tumor originated on the side of contour irregularity and has begun to spread circumferentially. The wall opposite the tumor is smooth and uninvolved by the tumor, but has been pulled inward by the desmoplastic tumor. The barium pool in Fig. 15-3A shows the contour of a luminal organ, but obscures mucosal detail. The air contrast image in Fig. 15-3B reveals the luminal contour in profile, as does the barium pool. The air contrast image also reveals the mucosal surface en face. In this case, the air contrast image shows the surface and the edge of the semiannular cancer.

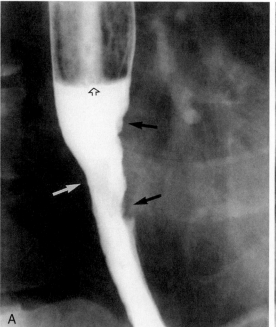
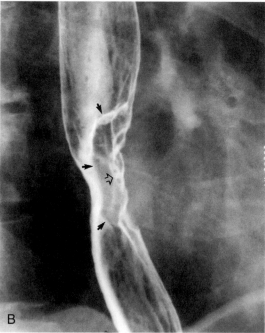

Figure 15-3. Air contrast versus the barium pool. **A,** Spot radiograph of the esophagus performed while the patient stands and drinks high-density barium shows a column of barium (with an air-barium level, *open arrow*) in the mid-esophagus. A region of focal circumferential narrowing, 3 cm in length, is present. The narrowing appears smooth on one wall (*white arrow*) and has an irregular contour on the opposite wall (*black arrows*). **B,** Spot radiograph performed seconds later after the barium column has passed through the esophagus shows the same circumferential narrowing with a smooth contour on one side and an irregular contour on the other. The mucosal surface is now seen en face as well, however, revealing focal mucosal nodularity (*open arrow*) and barium-coated lines (*arrows*) that disrupt the normal smooth surface of the esophagus and outline the outer margin of a mass.

8. What does *single contrast* mean?

A single-contrast study of a GI structure means that one contrast agent is used, such as a suspension of barium sulfate, an ionic water-soluble contrast agent such as diatrizoate meglumine (Gastroview/Gastrografin), or a nonionic water-soluble contrast agent such as iohexol (Omnipaque). Fig. 15-4 is an example of a single-contrast image obtained with the patient swallowing barium while lying in a prone position. A column of "thin" barium fills the distal esophageal lumen. The radiologist examines the luminal contour in profile for abnormalities that either protrude into the lumen or protrude outside of the expected luminal contour of the organ. The radiologist also looks for abnormalities en face. Large protrusions into the lumen displace the barium column, allow x-rays to pass through the esophagus, and appear as radiolucent "filling defects" in the barium column. Large protrusions outside the luminal contour fill with barium and, when seen en face, appear as a "double density" of barium.

In this patient, there is a small hiatal hernia (*h*). At the esophagogastric junction, a thin, smooth, symmetric ringlike narrowing, 3 mm in height, is seen in profile as a shelf-like indentation of the luminal contour (*white arrows*). En face, the ring is manifested as a thin radiolucent filling defect in the barium column (*open arrow*). This is a Schatzki ring, a narrowing that commonly causes dysphagia with solids.

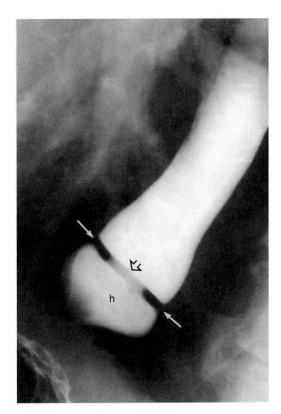

Figure 15-4. Schatzki ring shown by single-contrast esophagogram (see question 8 for explanation).

9. What does *double contrast* mean?

In a double-contrast study, the radiologist uses two contrast agents to examine the organs in question. A double-contrast upper GI series uses an effervescent agent that creates carbon dioxide to distend the luminal organs and high-density barium to "scrub and paint" the mucosa. This study is also known as an *air contrast upper GI series* or a *biphasic upper GI series*. Fig. 15-5 is a double-contrast image of the distal stomach. Rugal folds are seen as radiolucent filling defects in the barium pool (*white arrow*) and as parallel barium etched lines (*black arrows*). Rugal folds are composed of mucosa and submucosa and are most prominent along the greater curvature of the stomach. The normal gastric antrum (*A*) has few, if any, rugal folds in most patients.

10. What are clinical indications for performing an upper GI study?

Clinical indications for performing an upper GI study include heartburn, dysphagia, or odynophagia referred to a substernal location; upper abdominal pain or discomfort; upper GI bleeding; and vomiting.

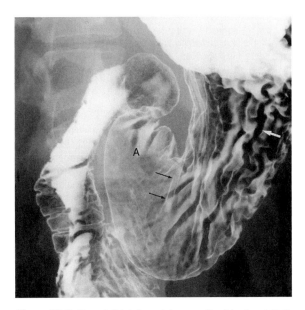

Figure 15-5. Normal distal stomach (see question 9 for description).

11. What are clinical indications for performing a video/DVD pharyngoesophagogram?

Clinical indications for performing a video/DVD pharyngoesophagogram include dysphagia or odynophagia referred to the head, neck, and suprasternal regions; history of globus sensation; chronic cough; aspiration pneumonia or cerebrovascular accident; dribbling from the mouth; abnormal tongue motions; and history of surgery or radiation of the tongue, palate, pharynx, or larynx.

> **Key Points: Radiology of the Upper GI Tract**
>
> 1. Single-contrast GI examinations
>   Use "thin barium" or water-soluble Gastroview (no gas used)
>   Are easier to perform in sick patients who cannot turn
>   Can detect bowel obstruction, perforation, or fistulas
> 2. Double-contrast GI examinations
>   Use high-density barium and air/carbon dioxide
>   Require patients to turn
>   Are more sensitive than single-contrast examinations for detecting
>   mucosal abnormalities

12. Describe the preparation for an upper GI study or pharyngoesophagogram.

Each hospital or outpatient facility has its own preparation routines for these studies. These preparations should be available from the radiologists in hard copy form or in an institutional document online. At our institution, a handout describing the examination and explaining the preparation (see the following) is available to all referring physicians:

1. Patients should have nothing by mouth after 9 PM.
2. Insulin-dependent diabetics should eliminate or decrease the dose of insulin the morning of the examination.
3. Patients should not take antacids or bismuth subsalicylate (Pepto-Bismol) on the morning of the examination
4. Patients should wear dentures or other swallowing appliances.
5. If patients have solid food dysphagia, they should bring a type of food that causes dysphagia.
6. After the examination, patients are encouraged to drink liquids and may take a laxative if additional radiologic tests are scheduled, or if there is a history of colonic hypomotility.

13. What are contraindications to a barium study of the upper GI tract?

Contraindications include:
- Known or suspected perforation (see question 14).
- Inability to swallow.

In the case of inability to swallow, an examination of the stomach and small bowel may be performed by sending the patient to fluoroscopy with a nasogastric tube placed in the stomach.

14. What type of contrast agent should be requested first in patients with suspected upper GI perforation?

In patients with known or suspected perforations of the pharynx, esophagus, or duodenum, an ionic water-soluble contrast agent such as diatrizoate meglumine (Gastroview or Gastrografin) should be used initially. This type of agent is readily absorbed from the soft tissues of the neck, mediastinum, and peritoneal cavity. This type of agent, if aspirated, has the theoretical potential of causing pulmonary edema because it is hyperosmolar and draws fluid into the lungs. If aspiration is a likely possibility, the radiologist may start with a nonionic water-soluble contrast agent that is either only mildly hyperosmolar (Iohexol [Omnipaque for Oral Use]) or iso-osmolar. Other radiologists start with barium if a perforation of the pharynx or esophagus is suspected, and there is a high risk of aspiration because barium in the soft tissues of the neck or mediastinum is relatively harmless. Barium entering the peritoneal cavity from a gastric or duodenal perforation can potentially cause mild barium peritonitis. This situation is not as serious, however, as barium entering the peritoneal space from a colonic perforation. The combination of barium and feces entering the peritoneal space during a barium enema has a much greater likelihood of causing peritonitis and has a high mortality rate.

15. When is a single-contrast upper GI series performed?

Double-contrast examinations focus on showing mucosal detail. Single-contrast examinations focus only on the big picture to detect obstruction, perforation, abnormal motility, or fistulas. A single-contrast examination is performed to detect a complication along a staple/suture line, at an anastomosis, or near a wound; to evaluate an organ as it passes through a surgically created tunnel; or to identify a rent in a mesentery. A single-contrast examination also may be performed to evaluate emptying of surgically created pouches after surgery for morbid obesity and in conjunction with a small bowel follow-through examination.

16. What portion of the GI tract is shown in Fig. 15-6?
For the answer, see the figure legend.

17. What portion of the GI tract is shown in Fig. 15-7?
For the answer, see the figure legend.

18. What are the indications for a small bowel follow-through?
A small bowel follow-through may be performed whenever small bowel disease is suspected. The patient drinks a large volume (750 to 1000 mL) of thin barium, and a single-contrast examination of the esophagus, stomach, and small intestine is performed. Barium filling of the small intestine is limited by gastric emptying at the pylorus. The radiologist is unable to distend all the loops of small intestine either quickly or at the same time. A small bowel follow-through is also limited by the normal 30- to 120-minute transit time from the pylorus to the ileocecal valve. The radiologist cannot stand in the fluoroscopic suite for 1 to 2 hours and watch the barium flow down the small intestine. The radiologist examines the patient at 15- to 30-minute intervals, palpating loops of small intestine when they are optimally distended with barium. A small bowel follow-through relies on fluoroscopically obtained spot films, not overhead images.

A water-soluble contrast agent is used if a perforation is strongly suspected. A water-soluble contrast study of the small bowel is often suboptimal, however, because the hyperosmolar water-soluble contrast agent draws fluid into the lumen and prevents fluid resorption. The water-soluble contrast agent is diluted, and the images are very difficult to interpret. If a gastric or proximal small bowel leak is suspected, a water-soluble contrast upper GI tract study and proximal small bowel follow-through usually suffice. If a mid to distal small bowel leak is suspected, a computed tomography (CT) scan may be the better initial test. If a very distal small bowel leak or anastomotic leak is suspected in a patient with an ileocolic anastomosis, a water-soluble contrast enema is probably the best examination.

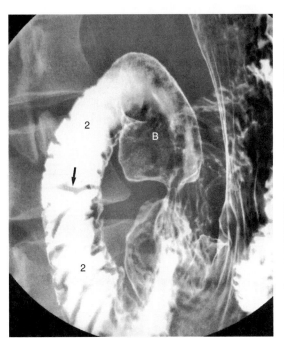

Figure 15-6. Spot radiograph of the duodenal bulb (*B*) and second portion of the duodenum (*2*) obtained during a double-contrast upper GI series. The folds of the duodenum (folds of Kerckring) (*arrow*) cross the duodenum except at the level of the papilla of Vater.

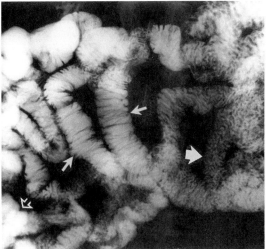

Figure 15-7. Close-up from an overhead view obtained during a small bowel follow-through examination. Many loops of small intestine are visible. Two loops are well distended (*thin arrows*) and show that the valvulae conniventes lie perpendicular to the longitudinal axis of the small bowel. Some loops are partially collapsed, and the valvulae conniventes overlap each other, giving the folds what has been described as a "feathery" (*thick arrow*) appearance. Some loops overlap, and no morphologic detail is visible (*open arrow*).

19. Fig. 15-8 is an overhead image obtained from what type of study? What organ is being imaged?
For the answer, see the figure legend.

20. What layers of the bowel wall comprise the valvulae conniventes?
Valvulae conniventes (plicae circulares, folds of Kerckring) are composed of mucosa and submucosa. These folds increase the surface area of the small bowel. The villi of the small intestine are about 1 mm in cross section and are just at the radiographic limits of resolution.

21. What are the indications for enteroclysis (small bowel enema)?
Small bowel enemas are difficult to perform and often are uncomfortable for the patient. They are superior, however, to small bowel follow-through examination for showing short lesions and the valvulae conniventes. Indications include the following:
- Unexplained anemia or GI bleeding; a patient should have a normal upper or lower endoscopy or normal double-contrast upper GI study and barium enema before enteroclysis
- Malabsorption
- Demonstration of skip lesions in a patient with known Crohn disease
- Suspected tumor of any kind

22. What is the preparation for enteroclysis?
Residual fluid and feces should be removed from the small intestine and right colon. The patient should not eat after 9 PM. Bisacodyl tablets are given with water at 10 PM the night before

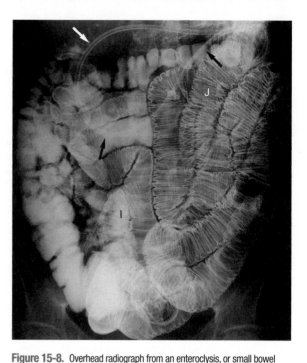

Figure 15-8. Overhead radiograph from an enteroclysis, or small bowel enema. During this examination, a tube is passed through the patient's mouth or nose, down the throat, through the esophagus, around the stomach, through the duodenum, and past the duodenal-jejunal junction. Passage of the tube (*arrows*) eliminates the pylorus as a rate-limiting factor of barium passage into the small bowel. In this particular case, the radiologist has injected medium-density barium to coat the mucosa and methylcellulose to distend the lumen. A double-contrast (but not air contrast) image is obtained. The jejunum (*J*) is in the left upper quadrant, and the ileum (*I*) is in the right lower quadrant. An enteroclysis may be performed as a single-contrast study with low-density barium or as a double-contrast study using barium to coat the mucosa and either air or methylcellulose to distend the lumen.

the examination to stimulate the right colon to contract. The patient does not drink fluids after midnight. Insulin-dependent diabetic patients do not take their morning dose of insulin. Other hospitals request that a full barium enema preparation be administered (see question 9 in Chapter 16).

23. Fig. 15-9 is a spot radiograph of the terminal ileum in a young man with chronic diarrhea. What disease does this patient have?
Fig. 15-9 is an image obtained during a *per-oral pneumocolon*. This is a specialized air contrast examination of the distal ileum, terminal ileum, cecum, and ascending colon. The patient undergoes a barium enema preparation the day before the examination to empty the terminal ileum and colon of feces. The patient then undergoes a routine small bowel follow-through examination. At the end of that examination, the per-oral pneumocolon study is performed. The patient receives 1 mg of glucagon intravenously to relax the colon, ileocecal valve, and small intestine. Air is insufflated into the rectum via a small soft catheter (e.g., Foley catheter). The radiologist distends the colon with air and attempts to reflux the terminal ileum with air. Air refluxes into the terminal ileum in most patients (85%), enabling double-contrast images of the terminal ileum that are superior to the images obtained during small bowel follow-through examination alone. A per-oral pneumocolon study may be valuable to show subtle mucosal changes of Crohn disease and to evaluate the right colon and ileocecal valve if these areas were not seen at either endoscopy or barium enema.

24. Fig. 15-10 is from a double-contrast esophagogram performed in an immunocompromised patient with acute odynophagia. What is your diagnosis?
For the answer, see the figure legend.

25. Fig. 15-11 is an image performed during an esophagogram while the patient lies prone and rapidly drinks thin barium. This patient had long-standing dysphagia for solids and chronic heartburn. What is your diagnosis?
Endoscopy and barium studies diagnose reflux esophagitis in about 40% of patients with biopsy-proven reflux esophagitis. Endoscopy has the ability to obtain biopsy specimens, whereas an upper GI series is more accurate in the

diagnosis of gastroesophageal reflux itself because only a small percentage of patients (10%) who have gastroesophageal reflux have reflux esophagitis. An upper GI study detects gastroesophageal reflux in about 50% to 70% of patients who have pH probe–proven gastroesophageal reflux. Barium studies are superior to endoscopy in the diagnosis of reflux-induced strictures because subtle tapered strictures are easily missed at endoscopy.

26. **Fig. 15-12 shows two images of the lesser curvature of the stomach from a double-contrast upper GI series performed in a young patient with 1 week of abdominal pain. What is your diagnosis?**
A double-contrast upper GI can be used to diagnose an ulcer confidently as a benign gastric ulcer in two thirds of patients with ulcers. In the remaining one third of patients, ulcers are either equivocally benign and need endoscopic biopsy or are frankly malignant.

27. **Fig. 15-13 is an image of the gastric antrum from a double-contrast upper GI series performed in a 52-year-old woman with anemia. What is your diagnosis?**
For the answer, see the figure legend.

28. **Fig. 15-14 is a close-up of the distal greater curvature of the stomach obtained during a double-contrast upper GI series performed in a patient with abdominal pain and rheumatoid arthritis. What is your diagnosis?**
For the answer, see the figure legend.

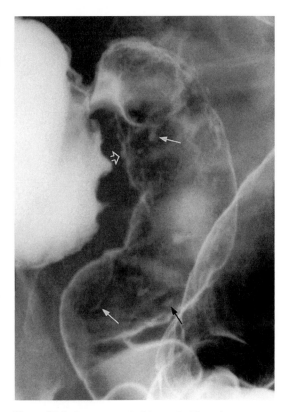

Figure 15-9. Spot radiograph of the terminal ileum shows numerous aphthoid ulcers en face as 2- to 5-mm punctate or slightly elongated collections of barium surrounded by radiolucent halos (*thin arrows*). In profile, the aphthoid ulcers appear as 2- to 4-mm punctate barium collections (*open arrow*) protruding outside the expected luminal contour. In patients with chronic diarrhea, aphthoid ulcers in the terminal ileum strongly suggests a diagnosis of Crohn disease. (From Rubesin SE, Bronner M, Radiologic-pathologic concept in Crohn's disease, Gastrointest Radiol 1 (1991) 27-55.)

29. **A coned-down image of the gastric fundus obtained during a double-contrast upper GI series is shown in Fig. 15-15. What is your diagnosis?**
For the answer, see the figure legend.

30. **A coned-down image of the gastric fundus obtained during a double-contrast upper GI series in shown in Fig. 15-16. What is your diagnosis?**
Fig. 15-16 shows the typical appearance of a submucosal mass. A smooth-surfaced tumor protrudes into the lumen. The tumor has an abrupt interface with the normal adjacent contour manifested, in profile, as sharp angulation with the lumen and, en face, as a ring shadow or sharp-edged barium pool. Central ulceration is shown in about 50% of submucosal masses. The most common submucosal mass in the stomach is a gastrointestinal stromal tumor (GIST). Lymphoma, granular cell tumor, and metastases are other common submucosal masses.

31. **Fig. 15-17 is an image of the gastric antrum from a double-contrast upper GI series performed in a 43-year-old man with anemia. What is your diagnosis?**
For the answer, see the figure legend.

32. **An elderly man complains of early satiety. A spot radiograph of the stomach from a double-contrast upper GI series is provided (Fig. 15-18). What is your diagnosis?**
For the answer, see the figure legend.

33. **Fig. 15-19 is a spot radiograph of the lower stomach obtained from a double-contrast upper GI series in a man who has had 4 months of abdominal discomfort. What is your differential diagnosis?**
For the answer, see the figure legend.

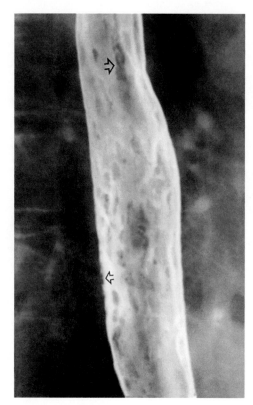 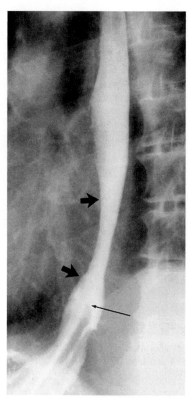

Figure 15-10. Spot radiograph of the esophagus obtained during a double-contrast upper GI examination shows numerous 1- to 4-mm, elongated radiolucent filling defects aligned longitudinally (*top arrow*). The intervening mucosa is smooth and normal. In profile, the filling defects are shown to be mildly elevated plaques (*bottom arrow*). These small, elevated plaques are almost pathognomonic for *Candida* esophagitis. A double-contrast esophagogram has 90% to 95% sensitivity for detecting *Candida* esophagitis in immunocompromised patients.

Figure 15-11. There is a long (4-cm), tapered narrowing of the distal esophagus (*thick arrows*) with an 8-mm luminal diameter. A small hiatal hernia is present; the *thin arrow* identifies the top of a gastric fold, and the esophagogastric junction is above the diaphragm. This is a classic reflux-induced stricture. Given the radiographic appearance of a benign distal esophageal stricture, the chance of Barrett esophagus is about 10% to 20%.

34. **A young man complains of acute right upper quadrant pain. Fig. 15-20 is a spot radiograph from a double-contrast upper GI series. What is your diagnosis?**
Ulcers in the duodenal bulb are invariably benign. Barium examinations are very effective (95%) at detecting acute duodenal bulb ulcers in patients who do not have scarring and sacculations related to chronic scarring. In about 20% of patients with recurrent ulcer disease, however, small ulcers may be missed in scarred or sacculated duodenal bulbs.

35. **Fig. 15-21A is a coned-down image of the mid-small intestine obtained in a man with unexplained heme-positive stool. Fig. 15-21B is an axial image from a CT scan that was performed several days later. What is your differential diagnosis?**
Enteroclysis (small bowel enema) is the best radiologic test for showing most small bowel tumors. Enteroclysis is poor at showing arteriovenous malformations, however. In patients with known metastatic melanoma, enteroclysis can be performed if there is a clinical question of small bowel metastases (Fig. 15-22).

36. **A young man complains of increasing abdominal distention and subacute right lower quadrant pain. Two images from a CT scan are presented (Fig. 15-23). Although a specific diagnosis is not possible, describe what is happening**
CT is an excellent first examination in patients with vomiting and abdominal distention and a suspected clinical diagnosis of small bowel obstruction. CT is a rapidly performed procedure compared with a small bowel follow-through in a patient with an obstruction. The radiologist looks for a transition zone between dilated,

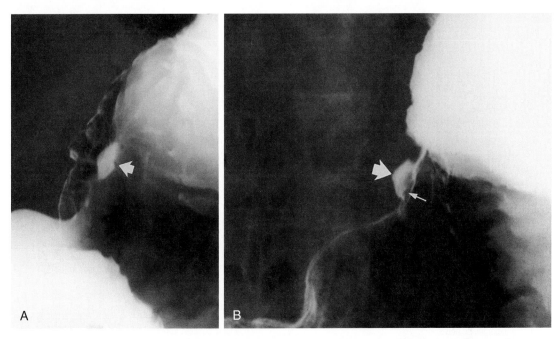

A

B

Figure 15-12. A, A 6-mm focal barium collection (*arrow*) is seen en face. No mass effect is seen. **B,** When the barium collection is viewed in profile, the collection protrudes from the expected luminal contour (*large arrow*). A thin lucency (*small arrow*) crosses the collection at its interface with the luminal contour. These are findings of a benign gastric ulcer. The ulcer niche (crater) is filled with barium (*large arrow*) and protrudes outside the expected contour of the stomach. No mass or mucosal nodularity is seen to indicate that a tumor is present. As the ulcer extends into the soft submucosal fat, it spreads laterally, burrowing under the mucosa. The undermined mucosa is manifested as the lucency (*small arrow*) crossing the edge of the ulcer, termed a *Hampton line*.

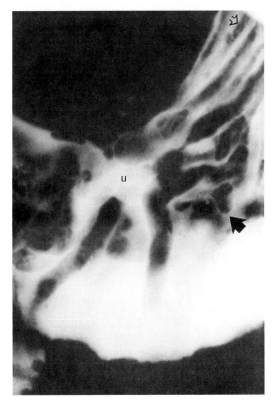

Figure 15-13. Coarsely lobulated, nodular folds radiate toward a central barium collection (*u*). Compare a normal-sized fold (*open arrow*) with an enlarged, lobulated fold (*black arrow*). The radiographic findings are that of a malignant tumor, proved at surgery to be an adenocarcinoma.

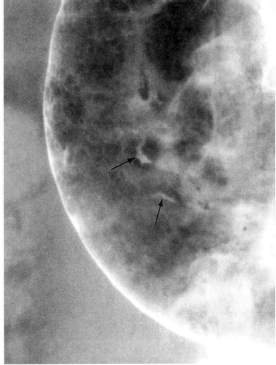

Figure 15-14. In the gastric antrum, there are two thin, serpentine barium collections (*arrows*) surrounded by radiolucent halos. These are the radiographic findings of erosive gastritis. Erosions are most commonly caused by nonsteroidal anti-inflammatory drugs (NSAIDs), but also may be caused by alcohol, viral infection, hypotension, or iatrogenic trauma (electrocautery). Linear erosions, as depicted in this figure, are usually related to NSAID use. This patient with rheumatoid arthritis was taking aspirin.

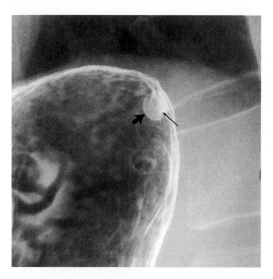

Figure 15-15. A small (6-mm) area of increased density is coated by barium (*thick arrow*). A subtle ring shadow (*thin arrow*) is seen centrally. These are the radiographic findings of a pedunculated polyp seen en face. The head of the polyp (*thick arrow*) is manifested as the outer barium-etched ring. The pedicle of the polyp (*thin arrow*) is etched in white and is seen toward the center of the polyp. The biopsy specimen showed this was a hyperplastic polyp.

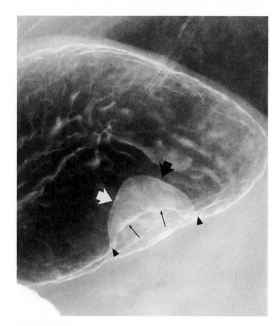

Figure 15-16. A 4-cm, smooth-surfaced mass (*large arrows*) is protruding into the stomach. The mass has sharp angles to the luminal contour (*arrowheads*). There is a sharp line between the obliquely oriented tumor and mucosal surface (*thin arrows*). These are the classic findings of a mass arising in the submucosa or muscularis propria, variably termed a *submucosal* or *extramucosal* mass. This proved to be a GIST.

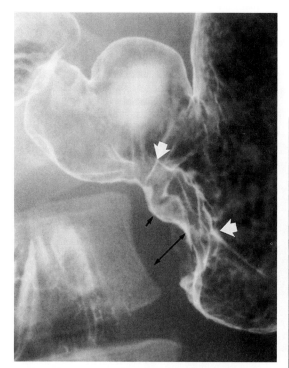

Figure 15-17. A mass is shown in profile as focal loss of the mucosal contour of the greater curvature of the gastric antrum with an area of soft tissue density (*double arrow*) protruding into the lumen. En face, the mass appears as numerous lobulated, barium-coated lines (*large arrows*) disrupting the mucosal surface. The mass has a central ulceration (*small arrow*) that is not filled with barium because the mass is located on the anterior wall of the stomach, and the barium has fallen into the dependent portion of the stomach—the gastric fundus. These radiographic findings are typical of a mass of mucosal origin, in this case an adenocarcinoma. Compare the nodular surface of this mucosal tumor with the smooth surface of the submucosal tumor in Fig. 15-16.

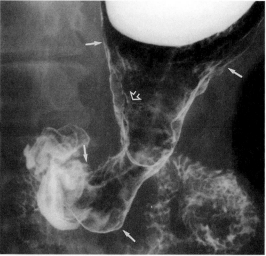

Figure 15-18. A long, circumferential, tapered narrowing of the distal gastric body and proximal gastric antrum is present (*between arrows on the greater and lesser curvatures*). The mucosal surface is only focally nodular (*open arrow*). These are the radiographic findings of linitis plastica, proved in this case to a signet-ring cell adenocarcinoma of the stomach broadly infiltrating the submucosa. Carcinomas of the stomach may spread longitudinally in the submucosal fat. If a desmoplastic (scirrhous) response occurs, large portions of the stomach may be narrowed. The most common causes of long gastric narrowing include adenocarcinoma, metastatic breast cancer, and corrosive ingestion.

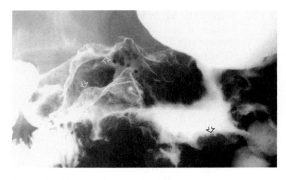

Figure 15-19. Rugal folds are composed of mucosa and submucosa. Rugal fold enlargement indicates a pathologic condition in the mucosa and submucosa. Radiographically, normal rugal folds are smooth, about 5 mm in size, and slightly more undulating along the greater curvature. Normal rugal folds also diminish in size from the gastric fundus to the antrum. A well-distended gastric antrum usually does not have rugal folds. In this image, the folds of the gastric antrum and body are markedly enlarged, lobulated, sometimes smooth (*white arrows*), and sometimes nodular (*black arrow*). The differential diagnosis includes tumor of the mucosa (adenocarcinoma) or the submucosa (lymphoma) or hyperplasia of a component of the mucosa (Ménétrier disease [i.e., hyperplasia of the surface foveolar cells]). This appearance cannot represent parietal cell hyperplasia seen in Zollinger-Ellison syndrome because parietal cells are not located in the gastric antrum, and the folds are larger than the folds typically seen in Zollinger-Ellison syndrome. This patient had lymphoma of the stomach.

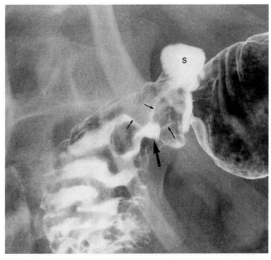

Figure 15-20. A 6-mm barium collection (*large arrow*) is seen in the duodenal bulb. Smooth folds (*thin arrows*) radiate to the margin of the collection. These are the radiographic findings of an acute, benign ulcer of the posterior wall of the duodenal bulb. Sacculation of the superior fornix of the duodenal bulb (*s*) reflects the scarring process radiating to the ulcer.

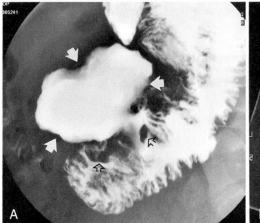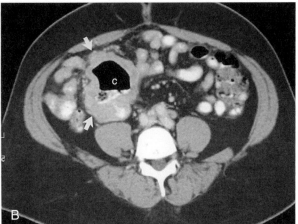

Figure 15-21. **A,** A large (6-cm) barium-filled cavity (*large arrows*) protrudes from the mesenteric border of the small intestine. Lobulated folds are seen on the mesenteric border of the bowel (*open arrows*). **B,** A mass (*arrows*) is seen in the right mid-abdomen. Centrally, a cavity (*c*) is filled with contrast agent, debris, and air. These are the radiographic findings of a cavitary tumor originating in the small intestine. Highly cellular tumors, such as lymphoma or metastatic melanoma, or highly vascular tumors, such as GIST, are the most common cavitary masses in the small intestine. This patient had a malignant GIST.

 fluid-filled bowel and collapsed bowel. CT can detect strictures related to Crohn disease, primary or metastatic tumors, internal or external hernias, and polypoid tumors causing intussusception. CT cannot directly show adhesions, the most common cause of small bowel obstruction in patients who previously have undergone surgery. CT diagnosis of adhesion is a diagnosis of exclusion; if an abnormality is not seen at the transition zone, a diagnosis of adhesion is made.

37. **A young man complains of diarrhea for 4 weeks. Fig. 15-24 is a spot image of the terminal ileum from a small bowel follow-through. What is your diagnosis?**
For the answer, see the figure legend.

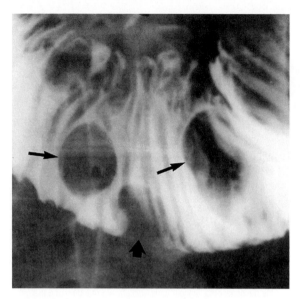

Figure 15-22. Metastatic melanoma to small intestine. Spot radiograph of the mid-small bowel obtained during the single-contrast phase of enteroclysis shows at least five, smooth-surfaced, round/ovoid radiolucent filling defects (*arrows*) in the barium column. These findings are typical of submucosal masses. The most common cause of multiple submucosal masses in the small bowel is metastatic melanoma. Disseminated lymphoma, other hematogenous metastases, or Kaposi sarcoma may have a similar appearance.

38. **A patient with known Crohn disease comes to the emergency department with abdominal pain. What radiologic test should be performed first?**
    A CT scan shows an unsuspected complication in about 25% of symptomatic patients with Crohn disease. Fig. 15-25 is such an example.

39. **A middle-aged woman has peripheral lymphadenopathy and heme-positive stool. Fig. 15-26 is an image of the terminal ileum and ileocecal valve from the single-contrast phase of a small bowel enema. What are the diagnostic possibilities?**
    For the answer, see the figure legend.

40. **A middle-aged woman has foul-smelling yellow stools. Fig. 15-27 is a spot image of the proximal jejunum obtained during enteroclysis. The *double arrows* represent 1 inch. What is your diagnosis?**
    Diseases that cause malabsorption usually involve the mucosa, submucosa, and lymphatics and mesenteric lymph nodes. Enteroclysis is superior to small bowel follow-through in the work-up of malabsorption because enteroclysis shows the mucosal surface and valvulae conniventes better than a small bowel follow-through.

41. **A 35-year-old woman has right lower quadrant pain and diarrhea. The results of the CT scan were normal. Fig. 15-28 is a spot radiograph of the distal ileum from a small bowel follow-through. What is your diagnosis?**
    Although CT is excellent at showing disease outside of the small bowel and markedly thickened bowel wall, CT cannot show the mucosal surface or subtle wall abnormalities, and it cannot be used to make specific diagnoses in most cases.

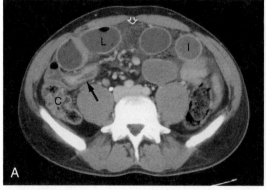
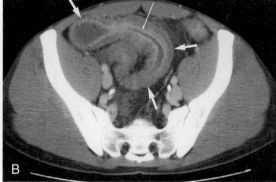

Figure 15-23. **A,** Axial image at the level of the iliac crests shows moderately dilated loops of ileum. Some ileal loops are completely filled with fluid (*I*) and are not visible on a plain film; other loops (*L*) have a small amount of intraluminal gas. A collapsed loop of ileum has a mildly thickened wall (*arrow*). A portion of the small bowel mesentery is hazy (*open arrow*) because of inflammatory stranding of the mesenteric fat. The cecum (*c*) is identified. **B,** Axial image caudal to **A** reveals a markedly thick-walled distal small bowel (*thick arrows*). The mucosal surface (*thin arrow*) is enhancing more than skeletal muscle. The submucosa is of low attenuation. This is a mural stratification pattern. A diagnosis of partial small bowel obstruction can be made, manifested as disproportionate dilation of proximal small bowel, but a specific diagnosis of the cause of bowel wall thickening cannot be made. The cause of the obstruction was shown on small bowel follow-through examination to be Crohn disease.

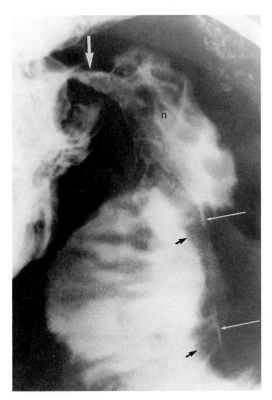

Figure 15-24. Note the long, thin barium collection (*thin white arrows*) on the mesenteric border of the terminal ileum. The collection is paralleled by a radiolucent mound of edema (*black arrows*). These are the radiographic findings of a mesenteric border ulcer, a radiographic finding that is almost pathognomonic of Crohn disease. Also present are thick, slightly nodular folds in the terminal ileum (*n*) and a mild stricture of the ileocecal valve (*thick white arrow*). (From Rubesin SE, Bronner M, Radiologic-pathologic concepts in Crohn's disease, Gastrointest Radiol 1 (1991) 27-55.)

42. A 44-year-old man had surgery for a persistent duodenal ulcer (Fig. 15-29). What operation was performed?

See the figure legend for the answer. Surgical treatment for peptic ulcer disease is reserved for complications such as perforation, severe hemorrhage, and obstruction. Vagotomy, in its various forms, denervates the body-type mucosa, reducing acid production. Acid secretion can be reduced further by resecting the gastric antrum, eliminating gastrin-secreting G cells. The remaining upper stomach is connected to the duodenum (termed *gastroduodenostomy/ Billroth I reconstruction*) or the jejunum (*gastrojejunostomy/ Billroth II reconstruction*). If an antrectomy is not performed, a pyloroplasty is done because vagotomy alters pyloric sphincter function, reducing gastric emptying.

43. What are the physiologic sequelae of gastric operations?

Truncal vagotomy accelerates liquid emptying from the stomach, but diminishes solid emptying. Truncal vagotomy diminishes pancreatic exocrine secretion and biliary secretion after a meal. A *dumping syndrome* may occur immediately or several hours after a meal. Dumping syndrome includes GI symptoms such as nausea or epigastric discomfort and systemic symptoms such as palpitations, dizziness, or syncope. *Alkaline reflux gastritis* is the term for gastritis induced by reflux of pancreaticobiliary secretions into the remaining stomach. This causes nausea, pain, or vomiting.

44. A 62-year-old man complains of abdominal pain 20 years after an antrectomy with gastroduodenostomy was performed for intractable duodenal ulcer disease (Fig. 15-30). What is your differential diagnosis?

Chronic reflux of pancreaticobiliary secretions (bile reflux) results in progression from chronic inflammation to development of mucosal hyperplasia, gastric

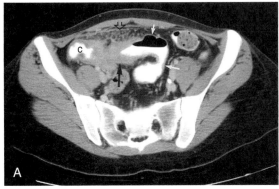

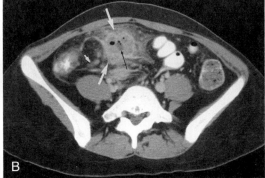

Figure 15-25. A, Axial image through the pelvis shows varying degrees of wall thickening in this patient with known Crohn disease. The thickness of the wall of the terminal ileum varies from normal (*short white arrow*) to mildly thickened (*long white arrow*) to markedly thickened (*long black arrow*). The wall of the cecum (*C*) is mildly thickened and has a mural stratification pattern. The omental fat (*open arrow*) anterior to the ileum has numerous linear soft tissue strands (so-called dirty fat). **B,** Axial image more cephalad in the pelvis shows an unsuspected abscess (*large white arrows*). A 5-cm inhomogeneous mass in the right lower quadrant has areas of soft tissue, fluid (*black arrow*), and air attenuation. The surrounding fat has soft tissue stranding. There also is local lymphadenopathy (*small white arrow*). These images are an example of the ability of CT to show serious complications in patients with known Crohn disease. (From Rubesin SE, Bartram CI, Laufer I, Inflammatory bowel disease, in: Levine MS, Rubesin SE, Laufer I [Eds], Double Contrast Gastrointestinal Radiology, third ed. Philadelphia, Saunders, 2000, pp. 417-470.)

metaplasia, and dysplasia, with the possible development of adenocarcinoma. Lack of eradication of *Helicobacter pylori* in the postoperative stomach can result in a similar cascade. If large, lobulated folds and nodular mucosa are seen long after gastric surgery, the differential diagnosis includes severe *H. pylori* gastritis or bile reflux gastritis complicated by hyperplasia, dysplasia, or adenocarcinoma. An adenocarcinoma was found in this patient.

45. A 45-year-old woman complains of vomiting. She had surgery for morbid obesity 2 years previously (Fig. 15-31). What operation did this patient have? Why is she vomiting?
For the answer, see the figure legend.

46. A 42-year-old woman has undergone surgery for morbid obesity (Fig. 15-32). What operation was performed?
For the answer, see the figure legend. Gastric bypass results in better weight loss than vertical banded gastroplasty. As a result, gastric bypass improves type 2 diabetes to a better degree than vertical banded gastroplasty. Gastric bypass has a greater incidence of immediate postoperative leaks. In the remote postoperative period, gastric bypass has a greater incidence of pouch ulceration, pouch outlet stenosis, vitamin B_{12} deficiency, and iron-deficiency anemia.

47. A 41-year-old woman had undergone surgery for morbid obesity (Fig. 15-33). What operation was performed?
For the answer, see the figure legend.

48. A 27-year-old woman underwent surgery for morbid obesity, and now presents with left upper quadrant pain and regurgitation. Fig. 15-34A is a spot radiograph from a study performed 14 months before the image in Fig. 15-34B. What has happened?
For the answer, see the figure legend. Complications of laparoscopic band surgery include port infections and inadequate weight loss. The stomach may form ulcers where the band compresses the upper gastric body, or the band may fully erode into the stomach. Slippage of the band in relationship to the stomach may result in obstruction.

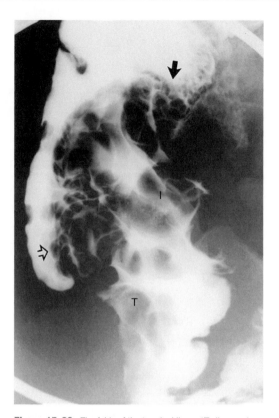

Figure 15-26. The folds of the terminal ileum (*T*), ileocecal valve (*I*), medial wall of the cecum (*open arrow*), and proximal ascending colon (*arrow*) are markedly thickened and slightly lobulated, but smooth-surfaced. There are no pathognomonic findings of Crohn disease (e.g., aphthoid ulcers, mesenteric border ulcers, cobblestoning, fissures, fistulas). The folds are much larger than would be seen in Crohn disease. The two most likely possibilities are lymphoma or carcinoma of the ileocecal valve invading the terminal ileum. This proved to be mantle cell lymphoma of the ileocecal region. This case shows that not all fold thickening in the terminal ileum during barium studies or wall thickening on CT is due to Crohn disease. Acute or semi-acute infections (e.g., *Yersinia* enterocolitis), tuberculosis in patients from endemic areas or patients with acquired immunodeficiency syndrome, and lymphoma can cause thick ileal folds. Unless the aforementioned pathognomonic findings of Crohn disease are present, biopsy, stool culture, or follow-up imaging is indicated.

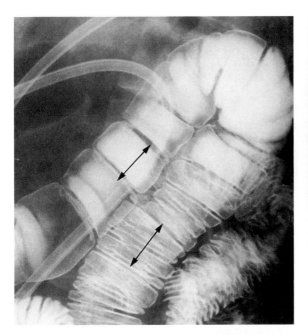

Figure 15-27. There are a diminished number of valvulae conniventes per inch in the more superior loop of the jejunum than in the inferior loop. Only two folds per inch are seen superiorly, whereas about five to six folds per inch are seen inferiorly (*double arrows*). Loss of valvulae conniventes indicates that there is a loss of mucosal surface area. These radiographic findings are the macroscopic correlate of villous atrophy seen in gluten-sensitive enteropathy (celiac disease, nontropical sprue). Celiac disease is underdiagnosed in adult patients. Currently, antibodies are found in 70% to 90% of patients with gluten-sensitive enteropathy and in about 1 in 200 adults. Diagnosis of celiac disease requires biopsy-shown improvement of villous atrophy after a trial of a gluten-free diet. The role of enteroclysis in symptomatic patients with celiac disease is to exclude development of a complication such as ulcerative jejunoileitis or adenocarcinoma or lymphoma of the small intestine.

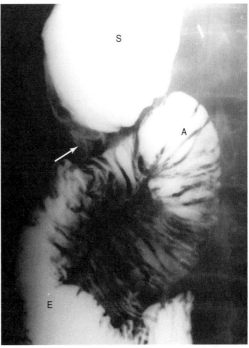

Figure 15-29. Antrectomy with gastrojejunostomy (Billroth II procedure). Spot radiograph from double-contrast upper GI series shows the remaining upper stomach (*S*) filled with barium. The gastrojejunal anastomosis (*arrow*), efferent limb (*E*), and afferent limb (*A*) are identified. In this patient, the afferent limb is on the left side of the anastomosis, but the loop curves back to the right to join the duodenum.

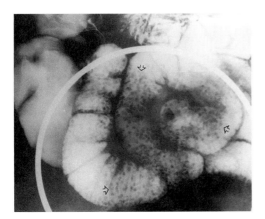

Figure 15-28. Innumerable uniformly round, radiolucent filling defects (1 to 2 mm in size) (*arrows*) are in the barium column of the distal-most three loops of ileum. Normal smooth mucosa separates these nodules. These findings are characteristic of extensive lymphoid hyperplasia. The causes of extensive lymphoid hyperplasia in the ileum include recent enteric infection and immunodeficiency states, such as common variable immunodeficiency and IgA deficiency. After the barium study, a diagnosis of common variable immunodeficiency was made.

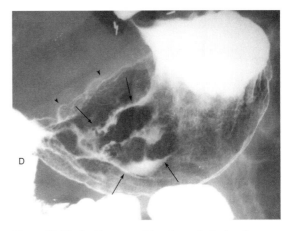

Figure 15-30. Gastric cancer arising after gastroduodenostomy (Billroth I procedure). Spot radiograph of the stomach shows large, lobulated folds (*arrows*) in the distal gastric body. The contour of the lesser curvature is undulating (*arrowheads*). The gastroduodenostomy is seen in overlap. The proximal duodenum (*D*) is identified.

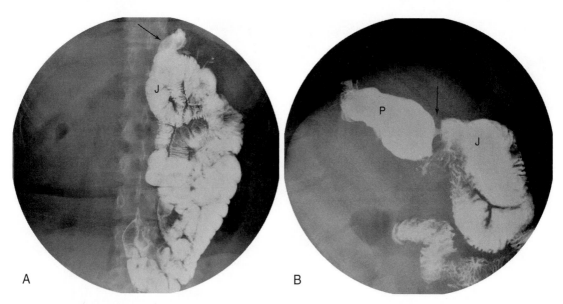

A   B

Figure 15-31. A, Spot radiograph of the abdomen obtained at low magnification shows a small portion of stomach (the gastric pouch—*arrow*). The remainder of the stomach, pylorus, and duodenum are not filled with barium. Barium enters the jejunum (*J*). **B,** Spot radiograph of left upper quadrant obtained with the patient in a left-side-down lateral position shows the gastric pouch (*P*), the gastrojejunal anastomosis (*arrow*), and the proximal jejunum (*J*). This patient had a gastric bypass procedure. Almost all of the stomach, all of the duodenum, and the first 50 to 150 cm of jejunum have been "bypassed." In normal postoperative patients, the gastric pouch is small, holding about 15 to 60 mL. In this patient, the gastric pouch is dilated because of chronic obstruction at the gastrojejunal anastomosis, resulting in vomiting. The gastrojejunal anastomosis (*arrow*) measures 5 mm in luminal diameter, but normally measures about 9 to 10 mm at our institution. The bypassed stomach, duodenum, and proximal jejunum are connected to the jejunum by a jejunojejunostomy. This author prefers the term *alimentary limb* for the portion of jejunum between the pouch and jejunojejunostomy, and the term *pancreaticobiliary limb* for the bypassed stomach, duodenum, and jejunum proximal to the jejunojejunostomy.

Figure 15-32. Vertical banded gastroplasty. Spot radiograph of the stomach from a single-contrast upper GI series is performed with the patient standing. The distal esophagus (*E*) is identified. An elongated gastric pouch (*P*) is present along the lesser curvature, separated from the upper stomach by a staple line (*arrowheads*). The pouch outlet (*arrow*) communicates with the gastric body. The gastric fundus is filled with air with the patient in an erect position. In a vertical banded gastroplasty, a hole is made by a staple gun about 5 cm inferior to the gastric cardia. A gastric pouch is constructed by firing a stapling device between the hole and the angle of His, creating a band of tissue between the cardia and the greater curvature (hence the term *vertical band*). The outlet of the pouch is formed by a mesh wrapped around the stomach, from the hole to the lesser curvature.

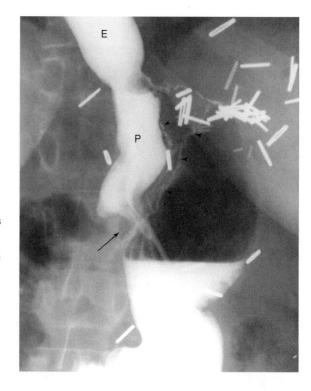

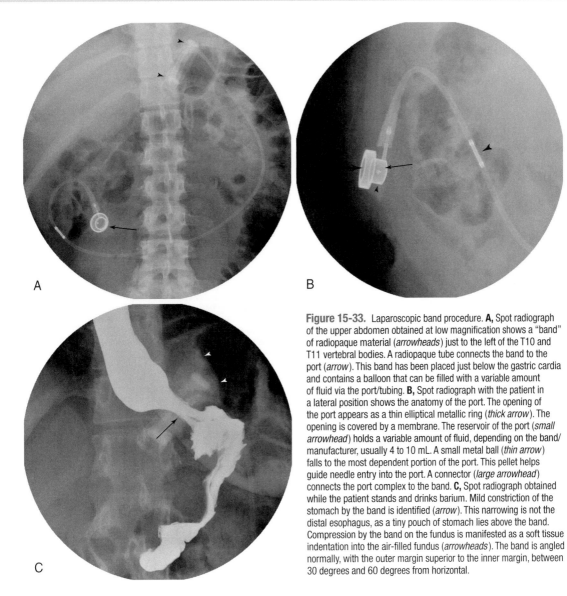

Figure 15-33. Laparoscopic band procedure. **A,** Spot radiograph of the upper abdomen obtained at low magnification shows a "band" of radiopaque material (*arrowheads*) just to the left of the T10 and T11 vertebral bodies. A radiopaque tube connects the band to the port (*arrow*). This band has been placed just below the gastric cardia and contains a balloon that can be filled with a variable amount of fluid via the port/tubing. **B,** Spot radiograph with the patient in a lateral position shows the anatomy of the port. The opening of the port appears as a thin elliptical metallic ring (*thick arrow*). The opening is covered by a membrane. The reservoir of the port (*small arrowhead*) holds a variable amount of fluid, depending on the band/manufacturer, usually 4 to 10 mL. A small metal ball (*thin arrow*) falls to the most dependent portion of the port. This pellet helps guide needle entry into the port. A connector (*large arrowhead*) connects the port complex to the band. **C,** Spot radiograph obtained while the patient stands and drinks barium. Mild constriction of the stomach by the band is identified (*arrow*). This narrowing is not the distal esophagus, as a tiny pouch of stomach lies above the band. Compression by the band on the fundus is manifested as a soft tissue indentation into the air-filled fundus (*arrowheads*). The band is angled normally, with the outer margin superior to the inner margin, between 30 degrees and 60 degrees from horizontal.

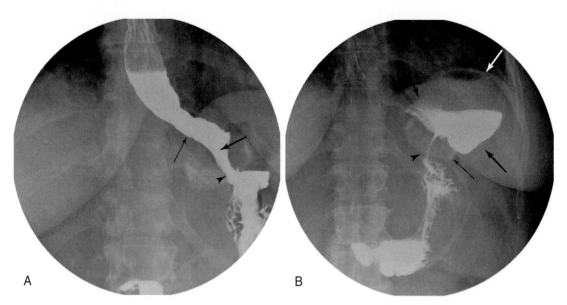

Figure 15-34. Slip of stomach through laparoscopic gastric band, resulting in high-grade gastric obstruction. **A,** "Baseline" spot radiograph performed while patient was asymptomatic shows a small pouch (*large arrow*) above the band. The esophagogastric junction is a thin indentation (*small arrow*). Note the width of the lumen of the stomach as it passes through the band (*arrowhead*) and the normal angle of the band. **B,** Spot radiograph performed 14 months later shows a large "pouch," including the gastric fundus and upper gastric body (*large arrows*) superior to the band. The lumen of the stomach is markedly narrow (about 1 mm) as it goes through the band (*arrowhead*). The band is now angled inferiorly (*thin arrow*). Residual fluid in the gastric fundus (note the air/fluid and fluid/barium levels) is also indicative of obstruction.

BIBLIOGRAPHY

[1] R.M. Gore, M.S. Levine (Eds.), Textbook of Gastrointestinal Radiology, second ed., Saunders, Philadelphia, 2000.
[2] H. Herlinger, D.D.T. Maglinte, B.A. Birnbaum (Eds.), Clinical Radiology of the Small Intestine, Springer-Verlag, New York, 1999.
[3] J.K.T. Lee, S.S. Sagel, R.J. Stanley, J.P. Heiken, Computed Body Tomography with MRI Correlation, third ed., Lippincott-Raven, Philadelphia, 1998.
[4] M.S. Levine, S.E. Rubesin, I. Laufer (Eds.), Double Contrast Gastrointestinal Radiology, third ed., Saunders, Philadelphia, 2000.
[5] M.A. Meyers, Dynamic Radiology of the Abdomen, fifth ed., Springer, New York, 2000.

ANATOMY

1. Identify the parts of the colon (numbers *1* through *8*) in Fig. 16-1. What structures are identified by the *open and white arrows*?
See the figure legend for answers.

2. What are haustra?
The longitudinal muscle layer of the colon is divided into three thick bands, termed the taeniae coli. There is a paucity of longitudinal muscle between the three tenial bands. Haustra are sacculations of colon protruding between the three rows of taeniae coli (Figs. 16-2 and 16-3). At the edges of the haustral sacculations, folds, termed *interhaustral folds,* radiate toward the taeniae coli. The colon is identified by its haustral sacculations and interhaustral folds on any radiologic study—whether plain radiograph, computed tomography (CT), magnetic resonance imaging (MRI), or barium enema. Rounded, air-filled pockets are seen in a nondependent (anterior) position. Fluid-filled or contrast-filled rounded sacculations are seen on the dependent (inferior) surface.

Haustra are relatively fixed structures in the right and transverse colon. Haustra are intermittently seen structures in the descending and proximal sigmoid colon, depending on the stage of colonic contraction. The left colon may intermittently appear "ahaustral," depending on the degree of colonic contraction. Although the edge of the colon has a sacculated appearance, the edge of the small bowel is relatively straight, altered only by its thin valvulae conniventes. Valvulae conniventes are thinner than interhaustral folds and cross the entire lumen of the bowel, whereas interhaustral folds cross about one third of the colonic diameter when seen in profile. Seen en face, the interhaustral folds may falsely appear to cross the entire lumen of the colon.

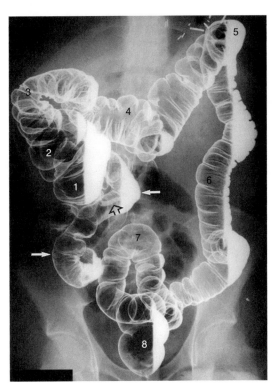

Figure 16-1. Overhead radiograph from double-contrast barium enema shows portions of the colon: *1* = cecum, *2* = ascending colon, *3* = hepatic flexure, *4* = mid-transverse colon, *5* = splenic flexure, *6* = descending colon, *7* = sigmoid colon, and *8* = rectum. The terminal ileum (*white arrows*) and the appendix (*open arrow*) are identified.

TECHNIQUE

3. Fig. 16-4 is from what type of examination?
A double-contrast (or air-contrast) barium enema uses two contrast agents to image the colon. A medium-density, medium-viscosity barium suspension is instilled into the colon via a rectal tube. This barium scrubs residual feces and fluid into the suspension, then coats the mucosal surface with barium. Air (or carbon dioxide) is insufflated via the rectal tube to distend the colon and render it "translucent." The end result is that the mucosal surface is "etched" in white by barium, and the colonic walls are widely separated. Spot radiographs and overhead images are then obtained. A colonic hypotonic agent (1 mg of intravenous glucagon) is routinely administered at our hospital. Other hospitals use glucagon only if there is colonic spasm, excessive patient discomfort, or inability to retain the contrast agent. In other countries, an anticholinergic agent (e.g., hyoscine-butylbromide [Buscopan]) may be used to induce colonic hypotonia.

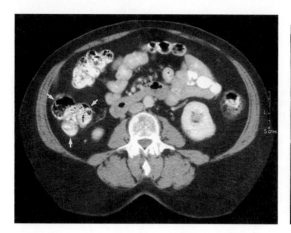

Figure 16-2. Haustra on CT. Axial image through the lower abdomen shows the three rows of haustral sacculations (*arrows*) in the ascending colon. The feces (*f*) in the ascending colon have a mottled appearance of air (*black*); soft tissue appears gray; the contrast agent appears white. Feces are not seen in the mid-small intestinal loops.

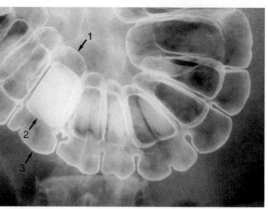

Figure 16-3. Spot radiograph of the transverse colon from a double-contrast barium enema shows three rows of haustral sacculations (edges of three haustral rows are identified by *black arrows*). The more dependent haustral row is partially filled with barium.

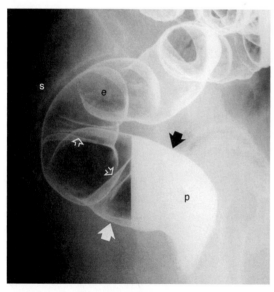

Figure 16-4. Spot radiograph of the rectum from a double-contrast barium enema study. The patient lies in a prone position, and the x-ray beam is "shot" across the patient; this is termed a *cross-table* image. The mucosal detail is seen en face in air contrast (*e*), but obscured by the barium pool (*p*). The radiologist looks at the contour of the colon in the barium pool (*black arrow*) and in the air (*white arrow*). Two of the valves of Houston are identified (*open arrows*). The proximal and mid rectum parallel the sacrum (*s*).

4. In what position is the patient lying tabletop of the fluoroscope in Fig. 16-1?

Air-barium levels are the clue to the patient's position. Barium is heavier than air; barium identifies the "down" side of the patient. The air-barium levels show that the patient is lying with his or her left side down. The x-ray tube is positioned in a *cross-table lateral position,* with the x-ray tube at one side of the tabletop, so the x-ray beam parallels the tabletop. A cassette is placed in an upright position, perpendicular to the tabletop, in front or in back of the patient. This image is termed a *left-side-down decubitus view.*

5. What type of patient is capable of undergoing a double-contrast barium enema?

A patient has to be able to hold the barium and air in his or her colon; anal sphincter tone must be normal. The patient must be able to roll around the tabletop of the fluoroscope; he or she must be strong enough to roll over in bed. The radiologist must be able to communicate with the patient. If the patient does not speak the same language as the radiologist, a translator must be provided. The patient must have enough mental acuity to be able to understand and respond to the following commands: "Don't breathe/breathe," "Turn left/turn right," and "Hold the barium in your rectum."

6. Fig. 16-5 is an image from what type of examination?

This is a spot radiograph from a single-contrast barium enema. This type of examination uses one contrast agent: low-density barium. Under fluoroscopic control, the colon is filled with barium. Spot radiographs and overhead images of the entire colon are obtained. Postevacuation spot radiographs or overhead images are also obtained.

7. What are the indications for a double-contrast barium enema?

Whenever colonic disease is suspected, and a patient has no contraindications for barium enema, this examination can be performed. Indications for double-contrast barium enema include rectal bleeding, diarrhea, abdominal pain, screening for colorectal neoplasia, or involvement of the colon by extracolonic inflammatory or neoplastic masses.

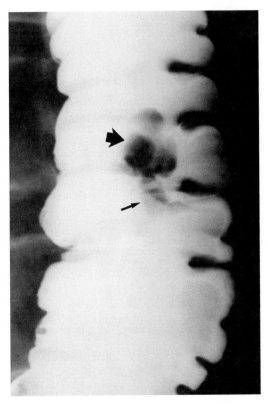

Figure 16-5. Spot radiograph of the ascending colon from a single-contrast barium enema. The radiologist evaluates the contour and the barium column. In this patient, the luminal contour has normal sacculations, but there is a 1.5-cm lobulated radiolucent filling defect (*thick arrow*) connected to a smooth tubular filling defect (*thin arrow*). This is the typical appearance of a pedunculated polyp in a single-contrast examination. Barium in the interstices of the lesion indicates its villous or tubulovillous nature. The polyp proved to be a tubulovillous adenoma. (From Rubesin SE, Stuzin N, Laufer I, Tumors of the colon. Semin. Colon. Rect. Surg. 4 (1993) 94-111.)

8. What are the indications for a single-contrast barium enema?

A single-contrast barium enema may be performed in patients with suspected fistula, high-grade colonic obstruction, or Hirschsprung disease. If a distal small bowel obstruction is suspected, a single-contrast barium enema with reflux of barium into the distal ileum to the point of obstruction may be performed as a complementary study to CT.

9. What is your hospital's preparation for a barium enema?

Each hospital has its own preparation for a barium enema that should be available from the Department of Radiology. Preparations generally include (1) a period during which solid food is limited in an effort to reduce undigested material reaching the colon, (2) an oral laxative, and (3) a medication that induces colonic contraction. The preparation at the Hospital of the University of Pennsylvania includes the following:

- Clear liquids only are allowed the day before the examination.
- At 5 PM the day before the examination, 10 to 16 oz of magnesium citrate is given.
- The patient should drink at least three to four 8-oz glasses of water throughout the day of the examination.
- At 10 PM the evening before the examination, four 5-mg bisacodyl tablets are taken with 8 oz of water.
- The patient should have nothing by mouth after midnight the night before until after the examination.
- The patient is given a bisacodyl suppository the morning of the examination.
- Insulin dose is reduced or eliminated the morning of the examination.
- After the examination, patients are encouraged to drink water and take laxatives if they have colonic hypomotility.

At our hospital, we do not use large-volume colonic lavage agents that are used for colonoscopy because they leave large amounts of fluid in the colon that degrade barium coating of the mucosa. Cleansing enemas are discouraged because they push fecal residue into the right colon and leave residual fluid in the colon.

10. What patients may require more than the standard barium enema preparation?

A 2-day preparation may be necessary in immobile or bedridden patients, patients with hypomotility disorders such as diabetes or hypothyroidism, postoperative patients, or patients taking opiates or drugs with anticholinergic side effects.

11. List the contraindications for a barium enema.

- Known or suspected colonic perforation. If a perforation is suspected, CT or an enema using a water-soluble contrast agent should be used.
- Fulminant colitis ("toxic megacolon") or any severe colitis (see Fig. 14-1).
- A recent procedure that has potentially created a hole in the colonic mucosa. A barium enema should be postponed for 1 week if a large forceps biopsy at rigid sigmoidoscopy, a snare polypectomy, or hot biopsy has been performed. A biopsy specimen taken with small forceps via a flexible endoscope is not a contraindication.

Also, the clinician should alert the radiologist if a patient has a latex allergy, so all products containing latex can be removed from the fluoroscopic suite, and the room can be cleaned before a procedure.

12. What are the contraindications for the use of intravenous glucagon?

Patients with known or suspected insulinoma or pheochromocytoma should not receive intravenous glucagon.

13. What patients should be scheduled early in the day?

Patients with latex allergy should be scheduled first in the day, after the room has been cleaned. Insulin-dependent diabetic patients, patients with hypoglycemia, or other patients who require breakfast should be scheduled as early in the day as possible.

14. What are the complications of a barium enema?

- The examination may fail to image the entire colon if the patient has colonic spasm or poor sphincter tone and is unable to retain barium or air.
- Distention of the colon may cause the patient to complain of cramps, but rarely produces syncope.
- Colonic perforation occurs in about 1 in 40,000 examinations. Perforation is usually retroperitoneal and related to distention of a rectal balloon. If a free intraperitoneal perforation occurs, it is usually in a patient who has severe colitis or ischemia. In contrast to the rarity of barium enema perforation, perforation occurs in about 1 in 1000 colonoscopies.
- Rarely, barium impaction occurs in patients who have colonic hypomotility, such as bedridden patients, patients taking narcotics or other drugs that cause hypomotility, and diabetic patients. Barium impaction can be prevented, in part, by having patients take oral laxatives after the procedure.
- Allergic reactions to the barium, glucagon, or colonic preparation are rare, but have been reported. Although allergic reactions to latex in barium enema balloons have previously occurred, the manufacturers have removed the latex from the balloons attached to the enema tips.
- Rarely, patients develop myocardial ischemia during barium enema.

15. Is antibiotic prophylaxis needed before administration of a barium enema?

There is conflicting evidence regarding bacteremia during barium enema. Routine antibiotic prophylaxis is probably unnecessary except in patients with susceptible cardiac lesions who have a history of endocarditis or a prosthetic valve.

16. What patients need a preparation for a CT scan?

Patients undergoing abdominal CT on an emergent basis do not have time to undergo an overnight preparation. Oral contrast agent is administered about 1 hour before CT in most patients. An effervescent agent (gas), water, or another fluid attenuation oral agent (e.g., methylcellulose or a barium suspension [VoLumen]) is administered to patients in whom the biliary tree or the head of the pancreas is the target region. In the future, if it is possible for patients with acute gastrointestinal bleeding to be studied with CT angiography, high-attenuation oral contrast agent will not be administered so that hypervascular lesions of the bowel can be more easily detected. Most hospitals do not require colonic and distal small bowel cleansing before nonemergent CT scans. Some patients undergoing nonemergent CT may benefit, however, from colonic cleansing before CT, including patients with weight loss, lower gastrointestinal bleeding, chronic abdominal pain, diarrhea, or abdominal distention.

17. What is the most important radiographic predictor of malignancy arising in a polyp?

Size is most important; the larger the polyp, the greater the chance of malignancy. The amount of villous change is a much less important factor. About 1% of tubular adenomas smaller than 1 cm are malignant (Fig. 16-6); 10% of tubular adenomas 1 to 2 cm are malignant, and 35% of

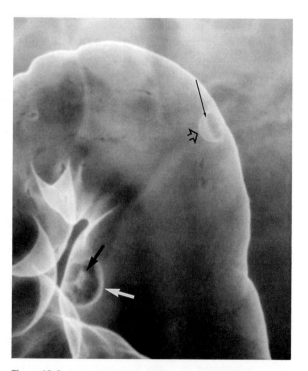

Figure 16-6. Spot radiograph of the splenic flexure shows two polyps. The small polyp resembles a hat. The top of the hat (*open arrow*) is the top of the polyp. The brim of the hat (*thin black arrow*) is barium trapped between the mucosa and the polyp as it is retracted by its stalk. This was a tubular adenoma. The second polyp has a more worrisome morphology—that of an umbilicated, sessile polyp. A small barium collection (*thick black arrow*) fills a central umbilication or ulceration. The edge of the polyp is coated by barium (or "etched in white") (*white arrow*). This polyp was a tubulovillous adenoma.

tubular adenomas larger than 2 cm are malignant. About 10% of villous adenomas smaller than 2 cm are malignant, and about 50% of villous adenomas larger than 2 cm are malignant. The presence of a pedicle longer than 1 cm means that a pedunculated polyp has a greater than 95% chance of benign behavior, regardless of the histology in the head of the polyp.

18. What does fine lobulation of the surface of a polyp mean?

Barium enters the interstices between fronds of a polyp (see Fig. 16-5), and the greater the number of lobules, the greater the amount of villous change in a polyp. A polyp with more than several lobules is in the spectrum of tubulovillous to villous adenoma (Fig. 16-7) and has a slightly greater risk of malignancy.

19. What percentage of colonic cancers is out of reach of the flexible sigmoidoscope?

Over the past 4 decades, the distribution of colon cancers has shifted toward the right colon (Fig. 16-8). About 40% to 50% of colonic cancers are out of reach of the flexible sigmoidoscope. This is why screening for colonic carcinoma requires a total colonic examination, either by colonoscopy or by double-contrast barium enema.

20. Which of the following morphologic shapes is the most common form of symptomatic colonic carcinoma: polypoid, carpet, plaquelike, or annular?

About 50% of advanced cancers in symptomatic patients are annular cancers. Obstructive symptoms result when annular lesions narrow the lumen. When an annular cancer is seen radiographically (Fig. 16-9), there is a 98% chance of serosal invasion, a 50% chance of lymph node metastasis, and about a 15% chance of liver metastasis.

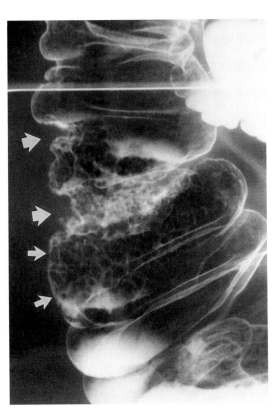

Figure 16-7. Adenocarcinoma arising in a villous adenoma of the ascending colon. Spot radiograph from a double-contrast barium enema shows a 4-cm area of polygonal nodules with barium filling the interstices between tumor lobules. The flat nature of the tumor is evident in profile where the luminal contour is neither pushed in nor excavated out (*small arrows*). Adenocarcinoma is present where the lesion disrupts the luminal contour (*large arrows*). This flat lesion has been called a "carpet lesion" by some authors. (From Rubesin SE, Laufer I, Pictorial glossary, in: Gore RM, Levine MS [Eds], Textbook of Gastrointestinal Radiology, second ed. Philadelphia, Saunders, 2000, pp. 44-65.)

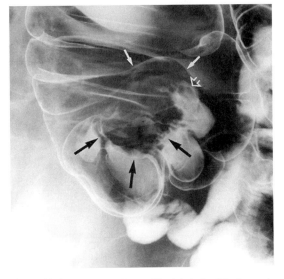

Figure 16-8. Polypoid carcinoma of the inferior lip of the ileocecal valve invading the terminal ileum. Spot radiograph of the cecum from a double-contrast barium enema shows a 3-cm, finely lobulated mass (*black arrows*) expanding the contour of the inferior lip of the ileocecal valve. The normal-sized and smooth superior lip of the ileocecal valve is labeled (*white arrows*) for comparison. The lumen of the ileocecal valve (*open white arrow*) is nodular, indicating tumor spread into the ileum.

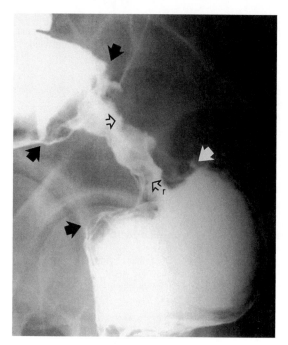

Figure 16-9. Annular adenocarcinoma of the rectum. Spot radiograph from the single-contrast phase of a double-contrast barium enema shows a 5-cm-long, circumferential narrowing of the proximal rectum. The lesion has abrupt shelf-like margins (*large black and white arrows*) and an irregular surface (*open arrows*). This has been called an "apple core" lesion, but this is a misnomer because the tumor represents the part of the apple that has been eaten away, and the lumen would be the "apple core."

Polypoid cancers are most commonly found in the rectum or cecum. Polypoid cancers may cause colonic bleeding, but do not usually result in obstructive symptoms unless intussusception occurs. Polypoid cancers have a better prognosis: 55% of patients have serosal invasion, and 25% have lymph node metastasis.

21. **What is the most common cause of colonic intussusception in adults?**
Colonic cancers are the most common cause of colonic intussusception in adults. Less likely causes include adenomas and lipomas.

22. **Hyperplastic polyps are found most commonly in what part of the colon?**
Hyperplastic polyps are small (<5 mm), smooth-surfaced polyps most commonly found in the rectum on the crest of folds. In contrast to adenomatous polyps, hyperplastic polyps are not premalignant.

23. **Fig. 16-10 is an image from a CT scan through the mid-abdomen. What is your diagnosis?**
The diagnosis is lipoma (see Fig. 16-10 legend for discussion). Lipomas are most commonly found in the right colon as a sessile or broadly pedunculated, smooth-surfaced mass (Fig. 16-11). On CT, the mass is shown to be composed of fat. These tumors change size and shape with palpation and varying degrees of colonic distention.

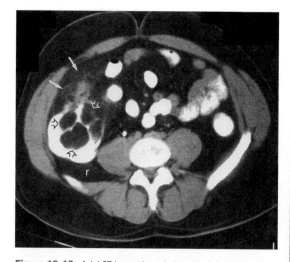

Figure 16-10. Axial CT image through the mid-abdomen shows a 4-cm polypoid mass in the right colon. Four lobules of fat attenuation (*open arrows*) are found in the contrast-filled lumen of the ascending colon. This is a lipoma, an incidental finding. (Compare the CT attenuation of the lipoma with the retroperitoneal fat [*r*].) The fat of the greater omentum (*white arrows*) and adjacent to the ascending colon shows stranding because of nearby right-sided diverticulitis. (From Rubesin SE, Laufer I, Tumors of the colon, in: Levine MS, Rubesin SE, Laufer I [Eds], Double Contrast Gastrointestinal Radiology, third ed. Philadelphia, Saunders, 2000, pp. 357-416.)

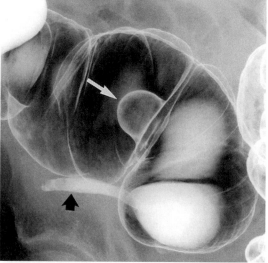

Figure 16-11. Spot radiograph of the cecum from a double-contrast barium enema shows a smooth-surfaced, 2-cm polypoid lesion (*white arrow*) arising from the superior lip of the ileocecal valve. This is the typical smooth appearance of a colonic lipoma on barium enema. The appendix is identified (*black arrow*).

24. What tumors commonly spread to the intraperitoneal space?

Ovarian cancer is the most common type of tumor that spreads to the peritoneal space in women. In men, cancers of the colon, pancreas, and stomach are the primary tumors that most frequently spread to the intraperitoneal space. Hepatocellular carcinomas spread to the peritoneal space, but they are less common in the United States compared with Asia or Africa.

25. What is the most common finding of intraperitoneal metastasis on CT?

Ascites is seen in about 70% of patients with intraperitoneal metastasis on CT (Fig. 16-12). Intraperitoneal implants are seen less commonly. Implants are more easily detected on the peritoneal surfaces of the diaphragm, liver, and omentum than in bowel. Barium enemas are helpful in determining the extent of colonic involvement and where to perform a colostomy in a patient with intraperitoneal implants.

26. What are the differences in distribution between ulcerative colitis and Crohn disease?

Ulcerative colitis (Table 16-1) is left-sided colonic disease, beginning at the anorectal junction and extending continuously and retrogradely a variable distance (proctosigmoiditis, left-sided colitis, pancolitis) (Fig. 16-13). Ulcerative colitis symmetrically involves a bowel segment (Fig. 16-14). Crohn disease involves the colon and terminal ileum in 55% of patients. Terminal ileal involvement alone is seen in 14% of patients. Terminal ileal and distal small bowel involvement alone is seen in 13% of patients. Pure colonic involvement is seen in about 15% of patients. Crohn disease is discontinuous, having patchy involvement locally and between loops, called skip areas. Crohn disease is asymmetric, first involving the mesenteric side of bowel.

27. Aphthoid ulcers are characteristic of which chronic inflammatory bowel disease?

In an American with long-standing symptoms, aphthoid ulcers are almost pathognomonic for Crohn disease (Fig. 16-15). They are also seen in patients with acute diarrheal states, such as yersiniosis, amebiasis, and viral (cytomegalovirus/herpes) infection. An aphthoid ulcer results from breakdown of the mucosa above an inflamed lymph aggregate in the lamina propria or submucosa. The other characteristic findings in Crohn disease include mesenteric border ulcers and crisscrossing knifelike clefts resulting in cobblestoning (see Table 16-1). Strictures, fissures, and fistulas are seen with transmural disease. Pathologically, granulomas are detected in 25% to 70% of patients. The characteristic radiographic findings in ulcerative colitis are granular mucosa (Fig. 16-16), ulcers on a background of inflammatory granularity, shortening of the colon, and loss of haustration.

28. What is the first radiographic study that should be performed in symptomatic patients with Crohn disease?

CT should be performed first, primarily to exclude an intra-abdominal abscess and to show the cause of separated bowel loops—whether abscess, inflammation, or fibrofatty proliferation. Fat does not creep or proliferate, so *fibrofatty proliferation* is a misnomer. Prominent fat may be related to retraction of fat secondary to inflammation spreading along lymphatic and venous channels.

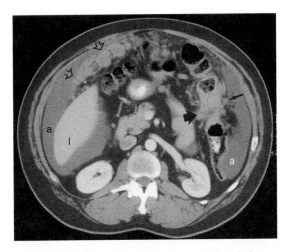

Figure 16-12. CT image shows adenocarcinoma of the splenic flexure with intraperitoneal metastasis. A 4-cm soft tissue mass (*thick arrow*) focally obliterates the lumen of the splenic flexure. Local lymphadenopathy is present (*thin black arrow*). Ascites (*black a*) surrounds the tip of the right lobe of the liver (*l*). Ascites is also present in the left paracolic gutter (*white a*). A soft tissue mass (*open arrows*) infiltrates the greater omentum, representing omental metastasis, the so-called omental cake.

Table 16-1. Comparison of Crohn Disease and Ulcerative Colitis

CROHN DISEASE	ULCERATIVE COLITIS
Right-sided	From rectum, extends proximally
Discontinuous	Continuous
Asymmetric	Symmetric
Terminal ileal changes in 85% of patients	Backwash ileitis in 10% of patients
Aphthoid ulcers	Mucosal granularity
Ulcers on background of normal mucosa	Ulcers on background of mucosal granularity
Severe perianal disease	Colon cancer in larger percentage of patients
Sinus tracks and fistulas	Sclerosing cholangitis in larger percentage of patients
Abscess	

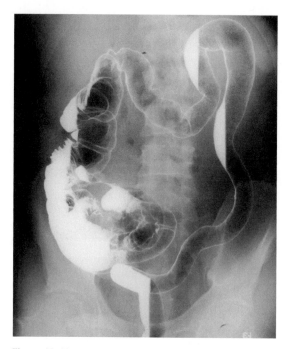

Figure 16-13. Ulcerative colitis. Overhead radiograph from double-contrast barium enema shows that the transverse, descending, and sigmoid colon and rectum have a tubular configuration. The colon is narrowed, and the haustral sacculations have disappeared. The rectum is narrowed, and the valves of Houston are gone. In this patient, the ascending colon appears normal. (From Rubesin SE, Bartram CI, Laufer I, Inflammatory bowel disease, in: Levine MS, Rubesin SE, Laufer I [Eds], Double Contrast Gastrointestinal Radiology, third ed. Philadelphia, Saunders, 2000, pp. 417-470.)

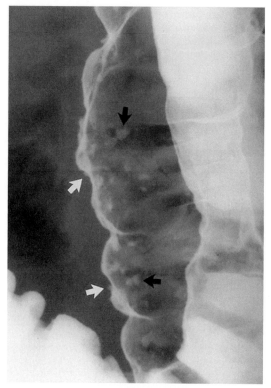

Figure 16-15. Aphthoid ulcers in Crohn disease of colon. Spot radiograph of the splenic flexure from a double-contrast barium enema shows numerous 2- to 3-mm punctate and stellate barium collections surrounded by radiolucent halos. Several aphthoid ulcers are identified in profile (*white arrows*) and en face (*black arrows*). A large portion of the mucosa is smooth and normal. (From Rubesin SE, Bartram CI, Laufer I, Inflammatory bowel disease, in: Levine MS, Rubesin SE, Laufer I [Eds], Double Contrast Gastrointestinal Radiology, third ed. Philadelphia, Saunders, 2000, pp. 417-470.)

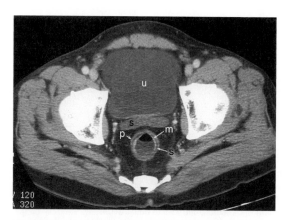

Figure 16-14. Ulcerative colitis on CT. Axial image through the pelvis shows that the rectum is narrow and has a "target sign." The mucosa enhances with intravenous contrast agent (*arrow m*); the submucosa is low attenuation (*arrow s*); the muscularis propria is soft tissue attenuation (*arrow p*). The urinary bladder (*u*) and seminal vesicles (*s*) are identified.

29. What is the most common form of colitis in an outpatient older than 50 years?

The most common form of colitis in an outpatient older than 50 years is ischemic colitis. The most common causes of ischemic colitis are low-flow states, such as congestive heart failure, shock, or arrhythmia. Occlusion of large vessels owing to atherosclerosis or embolism infrequently causes colonic ischemia because large collateral arterial arcs (arc of Riolan, marginal artery of Drummond) can compensate for central vascular occlusion.

Ischemia may occur in any part of the colon; however, it commonly involves the distal transverse colon and descending colon (Fig. 16-17) because these regions are the sites of transition between the blood supply from the superior mesenteric and inferior mesenteric arteries. The splenic flexure region is known as the "watershed" area of the colonic arterial supply.

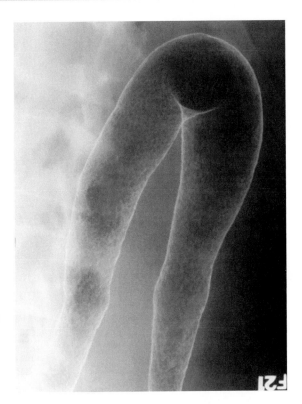

Figure 16-16. Ulcerative colitis. Spot radiograph of the splenic flexure from a double-contrast barium enema shows innumerable diminutive radiolucencies surrounded by linear and punctate barium collections. This very fine mucosal nodularity has been described as *granular mucosa*. It involves the entire surface of the bowel. The colon is tubular in shape without haustration. (From Rubesin SE, Bartram CI, Laufer I, Inflammatory bowel disease, in: Levine MS, Rubesin SE, Laufer I [Eds], Double Contrast Gastrointestinal Radiology, third ed. Philadelphia, Saunders, 2000, pp. 417-470.)

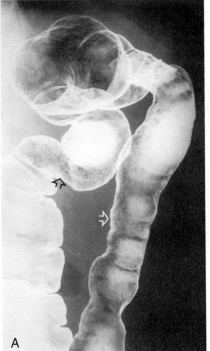

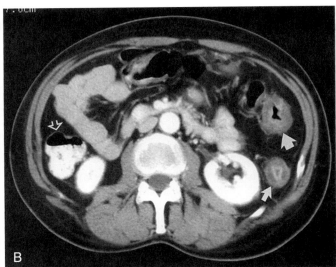

Figure 16-17. Ischemic colitis in a patient with 6 days of left upper quadrant pain and bleeding. **A,** Spot radiograph of the splenic flexure from a double-contrast barium enema shows diffuse narrowing of the lumen, loss of the normal haustral pattern, and fine nodularity of the mucosa (*arrows*). **B,** Axial CT image through the upper descending colon shows a mural stratification pattern in the splenic flexure (*thick arrow*) and descending colon (*thin arrow*). The low attenuation of the submucosa represents submucosal edema related to ischemia. Compare the thickness and attenuation of the wall in areas of ischemia with the wall of the normal ascending colon (*open arrow*). (**A,** From Rubesin SE, Bartram CI, Laufer I, Inflammatory bowel disease, in: Levine MS, Rubesin SE, Laufer I [Eds], Double Contrast Gastrointestinal Radiology, third ed. Philadelphia, Saunders, 2000, pp. 417-470.)

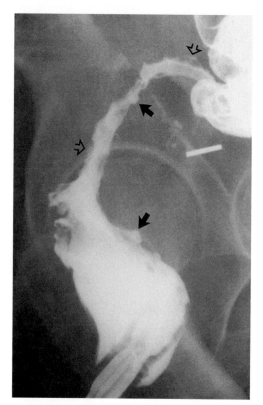

Figure 16-18. Spot radiograph of the rectum from the single-contrast phase of a double-contrast barium enema shows a 10-cm-long, focal narrowing of the distal sigmoid colon and proximal rectum. The margins of the stricture are tapered. The contour is irregular; the mucosa is nodular (*open arrows*), and focal ulceration (*black arrows*) is present. Clips present in the pelvis indicate prior surgery. In conjunction with the clinical history provided, a diagnosis of a radiation-induced stricture can be made. If no clinical history was available, a stricture resulting from Crohn disease, lymphogranuloma venereum, or a rare infiltrating carcinoma could give a similar radiographic appearance.

mesenteric side of the antimesenteric taeniae). The diverticula protrude into the pericolic fat, separated from the pericolonic fat by a thin layer of longitudinal muscle. *Diverticulum* is the singular form; *diverticula* is the plural form. "Diverticuli" and "diverticulae" are incorrect plural forms.

34. Describe the distribution of diverticula.
In patients with diverticulosis, diverticula are found in the sigmoid colon in 90% of patients, in the descending colon in 30%, and throughout the colon in 16%. Isolated right-sided diverticula, although uncommon in the United States (about 4% of patients), are common in Japan. Appendiceal diverticula are found in 0.2% to 2% of patients.

35. What is the primary muscle abnormality in diverticular disease?
The longitudinal muscle layer of the colon is primarily divided into three bands, termed the *taeniae coli*. In diverticular disease, elastin deposits

30. A woman with a history of cervical cancer now has rectal bleeding (Fig. 16-18). What is the most likely diagnosis?
Radiation-induced stricture is the most likely diagnosis (see Fig. 16-18 legend for discussion). Radiation acutely causes necrosis in the bowel walls. With time, blood vessels and lymphatics are obliterated, resulting in chronic ischemia with mucosal atrophy, fibrosis, and occasional stricture formation. Radiation-induced changes in the rectum, sigmoid colon, and pelvic ileum are common causes of gastrointestinal bleeding or obstruction. Radiation-induced colitis and enteritis are most commonly encountered in patients who have been irradiated for cervical or prostatic carcinoma.

31. What form of colitis is sometimes detected when CT is performed to exclude an intra-abdominal abscess in hospitalized patients with fever and leukocytosis?
Clostridium difficile colitis (pseudomembranous colitis) may be first detected on CT in patients with atypical clinical histories and nonspecific endoscopic findings, or when an abscess is to be excluded. The colonic wall has a thick, nodular contour (Fig. 16-19). Wall thickening may be of low attenuation with a mural stratification pattern.

32. Neutropenic colitis (typhlitis) most commonly involves what part of the colon?
CT may show typhlitis in the cecum and ascending colon or distal small intestine in neutropenic patients, in particular patients with right lower quadrant pain and diarrhea. Wall thickening, pericolic fat stranding/fluid, and focal perforation may be detected in neutropenic patients with leukemia, lymphoma, acquired immunodeficiency syndrome, organ transplants, or aplastic anemia.

33. What are colonic diverticula?
Colonic diverticula are protrusions of mucosa and submucosa through areas of colonic wall weakness (Fig. 16-20), primarily where the end arteries perforate the colonic wall (on the

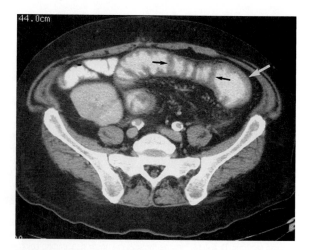

Figure 16-19. Colitis related to cytotoxin produced by *C. difficile*. Axial CT image through the upper pelvis in a febrile, postoperative patient reveals thickening of the walls (*white arrow*) and interhaustral folds (*black arrows*) of the descending and tortuous sigmoid colon.

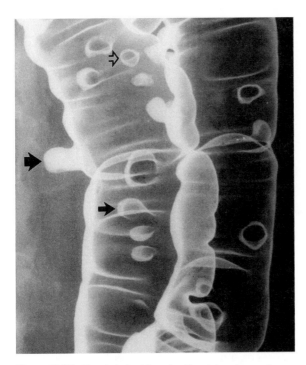

Figure 16-20. Diverticulosis of the colon. Coned-down image of the splenic flexure from a left-side-down decubitus overhead from a double-contrast barium enema reveals numerous diverticula. Some barium-filled diverticula are seen in profile (*thick black arrow*). Most diverticula seen en face have a small pool of barium on their dependent surface resembling a meniscus (*thin black arrow*). Other diverticula are devoid of a barium meniscus and are depicted only as barium-coated ring shadows (*open arrow*). The normal haustral sacculations and interhaustral folds are preserved.

between normal muscle fibers in the taeniae coli. Macroscopically, the taeniae coli are shortened and thickened, resulting in overall shortening and straightening of the colon and redundancy of the circular muscle fibers and mucosa. The circular muscle forms thick, 180-degree bands of muscle that cross the colon. This "bunching" together of the circular muscle layer and the mucosa of the colon occurs particularly in the sigmoid colon. The muscle abnormality is termed *myochosis.* The longitudinal muscle abnormality has also been termed *circular muscle thickening, hypertrophy,* or *bunching.* The term *diverticular disease* implies circular muscle bunching (Fig. 16-21). The term *diverticulosis* implies presence of diverticula with or without circular muscle bunching.

36. An elderly patient presents with acute left lower abdominal pain. The clinical concern is diverticulitis. What examination should be performed?

CT of the abdomen should be the first study performed in most adults with acute left lower abdominal pain. Ultrasound should be the first examination performed, particularly in women of childbearing age, if the clinician suspects disease originating in the ovaries or uterus.

37. Fig. 16-22 is an image from a CT scan in a patient with acute left lower quadrant abdominal pain is presented. What is your diagnosis?

An abscess abuts the sigmoid colon, a finding suggestive of diverticulitis. CT is superior to barium enema in the diagnosis of diverticulitis. CT shows the presence and size of the pericolic abscess and is superior in diagnosing other complications of diverticulitis (e.g., liver abscess, venous thrombosis, small bowel obstruction). CT is also slightly safer than contrast enema. Although most patients with diverticulitis have walled-off pericolonic inflammation or abscess formation, a small percentage (<1%) of patients with diverticulitis have free perforation into the peritoneal space. Barium enema would be potentially dangerous in this tiny subset of patients with free perforation.

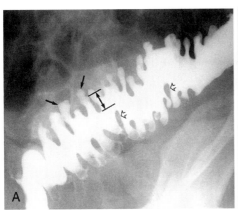
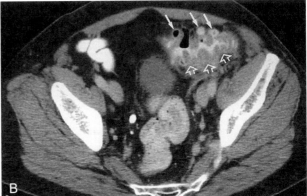

Figure 16-21. Diverticular disease of the sigmoid colon. **A,** Spot radiograph from a single-contrast barium enema shows circular muscle thickening and diverticulosis of the sigmoid colon. The lumen has a zigzag, accordion-like, or concertina-like appearance created by thick folds of circular muscle and redundant mucosa protruding into the lumen. The diverticula (*black arrows*) are small, barium-filled saccular protrusions outside of the expected luminal contour. Representative circular muscle folds are identified (*open arrows*). The height of one thick, circular muscle fold is identified by the *double arrow*. **B,** Axial CT image of a different patient with diverticular disease shows a thick, undulating wall (*open arrows*) in the sigmoid colon, the CT demonstration of circular muscle "bunching." Barium-filled and air-filled diverticula are present (*white arrows*).

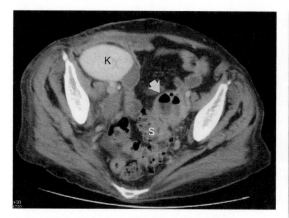

Figure 16-22. Axial CT image through the pelvis reveals a 3- × 4-cm heterogeneous mass (*arrow*) adjacent to the sigmoid colon (*S*). Fluid attenuation and air bubbles are seen centrally in the pericolic mass. A thick rind of soft tissue is at the periphery of the pericolic mass. The findings are that of a pericolic abscess in a patient with diverticulitis. No colonic wall thickening or intrinsic colonic mass is present to suggest a perforated colonic carcinoma. A right pelvic renal transplant (*K*) is also present.

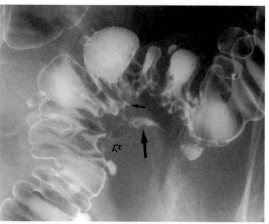

Figure 16-23. Diverticulitis. Spot radiograph of the sigmoid colon from a double-contrast barium enema shows several small barium-filled tracks (*open arrow*) forming a flame-shaped collection (*large arrow*) in the pericolic space. The wall of the adjacent sigmoid colon has a spiculated contour (spicule represented by *small arrow*). There is an extrinsic mass impression on the inferior wall of the sigmoid colon. Compare the asymmetric inflammatory changes with the normal contour of the opposite colonic wall. (From Rubesin SE, Laufer I, Diverticular disease, in: Levine MS, Rubesin SE, Laufer I [Eds], Double Contrast Gastrointestinal Radiology, third ed. Philadelphia, Saunders, 2000, pp. 471-493, Fig. 14-24.)

CT is inferior to barium studies in diagnosing a perforated colon cancer as the cause of the pericolic abscess. If CT shows focal colonic wall thickening, a mass, or pericolonic lymphadenopathy, endoscopy or barium enema may be indicated to exclude a perforated carcinoma, after the acute inflammatory process heals. Some patients with subacute abdominal pain undergo barium enema. The contrast findings of diverticulitis (Fig. 16-23) are the demonstration of air or contrast outside of the expected luminal contour and the extrinsic inflammatory effect the pericolic abscess has on the colon. CT and contrast enema are superior to endoscopy in the diagnosis of left lower quadrant pain.

38. A young woman complains of left lower quadrant pain (Fig. 16-24). What is your diagnosis?

The diagnosis is endometriosis involving the sigmoid colon. Disease in the peritoneal space descends to the rectovesical space in men and to the rectouterine space (pouch of Douglas) in women. This is most commonly seen with intraperitoneal metastases from the colon, pancreas, or stomach in men or ovarian cancer in women. Pelvic diseases can also invade the rectosigmoid colon—primary tumors from the ovary, cervix, or prostate or abscesses related to the ovaries, appendix, or colon. Barium studies and CT are superior to endoscopy in diagnosing extrinsic disease involving the colon.

39. What is defecography?

Defecography is an examination that records a patient defecating a thick, stool-like barium paste. This is a dynamic examination recorded on videotape or DVD recorder. Defecography is also known as *voiding proctography* and is often performed in conjunction with cystography.

40. What types of symptoms are indications for defecography?

Patients complaining of incontinence, painful defecation, incomplete defecation, or constipation may benefit from defecography.

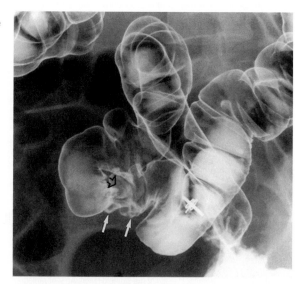

Figure 16-24. Spot radiograph from a double-contrast barium enema shows spiculation of the inferior border of the sigmoid colon (*white arrows*). The colon is tethered, manifested as smooth thin folds (*open arrow*), pulled toward the inferior contour. These are the findings of disease extrinsic to the colon. This young woman has endometriosis.

41. What happens to a patient during defecography?
The patient, if a woman, ingests a moderate volume of barium (500 mL) to opacify the small intestine. If the patient is a woman, a small amount (3 to 5 mL) of thick barium is instilled into the vagina to opacify the vagina. A tiny lead marker (e.g., a nipple marker used in chest radiography) is placed on the perineal body. Thick barium paste that mimics soft, formed stool is instilled into the rectum. The patient then sits on a commode and defecates. The radiologist takes images before, during, and after defecation. The images show the relationships between the small intestine, vagina, and rectum during defecation.

42. What abnormalities are detected during defecography that are not identified during endoscopy or barium enema?
Defecography can show rectocele, enterocele (Fig. 16-25), abnormal anal sphincter opening, abnormal "relaxation" of the puborectalis muscle of the pelvic floor, abnormal rectal squeeze, and varying degrees of prolapse of the rectal or anal tissue either through the anal canal or through the vagina (Fig. 16-26).

43. What study has been performed in Fig. 16-27? What is the diagnosis?
A *virtual colonoscopy* or *virtual colonography* examination has been performed. Carbon dioxide is insufflated into the colon. Volumetric data are collected at CT with the patient in a prone and supine position. Two-dimensional and three-dimensional images of colon are generated. The radiologist has the option to view the colon in various ways, using soft tissue and air windows. The colon can be viewed in any plane, especially axially (although Fig. 16-27A is a sagittal view). The colon can be viewed as a colonoscopist would view the colon—hence the term *virtual colonoscopy*. The CT data are reconstructed, and the computer guides the radiologist to "fly through" the colon as a virtual colonoscopist. The colon can be "splayed flat" and viewed as a pathologist would evaluate the colon at autopsy or surgical pathology.

Fig. 16-27 shows a 1.5-cm pedunculated polyp hanging from the posterior wall of the proximal rectum. This was a tubulovillous adenoma.

44. What are the advantages and disadvantages of virtual colonography?
Virtual colonoscopy is easier for a radiologist to perform. A technologist or nurse gives the patient intravenous glucagon and inserts a catheter into the rectum and insufflates carbon dioxide into the colon. A technologist performs the examination. The radiologist does not have to perform fluoroscopy, wear a lead gown, or take time to perform the procedure. The radiologist only reads the images. Virtual colonoscopy may be more comfortable for the patient than a barium enema because carbon dioxide is rapidly resorbed from the colon. Barium enema digital spot images are about 5 to 10 times the resolution as CT images. A CT scan is of higher radiation dose. CT is the equivalent of a three-dimensional single-contrast barium enema. It is not used to study the en face mucosal detail. During a barium study, the colonic mucosa is viewed in profile and en face. During a barium enema, the radiologist turns the patient to achieve proper luminal distention. Virtual colonoscopy is performed in prone and supine positions and does not achieve controllable optimal distention of each loop. Barium enema requires technical skill on the part of the radiologist. Virtual CT requires persistent diligence of the radiologist in reading the images.

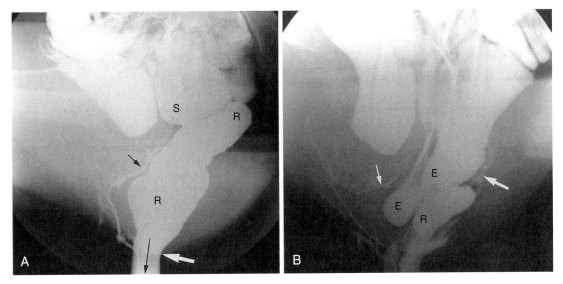

Figure 16-25. Development of enterocele during defecation. **A,** Lateral image of the pelvis at the beginning of defecation shows barium in the small bowel (*S*), rectum (*R*), and vagina (*short black arrow*). The anal sphincter (*white arrow*) is opening normally while the patient defecates paste (*long black arrow*). **B,** Lateral image of the pelvis at the end of defecation shows residual barium static in a small rectocele (*R*). Several barium-filled loops of small intestine (*E*) have dipped deep into the pelvis between the vagina (*thin arrow*) and collapsed rectum (*thick arrow*). This is an enterocele. Enteroceles typically appear at the end of defecation or during straining after defecation.

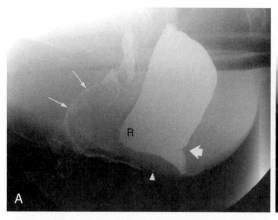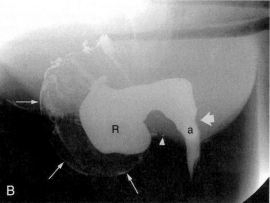

Figure 16-26. Development of rectocele prolapsing through the vagina during defecation. **A,** Lateral image of the pelvis at the beginning of defecation shows a mild bulging of the anterior wall of the rectum (*R*), representing the beginning of rectocele formation. The anal canal has not completely opened, and the impression of the puborectalis muscle (*thick arrow*) still is present. The vagina (*thin arrows*) bulges slightly forward. An *arrowhead* identifies a metallic marker on the perineal body. **B,** Lateral image of the pelvis at the end of defecation. The puborectalis impression has normally disappeared (*thick arrow*). The anal canal (*a*) remains open. The vagina (*long arrows*) and a large rectocele (*R*) now prolapse out of the vaginal introitus. An *arrowhead* identifies a metallic marker on the perineal body.

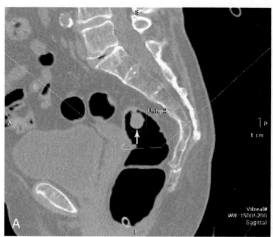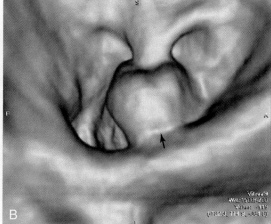

Figure 16-27. Adenoma detected at virtual colonography. **A,** Sagittal two-dimensional image from virtual colonography shows a 1.5-cm pedunculated polyp (*arrow*) arising in the proximal rectum. **B,** Endoluminal view of rectum shows the 1.5-cm pedunculated polyp (*arrow*). (Courtesy of Anna Lev-Toaff, MD, Hospital of the University of Pennsylvania.)

Double-contrast barium enemas are relatively inexpensive. Virtual colonoscopy is more expensive than barium enema and, as of 2009, was not reimbursable from insurance companies as a screening examination in most states. Virtual colonography is being used to evaluate patients immediately after incomplete colonoscopies.

45. What are the indications for a water-soluble contrast enema?
Water-soluble contrast agents use iodine as the x-ray absorber rather than barium. A water-soluble enema is used if there is concern for a colonic perforation because water-soluble contrast material is safer in the peritoneal space than barium. Water-soluble contrast agents are rapidly resorbed from the peritoneal cavity. The iodine is excreted by the kidneys. In comparison, if barium and feces spill into the peritoneal cavity, a severe, potentially life-threatening granulomatous peritonitis may ensue.

Some surgeons prefer that water-soluble contrast agents are used in patients with suspected colonic obstruction because the presence of residual barium in the colon would make spillage of colonic contrast agent at surgery more problematic. Water-soluble contrast agents may also be used in patients who may have a difficult time expelling barium from the colon before it forms concretions. These patients include debilitated, bedridden patients; patients on narcotic medications or medications with anticholinergic side effects; or patients in whom an oral preparation is contraindicated, such as patients with small bowel obstruction.

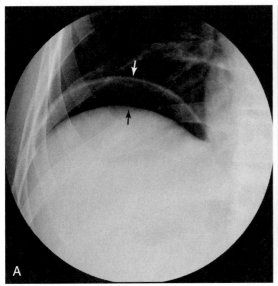 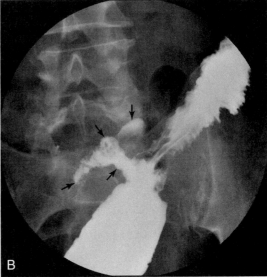

Figure 16-28. Leak at end-to-end colorectal anastomosis 11 days after partial colectomy for adenocarcinoma of the descending colon. **A,** Coned-down view of the right hemidiaphragm shows persistence of free peritoneal gas in a greater amount than would be expected 11 days after surgery. A lucent space separates the right hemidiaphragm (*white arrow*) from the superior edge of the liver (*black arrow*). **B,** Spot radiograph from a water-soluble contrast enema shows a 3-cm-long space (*arrows*) arising from the right lateral wall of the known end-to-end colorectal anastomosis. The space has an irregular contour inferiorly and a lobulated contour superiorly. This collection should not be mistaken for the colonic stump of a side-to-end colorectal anastomosis.

46. A water-soluble contrast enema is performed in a patient with a hand-sewn end-to-end colorectal anastomosis, after resection of a colonic adenocarcinoma. What is the diagnosis in Fig. 16-28?
See figure legend for explanation.

Key Points: Barium Enema

1. Know or have access to your institution's preparation instructions for barium enema.
2. Contraindications for barium enema include suspected perforation, fulminant colitis (toxic megacolon), recent polypectomy/deep biopsy, and latex or barium allergy.
3. A patient with latex allergy should be the first patient scheduled in the morning, after the fluoroscopic room has been cleaned; diabetic patients should be scheduled early in the day.
4. Know the difference between a double-contrast and single-contrast barium enema, and what types of patients are capable of undergoing a double-contrast barium enema.
5. A CT scan is the examination of choice in patients with suspected diverticulitis.

BIBLIOGRAPHY

[1] M.E. Cunnane, S.E. Rubesin, E.E. Furth, et al., Small flat umbilicated tumors of the colon: radiographic and pathologic findings, AJR Am J Roentgenol 175 (2000) 747–749.
[2] P.A. McCarthy, S.E. Rubesin, M.S. Levine, et al., Colonic cancer: morphology detected with barium enema examination versus histopathologic stage, Radiology 197 (1995) 683–687.
[3] S.E. Rubesin, C.I. Bartram, I. Laufer, Inflammatory bowel disease, in: M.S. Levine, S.E. Rubesin, I. Laufer (Eds.), Double Contrast Gastrointestinal Radiology, third ed., Saunders, Philadelphia, 2000, pp. 417–470.
[4] S.E. Rubesin, I. Laufer, Tumors of the colon, in: M.S. Levine, S.E. Rubesin, I. Laufer (Eds.), Double Contrast Gastrointestinal Radiology, third ed., Saunders, Philadelphia, 2000, pp. 357–416.
[5] S.E. Rubesin, I. Laufer, Diverticular disease, in: M.S. Levine, S.E. Rubesin, I. Laufer (Eds.), Double Contrast Gastrointestinal Radiology, third ed., Saunders, Philadelphia, 2000, pp. 471–494.

1. What sequences should be obtained when performing magnetic resonance imaging (MRI) of the liver?

A generic MRI protocol includes axial T1-weighted images, axial T2-weighted images (echo time [TE] range 80 to 120 ms), and heavily T2-weighted images (TE >180 seconds). T1-weighted images are ideally performed with a dual-echo gradient-echo sequence in which opposed-phase and in-phase images are obtained. Contrast-enhanced MR images are useful for characterizing indeterminate focal liver lesions, evaluating the hepatic vasculature, and detecting potential complications of liver cirrhosis.

2. Why does the liver have high signal intensity on T1-weighted images?

It is hypothesized that abundant intracellular protein and paramagnetic substances such as copper or zinc result in the relatively high T1 signal intensity of liver. Most focal liver lesions are hypointense to normal liver on T1-weighted images. T1-weighted images are useful for detection of liver lesions. Focal lesion characterization is usually established with the use of T2 and contrast-enhanced images.

3. Can T1-weighted MR images characterize focal liver lesions as hepatocellular in origin?

There are two ways that T1-weighted images can characterize focal liver lesions as hepatocellular in origin. First, if a focal liver lesion is isointense or hyperintense to surrounding liver parenchyma, it is likely hepatocellular in origin (Fig. 17-1 and Table 17-1). Nonhepatocellular focal liver lesions are usually hypointense to liver on T1-weighted images. Second, if chemical shift imaging reveals loss of signal intensity within a liver mass, the mass has been characterized as lipid-containing, and in almost all cases is also hepatocellular in nature.

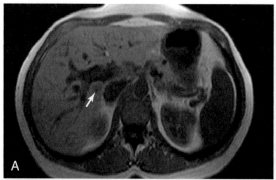
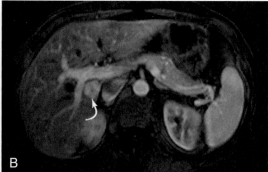
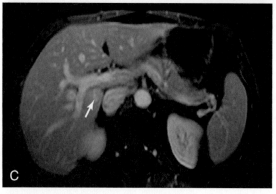

Figure 17-1. MRI depiction of focal nodular hyperplasia (FNH) in an asymptomatic woman. **A,** T1-weighted image shows well-circumscribed mass that has components that are isointense with surrounding liver. A central hypointense scar (*arrow*) is present. **B** and **C,** Arterial (**B**) and delayed phase (**C**) enhanced images show immediate marked enhancement of the FNH (*curved arrow* in **C**), whereas the delayed image reveals lesion washout and interval enhancement of the scar (*arrow*).

Table 17-1. MRI Appearance of Lesions of Hepatocellular Origin

	T1	T2 (TE = 80 ms)	T2 (TE = 180 ms)	POSTCONTRAST	OTHER
Focal fat/focal fatty sparing	Iso	Iso	Iso	Iso	Regions of fatty infiltration lose signal on chemical shift imaging
Focal nodular hyperplasia	Iso	Iso	Iso	↑↑↑ in arterial phase	Homogeneous for lesion size; central scar
Adenoma	Iso to ↑	Iso to ↑	Iso	↑↑ in arterial phase	Oral contraceptive use
Regenerative nodule	Iso to ↑	Iso	Iso	Iso	Cirrhosis
Hepatocellular carcinoma	Iso to ↓	Iso to ↑	Iso	↑↑ in arterial phase	Cirrhosis

Iso = roughly isointense to liver, ↑ = increased signal relative to liver, ↓ = decreased signal relative to liver.

Key Points: Differential Diagnosis of Hepatocellular Lesions

1. Focal nodular hyperplasia
2. Hepatic adenoma
3. Focal steatosis or focal sparing of steatosis
4. Regenerating nodule
5. Hepatocellular carcinoma

Key Points: Differential Diagnosis of Lipid-Containing Liver Lesions

1. Hepatic adenoma
2. Hepatocellular carcinoma (especially well-differentiated subtype)
3. Focal steatosis
4. All other conditions uncommon

---

4. What is the most commonly depicted benign hepatocellular lesion?

Focal nodular hyperplasia (FNH) is the most common benign hepatocellular lesion with a prevalence approaching 1% of the population. FNH is most often detected on computed tomography (CT) and MRI in younger asymptomatic women. FNH is not considered a neoplasm, but instead is defined as a regenerative lesion composed of benign hepatocytes. The etiology of FNH is not fully understood. It is hypothesized that FNH is a reactive response of normal liver parenchyma that forms around a vascular malformation.

5. What are the imaging findings of FNH?

The MRI findings of FNH can be divided into two regions: the peripheral regenerative tissue and the central scar (see Fig. 17-1). The peripheral portion of FNH has components that are isointense to liver on T1-weighted images in most lesions. On T2-weighted images, most FNH lesions have signal intensity in between that of liver and spleen. Isointensity to spleen on T2-weighted images is not diagnostic of malignancy (see question 16). During dynamic contrast-enhanced imaging, FNH shows marked arterial phase enhancement and variable rates of subsequent washout of contrast agent. The central scar of FNH shows low T1 signal intensity, shows high T2 signal intensity, and does not enhance during the arterial phase of contrast enhancement, but does variably enhance on delayed imaging.

The enhanced CT findings of FNH are similar to the MRI appearance. The lesion itself shows intense hyperattenuation during the arterial phase of enhancement with variable degrees of washout on subsequent phases. The central scar remains hypoattenuating on dynamic imaging, but fills in on delayed scanning. CT is less specific than MRI in being able to characterize focal lesions as hepatocellular based on relative attenuation.

Table 17-2. Differentiating Imaging Features of Hepatic Adenoma and Focal Nodular Hyperplasia

FEATURE	FOCAL NODULAR HYPERPLASIA	ADENOMA
Central scar	+++	—
Multifocality	+	+++
Intralesional fat	—	+++
Intralesional hemorrhage	—	+++
Marked arterial phase	+++	+
Enhancement	—	—
Oral contraceptive use	+	+++

6. What is the second most common benign hepatocellular mass?

Hepatic adenoma is the second most common benign hepatocellular lesion. Hepatic adenoma is a true neoplasm. Similar to FNH, hepatic adenoma is most commonly found in young women, especially women who take birth control pills. The incidence of hepatic adenoma has decreased in recent decades with modifications in the estrogen and progesterone content of oral contraceptives. Hepatic adenoma is treated with surgical resection because of the risk of bleeding, especially in lesions that are larger than 3 cm and located in the subcapsular portion of the liver.

7. How does one distinguish between hepatic adenoma and FNH at imaging?

Most FNH lesions reveal a central scar, whereas hepatic adenomas do not. FNH enhances to a greater extent and in a more homogeneous pattern compared with hepatic adenoma. On MRI, hepatic adenoma may show hyperintense components on T1-weighted images secondary to either intratumoral hemorrhage or lipid. Depicting loss of signal intensity on opposed-phase chemical shift imaging can show the presence of lipid. High signal intensity that persists on a fat-suppressed T1-weighted image represents intratumoral hemorrhage. FNH lesions do not hemorrhage and only rarely contain lipid. Hepatic adenomas are on average twice the size of FNH lesions and are more likely to be multiple. In questionable lesions, the use of a gadolinium agent that has delayed hepatocyte uptake (i.e., gadobenate dimeglumine) may be helpful: Most FNH lesions have delayed enhancement (1 to 3 hours after contrast agent administration), whereas most hepatic adenomas do not (Table 17-2).

8. What are the two most commonly encountered benign liver lesions?

Hepatic cysts and hemangiomas are the two most common benign liver lesions. Both lesions have been reported to be present in 15% to 20% of adults.

Key Points: MRI of the Liver

1. On T2-weighted images, liver metastases follow the signal intensity of spleen, whereas liver cysts and hemangiomas are hyperintense to spleen and relatively isointense to cerebrospinal fluid.
2. Most liver lesions are hypointense to liver on T1-weighted images. Lesion isointensity to liver on a T1-weighted image suggests that it is hepatocellular in origin.
3. Metastatic disease is rare in a cirrhotic liver. A focal liver lesion in a cirrhotic liver that shows arterial phase enhancement or is isointense to spleen on T2-weighted images should be considered hepatocellular carcinoma (HCC) until proved otherwise.
4. Chemical shift imaging of the liver is invaluable in diagnosing hepatic steatosis and depicting the presence of lipid within some hepatocellular neoplasms.

---

9. What are the CT and MRI features of hepatic cysts?

Most hepatic cysts are composed of simple serous fluid and have the CT and MRI signal intensity characteristics of simple fluid: very low signal intensity on T1-weighted images, very high signal intensity on T2-weighted images, and persistent high signal intensity on heavily T2-weighted (TE >180 ms) images. Cysts reveal fluid attenuation on CT. Cysts do not enhance after contrast agent administration on either CT or MRI.

Table 17-3. MRI Appearance of Nonhepatocellular Lesions

	T1	T2 (TE = 80 ms)	T2 (TE = 180 ms)	POSTCONTRAST	OTHER
Cyst	↓↓	↑↑↑	↑↑↑	No enhancement	
Hemangioma	↓↓	↑↑↑	↑↑	Interrupted peripheral nodular enhancement; progressive	
Metastasis	↓↓	↑↑	↑	Continuous rim enhancement	Multiplicity
Abscess	↓↓	↑↑	↑	Wall only; regional hyperemia or edema or both	Fever, chills

Iso = roughly isointense to liver, ↑ = increased signal relative to liver, ↓ = decreased signal relative to liver.

10. How are hemangiomas differentiated from cysts on MRI and CT?
Hemangiomas and cysts have similar T1 and T2 signal intensity. A simplified explanation is that as blood enters the enlarged cavernous vessels of a hemangioma, its velocity decreases, and it mimics stagnant fluid. Hemangiomas and cysts can have similar appearances on T1-weighted and T2-weighted images. On heavily T2-weighted images, hemangiomas remain hyperintense to liver and spleen, but become slightly hypointense relative to simple fluid (e.g., within hepatic cysts or cerebrospinal fluid). On dynamic enhanced CT or MRI, hemangiomas show discontinuous peripheral nodular enhancement that fills in centripetally with time (Table 17-3).

11. Are there atypical patterns of hemangioma enhancement on CT and MRI?
Yes. Smaller hemangiomas may appear homogeneously hyperintense during the arterial phase of enhancement. This appearance has been attributed to limitations of temporal resolution, not the spatial resolution, of CT and MRI. To differentiate such a smaller hemangioma from a hypervascular malignancy, one could perform a portal or delayed phase scan.

12. What is nonalcoholic fatty liver disease (NAFLD)?
NAFLD comprises a spectrum of disorders The most common subtype of NAFLD is uncomplicated steatosis, which affects 20% to 30% of adults in developed countries. Risk factors include obesity and diabetes. NAFLD is considered to be the hepatic manifestation of metabolic syndrome. Steatosis is defined histologically by the presence of excess lipid within hepatocytes. Patients with steatosis are usually asymptomatic, but may present with mild right upper quadrant pain or mildly elevated transaminases.

Approximately 10% of individuals with NAFLD may progress to develop nonalcoholic steatohepatitis (NASH). NASH is a histologic diagnosis and to date has not been characterized with noninvasive imaging. One third of patients with NASH may progress to cirrhosis. NASH is the leading cause of cryptogenic cirrhosis.

13. What are the imaging features of steatosis?
Unenhanced CT or chemical shift MRI can confirm the presence of hepatic steatosis (Fig. 17-2). A CT diagnosis is made when the unenhanced CT attenuation of liver is less than that of the spleen. The MRI diagnosis of steatosis is established by showing loss of signal intensity on an opposed-phase T1-weighted image compared with a corresponding in-phase image. CT is less sensitive than chemical shift MRI in the detection of lesser degrees of steatosis. MRI elastography is a new MRI technique that may allow one to distinguish between uncomplicated NAFLD and NASH.

14. What are the imaging features of liver cirrhosis?
Cirrhosis is defined as the presence of regenerating nodules and surrounding fibrosis. CT and MRI can show the presence of regenerating nodules. On MRI, benign regenerative nodules have relatively high signal intensity on T1-weighted images and low signal intensity on T2-weighted images—similar to normal liver. Preferential atrophy of the medial segment left lobe and anterior segment right lobe results in an appearance that has been described as the "empty gallbladder fossa sign." Caudate lobe and lateral segment left lobe hypertrophy can also be present in cirrhotic livers. Extrahepatic findings of cirrhosis that reflect the presence of portal hypertension include splenomegaly, varices, and ascites.

15. What are the imaging features of HCC?
Regenerative nodules obtain their blood supply from the portal vein. As regenerative nodules progress into dysplastic nodules and subsequently to HCC, the portal venous supply decreases, and the hepatic arterial supply increases.

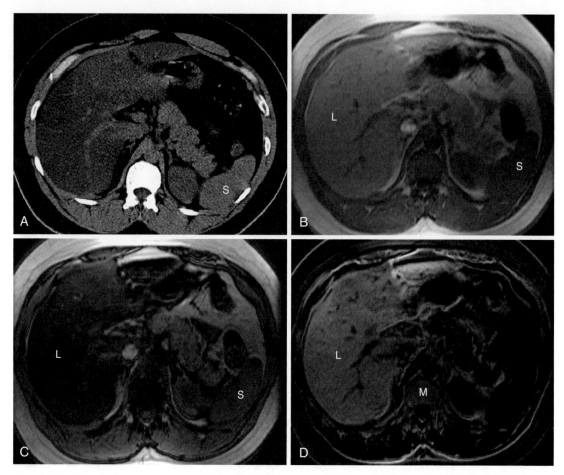

Figure 17-2. CT and MRI of hepatic steatosis. **A,** Nonenhanced CT image reveals that the liver has lower attenuation than the spleen (*S*).
B and **C,** Corresponding in-phase (**B**) and opposed-phase (**C**) T1-weighted gradient-echo MR images show normal high signal intensity liver
(*L*) and low signal intensity in spleen (*S*) in **B**, and variable loss of hepatic signal intensity in **C**, in keeping with steatosis. **D,** Subtraction image
(in-phase minus opposed-phase) depicts voxels that have lipid and water protons as high signal intensity. The variable signal within the liver (*L*)
reflects the distribution of steatosis. Normal vertebral body marrow (*M*) contains fatty and nonfatty elements and shows signal on this image.

A lesion that enhances during the arterial phase in a cirrhotic liver is suspicious for HCC. Focal arterial phase
enhancement is not specific for HCC, however. Hepatic "pseudolesions" have been reported that are depicted as small
foci of arterial phase enhancement. In contrast to HCC, on follow-up examinations they either disappear or become
smaller. These hepatic pseudolesions in the cirrhotic liver may be secondary to arterial-portal shunts or altered
intrahepatic flow dynamics or both.

Other imaging features that favor HCC include lesion multifocality, tumor thrombus in adjacent branches of the
portal vein, and the presence of contrast agent washout on the venous phase of imaging. An additional MRI
feature of HCC is lesion isointensity to spleen on T2-weighted images (Fig. 17-3). Although T2 isointensity to
spleen suggests metastatic disease in patients with established extrahepatic primary tumors, metastasis to a
cirrhotic liver is rare.

16. Describe the CT and MRI appearances of metastatic disease.

Suggestive imaging features of liver metastases include multifocality, internal heterogeneity, and ill-defined margins.
History of a known primary tumor or findings of extrahepatic metastatic disease would increase the likelihood
that coexistent liver lesions are malignant. Hepatic metastases commonly show rim enhancement on CT and MRI.
An insensitive but specific finding of hepatic malignancy on portal or delayed phase imaging has been termed the
peripheral washout sign. This sign refers to the appearance of decreased attenuation (CT), or signal intensity (MRI),
within the periphery of a lesion. Peripheral washout is hypothesized to occur because of increased tumor angiogenesis
with "leaky capillaries" within the growing outer margins of tumors that foster increased entry and egress of
extracellular contrast agents.

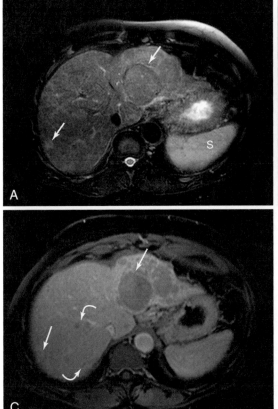

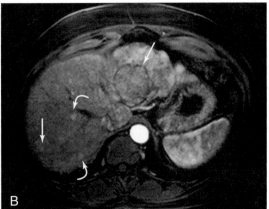

Figure 17-3. MRI depiction of multifocal HCC in a man with hepatitis C. **A,** T2-weighted fast spin-echo image reveals liver lesions (*arrows*) that have components that are isointense to spleen (*S*). **B** and **C,** Arterial (**B**) and portal phase (**C**) T1-weighted images show arterial phase enhancement and subsequent washout within the hepatomas (*straight arrows*). Additional hepatomas are revealed on **B** and **C** (*curved arrows*) that were not well depicted in **A**.

MRI can characterize many liver metastases without the use of a contrast agent. Metastatic disease appears isointense to spleen on moderate and heavily T2-weighted images (Fig. 17-4), whereas benign cysts and hemangiomas appear hyperintense to spleen. Gadolinium enhancement can help characterize indeterminate lesions further and evaluate for extrahepatic metastatic disease.

17. What MRI techniques are used to perform magnetic resonance cholangiopancreatography (MRCP)?
MRCP employs heavily T2-weighted sequences where bile and pancreatic juice have high signal intensity. These T2-weighted techniques do not selectively "enhance" the bile. Any other fluid within the same slice or volume (e.g., cerebrospinal fluid, urine, succus entericus) also is depicted as high signal intensity. T2-weighted MRCP techniques include thin-section imaging (usually obtained in the axial or coronal planes) or a single-projection coronal image that evaluates a 20- to 60-mm slab of tissue.

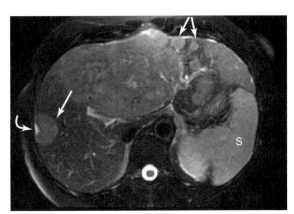

Figure 17-4. MRI of hepatic metastases in a woman with breast cancer. T2-weighted fast spin-echo image shows multiple liver lesions (*arrows*) that are isointense to spleen (*S*). The presence of capsular retraction along the margin of the right metastases is commonly identified in women with metastatic breast cancer who have been treated with chemotherapy. The presence of retraction is not predictive of therapeutic response, however.

The latter is an ideal technique to obtain a rapid overview image of the biliary system that can reveal the presence of duct dilation and or any suspect transition. The thin-section images can better reveal the presence of stones.

18. What are the advantages and disadvantages of MRCP compared with endoscopic retrograde cholangiopancreatography (ERCP)?
In contrast to ERCP, MRCP does not require sedation or bowel intubation, uses no ionizing radiation, and does not result in potential postprocedural pancreatitis. Potential advantages of ERCP include the ability to obtain biopsy specimens of suspect lesions, remove obstructing stones, and stent biliary strictures.

BIBLIOGRAPHY

[1] S.A. Anupindi, T. Victoria, Magnetic resonance cholangiopancreatography: techniques and applications, Magn. Reson. Imaging Clin. N. Am. 16 (2008) 453–466.

[2] R.J. Borra, S. Salo, K. Dean, et al., Nonalcoholic fatty liver disease: rapid evaluation of liver fat content with in-phase and out-of-phase MR imaging, Radiology 250 (2009) 130–136.

[3] G. Brancatelli, M.P. Federle, M.P. Vullierme, et al., CT and MR imaging evaluation of hepatic adenoma, J. Comput. Assist. Tomogr. 30 (2006) 745–750.

[4] Z.I. Carrim, J.T. Murchison, The prevalence of simple renal and hepatic cysts detected by spiral computed tomography, Clin. Radiol. 58 (2003) 626–629.

[5] F. Caseiro-Alves, J. Brito, A.E. Araujo, et al., Liver haemangioma: common and uncommon findings and how to improve the differential diagnosis, Eur. Radiol. 17 (2007) 1544–1554.

[6] J. Choi, Imaging of hepatic metastases, Cancer Control. 13 (2006) 6–12.

[7] C.A. Cuenod, L. Fournier, D. Balvay, J.M. Guinebretiere, Tumor angiogenesis: pathophysiology and implications for contrast-enhanced MRI and CT assessment, Abdom. Imaging 31 (2006) 188–193.

[8] F.M. Fennessy, K.J. Mortele, T. Kluckert, et al., Hepatic capsular retraction in metastatic carcinoma of the breast occurring with increase or decrease in size of subjacent metastasis, AJR Am. J. Roentgenol. 182 (2004) 651–655.

[9] L. Grazioli, G. Morana, M.A. Kirchin, G. Schneider, Accurate differentiation of focal nodular hyperplasia from hepatic adenoma at gadobenate dimeglumine-enhanced MR imaging: prospective study, Radiology 236 (2005) 166–177.

[10] R.F. Hanna, D.A. Aguirre, N. Kased, et al., Cirrhosis-associated hepatocellular nodules: correlation of histopathologic and MR imaging features, RadioGraphics 28 (2008) 747–769.

[11] K. Ito, D.G. Mitchell, E.S. Siegelman, Cirrhosis: MR imaging features, Magn. Reson. Imaging Clin. N. Am. 10 (2002) 75–92, vi.

[12] R.S. Rector, J.P. Thyfault, Y. Wei, J.A. Ibdah, Non-alcoholic fatty liver disease and the metabolic syndrome: an update, World J. Gastroenterol. 14 (2008) 185–192.

[13] A. Shimizu, K. Ito, S. Koike, et al., Cirrhosis or chronic hepatitis: evaluation of small (<or=2-cm) early-enhancing hepatic lesions with serial contrast-enhanced dynamic MR imaging, Radiology 226 (2003) 550–555.

[14] E.S. Siegelman, M.A. Rosen, Imaging of hepatic steatosis, Semin. Liver Dis. 21 (2001) 71–80.

[15] J.A. Talwalkar, M. Yin, J.L. Fidler, et al., Magnetic resonance imaging of hepatic fibrosis: emerging clinical applications, Hepatology 47 (2008) 332–342.

[16] T. Terkivatan, I.C. van den Bos, S.M. Hussain, et al., Focal nodular hyperplasia: lesion characteristics on state-of-the-art MRI including dynamic gadolinium-enhanced and superparamagnetic iron-oxide-uptake sequences in a prospective study, J. Magn. Reson. Imaging 24 (2006) 864–872.

[17] K. Yoshimitsu, Y. Kuroda, M. Nakamuta, et al., Noninvasive estimation of hepatic steatosis using plain CT vs. chemical-shift MR imaging: significance for living donors, J. Magn. Reson. Imaging 28 (2008) 678–684.

CT AND MRI OF THE SPLEEN

E. Scott Pretorius, MD

1. What are the magnetic resonance imaging (MRI) signal characteristics of the normal spleen?

The normal spleen is slightly hypointense to the liver on T1-weighted MR images, and slightly hyperintense to the liver on T2-weighted images.

2. What is the difference between white pulp and red pulp?

The spleen is composed of two tissue types, termed the *white pulp* and the *red pulp,* which are indistinguishable on unenhanced computed tomography (CT) or MRI. The white pulp represents lymphatic reticuloendothelial cells and lymphoid follicles. The vascular red pulp is composed of two distinct circulatory systems, one with slow flow and one with rapid flow. The open circulation of the spleen contains a slow flow filtration system through which abnormal and aged red blood cells, platelets, and granulocytes are cleared from the bloodstream. The closed, or direct, circulation supplies the splenic parenchyma that is exposed to more rapid blood flow.

3. Why does the normal spleen look so bizarre in the arterial phase?

During the arterial phase of contrast enhancement, the spleen appears as alternating, wavy bands of high and low CT attenuation or MRI T1 signal intensity. This has been termed the *arciform* enhancement pattern and is due to variable rates of flow within the two compartments of the red pulp. Variation from this pattern suggests diffuse splenic disease. After 1 minute, the distribution of contrast agent within the spleen rapidly equilibrates, and there is homogeneous, intense enhancement of the entire spleen (Fig. 18-1).

4. What is an accessory spleen?

An accessory spleen is a separate body of normal splenic tissue; CT attenuation and MRI signal are identical to the normal spleen. It is seen in 10% to 25% of patients, usually within the splenic hilum or near the pancreatic tail.

5. What is the differential diagnosis of splenomegaly?

The normal spleen is less than 13 cm in craniocaudad dimension. Splenic volume is a more accurate reflection of splenic size, and mean human adult splenic volume is approximately 215 mL. Causes of splenomegaly include cirrhosis with portal hypertension, leukemia/lymphoma, infections such as Epstein-Barr virus, thalassemia, granulomatous diseases including sarcoid, storage diseases such as Gaucher disease, and myeloproliferative diseases.

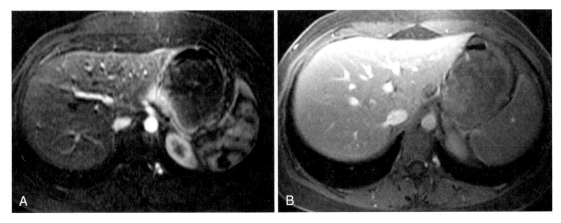

Figure 18-1. A and **B,** Axial postcontrast T1-weighted gradient-echo images in arterial phase (**A**) and portal venous phase (**B**) show normal splenic enhancement. In the arterial phase, the spleen displays alternating bands of high and low signal (or, on CT, high and low attenuation). In a more delayed phase, the spleen enhances homogeneously.

6. What is the most common cause of a small spleen?
Sickle cell disease resulting in splenic autoinfarction is the most common cause of a small or absent spleen. Autoinfarcted spleens of patients with sickle cell disease often appear as small, calcified structures in the left upper quadrant.

7. What does splenic iron deposition look like on MRI?
The presence of iron within the spleen results in low T1, low T2 signal relative to normal splenic tissue. Small foci of iron, termed *Gamna Gandy bodies*, result from intraparenchymal hemorrhage in cirrhotic patients with portal hypertension. Diffuse iron overload in the spleen is most commonly due to repeated transfusion. In contrast, genetic (primary) hemochromatosis, which results from a genetic abnormality that leads to excess iron absorption from the gut, classically affects the liver, pancreas, and myocardium, while sparing the spleen.

8. What are causes of splenic calcifications?
Histoplasmosis is the most common cause of splenic calcifications in the United States. Other causes include tuberculosis, brucellosis, infarct, cyst wall calcifications, and *Pneumocystis carinii* (*Pneumocystis jiroveci*) pneumonia.

9. What is the appearance of splenic segmental infarction on CT and MRI?
Splenic segmental infarction is depicted on contrast-enhanced CT or MRI as a wedge-shaped, peripheral region of marked hypoenhancement or nonenhancement. Causes of splenic infarction include bland emboli, septic emboli, pancreatitis, and sickle cell disease.

10. What abdominal organ is most commonly injured in blunt trauma to the abdomen?
The spleen is the most commonly injured organ in blunt abdominal trauma, followed by the liver, pancreas, and kidney. Splenic laceration generally can be managed conservatively in stable patients (Fig. 18-2).

11. What is a splenic cleft, and how can it be differentiated from a splenic laceration?
Splenic clefts (Fig. 18-3) are congenital, smooth infoldings of the splenic surface, which, in the setting of trauma, may potentially be confused with splenic laceration. Splenic clefts have gently curving, rounded margins, whereas lacerations tend to be associated with abrupt, straight margins and with nearby focal hemorrhage or hemoperitoneum.

12. What are some nontraumatic causes of splenic rupture?
Patients with mononucleosis, viral hepatitis, and coagulopathies all are at increased risk for splenic rupture.

Key Points: CT and MRI of the Spleen

1. On postcontrast images, the normal spleen displays alternating bands of high and low attenuation (CT) or signal (MRI) in the arterial phase. The spleen appears more homogeneous in a more delayed phase.
2. Splenic laceration can be differentiated from developmental splenic cleft. Patients with laceration have a history of trauma, display a low-attenuation defect with sharp edges, and have perisplenic hemoperitoneum.
3. MRI and CT are less specific in the characterization of splenic lesions than they are in characterization of liver, adrenal, or renal lesions.

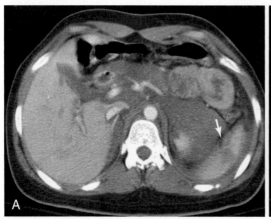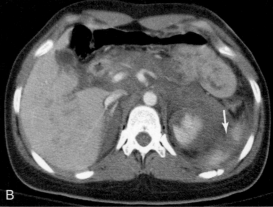

Figure 18-2. **A** and **B,** Axial postcontrast images in a trauma patient show splenic laceration. The hypoenhancing defect (*arrow*) in the spleen has "jagged" sharp edges, and is surrounded by high-attenuation hemoperitoneum. The left kidney is also lacerated.

13. What is the most common CT appearance of lymphoma involving the spleen?

The most common appearance is splenomegaly without focal lesion. If therapy would be altered by a positive result, splenic biopsy may be necessary to establish whether the spleen is affected by infiltrative lymphoma. In some lymphoma patients, one or more hypovascular splenic lesions may be seen, although in delayed postcontrast phases these lesions generally become isodense/isointense to the remainder of the spleen.

14. What is the role of imaging in the staging and management of Hodgkin disease and lymphoma?

Positron emission tomography (PET) and PET/CT are now considered to be the best imaging modalities for staging of Hodgkin disease and PET-avid lymphomas, and for follow-up examinations to evaluate response to treatment. The superiority of PET and PET/CT over contrast-enhanced CT in these diseases stems largely from the ability of PET-based modalities to detect disease in lymph nodes of normal size (Fig. 18-4).

PET and PET/CT are of greatest value in the three most common classes of lymphoma—Hodgkin lymphoma, diffuse large B-cell lymphoma, and follicular lymphoma—because these cell types are generally PET-avid. Some rarer lymphomas, such as marginal zone lymphoma, peripheral T-cell lymphoma, and MALT lymphoma, are less likely to be PET-avid and are generally staged with contrast-enhanced CT. MRI does not play a major role in the staging of lymphoma, largely because the focused nature of the MRI examination does not easily lend itself to imaging of this whole-body disease.

15. What is the differential diagnosis of a cystic lesion within the spleen?

Benign, post-traumatic splenic cysts are the most common focal splenic lesion in the United States. Also in the differential diagnosis are parasitic cyst (which is the most common cause worldwide), congenital epidermoid cyst, and abscess.

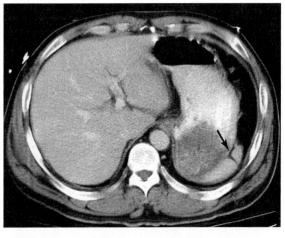

Figure 18-3. In contrast to Figure 18-2, this patient displays a developmental splenic cleft (*arrow*) with smooth, rounded edges and no surrounding hemoperitoneum.

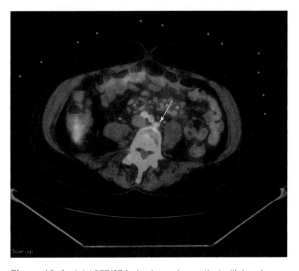

Figure 18-4. Axial PET/CT fusion image in a patient with lymphoma shows abnormal glucose uptake in a small left para-aortic node (*arrow*). The ability of PET/CT to show areas of disease such as this has resulted in the increased use of this modality in the staging of PET-avid lymphomas and in monitoring response to therapy.

16. What is the differential diagnosis of a noncystic lesion within the spleen?

Benign lesions include hemangioma, lymphangioma, splenic hamartoma, bacterial abscess, fungal abscesses, granuloma, lymphoma, and metastatic disease (Fig. 18-5).

17. Can CT or MRI reliably differentiate these noncystic splenic lesions from one another?

There is considerable overlap in the CT and MRI appearance of focal noncystic splenic lesions. History helps considerably, especially in diagnosing abscesses. In febrile patients, commonly patients with endocarditis, a focal splenic lesion with peripheral enhancement is likely to be a pyogenic abscess. Multiple, very small splenic lesions in an immunocompromised patient are likely to be fungal microabscesses, especially *Candida albicans*.

Metastatic disease to the spleen is uncommon. Hematogenous spread is the most common route of splenic involvement, and there is virtually always more than one lesion. Approximately one third of melanoma patients eventually develop splenic metastases. Although they do not go to the spleen as frequently, breast carcinoma and lung carcinoma, being more common tumors, cause the largest number of splenic metastases.

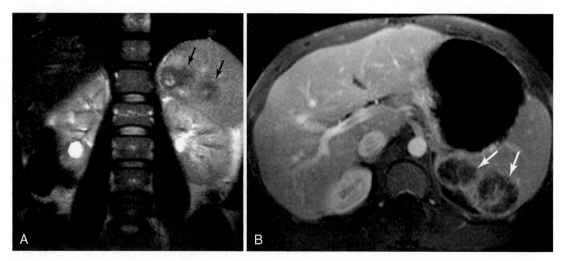

Figure 18-5. A, Coronal T2-weighted image in a patient with colon cancer shows multiple lesions (*arrows*) within the spleen. **B,** After contrast agent administration, these lesions (*arrows*) enhance heterogeneously. These lesions were metastatic carcinoma of the colon.

18. What is polysplenia?

Patients with polysplenia have 2 to 15 nodules of splenic tissue in the right or left upper quadrant. Polysplenia is found in patients with bilateral left-sidedness. Polysplenia is associated with cardiac septal defects (acyanotic), interruption of the inferior vena cava with azygous continuation, bilateral trilobed lungs, bilateral hyparterial bronchi (main stem bronchus lies below the artery, as is typically seen in the left lung), a midline liver, and a hypoplastic pancreatic body and tail.

19. What is asplenia?

Asplenia means absence of the spleen and is a feature of patients with bilateral right-sidedness. Asplenia is associated with more severe, cyanotic cardiac defects than is polysplenia. The inferior vena cava tends to be on the left side of the body, and the liver generally is found in the midline. Bilateral bilobed lungs and bilateral eparterial bronchi (main stem bronchus lies above the artery, as is typically seen in the right lung) are generally present.

BIBLIOGRAPHY

[1] R.M. Abbott, A.D. Levy, N.S. Aguilera, et al., From the archives of the AFIP: primary vascular neoplasms of the spleen: radiologic-pathologic correlation, Radiographics 24 (2004) 1137–1163.
[2] K.M. Elsayes, V.R. Narra, G. Mukundan, et al., MR imaging of the spleen: spectrum of abnormalities, Radiographics 25 (2005) 967–982.
[3] E.K. Fishman, J.E. Kuhlman, R.J. Jones, CT of lymphoma: spectrum of disease, Radiographics 11 (1991) 647–669.
[4] R.A. Novelline, J.T. Rhea, T. Bell, Helical CT of abdominal trauma, Radiol. Clin. North Am. 37 (1999) 591–612.
[5] F. Robertson, P. Leander, O. Ekberg, Radiology of the spleen, Eur. Radiol. 11 (2001) 80–95.

CHAPTER 19

CT AND MRI OF THE PANCREAS

Wendy C. Hsu, MD, and
E. Scott Pretorius, MD

1. **How does a pancreatic protocol computed tomography (CT) scan differ from a routine enhanced abdominal CT study?**

   A CT scan performed with pancreatic protocol images the pancreas with thin sections (1 to 4 mm) before intravenous contrast agent administration, in the arterial phase of contrast enhancement, and in the portal venous phase of contrast enhancement to detect and characterize focal pancreatic lesions. Immediately before the scan, the patient may be asked to drink water, which acts as a "negative" oral contrast agent (i.e., dark relative to the bowel wall and surrounding soft tissue). The water distends the duodenum to help to identify it as a structure separate from the pancreatic head.

   A routine enhanced abdominal CT scan is obtained in a single postcontrast phase (portal venous phase) of enhancement with axial section thickness of 5 to 8 mm. A positive oral contrast agent is used so that segments of fluid-filled small bowel are not mistaken for peripancreatic fluid collections. A routine abdominal CT scan is usually adequate for evaluation of diffuse pancreatic disease such as pancreatitis.

2. **What is the normal morphology of the pancreas on CT and magnetic resonance imaging (MRI)?**

   The pancreatic acini impart a slightly lobulated contour to the pancreas. The pancreas is not encapsulated. In anteroposterior dimension, the pancreatic head measures 2 to 2.5 cm; the pancreatic body and tail measure 1 to 2 cm. The maximal diameter of a normal main pancreatic duct is about 3 mm in adults, not to exceed 5 mm in elderly adults. The duct should taper slightly from head to tail. The main pancreatic duct of Wirsung empties into the duodenum via the major papilla of Vater (also known as the ampulla). In patients with pancreas divisum, the accessory duct of Santorini enters the duodenum via the minor papilla. The major papilla is located distal (caudal) to the minor papilla, along the medial aspect of the second portion of the duodenum.

3. **What blood vessels are found near the pancreas?**

   The splenic vein courses posterior to the body and tail of the pancreas. The portal vein confluence (where the splenic vein and superior mesenteric vein join to form the portal vein) lies immediately posterior and to the left of the pancreatic neck.

4. **What is the normal CT attenuation and MRI signal intensity of the pancreas?**

   - *CT density:* Soft tissue density is variable. Density may decrease with aging because of fatty replacement as part of the normal aging process.
   - *MRI signal intensity:* In the abdomen, the pancreas is the organ with the highest signal intensity on T1-weighted images because of its high protein content. T1-weighted images provide the most contrast between normal pancreas (high T1 signal intensity) and pancreatic disease processes (lower in T1 signal intensity). The addition of fat suppression on T1-weighted sequences eliminates signal of the peripancreatic fat and allows delineation of the contour of the pancreas.

5. **What is magnetic resonance cholangiopancreatography (MRCP), and how does it compare with endoscopic retrograde cholangiopancreatography (ERCP)?**

   MRCP (Fig. 19-1) consists of a series of heavily T2-weighted sequences that depict the pancreatobiliary ducts. Bile and secretions in the pancreatic duct are static or slow moving, and appear intrinsically very high in T2 signal. Signal from the surrounding tissues is markedly suppressed on these types of sequences. MRCP should be performed as part of a complete contrast-enhanced abdominal MRI study, so that important information about the surrounding soft tissues is also provided. MRCP is noninvasive and does not require sedation. ERCP has therapeutic applications, can directly visualize ampullary lesions, and has better resolution for fine detail.

   Gastroenterologists perform ERCP by passing an endoscope into the stomach and duodenum. The endoscope allows for visualization of the mucosa of the stomach. Contrast dye is injected into the pancreatic and common bile ducts to obtain

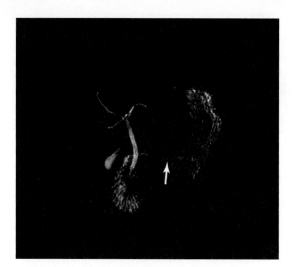

Figure 19-1. Normal coronal, heavily T2-weighted MRCP image. The normal-caliber pancreatic duct (*arrow*) and intrahepatic and extrahepatic bile ducts are well seen. Fluid in the stomach and duodenum also is apparent, which can be a limitation of this type of imaging.

cholangiographic images with an x-ray fluoroscope. Since the advent of MRCP, ERCP is performed less often, unless a therapeutic procedure is planned, such as stone removal, dilation of a sphincter, stent placement, or stricture dilation.

6. When is MRI/MRCP of the pancreas indicated?

General indications for MRI include (1) contraindications to contrast-enhanced CT, such as allergy to iodinated contrast agents or pregnancy, and (2) equivocal results on other imaging study. MRI/MRCP is particularly sensitive for assessment of various pancreatic disorders because of its superior soft tissue contrast, greater sensitivity for contrast enhancement, and direct multiplanar capability. Specific indications include evaluation of ducts and peripancreatic collections in chronic pancreatitis, identification of developmental abnormalities (pancreas divisum and annular pancreas), detection of small (<2 cm) adenocarcinomas including evaluation of a prominent pancreatic head without focal lesions seen on other imaging modality, characterization of a lesion as fat-containing (e.g., lipoma), evaluation of pancreatic transplant dysfunction and vascular complications, determination of the internal architecture of cystic lesions, detection of islet cell tumor, and assessment of organ involvement in genetic hemochromatosis.

7. What normal or normal variant structures may be seen in the portocaval space?

The uncinate process of the pancreas, the portocaval lymph node, and an accessory or replaced right hepatic artery (arising from the superior mesenteric artery) may be seen in the portocaval space.

8. What are the roles of CT in assessment of acute pancreatitis?

Contrast-enhanced CT is the imaging modality of choice for evaluation of complications of acute pancreatitis (Fig. 19-2). CT can detect peripancreatic inflammation, pancreatic edema, fluid collections (phlegmon, abscess, pseudocyst, hemorrhage, ascites), necrosis, splenic artery pseudoaneurysm, and splenic venous thrombosis. The presence of abscess or necrosis indicates need for intervention, specifically percutaneous drainage for the former and surgical débridement for the latter. A CT staging system for severity exists, but it has not been definitively shown to predict clinical outcome. (Prognosis is still best assessed using clinical staging such as the Ranson or APACHE II criteria.) CT is also used to guide percutaneous drainage procedures and to follow evolution or resolution of the disease. Diagnosis of acute pancreatitis remains a clinical one based on symptoms and laboratory values rather than imaging. A normal-appearing pancreas on CT does not exclude acute pancreatitis.

9. Is there an optimal time to perform the initial contrast-enhanced CT scan for assessment of complications of acute pancreatitis?

Yes. The optimal time seems to be 48 to 72 hours after acute onset of symptoms because the areas of liquefaction indicating pancreatic necrosis are better defined. Accurate assessment of the presence and extent of pancreatic necrosis has important implications because necrosis predicts high mortality and requires surgical débridement (see Fig. 19-5). Earlier scans may show areas of pancreatic heterogeneity that are not specific for necrosis in the setting of acute pancreatitis.

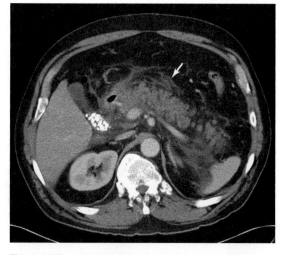

Figure 19-2. Axial CT image shows peripancreatic stranding (*arrow*), a finding of acute pancreatitis. There are multiple gallstones in the gallbladder, which were the cause of this patient's pancreatitis.

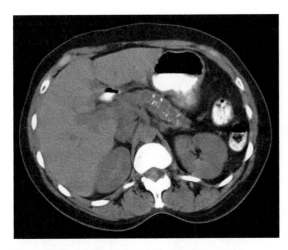

Figure 19-3. Axial unenhanced CT image shows multiple pancreatic calcifications, which are a common finding in chronic pancreatitis. The pancreatic duct is also dilated, although that is generally better appreciated on postcontrast images.

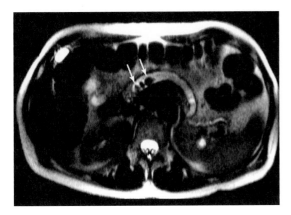

Figure 19-4. Axial T2-weighted MR image shows a greatly dilated pancreatic duct, with atrophy of the pancreatic parenchyma. Several stones (*arrows*) are seen in the duct in this patient with chronic pancreatitis.

10. What are imaging findings of chronic pancreatitis?

Chronic pancreatitis refers to irreversible damage from repeated episodes of pancreatitis. CT and MRI may reveal an atrophic pancreas with fatty replacement and areas of fibrosis and focal calcifications (Fig. 19-3). Irregular dilation of the main duct and side branches, with or without calculi or focal stricture, can also be seen (Fig. 19-4). Complications of pancreatitis that can be seen on CT and MRI include pseudocyst formation, splenic vein thrombosis, splenic artery pseudoaneurysm, pancreatic hemorrhage, and pancreatic necrosis.

11. *True or false*: Pancreatic adenocarcinoma enhances to a greater degree than normal surrounding pancreas during the arterial phase.

False. Pancreatic adenocarcinoma is a hypovascular tumor owing to its fibrotic nature (Figs. 19-5 and 19-6). During the arterial phase of enhancement, the tumor appears darker than the normal enhancing pancreas. This is true on CT, in which the tumor appears hypodense, and on MRI, in which the tumor appears hypointense on T1-weighted fat-suppressed postgadolinium imaging. During the portal venous phases, the tumor may become inconspicuous relative to the normal pancreas.

12. What CT and MRI findings determine unresectability of pancreatic adenocarcinoma?

Surgical excision would not be curative for pancreatic adenocarcinoma if the primary tumor extends directly into adjacent organs (stomach, spleen, colon, adrenal gland) or encases major blood vessels, including the celiac axis, hepatic artery, superior mesenteric artery, main portal vein, or superior mesenteric veins. Distant metastases to the liver or peritoneum also render a tumor unresectable (see Fig. 19-6).

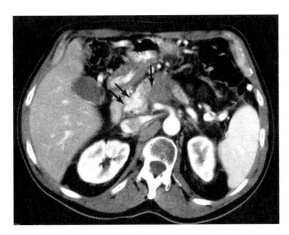

Figure 19-5. Axial contrast-enhanced CT image shows a mass in the body of the pancreas (*arrow*), which enhances less than the normal pancreatic head (*twin arrows*). This is the typical CT appearance of pancreatic adenocarcinoma.

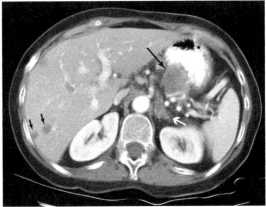

Figure 19-6. Axial postcontrast CT image shows hypoenhancing mass (*black arrow*) that arose from the tail of the pancreas. There is metastatic disease to the left adrenal gland (*white arrow*) and to the liver (*short black arrows*), which means that this patient's disease is unresectable.

Tumor invading the duodenum is considered resectable. Invasion of the gastroduodenal artery does not render a tumor unresectable because this vessel is removed in the Whipple procedure. Because of new surgical techniques such as venous graft interposition, limited short segment, nonocclusive involvement of the superior mesenteric vein may be considered resectable.

13. Why is the "double duct" sign important?

The *"double duct" sign* refers to obstruction and dilation of the common bile duct and the pancreatic duct (Fig. 19-7). It is highly suggestive of a pancreatic adenocarcinoma in the head of the pancreas. About 60% to 70% of adenocarcinomas occur in the head of the pancreas. The "double duct" sign is not entirely specific for malignancy because focal scarring from chronic pancreatitis can also create this appearance.

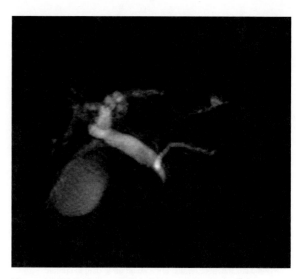

Figure 19-7. Coronal heavily T2-weighted MRCP shows dilation of the pancreatic duct and the common bile duct. This "double duct" sign can be caused ampullary lesions, distal common bile duct lesions, or pancreatic head masses.

Key Points: Pancreatic Adenocarcinoma

1. Pancreatic adenocarcinoma that encases the celiac axis and superior mesenteric artery (or portal vein) cannot be surgically resected.
2. On CT and MRI, pancreatic adenocarcinoma generally enhances less than the remainder of the pancreas.
3. Pancreatic islet cell tumors are usually hyperintense to the pancreas on T2-weighted images and tend to enhance more than the remainder of the pancreas after administration of CT or MRI contrast agents.

---

14. What are the three most common types of islet cell tumors?

The three most common types are insulinoma, gastrinoma, and nonfunctioning islet cell tumor.

15. How does an islet cell tumor typically enhance on CT and MRI?

Most islet cell tumors (about 70%) are hypervascular to the pancreas, enhancing greatest during the arterial phase (Fig. 19-8). Liver metastases, if present, are also hypervascular.

16. How do imaging findings at presentation differ for functioning versus nonfunctioning islet cell tumors?

Functioning islet cell tumors produce hormones allowing early diagnosis based on clinical manifestations and laboratory tests. Typically, they are small and homogeneous in CT density and MRI intensity at presentation. They tend to be hyperintense to the pancreas on T2-weighted images. Nonfunctioning tumors often grow to sizes greater than 5 cm with areas of necrosis before they become clinically apparent. These patients generally present with symptoms related to mass effect on the pancreatic duct and adjacent organs.

17. What is the differential diagnosis of a solid pancreatic mass?

When a solid pancreatic mass is identified, the two main considerations are pancreatic ductal adenocarcinoma and focal scar from chronic pancreatitis. Islet cell tumor, lymphoma, and metastatic disease are also in the differential diagnosis of a solid pancreatic mass.

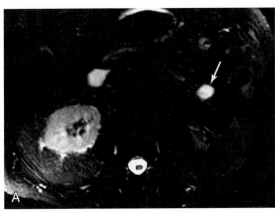 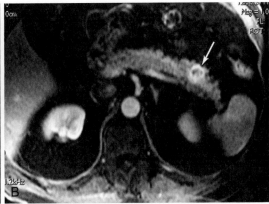

Figure 19-8. **A** and **B,** Axial T2-weighted image (**A**) and axial postcontrast T1-weighted gradient-echo image (**B**) show a lesion (*arrows*) in the pancreatic tail. Because the lesion is very hyperintense to the pancreas, it may be mistaken for a cyst on T2-weighted imaging. In contrast to a cyst, this lesion enhances markedly after contrast agent administration. This is an insulinoma, an islet cell neoplasm.

18. What causes diffuse fatty replacement of the pancreas?

Fatty replacement, either diffuse or patchy, can be a normal finding in older patients. Causes of premature fatty replacement include cystic fibrosis, obesity, steroids, and prior inflammation.

19. *True or false*: The pseudocyst is the most common cystic lesion of the pancreas.

True. The pseudocyst accounts for about 90% of all cystic lesions in the pancreas. Patients often, but not always, recall prior episodes of pancreatitis. In the absence of a clear history of pancreatitis, it may be impossible to distinguish the pseudocyst from a cystic pancreatic neoplasm.

20. What imaging features favor the diagnosis of serous cystadenoma versus a mucinous cystic neoplasm?

Serous cystadenomas (also known as *microcystic adenomas*) (Fig. 19-9) are benign neoplasms that are usually managed conservatively with follow-up imaging. Mucinous cystic neoplasms (also known as *macrocystic neoplasms*) (Fig. 19-10) must be surgically removed because mucinous cystadenocarcinomas are malignant, and mucinous cystadenomas have malignant potential. Serous cystadenomas generally have more than six locules of less than 2 cm each. They may have a central scar, and, if they calcify, they display central "sunburst" microcalcification of the scar. In contrast, mucinous cystic neoplasms generally have fewer than six locules of greater than 2 cm each. They do not have central scars, and if they calcify, it is peripheral mural calcification.

21. What is the most common congenital anomaly of the pancreas?

Pancreas divisum, which is found in 14% of patients on autopsy series, is the most common congenital anomaly of the pancreas. In this anomaly, the dorsal

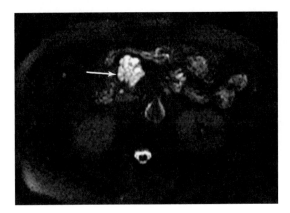

Figure 19-9. Microcystic adenoma. Axial T2-weighted image shows a lesion (*arrow*) of the pancreatic neck composed of numerous small cystic locules divided by fine septations. This is the MRI appearance of benign serous cystadenoma, also known as a microcystic adenoma.

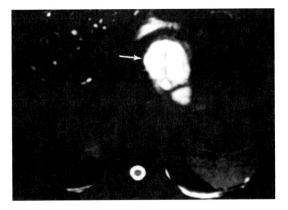

Figure 19-10. Axial T2-weighted image shows a lesion of the pancreatic body and tail (*arrow*). The locules are larger than the locules of the benign microcystic adenoma shown in Fig. 19-9. Macrocystic cystadenomas are considered to be tumors of low malignant potential.

anlage (body) fails to fuse with the ventral anlage (head) so that the larger dorsal duct empties via the smaller minor papilla. This anomaly may result in obstructive physiology related to poor drainage. The shorter ventral duct does not communicate with the dorsal duct and empties via the major papilla. Some authorities believe that pancreas divisum predisposes to recurrent pancreatitis, although others believe that the association is incidental.

22. What genetic disorder results in "bronze diabetes"?

Primary (genetic) hemochromatosis is an autosomal recessive disorder in which abnormal iron metabolism results in deposition of iron in various organs. Pancreatic iron deposition is a late finding in this disease and leads to diabetes. Hyperpigmentation imparts a bronze hue to the skin.

23. What are characteristic MRI findings in primary hemochromatosis?

Iron deposition in genetic hemochromatosis is responsible for diffuse low signal intensity on T2-weighted images of involved organs, in particular, the liver, heart, and pancreas. The pattern of organ involvement distinguishes primary hemochromatosis from secondary hemochromatosis (hemosiderosis), which is iron deposition owing to multiple blood transfusions. Iron in hemosiderosis is deposited in the reticuloendothelial system and involves the spleen, liver, and bone marrow.

24. Which pancreatic lesions are associated with von Hippel-Lindau disease?

Pancreatic epithelial cysts, islet cell tumors, and serous cystadenomas (microcystic adenomas) are associated with von Hippel-Lindau disease. Characteristic lesions in the central nervous system include cerebellar hemangioblastomas and retinal angiomas. Liver and renal cysts may be identified. Patients with von Hippel-Lindau disease are also at risk for developing renal cell carcinoma and pheochromocytoma.

25. Pancreatic epithelial cysts may be found in association with which three underlying diseases?

Pancreatic epithelial cysts may be found in association with von Hippel-Lindau disease, autosomal dominant polycystic kidney disease, and cystic fibrosis.

26. Which portions of the pancreas are most commonly injured in blunt trauma, and why?

The neck and body of the pancreas are most commonly injured (Fig. 19-11). Pancreatic injuries are uncommon, occurring in 0.5% of patients with abdominal trauma. The mechanism is typically blunt trauma to the mid-abdomen, which compresses the neck and body of the pancreas against the underlying spine.

27. What are CT imaging findings of pancreatic injury?

Contrast-enhanced CT is used as a screening modality in patients with abdominal trauma. Imaging findings of pancreatic injury may be subtle with an ill-defined area of low density in the organ and loss of the acini pattern because of edema. A linear hypodensity in the anteroposterior direction represents a laceration. Disruption of the pancreatic duct can be confirmed on ERCP, or increasingly MRCP, and may result in pseudocyst formation. Pancreatitis, abscess, necrosis, and fistula to other organs may develop. Pancreatic injuries have a high mortality rate because they are often associated with other life-threatening abdominal injuries. Imaging helps direct therapy, which may include partial pancreatectomy, pseudocyst drainage, or ductal stent placement.

28. What is an IPMT?

IPMT stands for *intraductal papillary mucinous tumor,* a type of pancreatic neoplasia in which large amounts of mucin are produced, resulting in dilation of the main pancreatic duct or affected side ducts or both. IPMT is most commonly depicted on CT and MRI as lobulated multicystic dilation of a branch duct or as diffuse dilation of the main pancreatic duct. Because of the large amount of mucin produced by the tumor, the ampulla of Vater often protrudes into the duodenum.

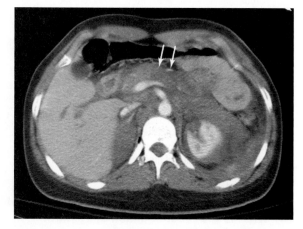

Figure 19-11. Axial CT image of a motor vehicle accident victim shows hypoenhancement of the pancreatic body (*arrows*) relative to the pancreatic neck. In this patient with hemoperitoneum, this represents traumatic pancreatic laceration.

BIBLIOGRAPHY

[1] E.J. Balthazar, R.M. Slone, A.J. Fisher, et al., Acute pancreatitis: assessment of severity with clinical and CT evaluation, Radiology 223 (2002) 603–613.
[2] A.M. Fisher, P.J. Pickhardt, Pancreas, in: R.M. Slone, et al. (Eds.), Body CT: A Practical Approach, McGraw-Hill, New York, 2000, pp. 145–158.
[3] J.N. Ly, F.H. Miller, MR imaging of the pancreas: a practical approach, Radiol. Clin. North Am. 40 (2002) 1289–1306.
[4] R.A. Semelka, L.R. Nagase, D. Armao, N.C. Balci, Pancreas, in: R.C. Semelka (Ed.), Abdominal-Pelvic MRI, Wiley-Liss, New York, 2002, pp. 373–489.
[5] E.P. Tamm, P.M. Silverman, C. Charnsangavej, D.P. Evans, Imaging in oncology from the University of Texas M.D. Anderson Cancer Center: diagnosis, staging and surveillance of pancreatic cancer, AJR Am. J. Roentgenol. 180 (2003) 1311–1323.

CT OF THE ACUTE ABDOMEN AND PELVIS

Drew A. Torigian, MD, MA

1. Why is computed tomography (CT) commonly used for diagnostic purposes in patients with an acute abdomen or pelvis?

Accurate and timely diagnosis of life-threatening disease involving the abdomen and pelvis is essential to decrease potential morbidity and mortality. Clinical evaluation is sometimes difficult, and laboratory analysis and plain film radiographic findings are not always useful in diagnosing the condition at hand. CT scanning of the abdomen and pelvis is a reliable, highly accurate, and fast imaging tool in the evaluation of symptomatic patients; it is most useful in patients with a clinical presentation that is unrevealing or confusing. CT allows for direct visualization of anatomic structures in the abdomen and pelvis, along with detection and characterization of the nature and extent of disease, when present.

2. How does CT work?

As a patient is passed through the large bore of the doughnut-shaped gantry of a CT scanner, an x-ray tube rapidly spins circumferentially around the patient while emitting a beam of x-ray radiation. At each point along the circumferential path of the tube, the x-ray beam is variably absorbed or attenuated, mainly owing to the density and chemical composition of the tissues encountered. The remainder of the beam that is not absorbed and passes through the patient is detected by x-ray detectors and contains data on tissue composition, density, and spatial distribution. This process is repeated at multiple points along the circumferential path of the x-ray tube as it moves around the patient, leading to multiple sets of projection data that all are acquired by the detectors. These raw data are sent to a computer that reconstructs the information into cross-sectional images of the body part scanned and displays information regarding tissue composition, density, and spatial localization.

3. When are oral and intravenous contrast materials for CT administered to patients with an acute abdomen?

Oral contrast material distends and opacifies bowel, allowing for better characterization of bowel pathologic conditions and separation of bowel structures from nonbowel structures. Intravenous contrast material aids in the characterization of pathologic lesions and allows for opacification and evaluation of vascular and urothelial structures. Both types of contrast material are generally administered in all patients with an acute abdomen. In patients with a history of intravenous contrast allergy or elevated creatinine level (generally ≥2 mg/dL), intravenous contrast material is generally not administered, unless the patient has received a corticosteroid preparation or is scheduled to undergo dialysis after the CT examination. In patients with suspected urolithiasis, unenhanced CT without oral or intravenous contrast material is generally performed because unenhanced images are often sufficient for making a diagnosis. In patients undergoing CT angiography evaluation of the arterial vasculature, oral contrast material is generally not administered because it can obscure normal vessels and vascular pathologic conditions during CT angiography image reconstruction.

4. What is the major differential diagnosis for acute abdominopelvic conditions diagnosable on CT?

This is a broad, but important differential diagnosis.
- Inflammatory/infectious causes of acute abdominopelvic pain include acute hepatitis, acute cholecystitis, acute cholangitis, acute pancreatitis, acute pyelonephritis, urolithiasis with hydro(uretero)nephrosis, peptic ulcer disease, infectious enteritis or colitis, diverticulitis, appendicitis, mesenteric lymphadenitis, typhlitis, peritonitis, epiploic appendagitis, and segmental omental infarction.
- Vascular causes include solid organ infarction (liver, spleen, kidney, uterine leiomyoma), bowel (mesenteric) ischemia/infarction, hemorrhage into a cyst (hepatic, renal, ovarian), abdominal aortic aneurysm (AAA) rupture, abdominal aortic dissection or penetrating aortic ulcer, and gonadal torsion.
- Traumatic causes include solid organ injury (spleen, liver, kidney, pancreas), hollow organ injury (bowel, bladder), and vascular injury.
- Other causes of acute abdominopelvic pain include bowel obstruction, bowel perforation, and ectopic pregnancy.

5. What is an abscess? What is its CT appearance?

An abscess is a loculated collection of pus that is typically surrounded by a thick rim of fibrous tissue. On CT, an abscess appears as a loculated fluid collection that may contain debris, protein, or hemorrhage with increased density, sometimes with gas bubbles or septations. An abscess often has a thick enhancing rim of fibrous tissue peripherally. When an abscess arises within a parenchymal organ, multiple small adjacent abscesses ("satellite lesions") are also commonly encountered.

6. What is acute appendicitis?

Acute appendicitis is inflammation of the appendix that occurs after luminal obstruction, and is one of the most common causes of acute abdominal pain. Patients commonly present with right lower quadrant pain and tenderness, nausea, vomiting, fever, and leukocytosis. Early and accurate diagnosis with CT helps to minimize morbidity and mortality owing to appendiceal perforation and prevents unnecessary surgery for nonsurgical conditions that may mimic the clinical presentation of appendicitis. The standard treatment for acute appendicitis is appendectomy.

7. Describe the CT findings related to acute appendicitis.

The most specific imaging finding is an abnormal appendix that is typically dilated 6 mm or more and is fluid-filled. A calcified appendicolith with periappendiceal fat stranding (appearing as ill-defined hazy increased density of the fat) is another highly specific CT finding (Fig. 20-1). Other findings include:

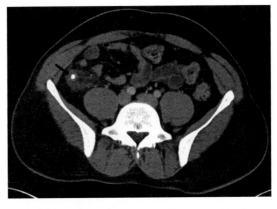

- Enhancement of the appendiceal wall
- Thickening of the appendiceal wall, sometimes with a low-density ring of submucosal edema in the wall ("target" sign)
- Reactive thickening of adjacent cecum or small bowel
- Arrowhead-shaped funneling of the cecal apex toward the occluded appendiceal lumen ("arrowhead" sign)
- A curved, soft tissue density between the cecal lumen and an appendicolith, which is representative of an inflamed cecal or appendiceal wall ("cecal bar" sign)
- Periappendiceal fluid
- Thickening and enhancement of the adjacent parietal peritoneum owing to focal peritonitis

Figure 20-1. Acute appendicitis on CT. Note thickened dilated tubular structure (*arrow*) containing radiodense appendicolith with associated periappendiceal fat stranding in right lower quadrant of abdomen owing to inflammation of appendix.

Complications include perforation with abscess formation, small bowel obstruction, and mesenteric venous thrombosis.

8. What is acute large bowel diverticulitis? What are the CT findings?

Acute diverticulitis involving the large bowel is inflammation/infection in the setting of large bowel diverticulosis (i.e., the presence of multiple blind outpouchings of the large bowel). This condition most commonly occurs in patients older than 65; patients present with fever, abdominal pain (often in the left lower quadrant), and leukocytosis. CT findings include pericolonic fat stranding (Fig. 20-2), thickening and enhancement of an inflamed diverticulum, pericolonic gas bubbles owing to bowel microperforation, and pericolonic fluid. Potential complications include abscess formation and fistula or sinus tract formation from the affected bowel segments to other bowel segments, pelvic organs, or skin surface.

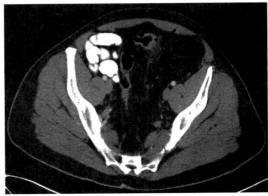

Figure 20-2. Acute large bowel diverticulitis on CT. Note hazy increased attenuation (*arrow*) representing pericolonic inflammatory fat stranding around loop of sigmoid colon and focal air-filled outpouching of colon representing diverticula.

9. **Describe acute mesenteric lymphadenitis and the associated CT findings.**

   Acute mesenteric lymphadenitis is a self-limited condition resulting from inflammation of ileal mesenteric lymph nodes, sometimes with associated terminal ileal and cecal inflammation. It often manifests with right lower quadrant pain and diarrhea, most often in children and young adults. The most common causative agents include the bacteria *Campylobacter jejuni* and *Yersinia* species. Characteristic CT findings include a cluster of enlarged right lower quadrant mesenteric lymph nodes, sometimes with thickening of the cecum or terminal ileum, and a normal-appearing appendix.

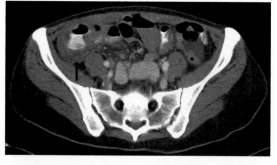

Figure 20-3. Neutropenic enterocolitis (typhlitis) on CT in setting of leukemia. Note wall thickening of ascending colon (*arrow*) associated with mild pericolonic inflammatory fat stranding.

10. **What is neutropenic enterocolitis (typhlitis)? What are the CT findings?**

    Neutropenic enterocolitis is acute inflammation of the cecum, sometimes with involvement of the ascending colon, terminal ileum, and appendix, typically seen in patients with immunosuppression, particularly in the setting of leukemia. Treatment is generally with antimicrobial therapy. CT findings include thickening of involved portions of the right colon, terminal ileum, and appendix, sometimes with a target sign from submucosal edema; inflammatory fat stranding or fluid around affected bowel loops; and gas in the bowel wall (pneumatosis) if there is bowel infarction (Fig. 20-3).

11. **Describe primary epiploic appendagitis (PEA) and segmental omental infarction. What are the CT findings?**

    PEA and segmental omental infarction are self-limited conditions that often manifest with focal, severe, acute abdominal pain and tenderness and are treated with conservative therapy (e.g., analgesics). PEA is related to torsion, inflammation, and ischemia of an epiploic appendage, and segmental omental infarction is related to spontaneous infarction of a portion of the omentum. CT findings of PEA include a small (1 to 5 cm), pedunculated, round or oval fat density structure

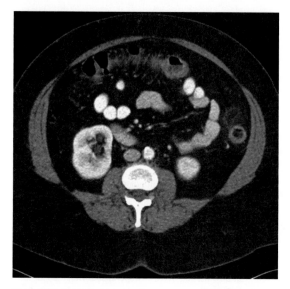

Figure 20-4. Primary epiploic appendagitis on CT. Note small pedunculated oval fat attenuation structure with associated hazy inflammatory fat stranding adjacent to serosal surface of descending colon (*arrow*).

with a soft tissue density rim located adjacent to the serosal surface of the colon (in the expected location of an epiploic appendage) (Fig. 20-4), commonly with a high-density central dot or line from hemorrhagic necrosis or thrombosis of a central vein. Associated inflammatory fat stranding and reactive bowel wall or peritoneal thickening may also be seen. CT findings of segmental omental infarction include a larger (5 to 10 cm), well-circumscribed focus of fat density with hazy inflammatory fat stranding. Typically, the infarction is located in the right anterolateral aspect of the abdomen between the colon and parietal peritoneum at or above the umbilical level (in the expected location of the greater omentum).

12. **What is acute cholecystitis?**

    Acute cholecystitis is inflammation of the gallbladder wall owing to obstruction of the cystic duct or gallbladder neck. This inflammation is most often caused by gallstones (calculous cholecystitis), although in 5% to 10% of cases, gallstones are not present (acalculous cholecystitis). Acalculous cholecystitis tends to occur in the setting of prolonged illness, such as with prior traumatic or burn injury or with a prolonged intensive care unit stay. Most patients present with right upper quadrant pain and tenderness (Murphy sign), although in the setting of severe advanced inflammation, diabetes mellitus, or elderly age, these clinical findings may be less severe or absent.

13. **List the CT findings related to acute cholecystitis.**

    CT findings include smooth or irregular gallbladder wall thickening, generally 3 mm or more in thickness (sometimes with decreased density because of edema); gallbladder distention; pericholecystic fat stranding; pericholecystic fluid; gallstones or gallbladder sludge; and adjacent increased enhancement of the liver parenchyma ("rim" sign) owing to the inflammatory process (Fig. 20-5). Only about 75% of gallstones are detected on CT, but CT has a sensitivity and specificity for the diagnosis of acute cholecystitis greater than 90%. Pericholecystic fat stranding is the most specific CT finding of acute cholecystitis.

14. What is gangrenous cholecystitis, and what are the CT findings?

Gangrenous cholecystitis is a severe, advanced form of acute cholecystitis with ischemic necrosis of the gallbladder wall, which is associated with a higher rate of gallbladder perforation. This cholecystitis occurs more commonly in elderly men and in individuals with preexisting cardiovascular disease. CT findings include marked gallbladder wall thickening and distention, intraluminal membranes, intraluminal hemorrhage (see Fig. 20-5), irregularity or absence of the gallbladder wall, and lack of gallbladder wall enhancement. Gas may also sometimes be seen within the gallbladder wall or lumen, and a pericholecystic abscess may be seen with perforation.

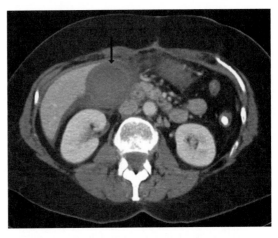

Figure 20-5. Acute gangrenous cholecystitis on CT. Note smooth gallbladder wall thickening (*arrow*), gallbladder distention, pericholecystic fat stranding, pericholecystic fluid, and high-attenuation hemorrhagic fluid within gallbladder lumen.

15. Describe emphysematous cholecystitis and its CT findings.

Emphysematous cholecystitis is a rare, rapidly progressive complication of acute cholecystitis, which is related to gas-forming infection (most often by *Clostridium welchii* and *Escherichia coli*) in the setting of gallbladder vascular insufficiency. Of cases, 75% occur in men, commonly in patients with diabetes mellitus, and are associated with a higher rate of gallbladder perforation. CT findings include gas within the gallbladder lumen or wall (sometimes with involvement of the pericholecystic tissues), along with other CT findings of acute cholecystitis previously described.

16. What is the treatment for acute, gangrenous, or emphysematous cholecystitis?

Urgent surgical resection is the treatment of choice before gallbladder perforation occurs. If gallbladder perforation occurs, typically seen on CT as gallbladder contour irregularity, complications of bacteremia, septic shock, bile peritonitis, or abscess formation may occur.

17. What is acute pancreatitis?

Acute pancreatitis is pancreatic inflammation resulting from autodigestion by activated pancreatic enzymes, most commonly a result of alcohol abuse and gallstones. Patients often present with nausea, vomiting, and mid-epigastric pain, and have a variable prognosis that is predominantly based on the severity of pancreatitis and the presence of complications.

18. Describe the CT findings related to acute pancreatitis.

The pancreas may appear normal in the setting of mild pancreatitis. Findings with increasing severity of pancreatitis include pancreatic enlargement (diffuse or focal); loss of the normal acinar pattern or decrease in density because of edema; haziness of the peripancreatic fat because of inflammation, edema, or peripancreatic fat necrosis (Fig. 20-6); peripancreatic fluid collections (sometimes with gas owing to fistula formation to adjacent bowel or superinfection); and pancreatic necrosis (seen as segmental or diffuse lack of enhancement of pancreatic parenchyma). Fluid collections are often present in the anterior pararenal space of the retroperitoneum, but may also commonly involve the lesser sac of the peritoneal cavity and the transverse mesocolon. Complications may include pseudocyst formation, hemorrhage, venous thrombosis (most commonly involving the splenic vein and superior mesenteric vein), and arterial pseudoaneurysm formation (often involving the splenic, gastroduodenal, pancreaticoduodenal, hepatic, and left gastric arteries) with subsequent rupture.

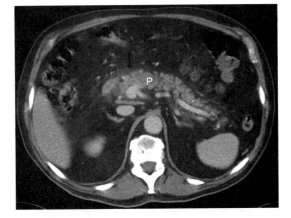

Figure 20-6. Acute pancreatitis on CT. Note mild peripancreatic fat stranding (*arrows*) around the entire pancreas (*P*).

19. What is the CT grading system for acute pancreatitis?

- *Grade A*: normal-appearing pancreas
- *Grade B*: pancreatic fullness or loss of the normal acinar pattern or both
- *Grade C*: peripancreatic fat stranding
- *Grade D*: one peripancreatic fluid collection
- *Grade E*: two or more peripancreatic fluid collections or retroperitoneal gas

20. Describe the normal phases of renal enhancement seen on CT.

The cortices of the kidneys enhance before the medullary pyramids do, and within about 30 to 45 seconds of intravenous contrast agent administration, the corticomedullary phase of enhancement is seen, in which only the renal cortices enhance. A short time later, homogeneous enhancement of the kidneys can be seen during the nephrographic phase of enhancement, when the cortices and medullary pyramids enhance. Finally, after a few minutes, contrast material that is excreted by the kidneys can be seen within the collecting systems, ureters, and bladder during the delayed or excretory phase of enhancement.

21. What is acute pyelonephritis, and what are the CT findings?

Acute pyelonephritis is infection of the kidney; patients often present with fever, chills, and flank pain and tenderness. It is most often due to ascending retrograde infection via the bladder, ureter, and collecting system with subsequent infection of the renal parenchyma. CT findings include a normal-appearing kidney; focal areas of striated or wedge-shaped hypoattenuation in the kidney, resulting in a heterogeneous nephrogram (Fig. 20-7); a "striated nephrogram" on delayed postcontrast images because of stasis of contrast material within edematous tubules; enlargement of the kidney; perinephric fat stranding; and renal pelvic and ureteral thickening with hyperenhancement. Sometimes, associated hydroureteronephrosis (dilation of the collecting system and ureter), renal infarction, or renal or perinephric abscess formation may be seen.

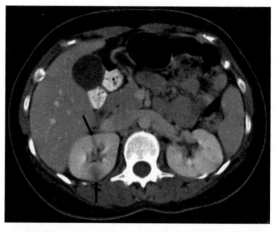

Figure 20-7. Acute pyelonephritis on CT. Note several focal areas of striated or wedge-shaped hypoattenuation (*arrows*) in the right kidney resulting in a heterogeneous right nephrogram.

22. What is emphysematous pyelonephritis? What is the CT appearance?

Emphysematous pyelonephritis is a severe, life-threatening infection of the renal parenchyma by gas-forming bacteria. This condition most often occurs in diabetic patients and is often seen when there is obstruction of the collecting system. Rapid progression to septic shock may occur, and the overall mortality rate may be 50%. The major CT finding is gas within the renal parenchyma, often with radial orientation within the renal pyramids, sometimes extending into the perinephric space, perinephric fascial planes, or collecting system. Associated findings of acute pyelonephritis, as previously described, are also commonly present, and treatment is typically with nephrectomy.

23. Describe the CT findings of urolithiasis along with its associated complications.

Urinary tract calculi (i.e., "liths" or stones) may vary in size from less than 1 mm to several centimeters ("staghorn" calculi) and are typically seen as round, oval, or polygonal foci of high radiodensity within the renal parenchyma (Fig. 20-8), collecting system, ureter, or bladder. Only calculi composed of protease inhibitors in patients with human immunodeficiency virus (HIV) infection who take such medications may be radiolucent on CT. When there is obstruction of the ureter by a calculus, which most often occurs at the ureteropelvic and ureterovesical junctions, CT findings may include dilation of the upstream ureter and collecting system, a thickened segment

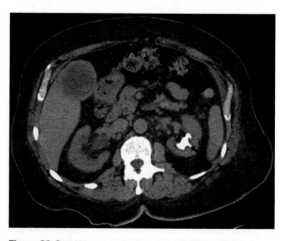

Figure 20-8. Left renal nephrolithiasis on CT. Note polygonal, very-high-attenuation structure (*arrow*) within left kidney owing to staghorn calculus. Mild left renal parenchymal atrophy is also present.

of ureter around the calculus ("rim" sign), delayed enhancement of the ipsilateral kidney ("delayed nephrogram"), perinephric or periureteral stranding, and perinephric fluid or urinoma formation (owing to rupture of a calyceal fornix with urine leak) that shows enhancement on excretory phase images. Scanning in the prone position may be useful in differentiating between a recently passed calculus within the urinary bladder and a calculus that is impacted within the ureterovesical junction because the former drops to the dependent surface of the bladder, and the latter remains trapped within the ureterovesical junction.

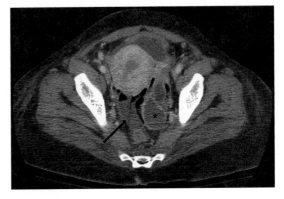

Figure 20-9. PID on CT. Note dilated fluid-filled and gas-filled tubular structure in left pelvis representing pyosalpinx (*), and loculated fluid and gas in cul-de-sac of pelvis representing pelvic abscess (*arrow*).

24. What is pelvic inflammatory disease (PID), and what are the CT findings?

PID is common and covers a spectrum of infectious diseases involving the reproductive tract of women, including endometritis, cervicitis, salpingitis, and oophoritis, along with some more advanced manifestations of disease. Patients typically present with vaginal discharge, pelvic pain, fever, and leukocytosis. CT findings include subtle mesenteric, omental, or pelvic fat stranding with obscuration of normal pelvic fascial planes; thickening of the uterosacral ligaments; pelvic peritoneal or endometrial fluid or gas; hyperenhancement or enlargement of the endometrium, cervix, fallopian tubes, or ovaries; thickening of the fallopian tubes, sometimes with dilation by fluid or pus (i.e., hydrosalpinx or pyosalpinx), and often with ovarian involvement (tubo-ovarian abscess [TOA]); abdominopelvic abscess formation (Fig. 20-9); and perihepatic fat stranding and fluid (Fitz-Hugh–Curtis syndrome). When an intrauterine device is present, infection by *Actinomyces israelii* is more likely and should be considered in the differential diagnosis.

25. List the major causes of bowel obstruction.

The most common cause of small bowel obstruction is adhesions secondary to prior surgery. Small bowel obstruction from hernia is the second most common cause. Other causes of small bowel obstruction are volvulus, malrotation, annular pancreas, endometriosis, foreign body, gallstone, bezoar, and Crohn disease. Major causes of large bowel obstruction include adhesions, hernia, colonic or rectal tumor, inflammatory bowel disease, sigmoid or cecal volvulus, intussusception, and fecal impaction.

26. Describe the CT findings associated with bowel obstruction.

The major finding is upstream dilation and downstream collapse of bowel with respect to the site of obstruction (i.e., the transition zone) (Fig. 20-10). Other findings may include focal bowel wall thickening; mass; luminal filling defect; luminal narrowing or angulation, tethering, or beaking of bowel at the transition zone; a mixture of particulate material and fluid within upstream dilated small bowel, mimicking the appearance of feces ("small bowel feces" sign); and gradual dilution of oral contrast material when passing from proximal to distal in dilated bowel upstream to the site of obstruction. Associated findings of bowel ischemia may also be present.

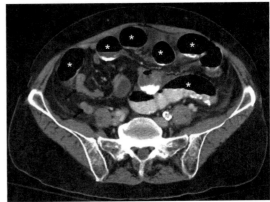

Figure 20-10. Small bowel obstruction on CT owing to nonvisualized adhesion. Note proximal dilated loops of small bowel (*) and distal collapsed loops of small bowel (*arrows*) indicating level of obstruction in small bowel.

27. Describe the CT findings associated with bowel ischemia.

If ischemic change of bowel is present (e.g., in the case of strangulation of herniated bowel), one may see bowel wall thickening often with a target sign, dilation of bowel, perienteric or pericolonic fat stranding or fluid, delayed hyperenhancement of bowel mucosa, lack of wall enhancement, pneumatosis (gas bubbles in the wall of the bowel) (Fig. 20-11), mesenteric or portal venous gas, or free intraperitoneal gas. If bowel ischemia is suspected, one should assess the patency of the celiac artery, superior mesenteric artery, inferior mesenteric artery, portal vein, superior mesenteric vein, and inferior mesenteric vein. When the central superior mesenteric vessels are affected, the entire small bowel, along with the large bowel proximal to the distal third of the transverse colon, tends to be affected. When the central inferior mesenteric vessels are affected, the distal third of the transverse colon, the descending colon, and the sigmoid colon are generally involved.

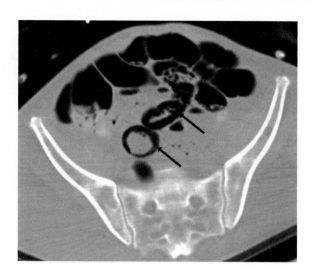

Figure 20-11. Small bowel ischemia on CT in the setting of sepsis and hypotension. Note presence of gas (*arrows*) in walls of several small bowel loops representing pneumatosis.

28. List the major causes of bowel ischemia.
- Arterial diseases that can result in bowel ischemia/infarction include embolic disease, arterial thrombosis, vasculitis, aortic dissection extending into a mesenteric artery, tumor encasement of an artery, and trauma.
- Venous causes of bowel ischemia/infarction include thrombosis, tumor encasement of a mesenteric vein, and trauma.
- Vessel hypoperfusion and systemic shock are also important causes of bowel ischemia/infarction.

Key Points: CT of the Acute Abdomen and Pelvis

1. If you visualize imaging findings of active arterial extravasation of contrast material, shock, or AAA rupture on CT, immediately check on the status of the patient, start intravenous fluids if needed, and get help from your clinical colleagues.
2. Whenever you see findings of bowel obstruction on CT, always evaluate the etiology at the transition zone, and exclude the presence of a closed loop obstruction because this constitutes a true surgical emergency.
3. Always evaluate patency of the mesenteric arterial and venous vessels on CT, particularly if the bowel is abnormal in appearance.
4. If traumatic injury to the kidneys, ureters, or bladder is suspected clinically or on the basis of CT findings, obtain images of these areas during the excretory phase of enhancement to detect urothelial perforation as leakage of contrast-opacified urine.

---

29. What is a closed loop bowel obstruction, and what are the CT findings?
A closed loop bowel obstruction is a surgical emergency and is due to obstruction of bowel at two separate locations along its course. This condition generally arises in the setting of volvulus, hernia, or adhesion formation, and can rapidly progress to ischemia, infarction, perforation, sepsis, and death. CT findings include C-shaped or U-shaped loops of dilated bowel, often with a radial configuration and convergence of mesenteric vessels toward a central focus; mesenteric haziness and fluid because of edema; prominent engorged mesenteric vessels; a swirling appearance of the mesentery and vessels adjacent to the transition zone ("whirl" sign); and beaking and tapering of bowel loops at the sites of obstruction ("beak" sign), often spatially located in close proximity to each other.

30. List the major causes of bowel perforation.
Major causes of bowel perforation include bowel infarction, obstruction (particularly closed loop obstruction), severe inflammatory bowel disease, peptic ulcer disease, diverticulitis, foreign body perforation, traumatic or iatrogenic injury, and involvement of bowel by tumor.

31. What are the CT findings associated with bowel perforation?
CT findings include direct visualization of a site of focal disruption in the wall of the bowel; free intraperitoneal air (when there is rupture of an intraperitoneal portion of bowel); free retroperitoneal air (when there is rupture of a retroperitoneal portion of bowel); gas bubbles, focal fluid, or inflammatory changes adjacent to the site of perforation; and leakage of fluid (bowel contents) and oral contrast material into the peritoneum or retroperitoneum (Fig. 20-12). If secondary peritonitis is present, thickening and enhancement of the peritoneum may be seen.

32. Describe the CT appearance of hemorrhage and active arterial hemorrhage.

Hemorrhage may occur in any portion of the abdomen and pelvis and generally appears as either a focal heterogeneous high-density region or a fluid collection, sometimes with a dependent high-density layer and a low-density nondependent layer related to settling of red blood cells ("CT hematocrit level"). The presence of focal high-density clotted blood in the abdomen or pelvis may serve as an indicator of the source of hemorrhage ("sentinel clot" sign). In patients with anemia, hemorrhage may have similar density to that of simple fluid, however. Active arterial hemorrhage appears as a round or linear focus of extraluminal contrast material with very high density, similar to that of contrast agent within arterial vessels, and is often surrounded by unenhanced high-density hemorrhage (Fig. 20-13).

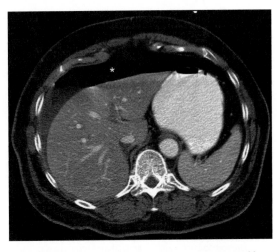

Figure 20-12. Bowel perforation on CT. Note large amount of free intraperitoneal air (*) in peritoneal space along with layering enteric fluid contents (*F*). An iatrogenic duodenal perforation was present more inferiorly (not shown).

33. Describe the CT findings related to AAA rupture and impending rupture.

CT findings of AAA rupture include periaortic and retroperitoneal hemorrhage, sometimes with hemoperitoneum, and active arterial hemorrhage, as previously described. Other CT findings of rupture or impending rupture include high-density hemorrhage within the thrombus or wall of an AAA ("crescent" sign); focal high density; irregular contour, defect, or interruption of atherosclerotic calcification of the aortic wall at the site of rupture; abnormal shape of an AAA; indefinable area of the posterior wall of an AAA that follows the vertebral contour of the spine ("draped aorta" sign); large size (40% of AAA >5 cm rupture within 5 years); and rapid increase in the size of an AAA.

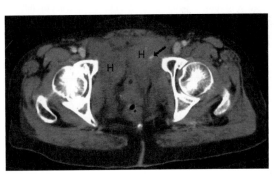

Figure 20-13. Pelvic hemorrhage on CT in the setting of trauma. Note extensive high-attenuation fluid within anterior pelvis representing hemorrhage (*H*) and linear focus of high-attenuation contrast material (*arrow*) that does not correspond with vascular structures, in keeping with active arterial hemorrhage.

34. What are the CT findings associated with shock, and what should one do on seeing these findings?

CT findings include a small caliber of the aorta and renal arteries (related to hypovolemia and compensatory vasoconstriction), a flattened inferior vena cava ("flat cava" sign), poor enhancement of a small spleen, persistent enhancement of the kidneys ("delayed nephrogram"), hyperattenuating adrenal glands, and diffuse thickening of the small bowel with dilation and patchy enhancement ("shock bowel"). Other findings may include hemorrhage, sometimes with active bleeding. When one sees findings of shock on CT, one should immediately check the patient's condition, start administering intravenous fluids, and call for assistance from other clinical staff as needed.

35. List the major CT findings associated with solid organ traumatic injury.

Contusions, lacerations, infarction, arterial pseudoaneurysm formation, and hemorrhage with or without active bleeding are findings that may be encountered on CT in the setting of solid organ injury. Contusions appear as focal regions of decreased enhancement, whereas lacerations appear as irregular linear, curvilinear, or branching foci of hypoattenuation within the parenchyma of a solid organ, sometimes containing gas or high-density hemorrhage (Fig. 20-14). Parenchymal infarction typically appears as focal or diffuse areas of hypoattenuation owing to lack of enhancement, often peripheral in location and wedge-shaped when focal, and commonly with a preserved peripheral rim of enhancement resulting from capsular collateral vascular supply. Arterial pseudoaneurysms generally appear as focal, round, or oval well-circumscribed structures that enhance and washout to a degree similar to that of other arterial vessels, such as the aorta, and may be treated through percutaneous interventional techniques.

36. Describe the major CT findings related to hollow organ traumatic injury.

With hollow organ injury, CT may show contusion; ischemia or infarction; hemorrhage, sometimes with active bleeding; and perforation. Contusion of a hollow organ generally appears as wall thickening with patchy enhancement, sometimes with increased density because of intramural hemorrhage, and often with adjacent mesenteric fluid, haziness, or hemorrhage when bowel is the hollow organ involved. The CT findings of bowel perforation have been described previously. With bladder rupture, fluid-density urine may be seen in the extraperitoneal space (with extraperitoneal bladder rupture) or in the peritoneal space (with intraperitoneal bladder rupture) that opacifies with renally excreted contrast material during the excretory phase of enhancement. With rupture of the collecting system or ureter, similar findings of extraluminal fluid-density urine with delayed contrast opacification during the excretory phase of enhancement may be seen in the retroperitoneum.

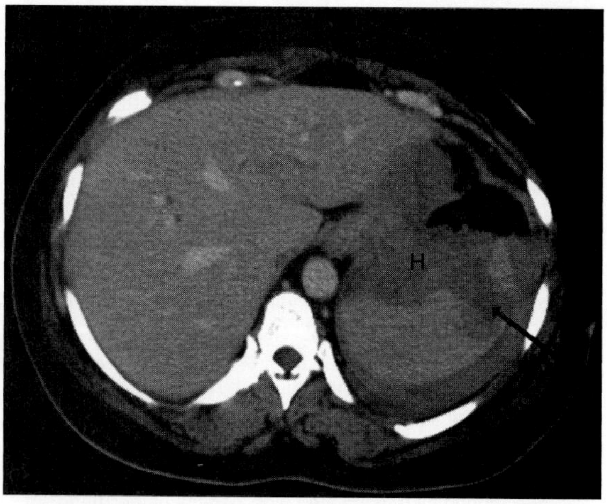

Figure 20-14. Splenic laceration on CT in setting of trauma. Note irregular linear focus of hypoattenuation (*arrow*) within parenchyma of spleen containing high-attenuation hemorrhage (*H*) (which also extends into peritoneal space).

37. What are the major CT findings associated with vascular traumatic injury?

CT findings of vascular injury include an abrupt caliber change of a vessel (indicative of contained rupture or pseudoaneurysm formation); an intimal flap within an arterial vessel; lack of luminal enhancement and enlargement of vessel caliber owing to acute thrombosis; active extravasation of contrast material owing to active bleeding; high-density hemorrhage either within the wall of a vessel (intramural hematoma) or surrounding a vessel; wall thickening, sometimes with an irregular contour; and secondary signs of solid organ infarction or bowel ischemia or infarction, as previously described.

38. What is Fournier gangrene? What is its CT appearance?

Fournier gangrene is necrotizing fasciitis of the perineal, genital, or perianal regions; it occurs most often in immunocompromised men and is due to gas-forming infection, most notably *Clostridium* species. CT findings include gas or fluid or both along fascial planes of the lower abdomen, pelvis, and perineum, often with extension into the subcutaneous fat, muscles, or deeper body wall layers; skin thickening or ulceration; inflammatory fat stranding; abscess formation; and lytic destruction of bone if osteomyelitis is present. Treatment is with aggressive fluid resuscitation, broad-spectrum antimicrobial therapy, and early surgical débridement to prevent septic shock and death. Adjuvant hyperbaric oxygen therapy may also be used in some cases.

BIBLIOGRAPHY

[1] E.J. Balthazar, Staging of acute pancreatitis, Radiol. Clin. North Am. 40 (2002) 1199–1209.
[2] G.L. Bennett, E.J. Balthazar, Ultrasound and CT evaluation of emergent gallbladder pathology, Radiol Clin North Am 41 (2003) 1203–1216.
[3] G.L. Bennett, C.M. Slywotzky, G. Giovanniello, Gynecologic causes of acute pelvic pain: spectrum of CT findings, Radiographics 22 (2002) 785–801.
[4] B.A. Birnbaum, S.R. Wilson, Appendicitis at the millennium, Radiology 215 (2000) 337–348.
[5] M. Boudiaf, P. Soyer, C. Terem, et al., CT evaluation of small bowel obstruction, Radiographics 21 (2001) 613–624.
[6] L.B. Ferzoco, V. Raptopoulos, W. Silen, Acute diverticulitis, N. Engl. J. Med. 338 (1998) 1521–1526.
[7] D.E. Grayson, R.M. Abbott, A.D. Levy, P.M. Sherman, Emphysematous infections of the abdomen and pelvis: a pictorial review, Radiographics 22 (2002) 543–561.
[8] A. Kawashima, C.M. Sandler, S.M. Goldman, et al., CT of renal inflammatory disease, Radiographics 17 (1997) 851–866.
[9] M. Macari, E.J. Balthazar, The acute right lower quadrant: CT evaluation, Radiol. Clin. North Am. 41 (2003) 1117–1136.
[10] J.W. Sam, J.E. Jacobs, B.A. Birnbaum, Spectrum of CT findings in acute pyogenic pelvic inflammatory disease, Radiographics 22 (2002) 1327–1334.
[11] M. Sirvanci, M.H. Tekelioglu, C. Duran, et al., Primary epiploic appendagitis: CT manifestations, Clin. Imaging 24 (2000) 357–361.
[12] B.A. Urban, E.K. Fishman, Tailored helical CT evaluation of acute abdomen, Radiographics 20 (2000) 725–749.

V

GENITOURINARY TRACT

CHAPTER 21

INTRAVENOUS UROGRAPHY

Parvati Ramchandani, MD

1. What is an intravenous urogram (IVU)?

An IVU is a radiographic study that provides anatomic and functional information about the urinary tract. Radiographic contrast agent is injected intravenously, and a series of films are performed to show the kidneys, ureters, and urinary bladder. Other synonyms used for this study are *intravenous pyelogram (IVP)* and *excretory urogram.* Although IVP is probably the most commonly used term for this study, it is inaccurate because pyelogram literally means "a study of the renal pelvis." An IVU provides far more information than just an anatomic depiction of the renal pelvis alone. The term *pyelogram* is reserved for retrograde studies in which only the collecting system is visualized.

2. In what clinical situations is IVU useful?

The major indications for IVU are to evaluate patients with gross or microscopic hematuria, transitional cell carcinoma (TCC), urinary tract stones, and suspected postsurgical or post-traumatic ureteral leaks.

3. The patient I am seeing in the clinic has gross hematuria. Can I send him to the radiology department for IVU today?

Good-quality IVU requires preprocedural preparation. For most of the indications previously listed, it is better to schedule the study so that the patient can receive a bowel preparation. In emergent situations, such as a suspected ureteral leak, the study can be performed without preprocedural preparation, recognizing that the evaluation of the collecting systems for subtle abnormalities may be suboptimal without the bowel preparation.

4. What preprocedural preparations are necessary for IVU?

Preprocedural preparations are aimed at cleansing the colon so that overlying bowel contents do not obscure the upper urinary tract. Colon cleansing generally consists of laxatives taken the evening before the study. Patients are also asked to avoid solid food the day before the study and consume a clear liquid diet instead.

5. When is IVU contraindicated?

- IVU requires the administration of an intravenous contrast agent and should not be performed in patients who have a history of severe allergy to radiographic contrast agents. Severe reactions include bronchospasm, laryngeal edema, or anaphylactic shock. In patients with a history of minor allergic reactions to contrast agents, such as hives, IVU can be performed after preprocedural preparation with steroids and antihistaminic agents (e.g., diphenhydramine). Steroid administration should optimally be started at least 12 hours before the procedure for maximal efficacy.
- Patients with renal insufficiency may have further deterioration in renal function after intravenous contrast agent administration. IVU is best avoided in such patients, and alternative imaging techniques should be used to evaluate the urinary tract.
- Pregnancy is a relative contraindication, with the primary concern being radiation exposure to the fetus, particularly in the first and second trimesters of pregnancy. All women of childbearing age are directly questioned to determine the date of the last menstrual period and to ascertain whether the patient could be pregnant. If there is concern, a pregnancy test is obtained before performing the study. If IVU is unavoidable in a pregnant patient, efforts are made to minimize the number of films obtained and limit the radiation exposure.
- Patients taking oral hypoglycemic agents, such as metformin (Glucophage), should stop taking the medication at the time of IVU and not resume it until renal function has been confirmed as being normal to avoid the risk of lactic acidosis. Current guidelines do not require the patient to stop taking the medication before contrast agent administration.

6. What radiographic contrast agents are used for IVU?

The choice of contrast agent is primarily between older ionic contrast agents and newer nonionic contrast agents. Nonionic contrast agents are iso-osmolar and have fewer minor side effects. It is controversial whether major contrast agent reactions occur less often than with ionic contrast agents. Because of their iso-osmolar nature, nonionic contrast agents cause less hemodynamic alteration and are better tolerated by patients with cardiac disease.

Ionic contrast agents are older agents and are two to three times less expensive than nonionic contrast agents. The hyperosmolar character of these agents leads to a higher incidence of minor reactions, however, such as nausea, hives, and skin flushing. In patients with cardiac disease, there is greater potential for precipitating fluid overload and heart failure with these agents. At present, most radiology departments in the United States and Europe favor the use of nonionic contrast agents for intravascular use in all patients.

7. What is the sequence of radiographs for IVU?

The procedure begins with two plain radiographs, known as the *preliminary* or *scout films,* which are used to examine the soft tissues, bones, and bowel gas pattern. One radiograph is centered over the kidneys, and the second radiograph views the entire abdomen to the level of the pubic symphysis. Scout radiographs are particularly important for detecting radiopaque urinary tract stones because these stones have the same radiographic density as excreted contrast agent and are often difficult to visualize when the collecting system is opacified with contrast agent (Fig. 21-1). In addition to calculi, the scout radiographs are also used to detect renal masses (Fig. 21-2A).

The filming sequence of IVU is aimed at evaluating the parenchyma for masses and the collecting system for urothelial neoplasms and other abnormalities, such as papillary necrosis. Parenchymal evaluation is performed with a series of films called *nephrotomograms,* in which the x-ray tube moves over the patient in an arc with a fixed focal plane that is in sharp focus (Fig. 21-2B). Structures anterior or posterior to the focal point are blurred.

Evaluation of the collecting systems for subtle abnormalities is aided by distention of the collecting system. This requires compressing the abdomen with inflatable balloons so that the ureters are obstructed (Fig. 21-2C). When the compression is released, contrast agent floods the ureters, allowing visualization of the entire length of the ureters. A film is also obtained in the upright position, which is very sensitive for showing low grades of obstruction (Fig. 21-2D). An unobstructed collecting system should drain nearly completely on an upright film. Films of the urinary bladder are obtained with the bladder distended and then after the patient voids. The latter film allows a rough estimate of bladder function and is a sensitive film for showing bladder masses.

8. How should a patient with hematuria be evaluated?

The upper and lower urinary tract of a patient with hematuria should be evaluated for stones, neoplasms, and other abnormalities that may cause hematuria. The upper urinary tract is usually evaluated with IVU, although there is now growing interest in using computed tomography (CT) for this purpose. The sensitivity and specificity of CT urography compared with conventional IVU in diagnosing collecting system abnormalities are still unclear and the subject of avid research. CT is much more sensitive than IVU in diagnosing renal parenchymal abnormalities and in detecting small renal masses. Currently, IVU is the best study to evaluate the renal parenchyma and the collecting system in a patient

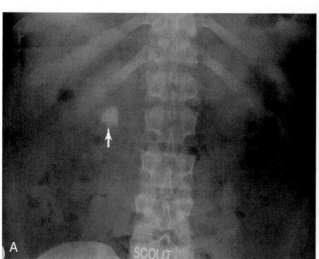
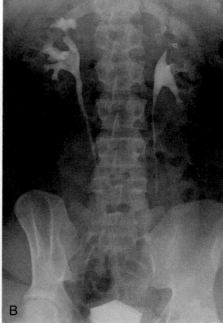

Figure 21-1. Right renal calculus. **A,** Preliminary radiograph centered over the kidneys shows an opaque calculus in the right kidney (*arrow*). **B,** Image from IVU. The stone is largely obscured by the contrast material in the right renal pelvis.

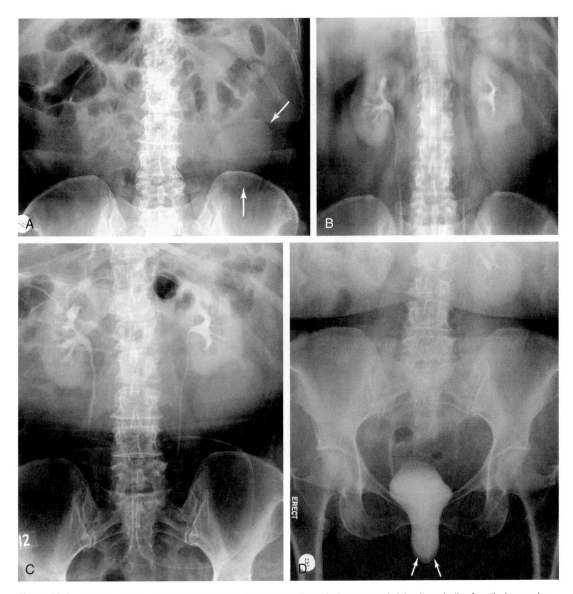

Figure 21-2. Films from IVU in a 78-year-old woman. **A,** Preliminary radiograph shows a rounded density projecting from the lower pole of the left kidney (*arrows*), suggesting the presence of a left renal mass. **B,** Nephrotomogram shows the right kidney to be normal. A mass in the left lower pole is seen well. US subsequently showed this to be a simple renal cyst (not illustrated). **C,** Film at 12 minutes after injection with abdominal compression. Note the well-distended collecting systems and ureters, with the ureteral contrast column obstructed by the compression balloons. Urothelial abnormalities are difficult to detect in underdistended collecting systems. **D,** Erect radiograph. There is near-complete drainage of the collecting systems. Note the descent of the bladder below the symphysis pubis (*arrows*) in this elderly woman with a cystocele caused by pelvic floor laxity.

with microscopic hematuria. The urinary bladder is best evaluated with cystoscopy; all imaging studies are much less sensitive in showing pathologic conditions of the bladder.

9. What should be done if IVU suggests the presence of a renal mass?

It is difficult to distinguish whether a renal mass represents a benign renal cyst (an extremely common occurrence in patients >50 years old) or a renal cell carcinoma on IVU. Any masses detected on IVU should be evaluated further and definitively characterized with a cross-sectional technique, such as renal ultrasound (US), precontrast and postcontrast CT, or renal magnetic resonance imaging (MRI).

10. My patient has presented with diffuse lung metastases and gross hematuria. Should I evaluate him with IVU to look for a renal malignancy?

When looking for a primary renal tumor, CT or MRI is preferable to IVU because they are more sensitive in detecting small masses. Lesions less than 2 to 3 cm in size are difficult to detect on IVU.

11. Why is IVU necessary in patients with TCC of the urinary bladder?

TCC is 50 times more common in the urinary bladder than in the upper urinary tract. TCC is a multifocal process, however, and upper urinary tract involvement occurs in 3% to 4% of patients with bladder TCC, either synchronously at the time of bladder cancer diagnosis or in a metachronous fashion. The upper urinary tract of patients with bladder cancer must be kept under close surveillance, usually with periodic IVUs. Patients with upper urinary tract TCC have a 30% to 40% incidence of TCC involving the opposite side.

12. What does TCC look like on radiographic studies?

Persistent filling defects in the pyelocalyceal system or the ureters are the most common finding (Fig. 21-3). With larger lesions, there may be obstruction of the ipsilateral collecting system by the tumor mass or blood clot.

13. What do stones look like on IVU?

Approximately 85% of urinary tract stones are composed of calcium oxalate and are radiopaque on plain abdominal films (see Fig. 21-1A). Ten percent of stones are composed of uric acid and are either nonopaque or very faintly opaque on abdominal films. Nonopaque stones are invisible on plain radiographs, but are seen as filling defects in the contrast-opacified collecting system. Stones associated with chronic or recurrent infection can grow to fill the entire collecting system (known as "staghorn stones") (Fig. 21-4). Other stone compositions, such as cystine and xanthine, are less common. All stones, regardless of their composition, are dense on CT and echogenic on US. The terms *radiopaque* and *nonopaque,* when used to describe urinary stones, apply only to the appearance of stones on plain abdominal radiographs.

14. Is a filling defect in the collecting system diagnostic of TCC?

No. Other pathologic conditions that can cause a filling defect are nonopaque stones, blood clots, fungus balls in patients with a fungal urinary tract infection (UTI), and subepithelial cysts associated with chronic infection or inflammation.

15. How do I distinguish between these different pathologic conditions?

If a filling defect is detected in the collecting system, a brush biopsy is the next step, so that cytopathologic analysis can be performed. Nonopaque stones are mobile, whereas blood clots are always associated with gross hematuria. Fungus balls occur in immunocompromised patients with a fungal UTI.

Key Points: Intravenous Urogram

1. All urinary stones are dense on CT scans, including stones that are radiolucent (and undetectable) on plain radiographs.
2. A renal mass detected on IVU should be characterized further by cross-sectional imaging.
3. Patients with suspected acute renal colic are best evaluated with noncontrast CT rather than IVU.

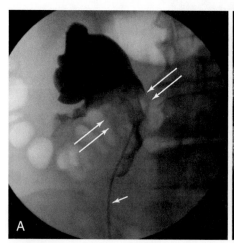
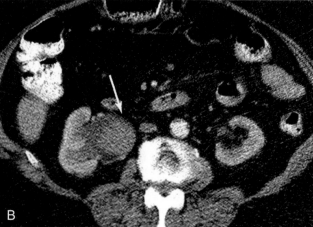

Figure 21-3. TCC in the right kidney. **A,** Image from a retrograde pyelogram shows an irregular filling defect in the right renal pelvis and proximal ureter (*arrows*). The collecting system above the mass is dilated. Note the right retrograde catheter (*single arrow*) in place for the contrast agent injection. A brush biopsy was performed using this catheter later in the study. **B,** CT scan in the same patient shows a large mass in the right renal pelvis (*arrow*) that corresponds to the abnormality seen on the retrograde pyelogram.

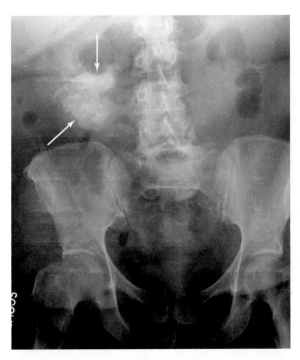

Figure 21-4. Staghorn calculus within the right kidney, occupying a large part of the collecting system (*arrows*). These stones are usually related to chronic UTI and are composed of ammonium magnesium calcium phosphate.

16. My patient has severe flank pain after hiking all day in 100° F weather. What study should I order to exclude renal colic as a cause of his flank pain?
CT is the diagnostic modality of choice in evaluating patients who are suspected to have acute renal colic resulting from a stone. No intravenous or oral contrast administration is necessary. Nearly all stones larger than 2 to 3 mm are visible on CT.

17. What abnormalities are seen on IVU in a patient with acute renal colic?
A stone may be visible on the scout radiograph, although calcified phleboliths in the pelvis can be confounding (Fig. 21-5A). Phleboliths are small calcifications in pelvic veins that may be difficult to distinguish from ureteral stones on plain radiographs (and noncontrast CT), but should lie outside the opacified ureter on IVU and excretory phase CT. Obstruction resulting from a stone causes a delay in excretion of contrast agent and delayed drainage of contrast agent from the collecting system and ureter (Fig. 21-5B-D).

18. Because CT detects all stones, when is IVU necessary in patients with urinary tract stones?
IVU is helpful in showing the anatomy of the urinary tract in patients with recurrent stones, in patients in whom stone passage is arrested in the ureter, and in patients in whom surgical intervention is being considered to treat the stones. In such cases, IVU helps identify congenital or acquired abnormalities that may be potentiating stone formation, collecting system damage related to chronic stone disease, and ureteral strictures that may prevent spontaneous passage of stones. Stones that are smaller than 5 to 6 mm almost always pass spontaneously, whereas larger stones may require surgical intervention.

IVU may also show abnormalities, such as medullary nephrocalcinosis, that may be contributing to recurrent stone disease. Clustered calcifications are present in the medullary pyramids in patients with medullary nephrocalcinosis, which can be due to medullary sponge kidney, renal tubular acidosis, or hyperparathyroidism—the latter two diagnoses are made on clinical grounds, but medullary sponge kidney, in which the collecting ducts are dilated and prone to form stones, can be diagnosed only by IVU.

19. My patient is 2 days postsurgery for an abdominal tumor, and the surgical drains are putting out a lot of yellow fluid. What should I do?
Collecting system or ureteral injury can be iatrogenic or related to blunt or penetrating abdominal trauma. This patient can be evaluated either with IVU or contrast-enhanced CT with imaging in the excretory phase. Both studies would show contrast leakage from the collecting system into the retroperitoneal tissues in the region of injury.

20. Is there a role for IVU in evaluating patients with abdominal masses?
IVU offers information about the retroperitoneum only in an indirect manner. Displacement of the kidney or ureter may suggest the presence of a mass. A cross-sectional study such as CT or MRI is preferable when a potential mass is being investigated. Retroperitoneal masses may be detected, however, on IVU performed for other reasons (Fig. 21-6). Careful attention should be paid to the course and position of the kidneys and ureters when evaluating IVU.

21. What is the role of IVU in a patient with suspected urinary tract obstruction?
If the patient has renal insufficiency with elevation in the serum creatinine level, administration of a contrast agent is contraindicated. Renal US is the best study to evaluate such a patient for a dilated collecting system, which would indicate obstruction. Isotope renal scan may also be useful in this clinical scenario. Nondilated obstructive uropathy is rare. In patients with normal renal function and suspected obstruction, renal US and isotope renal scan remain the mainstays for evaluation. In an occasional patient with equivocal results from other diagnostic tests, IVU may help. Prompt and symmetric excretion on the two sides and complete drainage of the collecting systems on an erector postvoid radiograph effectively exclude significant urinary obstruction. In postoperative patients in whom urinary diversion has been performed, a study in the first few months after surgery serves as a baseline to exclude strictures at the ureteral anastomosis site.

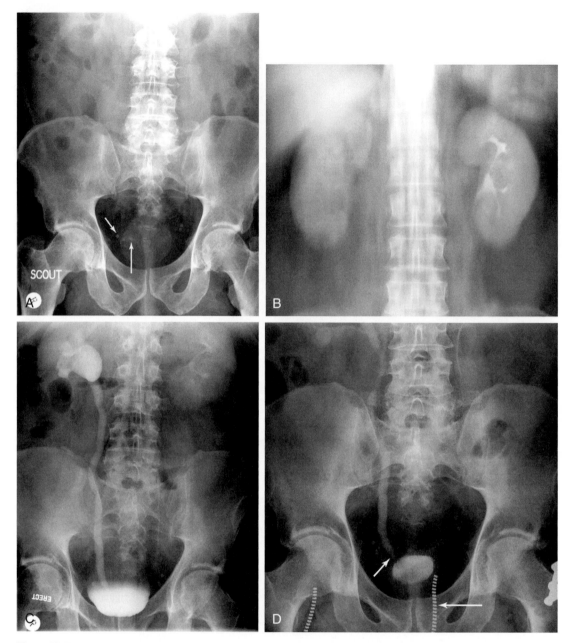

Figure 21-5. Right ureteral calculus with partial obstruction. **A,** Preliminary radiograph. Multiple calcific densities are seen in the pelvis in this patient with right flank pain. The *long arrow* marks the irregular, right distal ureteral stone. The other densities, including the one marked by the *short arrow,* represent smoothly rounded calcified phleboliths. **B,** Nephrotomogram shows delayed excretion from the right kidney. The left kidney is normal in appearance (compare with Fig. 21-2B with symmetric excretion on both sides). **C,** Erect radiograph shows a column of contrast material in the dilated right collecting system and ureter to the level of the bladder. The stone seen on the preliminary film is obscured on this image. Note the near-complete drainage of contrast material from the normal left collecting system. **D,** Postvoid radiograph shows continuing ureteral dilation to the level of the stone (*short arrow*). The other densities seen on the preliminary image are outside of the contrast-filled ureter, indicating that they are phleboliths. Note trouser zipper (*long arrow*).

22. Is IVU useful in patients with UTIs?

In patients with clinically suspected acute pyelonephritis, IVU has no role in diagnosis because the study results are usually normal, and neither confirm nor refute the clinical suspicion. In patients with chronic or recurrent UTIs, IVU may show a congenital abnormality or an obstructive lesion such as a stricture that may be contributory to the refractory UTI. Scarring of the parenchyma and calyces may confirm the diagnosis. Reflux nephropathy typically results in polar parenchymal scarring, particularly in the upper poles. In infections such as tuberculosis, cavitary changes may be seen in the renal papillae in association with strictures in the infundibula and parenchymal calcifications, which clinch the diagnosis.

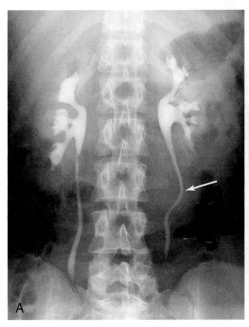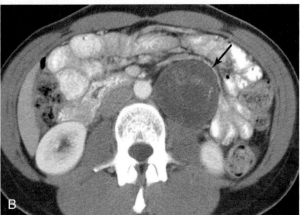

Figure 21-6. Left ureteral deviation by a retroperitoneal mass. **A,** Image from IVU shows focal lateral deviation of the left lumbar ureter (*arrow*). This deviation indicates the presence of a retroperitoneal mass and should prompt further imaging with CT or MRI to evaluate the retroperitoneum. **B,** Contrast-enhanced CT scan shows a large retroperitoneal mass (*arrow*) that proved to be a paraganglioma.

BIBLIOGRAPHY

[1] P.L. Choyke, H. Hricak, P.J. Kenney, et al., The future of research in genitourinary radiology: through the looking glass—a view from the Society of Uroradiology, Radiology 207 (1998) 3–6.

[2] R.B. Dyer, M.Y. Chen, R.J. Zagoria, Intravenous urography: technique and interpretation, Radiographics 21 (2001) 799–824.

[3] R.C. Smith, M. Verga, S. McCarthy, A.T. Rosenfield, Diagnosis of acute flank pain: value of unenhanced helical CT, AJR Am. J. Roentgenol. 166 (1996) 97–101.

CHAPTER 22

GENITOURINARY FLUOROSCOPIC EXAMINATIONS

Parvati Ramchandani, MD

1. What are genitourinary fluoroscopic examinations?

Genitourinary fluoroscopic examinations are studies that require "real-time" observation using fluoroscopy so that maximal information is obtained about the anatomy of the structure being studied; some studies also provide physiologic information about function. Contrast agent is injected into the various portions of the urinary tract for these examinations. Examples are retrograde pyelograms for evaluation of the upper urinary tract, cystogram or voiding cystourethrogram (VCUG) to evaluate the lower urinary tract, retrograde urethrogram (RUG) to evaluate the urethra, and hysterosalpingogram to evaluate the uterus and fallopian tubes.

2. How are retrograde pyelograms and intravenous urograms (IVUs) different? Do they provide the same information?

For a retrograde pyelogram, cystoscopy is performed (most often by a urologist), and a catheter is placed into the renal pelvis. Contrast agent is injected through this catheter under fluoroscopic guidance to evaluate the lumen of the pyelocalyceal system and the ureter for mucosal abnormalities, such as transitional cell carcinoma.

As discussed in Chapter 21, IVU requires intravenous administration of contrast agent, and it provides physiologic information about the function of the kidney, in addition to depicting the anatomy of the renal parenchyma and the collecting systems. A retrograde pyelogram provides only anatomic information about the lumen of the collecting system, but the depiction of the anatomy is superior to that seen with IVU.

A retrograde pyelogram is performed if the patient cannot receive an intravenous contrast agent because of renal insufficiency or a history of severe contrast agent allergy. Retrograde examination can also be performed if IVU fails to show the entire pyelocalyceal system or ureter or to evaluate further an abnormality seen on IVU.

3. What is the difference between a cystogram and VCUG?

A cystogram is tailored to evaluate the urinary bladder alone, whereas VCUG includes evaluation of the bladder neck and urethra under fluoroscopic observation. Both studies require injection of radiographic contrast agent into the urinary bladder through either an indwelling bladder drainage catheter or a catheter placed in the urinary bladder solely for the procedure. A cystogram is limited to images of the bladder, whereas in VCUG, the catheter is removed after the bladder has been distended with contrast agent, and the patient voids under fluoroscopic observation so that the bladder neck and urethra can also be evaluated.

4. What are the indications for cystogram and VCUG?

These studies can be performed to evaluate the anatomy of the bladder and urethra in patients with voiding dysfunction or recurrent urinary tract infections (UTIs) (Fig. 22-1), to look for a leak or fistula from the bladder after surgery or abdominal trauma (Fig. 22-2),

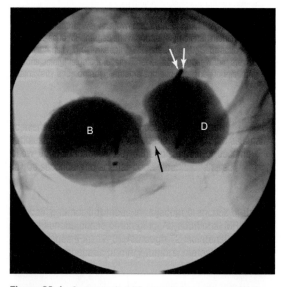

Figure 22-1. Cystogram in a 70-year-old man with complaints of incomplete emptying. There is a large bladder diverticulum (*D*) arising from the left side of the urinary bladder (*B*) with a wide neck (*single arrow*). When the patient voids, contrast agent (and urine) fills the diverticulum and then flows back into the urinary bladder when voiding stops, accounting for the patient's symptoms of incomplete emptying. The urine stasis in a bladder diverticulum can be associated with the formation of stones or recurrent UTIs. The *double arrows* point to a surgical clip in the pelvis from a previous surgery.

to evaluate vesicoureteral reflux (VUR), or to evaluate urinary incontinence.

5. Is a cystogram sensitive in excluding a leak from the bladder?

Yes, but only if the study is performed in the correct manner. It is important to distend the urinary bladder with contrast agent until a detrusor contraction occurs, which indicates that the bladder capacity has been reached. Otherwise, small leaks may not be shown. There is a great deal of variation in the amount of bladder filling required to produce a detrusor contraction, but most patients require 300 to 600 mL of contrast agent to reach this point. A detrusor contraction is recognized by one of the following: (1) the patient voids, (2) there is resistance to injection of contrast agent through a hand-held syringe so that the barrel of the syringe starts to move back, or (3) flow through a contrast agent–filled bag 35 to 40 cm above the fluoroscopy table stops or reverses.

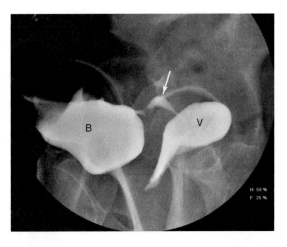

Figure 22-2. VCUG in a 40-year-old woman with vaginal leakage after hysterectomy. There is a fistula (*arrow*) between the posterior aspect of the urinary bladder (*B*) and the vagina (*V*). Vesicovaginal fistulas can be a complication of hysterectomy; difficult vaginal delivery, particularly if forceps are used; cesarean section; and gynecologic neoplasms, such as cervical cancer.

6. A patient is brought to the emergency department with blunt abdominal trauma and pelvic fractures. Does this patient need both an abdominopelvic computed tomography (CT) scan and a fluoroscopic cystogram?

No. The bladder can be distended with contrast agent on the CT table (termed *CT cystogram*) to evaluate for a leak. CT cystogram is as sensitive as a fluoroscopic cystogram, if not more so, in excluding a leak from the urinary bladder. Before placing a catheter in the urinary bladder in a patient with pelvic fractures, however, the urethra should be evaluated with RUG, and a catheter should be advanced through the urethra only if there is no urethral injury. Failure to follow this sequence could cause a partial urethral injury to become a complete urethral disruption.

7. Why is VUR important? How is it shown?

VUR in children can cause recurrent UTIs and lead to permanent renal scarring, termed *reflux nephropathy*. This condition can cause complications such as hypertension and renal insufficiency; 10% to 30% of all cases of end-stage renal disease may be related to reflux nephropathy. In adults, VUR has less clinical significance, although it can be associated with recurrent UTI and, rarely, even flank pain. VUR is reliably shown by fluoroscopically monitored VCUG. If the bladder is not distended to the point of voiding, VUR may not be shown. In children, radionuclide cystography is an alternative study to minimize the radiation exposure to pelvic organs.

8. What is RUG?

RUG is a study used primarily to evaluate the anterior urethra in men (Fig. 22-3). The male urethra is divided into two portions: the posterior urethra, consisting of the prostatic and membranous urethra, and the anterior urethra, consisting of the bulbar and pendulous urethra. The external urethral sphincter, located in the urogenital diaphragm, demarcates the posterior urethra from the anterior urethra. The posterior urethra has smooth muscle that relaxes when the detrusor muscle contracts during voiding and is best seen on VCUG. Although visualized on VCUG, the anterior urethra is better evaluated by RUG, which is performed by placing a Foley catheter in the tip of the penis and injecting contrast agent under fluoroscopic guidance. The urethra is usually opacified only to the level of the external sphincter on RUG because the sphincter is contracted in the nonvoiding state, and contrast agent cannot flow proximal to it.

9. How is the female urethra evaluated?

The entire female urethra is well shown on VCUG (Fig. 22-4). The short length of the female urethra makes RUG a difficult and unnecessary procedure in women.

10. What is a loopogram?

In patients who have undergone cystectomy (usually performed for muscle-invasive bladder cancer), the ureters are connected to a loop of ileum known as an ileal conduit. The ileal conduit is excluded from the intestinal stream and is connected to the anterior abdominal wall through a stoma; a urinary drainage bag is usually applied to the stoma site. A loopogram is performed to evaluate the conduit and the upper urinary tracts. A catheter is placed in the ileal conduit, and contrast agent is injected under fluoroscopic guidance until it refluxes in a retrograde fashion into the ureters and the pyelocalyceal systems.

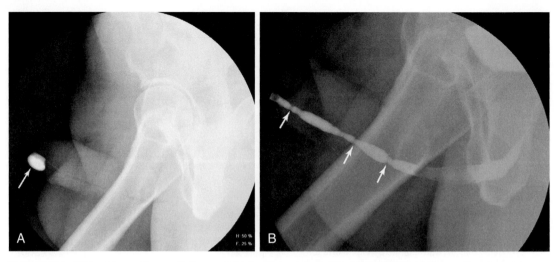

Figure 22-3. RUG in a 30-year-old man with history of gonorrhea. **A,** The balloon of the Foley catheter (*arrow*) is in the tip of the penis and has been distended with contrast agent. The balloon is usually placed in the fossa navicularis, which is an area of natural widening in the glans penis. **B,** The anterior urethra is opacified with contrast agent. Multiple strictures (*arrows*) in the penile urethra are typical of inflammatory disease. The bulbar urethra is the urethral segment proximal to the *arrows*. The wide caliber of the proximal bulbar urethra is the normal appearance of this segment of the bulbar urethra.

11. What is a hysterosalpingogram?
A hysterosalpingogram is a study to evaluate the uterine cavity and the fallopian tubes (Fig. 22-5). After sterile cleansing of the vaginal canal and the exocervix, a cannula is placed in the external cervical os, and contrast agent is injected under fluoroscopic guidance. The procedure is performed in women with primary or secondary infertility and in women with recurrent miscarriages.

12. Does magnetic resonance imaging (MRI) or ultrasound (US) examination of the pelvis provide the same information as hysterosalpingogram?
MRI and US are excellent at showing the uterus, but both studies are poor at showing the normal fallopian tubes. Dilated fallopian tubes (hydrosalpinx) can be identified on MRI and ultrasound, but abnormality in nondilated tubes is best seen on a hysterosalpingogram (Fig. 22-6).

13. If I have a female patient with a pelvic mass, what study would be helpful in further evaluation?
Either MRI or US would be useful to determine the organ of origin of the mass (gynecologic vs. nongynecologic mass, uterine vs. ovarian origin) and to characterize it further. Hysterosalpingogram has no role in this situation.

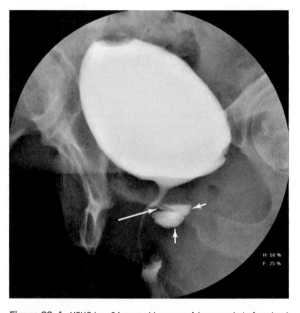

Figure 22-4. VCUG in a 34-year-old woman. A large pocket of contrast agent on the posterior aspect of the urethra represents a urethral diverticulum (*arrows*). A urethral diverticulum is usually the result of infection in periurethral glands, which decompress into the urethra and result in a communicating cavity. Patients present with postvoid dribbling, perineal discomfort, or recurrent UTIs.

14. What about a postmenopausal patient with vaginal bleeding? Would hysterosalpingogram be helpful in evaluating the endometrium in this patient?
Endometrial abnormalities, such as endometrial hyperplasia or endometrial cancer, can cause perimenopausal/postmenopausal bleeding and are best evaluated by transvaginal US or pelvic MRI.

Key Points: Genitourinary Fluoroscopic Examinations

1. Diagnosing small leaks from the urinary bladder requires adequate distention until a detrusor contraction occurs, regardless of whether the evaluation is performed with CT or fluoroscopy.
2. The anterior urethra in men is better evaluated on RUG. The posterior urethra in men is better evaluated on VCUG.
3. In a man with pelvic trauma, the urethra should be evaluated with RUG before placement of a bladder drainage catheter.
4. A retrograde pyelogram is an alternative study to IVU to evaluate the urothelium in patients in whom intravenous contrast administration is contraindicated.
5. A hysterosalpingogram is the most useful imaging study to evaluate the uterus and the fallopian tubes in patients with infertility.

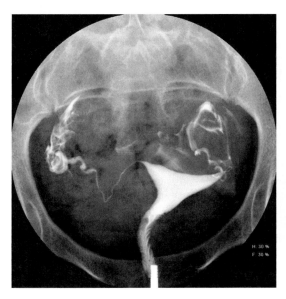

Figure 22-5. Normal hysterosalpingogram in a young woman with primary infertility. The metal cannula within the external os is seen at the bottom of the figure. The uterine cavity and both fallopian tubes appear normal. There is contrast agent spilling from both tubes into the pelvic peritoneal cavity, which is a normal finding.

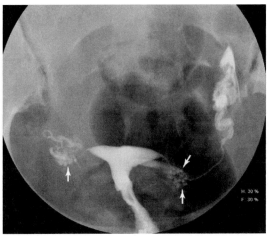

Figure 22-6. Hysterosalpingogram in a woman with a history of pelvic inflammatory disease. Outpouchings of contrast agent (*arrows*) are seen in the proximal portions of both fallopian tubes, a sequela of prior pelvic inflammatory disease. This condition is termed *salpingitis isthmica nodosa,* and it is associated with tubal dysmotility and infertility. This diagnosis would be difficult to make with any other imaging modality. The patient was advised to consider in vitro fertilization.

BIBLIOGRAPHY

[1] N.R. Dunnick, C.M. Sandler, J.H. Newhouse, E.S. Amis (Eds.), Textbook of Uroradiology, third ed., Lippincott Williams & Wilkins, Philadelphia, 2001.
[2] C.M. Sandler, S.M. Goldman, A. Kawashima, Lower urinary tract trauma, World J. Urol. 16 (1998) 69–75.
[3] J.P. Vaccaro, J.M. Brody, CT cystography in the evaluation of major bladder trauma, Radiographics 20 (2000) 1373–1381.

1. What computed tomography (CT) protocol should be used to characterize a focal renal mass?
A dedicated renal CT scan includes precontrast and postcontrast images because it is by comparing the appearance of a lesion on these two sets of images that the radiologist determines whether or not a lesion displays enhancement. Most CT examinations of the abdomen include only postcontrast images and are not optimal for characterizing a renal mass.

2. What magnetic resonance imaging (MRI) protocol should be used to characterize a focal renal mass?
Our preferred protocol for characterization of a renal mass is (1) breath-hold T1-weighted gradient-echo images, in-phase and out-of-phase; (2) axial fat-saturated fast spin-echo T2-weighted images; (3) coronal fat-saturated three-dimensional T1-weighted gradient-echo images obtained before, during, and after injection of intravenous gadolinium contrast agent; and (4) axial delayed phase T1-weighted gradient-echo images of the entire abdomen.

In the kidneys and elsewhere in the body, it is imperative that if intravenous contrast agent is administered, a set of precontrast images must be acquired with parameters (e.g., TR, TE, flip angle) that are *exactly* the same as those of the postcontrast acquisition. This is the only way that one can determine whether or not a lesion enhances on postcontrast images.

3. What is the normal enhancement pattern of the kidneys on CT and MRI?
Because kidneys receive approximately 25% of cardiac output, the kidneys enhance avidly and rapidly after contrast agent administration. Early renal enhancement on CT and MRI is termed the *corticomedullary phase,* in which the peripheral renal cortex is seen to enhance more than the central renal medulla (Fig. 23-1A). The corticomedullary phase

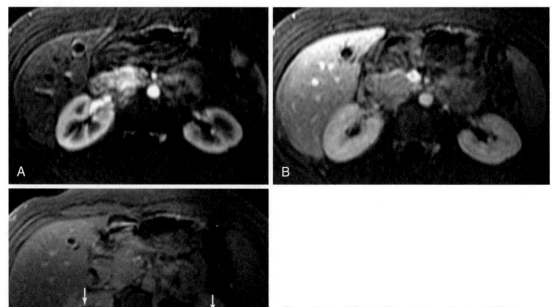

Figure 23-1. **A-C,** Axial T1-weighted gradient-echo MR images with fat saturation in the corticomedullary (**A**), nephrographic (**B**), and excretory (**C**) phases after administration of intravenous gadolinium chelate contrast agent. Excreted gadolinium chelate (*arrows*) may appear either bright on T1 (if dilute urine) or, as in this case, dark on T1 (if concentrated urine).

is followed by the nephrographic phase (Fig. 23-1B), in which the renal cortex and medulla have enhanced to roughly the same degree. This is generally the best phase in which to detect renal neoplasms. Finally, in the excretory phase, a functioning kidney excretes the injected contrast material. This phase is bright in the renal collecting system on CT. The T1 appearance of excreted gadolinium chelates depends on whether the kidney is making a dilute or concentrated urine. More dilute gadolinium chelates in urine are bright on T1, owing to T1 shortening effects. At higher concentrations, gadolinium chelates may appear very dark on T1-weighted images because T2 effects predominate (Fig. 23-1C).

4. What are the expected CT and MRI findings of renal cell carcinoma (RCC)?

Because of the presence of internal necrosis or hemorrhage, the appearance of RCC is variable. The common finding on CT and MRI of RCCs is that they enhance after the administration of intravenous contrast agents, and, in contrast to benign angiomyolipomas, they do not contain macroscopic fat. A solid renal lesion that enhances and that does *not* contain macroscopic fat is RCC until proved otherwise (Figs. 23-2 and 23-3).

5. What are risk factors for RCC?

Known risk factors for RCC include cigarette smoking, exposure to petroleum products or asbestos, hypertension, and obesity. It is approximately twice as common in men as women, and slightly more common in blacks than in whites of European descent. Most patients are older than 40 years, and individuals in the seventh and eighth decades of life are most commonly affected. Patients with acquired cystic kidney disease, von Hippel-Lindau disease, hereditary papillary renal cancer, and possibly tuberous sclerosis are also at increased risk.

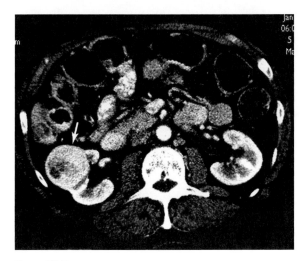

Figure 23-2. Axial postcontrast CT scan shows large, solid, enhancing renal lesion (*arrow*) that does not contain macroscopic fat. Such lesions should be removed. This lesion was RCC.

6. What is the Bosniak system for cystic renal lesions?

This important classification system describes features of cystic renal lesions and indicates recommendations for management. Although developed for CT, the morphologic features can be applied to MRI as well. Calcifications within a lesion are likely to be best seen on unenhanced CT. Internal soft tissue architecture within a cystic lesion is likely to be best depicted on multiplanar MRI.

- Bosniak class 1 lesions are simple cysts. On CT or MRI, they have a thin or imperceptible wall, have no internal architecture, and do not enhance after contrast   agent administration.
- Bosniak class 2 lesions may have a single thin septation or fine mural calcification. Also in class 2 are CT "hyperdense" cysts, which contain internal protein or hemorrhage, and which are hyperintense to normal renal parenchyma on T1-weighted images. These benign cysts do not enhance after contrast agent administration and have variable T2 signal intensity depending on their protein content.

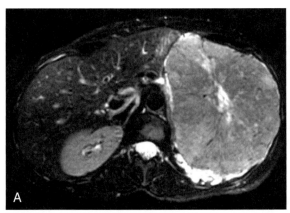
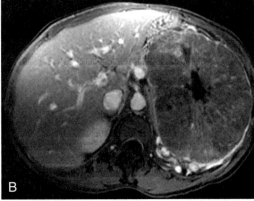

Figure 23-3. A and **B,** Axial T2-weighted image (**A**) and postcontrast T1-weighted gradient-echo image (**B**) show large enhancing left retroperitoneal mass that arose from the left kidney. This lesion, which did not contain macroscopic fat, was RCC.

- Bosniak class 3 lesions have thicker septations, multiple septations, or bulky mural calcifications. These lesions should be excised.
- Bosniak class 4 lesions display enhancing mural solid nodules that should be excised. Most of these lesions are cystic RCCs (Fig. 23-4).

7. What if I cannot tell whether a septation is thin or thick, or if the mural calcification is fine or bulky?

Deciding whether a cystic renal lesion is class 2 or class 3 can often hinge on whether an internal septation is judged to be thin (class 2) or thick (class 3), or on whether mural calcification is fine (class 2) or bulky (class 3). For the rare lesions that are truly indeterminate, class 2F may be assigned. These lesions are followed with CT or MRI, usually at an interval of 4 to 6 months.

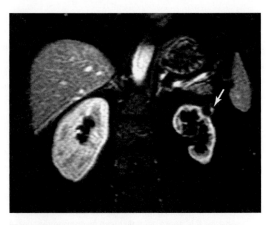

Figure 23-4. Coronal postcontrast T1-weighted gradient-echo image with fat saturation shows a cystic left renal lesion with an enhancing mural nodule (*arrow*). This is a Bosniak class 4 cystic RCC.

8. Is CT or MRI better for characterizing cystic renal lesions?

This is a question without a simple answer. Both modalities have proven to be very good at characterizing renal masses. A high-quality MRI performed on a high field (1.5-Tesla) scanner is, overall, probably better than CT for characterizing renal masses because of the high soft tissue contrast of MRI. High-quality MRI is difficult to perform, however, because it requires considerable experience on the part of the technologist and radiologist. A good MRI examination also requires a cooperative patient because the examination requires that the patient remain motionless during imaging, and requires that the patient perform several breath-holds. If a patient is incapable of remaining motionless or of performing multiple breath-holds, a CT examination is likely to be much better than a motion-filled MRI.

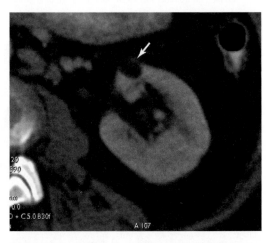

Figure 23-5. Axial unenhanced CT image shows a fat-density mass (*arrow*) in the left anterior interpolar region. Because this renal lesion contains material that is of fat attenuation, it is a benign angiomyolipoma.

9. What is an angiomyolipoma?

An angiomyolipoma is a benign hamartoma that, as its name suggests, contains elements of blood vessels (*angio*-), muscle (*myo*-), and fat (*lipoma*). Because of their solid nature and enhancement, they may be confused with enhancing RCCs. A CT (Fig. 23-5) or MRI (Fig. 23-6) diagnosis of angiomyolipoma is made by identifying macroscopic fat (a region of negative Hounsfield values on CT, or tissue that follows the signal intensity of body wall fat when the same MRI sequence is performed with and without frequency-selective fat saturation).

10. What syndrome is associated with angiomyolipomas?

Tuberous sclerosis is associated with angiomyolipomas. This syndrome can cause renal cysts or renal angiomyolipomas. Tuberous sclerosis probably also puts a patient at a slightly higher risk of RCC. Angiomyolipomas can also occur sporadically, in patients without tuberous sclerosis.

11. How are angiomyolipomas treated?

They are usually embolized—deprived of their blood supply—when they grow to be 4 cm or greater. Embolization is performed because larger lesions are at greater risk of hemorrhage.

12. I see an enhancing renal mass that does not have fat attenuation on CT, and that does not have fat signal on MRI. What is the differential diagnosis?

This lesion would be presumed to be RCC until proved otherwise. Other lesions that could have this appearance include oncocytoma, transitional cell carcinoma (TCC), angiomyolipoma without detectable fat, or renal lymphoma.

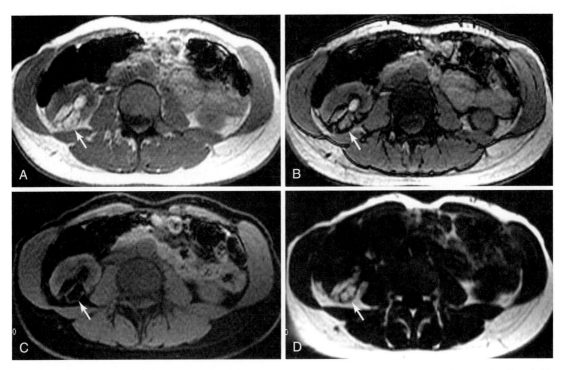

Figure 23-6. A-D, Axial T1-weighted gradient-echo images obtained in-phase (**A**), out-of-phase (**B**), with explicit fat saturation (**C**), and with explicit water saturation (**D**). The right-sided renal lesion (*arrows*) follows the signal of the body wall fat on all pulse sequences, indicating the presence of macroscopic fat within the lesion. This is diagnostic of benign angiomyolipoma.

13. How is RCC staged by CT and MRI?

RCC is most commonly staged using the Robson classification. Stage 1 includes tumors that are confined entirely to the kidney. Stage 2 lesions invade the perinephric fat or the adrenal gland on the same side. Stage 3a has tumor thrombus in the renal vein or inferior vena cava; stage 3b has tumor in regional lymph nodes; stage 3c involves regional lymph nodes and the renal vein, inferior vena cava, or both. Stage 4 RCCs involve distant metastases, such as the lung, liver, or bones.

> **Key Points: CT and MRI of the Kidney**
>
> 1. An enhancing renal mass that does not contain macroscopic fat is RCC until proved otherwise.
> 2. An enhancing renal lesion with macroscopic fat is a benign angiomyolipoma.
> 3. Cystic renal lesions that contain thick internal septations, thick mural calcification, or enhancing mural nodules are suspicious for cystic RCCs and should be excised.

14. What does renal infarction look like on CT or MRI?

Patients who have embolic disease, or who have injury to the aorta, renal artery, or a renal artery branch can develop segmental renal infarctions. These are wedge-shaped areas of hypoenhancement, broader at the periphery of the kidney and narrow near the center of the kidney. In segmental renal infarction, there is often a thin rim of preserved enhancement at the edge of the kidney because this region has a separate arterial supply via the renal capsular artery.

15. What does renal laceration look like on CT?

Laceration of the kidney complicates 10% to 25% of blunt abdominal trauma cases. In patients with renal cortical laceration, CT shows interruption of the renal cortex, with associated subcapsular hematoma.

16. **What findings on a trauma CT scan indicate that a kidney would need to be surgically repaired?**

Superficial renal lacerations in stable patients can be managed conservatively, without surgery. Surgical repair is indicated for deep lacerations with disruption of the collecting system, for comminuted renal fractures, and for vascular pedicle injuries. Vascular pedicle injuries may include arterial/venous avulsion, intimal flap dissection, or traumatic vessel occlusion.

17. **What is autosomal dominant polycystic kidney disease (ADPKD)? Is it associated with RCC?**

As the name implies, ADPKD is a slowly progressive, single-gene inherited condition that leads to formation of multiple renal cysts in the kidneys. Although many individuals present as adults with symptoms of renal enlargement and renal insufficiency (with associated hypertension and anemia), affected individuals may begin to develop cysts in childhood. Patients with ADPKD often also develop multiple liver cysts, and are at increased risk for development of intracerebral aneurysms. There is no increased risk for RCC.

18. **What is autosomal recessive polycystic kidney disease (ARPKD)? Is it associated with RCC?**

ARPKD usually manifests on prenatal sonography, or in early childhood. The disease may be fatal in very early childhood, but some patients survive in to adolescence. ARPKD is associated with congenital hepatic fibrosis. There is no increased risk for RCC.

19. **What are two genetically inherited syndromes that *are* associated with RCC?**

Von Hippel-Lindau disease and the very rare hereditary papillary RCC syndrome are autosomal dominantly inherited and associated with development of multiple RCCs. A diagnosis of one of these syndromes often leads to screening of first-degree relatives because they may also carry the disease gene.

20. **What is acquired cystic renal disease? Is it associated with RCC?**

Acquired cystic renal disease is the term applied to patients who have end-stage renal disease, are on dialysis, and have very small kidneys with multiple cysts. These patients are at approximately six to seven times normal risk of developing RCC.

21. **Should patients on dialysis be screened for RCC?**

This is controversial. RCCs found in patients with the acquired cystic renal disease are often low-grade neoplasms, and are of relatively little clinical significance in patients with short expected life spans and multiple comorbid diseases. If screening is performed, it is probably best reserved for younger patients or for patients who, other than their renal disease, are in good health.

22. **What are some features that suggest oncocytoma on CT and MRI?**

Oncocytomas are solid, enhancing lesions. Oncocytomas may display a central, hypoenhancing scar, and they tend to be relatively homogeneous for lesion size. Because these findings can also be seen in RCC, oncocytomas cannot be reliably differentiated from RCCs on CT or MRI. Although most exhibit benign behavior, there have been reports of rare metastases from oncocytomas. They are perhaps best thought of as lesions of low malignant potential, and most can be excised by partial nephrectomy.

23. **What are the findings of pyelonephritis on CT or MRI?**

The affected kidney is usually enlarged, and there may be stranding in the fat surrounding the kidney. The enhancement of the kidney often is delayed, relative to the unaffected contralateral kidney. A "striated nephrogram" can usually be seen, especially on delayed phase images, where the kidney displays alternating bands of high and low CT attenuation or MRI signal intensity (see Fig. 20-7).

24. **A multiloculated cystic lesion looks like it has herniated into the renal collecting system. What could this be?**

This is likely a multilocular cystic nephroma. This unusual lesion is found in young boys and in older women. As its name suggests, it appears as an agglomeration of multiple cystic spaces. In approximately one third of cases, the lesion can herniate into the renal collecting system. Although considered benign, multilocular cystic nephroma undergoes sarcomatous degeneration in approximately 7% of cases. These lesions are excised.

25. **Are CT and MRI useful in imaging TCC?**

TCC may arise in the epithelium of the renal collecting systems, the ureters, the urinary bladder, and portions of the urethra. CT and MRI can detect large masses, but both modalities have difficulty identifying small, flat tumors that do not result in proximal hydroureteronephrosis. Intravenous urogram (IVU) remains superior to CT and

MRI for detecting this type of lesion, although multidetector CT urography and gadolinium-enhanced magnetic resonance urography (MRU) are rapidly gaining acceptance as viable alternatives to IVU in imaging patients for suspected TCC.

26. What are the MRI signal characteristics typical of TCC?
TCC is hyperintense on T1-weighted and hypointense on T2-weighted images compared with surrounding urine.

27. What does renal lymphoma look like on CT and MRI?
Renal lymphoma is usually B-cell lymphoma and is generally a manifestation of widespread systemic disease. The most common initial presentation is that of a larger retroperitoneal mass, surrounding one or both kidneys and possibly the inferior vena cava and aorta. It is of low intermediate signal on T1-weighted and T2-weighted images, similar to the spleen or lymph nodes. It enhances weakly after contrast agent administration. After treatment for lymphoma, renal involvement by the disease is often seen as multiple, focal rounded intraparenchymal masses.

28. Does metastatic disease go to the kidneys? What does it look like on CT and MRI?
Yes, metastatic disease can go to the kidneys, although these lesions are usually very small and not clinically significant. They are seen often on autopsy, but usually do not cause clinical morbidity on their own. On CT or MRI, they are seen as multiple bilateral renal lesions with infiltrative margins.

29. What protocol should be used for performing CT or MRI on a patient who is a potential renal donor?
Either CT or MRI may be used to evaluate a potential renal donor. On CT, a precontrast topogram may be used to evaluate for the presence of renal stones. Multidetector thin-section imaging through the kidneys is performed to detect and evaluate the renal arteries. Delayed phase imaging may be performed to evaluate venous morphology. Finally, excretory phase topogram can be performed to visualize the renal collecting system and ureters.

On MRI, precontrast T1-weighted gradient-echo and T2-weighted images are acquired, followed by coronal, three-dimensional T1-weighted gradient-echo images acquired in the arterial and venous phases of enhancement. Furosemide, 10 mg, may be given with the gadolinium chelate, and MRU may be obtained approximately 5 minutes later.

30. What kinds of things should be included in the CT or MRI report on a patient who is a potential renal donor?
Important information includes renal size; the presence or absence of renal mass or other renal abnormality; and the number, size, and position of renal arteries, renal veins, and ureters for each kidney. Renal artery duplication is common and is found in approximately 30% of all kidneys. The presence or absence of prehilar arterial branching should be noted; in particular, the distance between the aorta and first arterial branch is surgically relevant. The morphology of the left renal vein is more variable than the right. The left renal vein usually passes anterior to the aorta before joining the inferior vena cava. It may pass posterior to the aorta (retroaortic left renal vein) however, or there may be two left renal veins—one anterior to the aorta and one posterior—which is called a circumaortic left renal vein.

31. I have an emergency department patient with flank pain. What is the best radiologic test to find renal and ureteral calculi?
Unenhanced multidetector CT has replaced IVU as the examination of choice for identifying renal and ureteral stones (Fig. 23-7). If a cause for the patient's pain is not found, or if a calcific density is identified, and it is

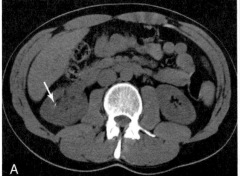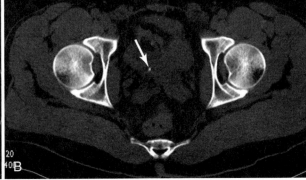

Figure 23-7. A and **B,** Axial unenhanced CT images of the kidneys (**A**) and pelvis (**B**) show the presence of a 1-mm right renal calculus (*arrow*). The patient's flank pain was due to the right distal ureteral calculus (*arrow* in **B**).

uncertain whether that density lies within the ureter, contrast agent may be given, and the abdomen and pelvis may be scanned again.

32. What is post-transplant lymphoproliferative disorder (PTLD)?

PTLD is a spectrum of diseases ranging from benign lymphoid proliferation to malignant lymphoma. PTLD is caused by Epstein-Barr virus and is seen in transplant patients receiving immunosuppressive medications, such as azathioprine (Imuran), muromonab-CD3 (Orthoclone OKT3), and cyclosporine. Greater amounts of immunosuppression are associated with higher rates of incidence of PTLD. Liver transplant recipients are at greater risk than renal transplant recipients.

33. Other than PTLD, what are some things that can go wrong with a renal transplant?

Things can go wrong with any of the surgical anastomoses—arterial, venous, and ureteral. Complications include renal artery stenosis, renal artery thrombosis, renal vein thrombosis, and ureteral leak. Patients may also develop pelvic "masses," including urinoma, hematoma, and lymphocele. Finally, the transplant may not function well and may develop acute tubular necrosis or rejection.

34. What is a horseshoe kidney?

When the lower poles of the left kidney and right kidney are attached to one another, this is termed a *horseshoe kidney*. The region of connection, termed the *isthmus,* may be composed of fibrous tissue or functioning renal parenchyma. Horseshoe kidney is more common in patients with Turner syndrome.

35. For what diseases are individuals with horseshoe kidneys at increased risk?

Individuals with horseshoe kidney are at increased risk for ureteropelvic junction obstruction, stone formation, vesicoureteral reflux, infection, trauma, Wilms tumor, TCC, and RCC.

36. What is CT urography, and how is it performed?

CT urography is an examination that is generally performed for hematuria. It involves acquisition of unenhanced images (for identification of renal or ureteral calculi), nephrographic phase images (at approximately 110 seconds postinjection, for renal masses), and excretory phase images (at approximately 6 to 8 minutes postinjection, for evaluation of renal collecting systems and ureters). Reformatted images of the excretory data are generated in multiple projections, to create images of the renal collecting systems and ureters that are analogous to conventional urograms.

37. What is MRU? What are the relative strengths and weakness of CT urography and MRU?

MRU is performed similarly to CT urography, using precontrast images, nephrographic images, and excretory phase images. Coronal, three-dimensional, T1-weighted gradient-echo images are used for all acquisitions, and gadolinium chelates are injected rather than iodine-based compounds (Fig. 23-8).

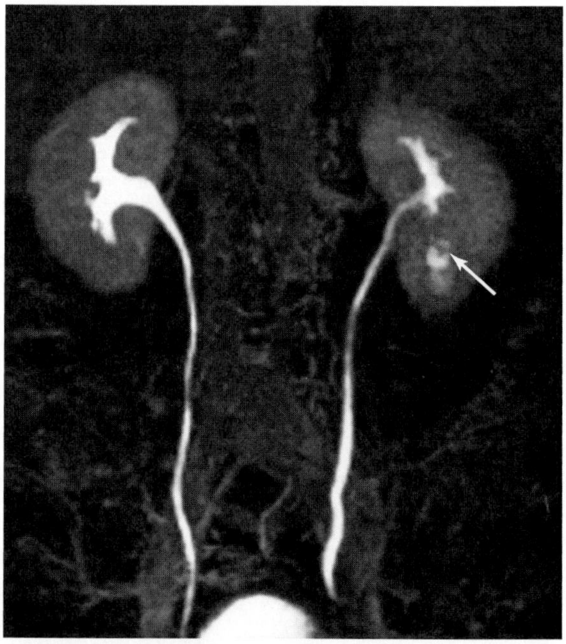

Figure 23-8. Coronal, excretory-phase MRU performed 8 minutes after administration of intravenous contrast agent shows a filling defect in the lower pole of the left kidney, representing TCC (*arrow*). The right renal collecting system is normal.

Two major advantages of MRU versus CT urography are the lack of ionizing radiation in MRU and the ability to acquire multiple excretory phase datasets rather than just one, which is especially useful if renal excretion is delayed. Advantages of CT urography over MRU include the much greater sensitivity of CT for detection of renal calculi, and the superior spatial resolution of multidetector row CT relative to MRI.

BIBLIOGRAPHY

[1] G.M. Israel, G.A. Krinsky, MR imaging of the kidneys and adrenal glands, Radiol. Clin. North Am. 41 (2003) 145–159.

[2] E.S. Pretorius, M.L. Wickstrom, E.S. Siegelman, MR imaging of renal neoplasms, Magn. Reson. Imaging Clin. N. Am. 8 (2000) 813–836.

[3] S. Sheth, J.C. Scatarige, K.M. Horton, et al., Current concepts in the diagnosis and management of renal cell carcinoma: role of multidetector CT and three-dimensional CT, Radiographics 21 (2001) S237–S254.

[4] J.M. Teichman, Clinical practice: acute renal colic from ureteral calculus, N. Engl. J. Med. 350 (2004) 684–693.

CT AND MRI OF THE ADRENAL GLANDS

E. Scott Pretorius, MD

1. Where are the adrenal glands located?

The adrenal glands lie superior to the upper poles of the kidneys and are contained, with the kidneys, within Gerota fascia. The right adrenal gland lies posterior to the inferior vena cava, medial to the right lobe of the liver, and lateral to the right diaphragmatic crus. The left adrenal gland lies slightly inferior to the right adrenal gland. It can be found to the left of the aorta and the left diaphragmatic crus, posterior to the splenic vessels.

2. What do normal adrenal glands look like on computed tomography (CT) and magnetic resonance imaging (MRI)?

On CT, the adrenal glands are of soft tissue attenuation and are denser than the surrounding fat. On MRI, the normal adrenal gland has similar signal intensity to that of the kidney on T1-weighted and T2-weighted images. Both adrenal glands are most commonly shaped like an inverted letter "Y" or an inverted letter "V." Each adrenal gland has a body, medial limb, and lateral limb. Each limb is most commonly 4 to 6 mm in thickness and should be less than 10 mm in thickness (Fig. 24-1).

3. What is the differential diagnosis of an adrenal lesion seen on CT or MRI?

The differential diagnosis of an adrenal lesion includes benign and malignant entities. Benign lesions include adrenal cortical adenomas (which are very common), adrenal cysts, and myelolipoma. Adrenal hemorrhage may mimic a solid lesion. Malignant causes include metastatic disease, which is very common, and adrenal cortical carcinoma. Adrenal pheochromocytomas may exhibit either benign (approximately 90%) or malignant (approximately 10%) behavior. In the absence of a known malignancy, a small (≤1 cm), well-circumscribed adrenal lesion is virtually always benign.

4. What is chemical shift imaging?

Chemical shift imaging is an MRI technique that is used to determine whether lipid and water protons are present with the same small voxel (three-dimensional pixel) of space (Fig. 24-2). T1-weighted gradient-echo images are obtained "in phase" (meaning that the signals of lipid and water protons are additive, and both contribute to the observed signal intensity) and "out of phase" (meaning that the signals of lipid and water protons are destructive to one another; if both are present in a voxel, their signals tend to cancel each other out). If one compares an in-phase image with an out-of-phase image, there would be less signal on the out-of-phase image in areas that contain lipid and water protons. In areas that contain all lipid protons and in areas that contain all water protons, the signal would not change between the two images. To see the effect of destructive interference on the out-of-phase image, both kinds of protons must be present.

5. How can I tell which is the out-of-phase image?

The out-of-phase image can be identified by the dark outlines seen at fat-water interfaces (see Fig. 24-2B). This outline is seen where the kidneys meet the fat that surrounds them. This is termed "etching" artifact or "India ink" artifact. The TR of the in-phase image and the out-of-phase image should always be the same, so that valid signal comparisons can be made between the two images. At 1.5-Tesla, a TE of 4.4 ms is in-phase, and multiples of this time (2 × 4.4 = 8.8 ms) are also in-phase. Other TEs are out-of-phase. In this example, a TE of 2.2 ms is directly out-of-phase, and it is here that the maximum chemical shift effect is observed.

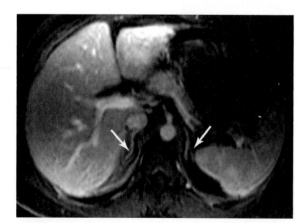

Figure 24-1. Axial T1-weighted gradient-echo MR image after gadolinium administration shows the normal appearance of the adrenal glands (*arrows*). The limbs of the normal adrenal are less than 10 mm in thickness.

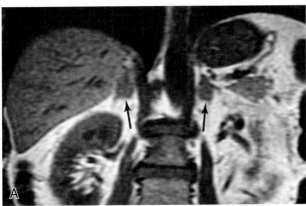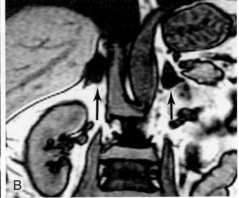

Figure 24-2. A and **B,** Coronal T1-weighted gradient-echo images in-phase (**A**) and out-of-phase (**B**) show dramatic signal loss in bilateral adrenal lesions (*arrows*) on the out-of-phase image relative to the in-phase image. This finding indicates the presence of fat and water protons in the lesions and is diagnostic of benign adrenal adenomas.

6. How can MRI be used to show that an adrenal lesion is an adenoma?

The presence of intracytoplasmic lipid is very specific for the diagnosis of benign adenoma. About 70% of all adrenal adenomas exhibit the presence of this lipid and are termed *lipid-rich* adenomas. The remainder are termed *lipid-poor* adenomas. MRI is very sensitive at detecting intracytoplasmic lipid. T1-weighted gradient-echo images can be obtained in-phase and out-of-phase. If the signal intensity within the adrenal lesion on the out-of-phase image is 20% less than the signal within the lesion on the in-phase image, this shows that there is intracytoplasmic lipid present, and the lesion is a benign adenoma (see Fig. 24-2).

7. How can unenhanced CT be used to show that an adrenal lesion is an adenoma?

Thin-section (≤5 mm) unenhanced CT is performed. If the adrenal lesion measures less than 10 HU on unenhanced CT, this is generally accepted as indicating the presence of intracytoplasmic lipid within a benign adenoma (Fig. 24-3A).

8. Are there any malignant adrenal lesions that can contain intracytoplasmic lipid?

Clear cell renal cell carcinomas often have detectable intracytoplasmic lipid, are of low CT attenuation, and display signal loss on chemical shift MRI. If these tumors metastasize to the adrenal gland, the adrenal metastases mimic adenomas on unenhanced CT and chemical shift MRI.

9. How can enhanced CT be used to show that an adrenal lesion is an adrenal cortical adenoma?

If unenhanced CT does not characterize the adrenal lesion, intravenous contrast agent can be given. CT imaging of the adrenal gland is performed 80 seconds and 10 minutes after contrast agent administration. Region-of-interest measurements are taken of the adrenal lesion on the 80-second and the 10-minute scan, and a percentage of *washout* is calculated. The percentage of contrast agent washout is equal to [1 − (attenuation at 10 minutes/attenuation at 80 seconds)] × 100%.

Washout that is greater than 50% is very specific for benign adrenal adenoma. Metastatic disease characteristically displays washout of less than 50% (Fig. 24-3B and C). The presence or absence of intracytoplasmic lipid within an adenoma does not make a lesion more or less likely to display washout.

10. Which is better for imaging the adrenal glands, CT or MRI?

This is controversial. It depends a great deal on institutional experience and the level of expertise exhibited by the technologist and radiologist. Chemical shift MRI is easily performed, but some centers may lack experience with this technique. Many adrenal lesions are incidentally discovered on CT, but because neither thin-section unenhanced images nor 10-minute delayed images are part of most abdominal CT protocols, the patient often has to return for a second study.

11. What is the difference between a functioning and a nonfunctioning adenoma? Can CT or MRI differentiate these?

CT and MRI cannot differentiate functioning adenomas (adenomas that have endocrine activity) from adenomas that are nonfunctioning. Functioning adenomas may result in hyperaldosteronism (Conn syndrome) or hypercortisolism (Cushing syndrome).

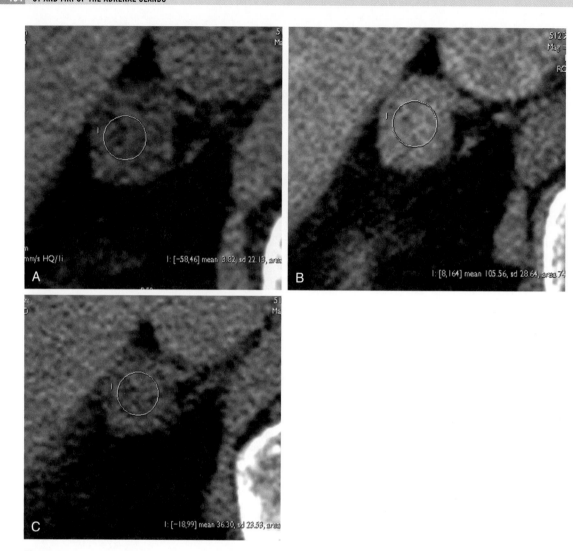

Figure 24-3. A, Axial, unenhanced CT scan performed in a 73-year-old woman with lung cancer and an adrenal lesion shows that the adrenal lesion measures 3.82 HU. Because this lesion is less than 10 HU, it is a benign adenoma. **B** and **C,** Postcontrast CT images obtained at 80 seconds (**B**) and 10 minutes (**C**) after contrast agent administration show that the lesion measures 105.56 HU at 80 seconds postcontrast and 36.30 HU at 10 minutes postcontrast. Because the washout is greater than 50%, this lesion is confirmed to represent a benign adenoma.

12. What is a myelolipoma, and how can CT and MRI be used to show that an adrenal lesion is a myelolipoma?

Adrenal myelolipomas are benign adrenal neoplasms composed of fatty tissue and variable amounts of hematopoietic elements. On CT, internal attenuation values of −20 to −30 are detected within the fatty portions of the lesion. On MRI, there are elements within the lesion that follow the signal of body wall fat on all pulse sequences. On MRI, it is useful to perform the same sequence (either T1 or fast spin-echo T2) with and without explicit fat saturation. If the tissue in question is fat, it is very bright on the non–fat-saturated sequence and becomes dark on the fat-saturated sequence.

13. On MRI, I see an adrenal lesion that does not lose signal on chemical shift imaging. Could it still be an adenoma?

Yes. It could be a lipid-poor adenoma. Metastatic disease and other adrenal lesions cannot be excluded in this situation, however.

14. What is a collision tumor?

A collision tumor is a metastasis to an adrenal gland that also contains an adrenal cortical adenoma. These are uncommon; however, in patients with known malignancies, one should be careful about calling a lesion an adenoma if the lesion contains two distinct parts that display very different CT and MRI characteristics.

15. How commonly do malignancies spread to the adrenal glands?

About 50% of melanomas metastasize to the adrenal glands, and 30% to 40% of breast and lung cancers and 10% to 20% of renal and gastrointestinal tumors have adrenal metastases.

16. How do adrenal cysts form, and what do they look like on CT and MRI?

Most adrenal cysts are pseudocysts and form after adrenal hemorrhage. As fluid-containing structures, adrenal cysts are of fluid density on CT and are of high T2-signal intensity on MRI. They do not enhance after administration of contrast agent.

17. What causes adrenal hemorrhage?

Adrenal hemorrhage can be secondary to extreme stress, trauma, or coagulopathic states. Common causes of coagulopathy include anticoagulant and thrombolytic agent use, systemic malignancies, and sepsis.

18. How can CT or MRI be used to tell the difference between adrenal hemorrhage and an adrenal mass?

Compare precontrast and postcontrast images. Masses are living tissue and enhance on CT and MRI. Adrenal hemorrhage does not enhance.

19. What does pheochromocytoma look like on CT?

If the patient has laboratory values indicating an elevated catecholamine level, unenhanced CT is often the first imaging study performed. If an adrenal lesion is identified, this is presumed to represent pheochromocytoma. Approximately 10% of adrenal lesions are calcified on unenhanced CT.

If an adrenal lesion is not found on unenhanced CT, intravenous contrast agent can be given. Pheochromocytomas enhance very avidly after contrast agent administration. Some centers prefer not to perform contrast-enhanced CT if pheochromocytoma is suspected because of reported cases of precipitation of hypertensive crisis after administration of iodine agents. MRI can be performed as an alternative.

20. What is the differential diagnosis of T2-hyperintense adrenal lesions on MRI?

Adrenal cysts and pheochromocytoma can be markedly hyperintense on T2-weighted MR images, although many pheochromocytomas contain regions that are not T2-hyperintense. These two lesions are easily differentiated by administration of intravenous gadolinium chelate. Cysts do not enhance, and pheochromocytomas enhance avidly on CT and MRI (Fig. 24-4).

21. My patient has an elevated urine catecholamine level and hypertension, but there is no adrenal lesion on CT (or MRI). Where else should I look for a pheochromocytoma?

Pheochromocytoma can occur anywhere along the sympathetic chain. The organ of Zuckerkandl (near the aortic bifurcation) and the urinary bladder are also important places to look.

22. What is the pheochromocytoma "rule of tens"?

Approximately 10% of pheochromocytomas are bilateral, 10% occur outside of the adrenal gland, 10% are calcified, and 10% are malignant. It is perhaps more useful to remember the "rule of 90s" that this implies. Most pheochromocytomas are unilateral, in the adrenal gland, not calcified, and benign.

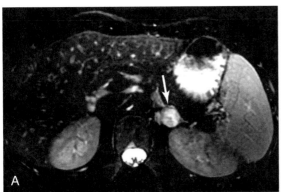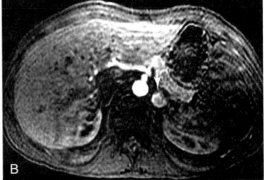

Figure 24-4. A, Axial T2-weighted MR image shows a left adrenal lesion (*arrow*) that is of high T2 signal. This could represent a cyst or pheochromocytoma. **B,** Arterial phase postcontrast T1-weighted gradient-echo MR image shows that the lesion (*arrow*) enhances avidly. These are MRI findings of pheochromocytoma.

23. My patient has lung cancer. What are the odds that there would be an adrenal lesion at time of presentation?

About 10% of patients with carcinoma of the lung have adrenal metastases at the time the primary tumor is diagnosed.

24. How can I tell whether a lesion is in the adrenal gland or in the upper pole of the kidney?

This can be surprisingly difficult, especially when the lesion is large. MRI has the ability to image directly in any plane, and sagittal or coronal images are often helpful in differentiating an adrenal lesion from a renal lesion. If CT has been performed, reformatting the data into a sagittal or coronal plane on a workstation is usually helpful.

25. Where do the adrenal arteries arise?

There are usually three main arteries. The superior adrenal artery originates from the inferior phrenic artery, the middle adrenal artery arises directly from the aorta, and the inferior adrenal artery is a branch of the renal artery.

26. Where do the adrenal veins drain?

The right adrenal vein enters directly into the inferior vena cava. The left adrenal vein drains into the inferior phrenic vein and then to the left renal vein.

27. On CT and MRI, I see an adrenal mass that extends into the left renal vein. Does that help narrow the differential diagnosis?

Yes. This is a common finding in adrenal cortical carcinoma. Adrenal cortical carcinomas are generally large tumors (>5 cm) that display avid enhancement, particularly at their periphery. Because of internal necrosis and hemorrhage, they often display great internal heterogeneity on CT and MRI.

Key Points: CT and MRI of the Adrenal Glands

1. The differential diagnosis of a lesion in the adrenal gland includes adrenal cortical adenoma, adrenal cyst, myelolipoma, pheochromocytoma, metastatic disease, and adrenal cortical carcinoma.
2. There are three ways to show that an adrenal lesion is a benign adenoma: attenuation of less than 10 HU on unenhanced CT, washout of greater than 50% on 10-minute delayed CT, or signal loss of 10% to 15% on chemical shift MRI.
3. Most pheochromocytomas occur in the adrenal glands and enhance avidly on CT and MRI.
4. CT and MRI cannot differentiate functioning (endocrinologically active) adenomas from nonfunctioning adenomas.

---

28. What are the causes of Conn syndrome?

Conn syndrome, or primary hyperaldosteronism, is caused by an adrenal adenoma in 80% of cases. In the remaining 20% of cases, the cause is adrenal hyperplasia. Patients have hypertension, an elevated aldosterone level, and low potassium and renin levels. Patients with high aldosterone and renin levels likely have secondary hyperaldosteronism, which is secondary to renal artery stenosis.

Among patients with primary hyperaldosteronism, it is important to differentiate between patients with adenomas and patients with adrenal hyperplasia. Aldosteronomas are treated surgically. Hyperplasia is managed medically. If CT and MRI do not reveal an adrenal lesion, adrenal vein sampling can be performed to exclude the presence of a unilateral, hyperfunctioning aldosteronoma.

29. What are the causes of Cushing syndrome?

Cushing syndrome is most commonly (80%) caused by an adrenocorticotropic hormone (ACTH)–producing pituitary adenoma that stimulates excessive cortisol production from the adrenal glands. About 15% of all cases of Cushing syndrome involve autonomous, cortisol-producing adenomas. The remaining cases involve cortisol-producing adrenal cortical carcinomas or ACTH-producing small-cell carcinomas of the lung.

30. Both adrenal glands look thick, but I do not see a focal mass. What does this mean?

This is likely adrenal hyperplasia. In adults, this can be seen in any "stress" situation that requires the body to make more cortisol. Congenital adrenal hyperplasia can be seen in neonates. It is a manifestation of many genetic disorders that result in an inability to make sufficient cortisol or aldosterone. Affected neonates and infants develop adrenal hyperplasia and often overproduce sex hormones, leading to virilization.

31. Which of the multiple endocrine neoplasia (MEN) syndromes involve the adrenal glands?

MEN types IIa and IIb involve pheochromocytomas.

- MEN I (Wermer syndrome) is characterized by parathyroid hyperplasia, pituitary tumors, and pancreatic islet cell tumors.
- MEN IIa (Sipple syndrome) is characterized by pheochromocytoma, medullary thyroid carcinoma, and hyperparathyroidism.
- MEN IIb is similar to MEN IIa, but without parathyroid involvement and with the presence of multiple mucosal neuromas and ganglioneuromas throughout the gastrointestinal tract.

BIBLIOGRAPHY

[1] M. Korobkin, CT characterization of adrenal masses: the time has come, Radiology 217 (2000) 629–632.
[2] W.W. Mayo-Smith, G.W. Boland, R.B. Noto, M.J. Lee, State-of-the-art adrenal imaging, Radiographics 21 (2001) 995–1012.
[3] P. Otal, G. Escourrou, C. Mazerolles, et al., Imaging features of uncommon adrenal masses with histopathologic correlation, Radiographics 19 (1999) 569–581.
[4] C.S. Pena, G.W. Boland, P.F. Hahn, et al., Characterization of indeterminate (lipid-poor) adrenal masses: use of washout characteristics at contrast-enhanced CT, Radiology 217 (2000) 798–802.
[5] E.S. Siegelman, MR imaging of the adrenal neoplasms, Magn. Reson. Imaging Clin. N. Am. 8 (2000) 769–786.

ULTRASOUND OF THE FEMALE PELVIS

Jeffrey Scott Friedenberg, MD, and
Susan E. Rowling, MD

1. What are the main indications to perform an ultrasound (US) examination of the female pelvis?

US is useful in the evaluation of pelvic masses, pelvic pain, and abnormal bleeding. A pelvic US can also be performed to evaluate for uterine anomalies or to monitor for the development of ovarian follicles in infertility patients.

2. How is a pelvic US performed?

The typical scanning techniques are transabdominal and endovaginal. We typically begin with a transabdominal scan, which is performed with the patient's bladder full. If we are satisfied with the images and have answered the clinical question, the study is complete. If additional information can be obtained with an endovaginal examination, the patient is asked to empty her bladder before the examination is performed. Transperineal US is seldom performed, but can be useful in the evaluation of the urethra, vagina, and cervix.

3. What is the normal US appearance of the uterus?

The uterus has a homogeneous myometrium of moderate echogenicity with a central echogenic band representing the endometrial stripe complex. Peripheral arcuate vessels may also be identified. A thin hypoechoic layer may surround the endometrium, particularly in postmenopausal women, and represents the innermost layer of myometrium. During the late proliferative (periovulatory) phase of the menstrual cycle, the endometrial stripe may have a trilaminar appearance, with an echogenic outer layer surrounding two hypoechoic layers separated by a thin echogenic line that represents apposition of the two endometrial layers.

4. How is the endometrial stripe routinely measured?

The endometrial stripe complex is measured in the sagittal plane at its widest point, including both layers, from the most anterior to the most posterior echogenic portions of the stripe. If there is fluid within the endometrial cavity, the fluid is not included in the measurement. Endovaginal US is the most accurate way to measure the endometrium.

5. What is the normal thickness of the endometrium?

Endometrial stripe thickness varies depending on the timing of the patient's menstrual cycle. During the menstrual phase, the endometrium typically measures 1 to 4 mm. In the proliferative phase, the endometrial stripe may measure 4 to 8 mm, and in the secretory phase, the endometrial stripe may measure 8 to 16 mm. These numbers do not apply for a postmenopausal woman, in whom a thickness of 8 mm is considered normal if she is asymptomatic. Abnormal thickening of the endometrium can be a sign of endometrial cancer.

6. What is the name of the simple cysts identified within the cervix? What is their clinical significance?

Cysts within the cervix are called *nabothian cysts*. They represent dilated or obstructed endocervical glands. They are very common in women of reproductive age and are usually of no clinical significance. Occasionally, the cysts appear complicated, secondary to hemorrhage or infection. Nabothian cysts can be a cause of benign cervical enlargement if they are large or multiple.

7. What is the most common tumor of the uterus?

The most common uterine tumors are fibroids (leiomyomas), which are seen in approximately 25% of women. Fibroids are benign tumors of smooth muscle origin that can enlarge under hormonal influence. They are typically heterogeneous masses with posterior shadowing and may contain coarse calcifications or, rarely, central fluid secondary to necrosis. Fibroids can be subserosal, intramural, or submucosal in location. Large subserosal or intramural fibroids may cause symptoms by exerting pressure on adjacent organs. Submucosal leiomyomas are common causes of abnormal uterine bleeding and may become pedunculated within the endometrial cavity.

8. What are the most common causes of vaginal bleeding in a postmenopausal woman?

Postmenopausal bleeding can occur for numerous reasons, the most ominous of which is endometrial carcinoma. Other causes include endometrial hyperplasia, endometrial atrophy, submucosal fibroids, and endometrial polyps

(Fig. 25-1). Although US may not definitively diagnose endometrial carcinoma, the purpose of the study is to determine which women need more invasive testing, such as an endometrial biopsy or hysteroscopy.

9. What are the US findings related to endometrial carcinoma?

The main finding of endometrial carcinoma is an abnormally thickened endometrium. Other findings include increased vascularity with multiple feeding vessels and an indistinct interface between the endometrium and the myometrium. These findings are not specific for endometrial carcinoma, however, and further imaging or tissue sampling, or both, is necessary. In an asymptomatic postmenopausal woman not undergoing hormone replacement therapy, the endometrial stripe should not exceed 8 mm. In a woman with postmenopausal bleeding, a biopsy should be considered if the endometrium measures greater than 5 mm. When the endometrium measures 4 mm or less, endometrial atrophy is the most likely diagnosis, and no further work-up is necessary.

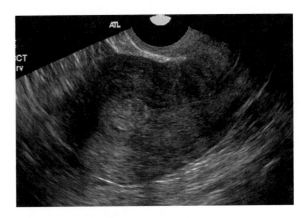

Figure 25-1. Endometrial polyp. Sagittal view of the uterus shows focal echogenic thickening of the endometrial stripe. Doppler interrogation showed a single feeding vessel in this lesion, which turned out to be an endometrial polyp.

10. How can US help differentiate an endometrial polyp from other causes of endometrial thickening?

The most reliable technique to distinguish between these entities is sonohysterography, in which a catheter is introduced into the endometrial canal, and approximately 5 mL of saline is infused into the endometrial cavity during endovaginal US. An endometrial polyp is a focal endocavitary mass that most commonly appears homogeneous and echogenic in texture, but may contain internal cysts, and has either a narrow or broad-based attachment to the endometrium. On color or power Doppler interrogation, the most specific finding of an endometrial polyp is a single central feeding vessel entering from the endometrium.

11. What is the US appearance of endometrial hyperplasia?

Endometrial hyperplasia is commonly a diffuse process with diffuse thickening of the endometrium, but it may occasionally be asymmetric or focal. The thickening is homogeneous or contains small cysts. On color Doppler, hyperplasia is relatively hypovascular, in contrast to cancer, which is typically markedly hypervascular. Sonohysterography helps confirm the diffuse nature of the thickening, which can be adequately sampled with blind biopsy or dilation and curettage. Alternatively, if a focal abnormality is identified at sonohysterography, hysteroscopy is necessary for biopsy or resection because focal lesions may be missed at the time of blind endometrial biopsy or dilation and curettage.

12. Describe the major congenital uterine anomalies.

The uterus, cervix, and upper portion of the vagina develop from the fused ends of the müllerian ducts. Multiple uterine anomalies result from various degrees of arrested development of the müllerian ducts (agenesis, hypoplasia, or unicornuate uterus), failure of fusion of the müllerian ducts (bicornuate or didelphys uterus) (Fig. 25-2), or failure of resorption of the median septum (septate uterus). When a uterine anomaly is identified, it is important to evaluate the kidneys because associated anomalies, such as renal agenesis or renal ectopia, are common.

13. What is the role of US in the diagnosis of uterine anomalies?

Some uterine anomalies can be accurately diagnosed with US, such as absent uterus or didelphys uterus, in which there are two widely separated uterine horns and two cervices. Two-dimensional US may not be accurate, however, in the diagnosis of other uterine

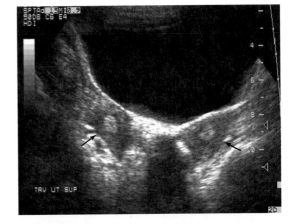

Figure 25-2. Uterine didelphys. Transabdominal transverse view of the pelvis shows two distinct, widely separate uterine horns (*arrows*).

anomalies. It is difficult to distinguish a bicornuate uterus from a septate uterus because it may be impossible to assess the external fundal contour of the uterus. A bicornuate uterus should have a deep fundal indentation of 1 cm or greater, whereas a septate uterus has a normal outer fundal contour. Magnetic resonance imaging (MRI) or three-dimensional US is more accurate in making the appropriate diagnosis and guiding treatment planning.

14. What are the findings associated with adenomyosis on US?
Adenomyosis occurs when there are ectopic endometrial glands within the myometrium. It is a common cause of pelvic pain, menorrhagia, or uterine enlargement (Fig. 25-3). Although MRI is more accurate in the diagnosis of adenomyosis, some US findings are suggestive, such as globular uterine enlargement with asymmetric thickening of the myometrium, heterogeneous myometrium with streaky shadowing, and small myometrial cysts. Compared with fibroids, adenomyosis is more ill-defined, is noncalcified, and is tender to palpation with the vaginal probe.

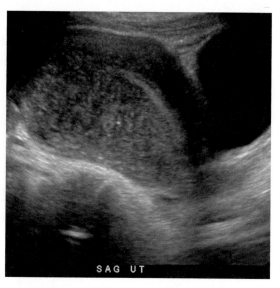

Figure 25-3. Adenomyosis. There is marked thickening and heterogeneity of the posterior wall of the uterus. No discrete mass is identified to suggest fibroids.

15. What is the normal US appearance of the ovary in a premenopausal woman?
The ovaries appear as ovoid soft tissue structures in the adnexa with a volume of approximately 10 mL. During the follicular phase of the cycle, the ovaries contain a varying number of anechoic follicles, which can vary in size depending on the phase of the cycle. During the periovulatory phase, there is commonly a dominant follicle that may measure 2.5 to 3 cm. After ovulation, in the luteal phase, there is commonly a hemorrhagic corpus luteum with internal echoes and a characteristic rim of increased peripheral blood flow.

Key Points: Ultrasound of the Female Pelvis

1. US is useful in evaluating women with pelvic pain, pelvic masses, and dysfunctional uterine bleeding. US can also help in the diagnosis of congenital uterine anomalies and the evaluation of ovarian follicles in infertility patients.
2. Thickening of the endometrial stripe may be a sign of endometrial carcinoma, and further evaluation with hysteroscopy or endometrial biopsy should be performed.
3. Ovarian cysts are very common in premenopausal women, and follow-up of these lesions should be based on their size and morphology.
4. Features that can suggest a benign versus malignant etiology of an ovarian mass depend on the age of the patient, morphology of the lesion, size of the mass, and resistive index.

---

16. Describe the management of simple ovarian cysts in premenopausal women.
Simple cysts within the ovary that are anechoic, thin-walled, and without septations or solid components are managed based on their size. Because the normal dominant follicles can range up to 3 cm (or sometimes greater), simple ovarian cysts smaller than 3 cm in premenopausal women need no follow-up and typically resolve spontaneously. Cysts greater than 3 cm generally require a 6-week follow-up, which places the patient at a different phase in her cycle. If the cyst is large or shows interval growth or lack or regression, further evaluation with laparoscopy may be warranted because many of these lesions represent cystic ovarian neoplasms, such as a benign serous cystadenomas.

17. What are the US findings associated with a hemorrhagic cyst?
A hemorrhagic cyst is a common finding in a premenopausal woman, particularly in the luteal phase of the menstrual cycle, and is often associated with acute onset of pelvic pain. The appearance of the internal blood products varies with the age of the hemorrhage. Acute hemorrhage may mimic an echogenic mass, but can be distinguished from a soft tissue mass by increased through-transmission and lack of internal blood flow. As the clot lyses and retracts, there may be an internal reticular pattern of lacelike septations, an internal fluid-fluid level, or a retracting avascular clot adherent to the wall (Fig. 25-4).

18. What features of an ovarian mass suggest a benign versus malignant etiology?

Patient age is important because benign lesions predominate in premenopausal women. The size of mass is important, too, because masses smaller than 6 cm are typically benign, whereas malignant masses may be very large, often greater than 10 cm. Lesion morphology may be assessed on US. Benign lesions tend to be simple cystic masses with thin, smooth walls. Solid masses or complex cystic masses with thick, irregular septations or mural nodules are typically malignant. Finally, Doppler US findings should be assessed. Malignant masses commonly have increased blood flow to their septations and mural nodules, and they display relatively high diastolic flow, with low resistive indices (<0.4) on pulsed Doppler.

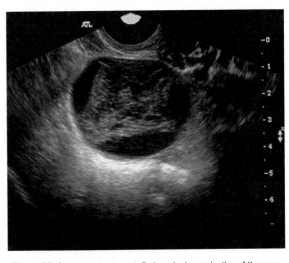

Figure 25-4. Hemorrhagic cyst. Endovaginal examination of the ovary shows a complex cystic mass with increased through-transmission, a lacelike pattern, and a retractile clot adherent to the wall. Color Doppler showed the lesion to be avascular.

19. If a woman presents with a palpable mass in the pelvis, but no abnormality is identified on US, which lesion should be considered? (*Hint:* This is the most common ovarian neoplasm to occur in women younger than 50 years old.)

The palpable mass may represent a dermoid cyst, also known as a *mature teratoma* (Fig. 25-5). Dermoids may be bilateral in 10% to 15% of patients. They have a variety of appearances on US, owing to components arising from any of the three germ layers. They range from completely cystic to completely echogenic with shadowing. The most specific finding is a cystic mass with an echogenic mural nodule, termed the *dermoid plug,* which often contains bone or teeth. Other dermoids have fat/fluid levels or a mesh of floating linear echoes owing to hair. Dermoid cysts with prominent posterior shadowing can be difficult to detect with US because they mimic the appearance of bowel gas, or they may be much larger than what is visible on US, which is known as the "tip-of-the-iceberg" sign.

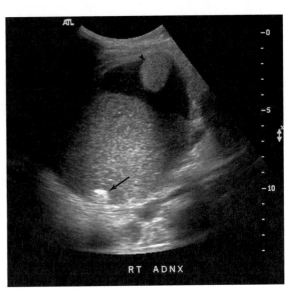

Figure 25-5. Ovarian dermoid—a complex adnexal mass containing cystic and solid components. Anteriorly, there is a solid nodule (*arrowhead*) within the cystic portion of the lesion; this represents the dermoid plug. Posterior is an echogenic structure with shadowing (*arrow*) that represents a tooth.

20. What findings are associated with pelvic inflammatory disease on US?

The findings related to pelvic inflammatory disease depend on the severity of the infection. The US findings may be normal in mild infections or show fluid within the cul-de-sac, mild uterine enlargement, or endometrial fluid. More severe ascending infections result in salpingitis with pyosalpinx (dilated fallopian tube with internal debris and thickened hyperemic fallopian tube wall). The diagnosis of tubo-ovarian abscess is made when the dilated, inflamed tube is inseparable from the ovary, forming a complex hypervascular cystic mass.

21. What is the imaging modality of choice in a patient with suspected endometriosis?

MRI is the best modality to evaluate for endometriosis. US provides little information in cases with disseminated endometriosis. In the focal form of the disease, US can detect endometriomas, which often appear as complex cystic adnexal masses with diffuse, homogeneous, low-level echoes; increased through-transmission; and calcification in the wall (Fig. 25-6).

22. If a woman presents with infertility, hirsutism, and oligomenorrhea, and pelvic US displays large ovaries with multiple, peripherally based follicles, what is the diagnosis?

The diagnosis is Stein-Leventhal syndrome (polycystic ovarian disease) (Fig. 25-7). Although this diagnosis is made clinically, the US finding of enlarged ovaries (e.g., with a volume >18 mL) supports the diagnosis. The ovaries are often rounded in shape, with increased central stroma and multiple, small, peripheral follicles of uniform size, owing to the lack of maturation of a dominant follicle and anovulation. Normal ovaries also often have numerous follicles, but the follicles are typically of varying sizes.

23. What are the US findings associated with ovarian torsion?

Although suspected ovarian torsion is a common indication given by emergency department

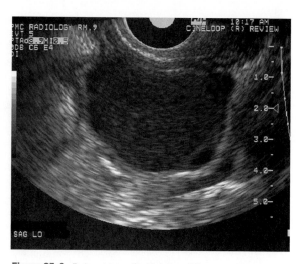

Figure 25-6. Endometrioma. Sagittal view of the ovary shows a mass with diffuse, low-level echoes and increased through-transmission.

clinicians for emergent pelvic US, the incidence is rare, and the diagnosis often must be made clinically. Certain US findings suggest ovarian torsion, however. In the absence of an underlying cyst or mass, the torsed ovary appears enlarged, edematous, and echogenic with small cortical cysts and absent or diminished blood flow, particularly venous. There may be preserved arterial flow because of the dual blood supply or incomplete occlusion of the artery. Severe pain and free fluid are common.

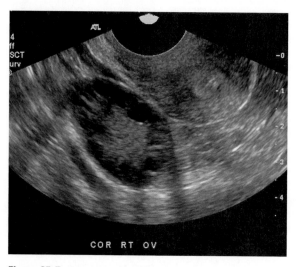

Figure 25-7. Polycystic ovarian disease. US shows an enlarged ovary with multiple peripheral follicles and echogenic central stroma.

BIBLIOGRAPHY

[1] K.G. Davidson, T.J. Dubinsky, Ultrasound evaluation of the endometrium in postmenopausal vaginal bleeding, Radiol. Clin. North Am. 41 (2003) 769–780.

[2] D. Levine, Female pelvis, in: J.P. McGahan, B.B. Goldberg (Eds.), Diagnostic Ultrasound: A Logical Approach, Lippincott-Raven, Philadelphia, 1998, pp. 935–964.

[3] D. Levine, Postmenopausal pelvis, in: J.P. McGahan, B.B. Goldberg (Eds.), Diagnostic Ultrasound: A Logical Approach, Lippincott-Raven, Philadelphia, 1998, pp. 965–985.

[4] K.T. Nguyen, The ovaries and adnexae, in: E.E. Sauerbrei, K.T. Nguyen, R.L. Nolan (Eds.), A Practical Guide to Ultrasound in Obstetrics and Gynecology, Lippincott-Raven, Philadelphia, 1998, pp. 71–103.

[5] M.J. O'Neill, Sonohysterography, Radiol. Clin. North Am. 41 (2003) 781–797.

[6] E.E. Sauerbrei, The non-gravid uterus, vagina, and urethra, in: E.E. Sauerbrei, K.T. Nguyen, R.L. Nolan (Eds.), A Practical Guide to Ultrasound in Obstetrics and Gynecology, Lippincott-Raven, Philadelphia, 1998, pp. 33–70.

MRI OF THE FEMALE PELVIS

Gautham Mallampati, MD

1. Describe the normal location and normal magnetic resonance imaging (MRI) appearance of the ovaries.

Each ovary is located within the ovarian fossa. Anteriorly, the ovarian fossa is bounded by the external iliac vessels. Posteriorly, the ovarian fossa is bounded by the internal iliac vessels and ureter. The ovaries show intermediate signal on T1-weighted MR images. On T2-weighted images, the ovaries are mildly hyperintense to the uterine myometrium. The zonal anatomy of the ovary can often be delineated on T2-weighted images, with the peripheral cortex mildly hypointense to the higher signal central medulla. Uncomplicated functional cysts located within the ovary have high T2-weighted and low T1-weighted signal relative to the ovarian stroma.

2. How can uncomplicated functional cysts be distinguished from cystic ovarian malignancy?

Uncomplicated functional (physiologic) cysts do not contain internal solid components or complex fluid. Physiologic cysts have a thin wall and display no internal architecture. Functional cysts usually measure less than 4.5 cm. Features of cystic ovarian malignancy include solid internal components, such as mural nodules (Fig. 26-1). Ovarian malignancies may display internal hemorrhage and necrotic material, and generally have more heterogeneous signal characteristics than do physiologic cysts.

3. What is the significance of a papillary projection with a cystic ovarian structure?

A papillary projection is a frondlike structure projecting from the cyst wall into the lumen. Its presence indicates that the cyst is neoplastic (as opposed to a physiologic, functional cyst). Ovarian neoplastic cysts may be either benign or malignant.

4. What are four benign masses of the ovary that exhibit characteristic MRI features?

One of the advantages of MRI is its ability to characterize the internal content of masses and narrow the differential diagnosis of masses more precisely than computed tomography (CT) or ultrasound (US). Mature teratomas (also termed *dermoid cysts*), endometriomas, hemorrhagic cysts, and ovarian fibromas can exhibit MRI features that permit benign diagnoses to be made noninvasively.

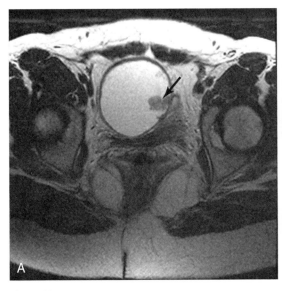 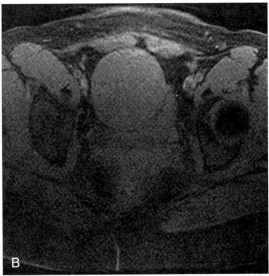

Figure 26-1. Serous cystadenocarcinoma. **A,** T2-weighted MR image shows midline cystic mass with left-sided solid component (*arrow*). **B** and **C,** Precontrast (**B**) and postcontrast (**C**) fat-saturated T1-weighted images show enhancement of the solid component (*arrow*) of a left ovarian serous cystadenocarcinoma.

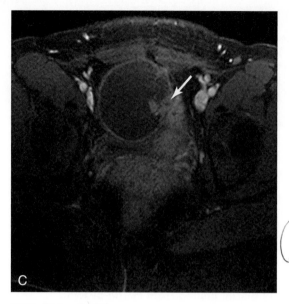

Figure 26-1.—Cont'd

5. Describe the content of mature teratomas that gives them a characteristic MRI appearance.

The diagnosis of mature teratoma is made by identifying macroscopic fat within an ovarian lesion (Fig. 26-2). Fat within an ovarian lesion can be conclusively identified by performing the same T1-weighted sequence with and without explicit fat saturation. Macroscopic fat follows the signal intensity of the body wall fat on all pulse sequences. It is very bright on T1-weighted images performed without fat saturation and dark on T1-weighted images performed with fat saturation. Mature teratomas, although benign, are resected because of potential complications, including ovarian torsion, chemical peritonitis if ruptured, and a very low risk for malignant degeneration.

6. What imaging characteristics does a hemorrhagic ovarian cyst share with a dermoid?

Both of these lesions most commonly reveal high signal intensity on T1-weighted images. In contrast to a fat-containing mature teratoma, the hemorrhagic cyst retains its bright signal intensity on T1-weighted images acquired with fat saturation. The hemorrhagic cyst is a functional cyst, such as a follicular cyst or corpus luteal cyst, that has been complicated by internal hemorrhage. These lesions, in contrast to dermoids, tend to resolve with follow-up.

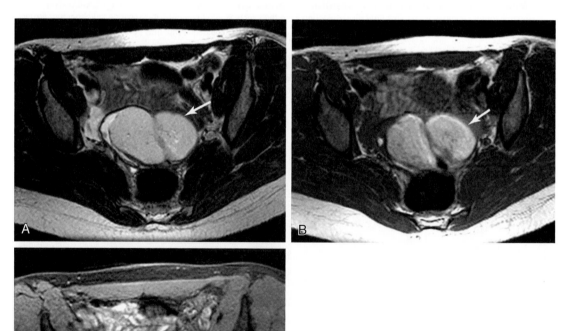

Figure 26-2. Mature ovarian teratoma. A, T2-weighted signal-shot fast spin-echo (FSE) image reveals high signal intensity mass in the posterior pelvis (*arrow*). B, T1-weighted image reveals high signal intensity (*arrow*) within this mass, correlating to either lipomatous or hemorrhagic/proteinaceous content. C, T1 sequence with explicit fat saturation. The region (*arrow*) that was hyperintense in B is now hypointense, indicating that the tissue is fat and not hemorrhage or protein. Fat within an ovarian lesion is diagnostic of a germ cell neoplasm—in this case a benign mature teratoma.

7. Can MRI be used to distinguish between hemorrhagic cysts and endometriomas?
Yes. Although both of these lesions may have similar appearances on T1-weighted images and fat-saturated T1-weighted images because they both contain blood products, the lesions can often be distinguished with the use of T2-weighted images, which are sensitive to internal fluid content. Endometriomas tend to show low signal intensity on T2-weighted images, a characteristic that has been referred to as "shading" (Fig. 26-3). They are also more commonly multiple and bilateral than hemorrhagic cysts.

8. How can MRI aid with the diagnosis of ovarian torsion?
Although US is the first-line imaging method for the evaluation of suspected ovarian torsion, MRI is helpful if US is nondefinitive. MRI findings of torsion include increased ovarian size, increased ovarian T2 signal intensity, deviation of the uterus toward an ipsilateral adnexal mass, and the presence of ascites. A torsed, necrotic ovary fails to enhance after gadolinium administration.

9. From what cell types can primary ovarian tumors originate? What are some collective features of ovarian malignancy?
Cells of epithelial origin account for 85% of ovarian malignancies and 60% of ovarian neoplasms. Sex cord stromal tumors and germ cell tumors account for the remaining malignancies. The presence of solid internal elements is a common feature of malignancy. Thick (>3 mm) internal septations and papillary projections are findings that indicate a cystic structure is more likely a cystic neoplasm rather than a physiologic cyst. Solid, nonfatty mural nodules; peritoneal metastasis; and ascites all are common features of ovarian malignancy.

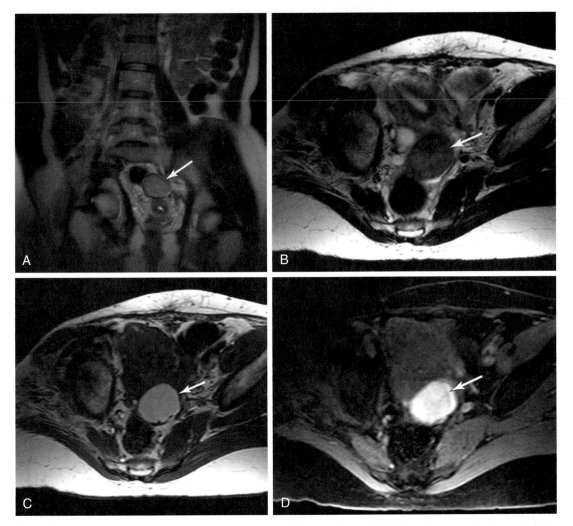

Figure 26-3. Endometrioma. **A** and **B,** Coronal T2-weighted single-shot FSE image (**A**) and axial FSE T2-weighted image (**B**) of the pelvis show a mass posterosuperior to the uterus (*arrows*) that exhibits relatively low signal; this has been termed *shading.* **C,** T1-weighted image shows high signal intensity within this mass (*arrow*). In the ovary, this could be due to either lipomatous or hemorrhagic content. **D,** Fat-saturated T1-weighted image shows preserved high signal intensity of this endometrioma (*arrow*); this represents hemorrhagic contents rather than fat.

10. What is the role of MRI in pregnancy?

US is the imaging technique of choice for the assessment of the fetus. MRI is thought to be safe for the fetus; however, it is avoided in the first trimester unless it offers a large advantage over other studies and is medically necessary. MRI can be useful for the evaluation of fetal anomalies—most commonly cerebral malformations and complex malformations that are difficult to characterize with US. Maternal lesions, such as ovarian malignancies, can also be evaluated with MRI. The administration of gadolinium contrast agents is avoided in pregnant patients because they may cross the placental barrier, and their effect on the fetus is unknown.

11. What is the MRI appearance of the normal uterus?

The uterus comprises the fundus, corpus, and cervix. The corpus and fundus are composed of the endometrium, myometrium, and serosa. The endometrium displays a very high T2-weighted signal. The inner portion of the myometrium, also referred to as the "junctional zone," shows a low signal on T2-weighted images. The outer myometrium and serosa are of intermediate signal intensity. These distinctions become less clear in postmenopausal women. On CT and MRI, the normal cervix enhances less than the uterine corpus and fundus.

12. Describe the types of congenital uterine abnormalities and the role of MRI in detecting them.

Failure of the müllerian ducts to develop properly can result in several different types of uterine anomalies (Fig. 26-4). Septate uterus and bicornuate uterus are the most common abnormalities, and are also the most common types to result in infertility. Septate uterus causes spontaneous abortion more commonly than bicornuate uterus. The treatment for these two abnormalities also differs. Septate uterus can be treated with hysteroscopic resection of the septum. Bicornuate uterus is treated with open surgery. MRI can generally distinguish between these two abnormalities. A septate uterus has a smooth outer contour and a fibrous septum. A bicornuate uterus displays a depression (≥1 cm) of the outer contour of the fundus and a thicker, more muscular septum.

13. Name two benign diseases of the uterine myometrium.

Uterine leiomyomas (fibroids) and adenomyosis are benign diseases of the uterine myometrium. US is the primary modality for evaluation of leiomyoma, although MRI can generally provide more definitive lesion characterization and localization. Leiomyomas can occur in submucosal, intramural, and subserosal locations. Submucosal lesions abut the endometrial canal. Intramural lesions are located entirely within the muscular wall of the uterus. Subserosal lesions lie more peripherally, just deep to the outermost layer of the uterus, and can become pedunculated.

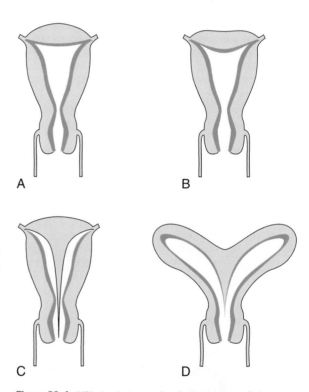

Figure 26-4. Müllerian duct anomalies. **A,** Normal uterus. **B,** Arcuate uterus, with a small (<1 cm) depression of the outer contour of the uterine fundus. **C,** Septate uterus, with a thin internal septum, but a normal outer contour to the uterine fundus. **D,** Bicornuate uterus, with a deep depression of the outer contour of the fundus; this results from a partial failure of fusion of the müllerian ducts.

Leiomyomas are well-demarcated lesions with low signal intensity on T1-weighted and T2-weighted images. Leiomyomas usually show some degree of enhancement after the administration of gadolinium contrast material. Avid leiomyoma enhancement is correlated with favorable symptomatic response of fibroid-related pelvic pain after uterine arterial embolization therapy. Adenomyosis occurs when there is invasion of the myometrium by endometrial tissue. It is manifested by either focal or diffuse areas of junctional zone thickening.

14. What degree of junctional zone thickness is indicative of adenomyosis?

The normal junctional zone is less than 8 mm in thickness (Fig. 26-5). When the junctional zone is either focally or diffusely greater than 12 mm in thickness, adenomyosis can be diagnosed (Fig. 26-6). In adenomyosis, the normally low

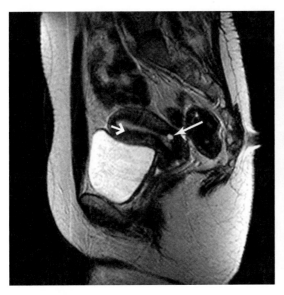

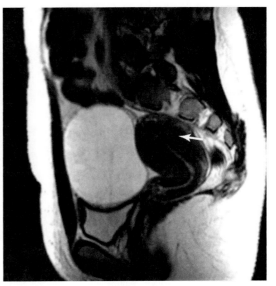

Figure 26-5. Normal uterine junctional zone. The junctional zone (*short arrow*) in this patient measures 7 mm and is normal in appearance. Note the small benign nabothian cyst in the cervix (*long arrow*).

Figure 26-6. Adenomyosis. The junctional zone (*arrow*) in this patient measures 16 mm, indicating diffuse adenomyosis. Also note the cystic lesion anterior to the uterus and superior to the bladder, which is a pathologically proven serous cystadenoma.

T2 signal intensity junctional zone can contain islets of focally increased T2-weighted signal intensity. The presence of these areas of signal discrepancy can be used to suggest adenomyosis with an intermediate junctional zone thickness of 8 to 12 mm.

15. If focal adenomyosis and leiomyomas are both of low-signal intensity on T1 and T2 images, how are they distinguished?
Adenomyosis generally displays ill-defined borders, whereas leiomyomas are more commonly well defined on MRI. Focal areas of adenomyosis, or adenomyomas, are usually oval, with the long axis of the lesion parallel to the endometrium. Adenomyomas also show little mass effect.

16. Name three malignant uterine neoplasms.
Endometrial cancer, uterine sarcoma, and cervical carcinoma are three malignant uterine neoplasms. Endometrial cancer is the most common type of female genital tract cancer. Cervical cancer is the third most common type, after ovarian carcinoma. Uterine sarcomas are rare.

17. What is the role of MRI in endometrial carcinoma?
MRI is not used in screening for endometrial diseases because benign entities such as endometrial polyps and hyperplasia have a similar MRI appearance to early endometrial cancer. MRI can be helpful for the staging of endometrial cancer. Endometrial cancer most commonly appears as widening of the endometrial stripe. Extension into the myometrium, extension toward the cervix, regional nodal spread, and distant metastases all can be characterized with MRI.

18. What is the normal appearance of the uterine cervix on MRI?
The zonal anatomy of the cervix is best appreciated on T2-weighted images. The epithelium and mucus within the endocervical canal are of high T2 signal. Immediately peripheral to the epithelium is a layer of T2-hypointense stroma. A more intermediate T2 signal layer of smooth muscle is located outside of the fibrous stroma. This layer is contiguous with the outer myometrium of the uterus (Fig. 26-7).

19. Describe the role of MRI in the evaluation of cervical cancer.
Similar to its role in endometrial cancer, MRI is not used for the diagnosis of cervical cancer, but for the staging of disease. MRI can assess for the presence of parametrial invasion and distinguish between early stage and advanced stage cancer. Early stage cancer can be treated with hysterectomy; advanced cancer is initially treated with a combination of chemotherapy and radiation therapy. The presence of parametrial invasion is represented on T2-weighted images by spread of tumor through the low-intensity fibrous stroma, described previously. MRI is also useful for the diagnosis of recurrent cervical cancer.

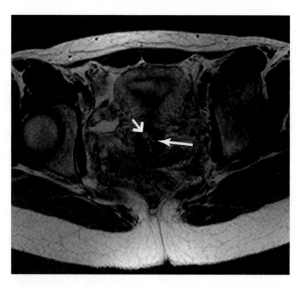

Figure 26-7. Normal cervical anatomy. The endocervix is hyperintense on this T2-weighted image (*long arrow*) and is surrounded by T2-hypointense cervical stroma and, more peripherally, a more intermediate signal layer of smooth muscle. Note the benign nabothian cyst (*short arrow*).

20. What term is given to the cystic outpouchings of the anterior urethra into the vaginal canal? How do these outpouchings appear on MRI?

Cystic outpouchings of the urethra are termed *urethral diverticula.* These diverticula are caused by obstruction of the periurethral glands secondary to recurrent infections. Similar to other cystic lesions on MRI, these lesions show bright T2 signal and low T1 signal. MRI is superior to other imaging methods for the evaluation of these lesions when they become symptomatic because it offers valuable anatomic information for surgical planning.

Key Points: MRI of the Female Pelvis

1. MRI can accurately characterize many benign lesions of the ovary, including physiologic cysts, mature teratomas (also known as dermoid cysts), endometriomas, fibromas, and hemorrhagic cysts.
2. Findings used to distinguish ovarian cystic neoplasms from simple, physiologic ovarian cysts include thick internal septations; papillary projections; and solid, enhancing, mural nodules.
3. MRI is useful for the staging of ovarian, endometrial, cervical, and vaginal cancers.
4. Uterine leiomyomas and adenomyosis are two benign diseases that have characteristic MRI appearances.
5. Cystic lesions of the female pelvis include ovarian cysts, Bartholin cysts, Gartner duct cysts, and urethral diverticula. All show high T2-weighted signal because they contain fluid. The T1 signal may be variable because of the presence of variable amounts of internal hemorrhage or protein.

---

21. What is the difference between the MRI appearance of Bartholin cysts and Gartner duct cyst?

Bartholin cysts arise from obstruction of the Bartholin glands, which are located in the distal (inferior) posterolateral vagina. Gartner duct cysts are congenital lesions located in the anterolateral aspect of the proximal (superior) vagina. Both of these lesions show the typical high T2-weighted signal of cysts. The T1-weighted signal may vary if the cysts are complicated with infection or proteinaceous content.

22. What is the most common primary vaginal malignancy?

Squamous cell carcinomas constitute most vaginal malignancies. MRI is primarily used for tumor staging. The normal vagina shows a normal central area of high T2 signal and low T1 signal that correspond to the mucosal layer and fluid within the canal. Moving outward from the lumen, the second layer of the vagina is of low signal on T1-weighted and T2-weighted images and includes the submucosa and muscularis. The most peripheral layer consists of the adventitia, which is of high T2 signal and low T1 signal intensity. Vaginal cancer is best appreciated on T2-weighted images, where the tumors are generally hyperintense to the normal vaginal muscularis. Vaginal malignancies generally show enhancement.

23. When is MRI of the female pelvis performed with and without the patient engaging in the Valsalva maneuver?

MRI of the female pelvis is performed with and without Valsalva maneuver routinely for the assessment of pelvic floor laxity. The descent of pelvic organs below the pubococcygeal line, which connects the last joint of the coccyx to the inferior portion of the pubic symphysis, is indicative of pelvic floor laxity.

BIBLIOGRAPHY

[1] S. Chaudhry, C. Reinhold, A. Guermazi, et al., Benign and malignant diseases of the endometrium, Top. Magn. Reson. Imaging 14 (2003) 339–357.
[2] E.S. Pretorius, E.K. Outwater, J.L. Hunt, E.S. Siegelman, Magnetic resonance imaging of the ovary, Top. Magn. Reson. Imaging 12 (2001) 131–146.
[3] J. Ryu, B. Kim, MR imaging of the male and female urethra, Radiographics 21 (2001) 1169–1185.
[4] K. Togashi, MR imaging of the ovaries: normal appearance and benign disease, Radiol. Clin. North. Am. 41 (2003) 799–811.

MRI AND ULTRASOUND OF THE MALE PELVIS

Lisa Jones, MD, PhD, and
E. Scott Pretorius, MD

1. What is the anatomy of the prostate gland?
The prostate consists of a peripheral gland and a central gland (Fig. 27-1). The central gland is located anterior and superior to the peripheral gland and is the portion of the prostate gland that is most intimate to the urethra. Benign prostatic hyperplasia (BPH) affects the central gland. The peripheral gland comprises the posterior and inferior aspects of the prostate. Although cancer can occur in the central gland, most cancers occur in the peripheral gland. Perhaps counterintuitively, the more cranial portion of the prostate is termed the *base*. The more caudal portion is termed the *apex*.

2. What is the normal size of the prostate gland?
Radiologists often estimate the volume of objects by multiplying the anteroposterior, transverse, and longitudinal measurements by one another and then multiplying that result by 0.52, which is π/6. This is an estimation of the volume of an elliptical object. Expected prostate volume increases with advancing age. A prostate with a volume of greater than 40 mL is considered to be enlarged.

3. What values of prostate-specific antigen (PSA) are considered normal and abnormal?
A normal PSA value is less than 4, and an abnormal value is greater than 10. Values between 4 and 10 are borderline.

4. Other than prostate cancer, what can elevate PSA?
Prostatitis, BPH, prostate infarcts, and biopsy can cause an elevated PSA.

5. Where does BPH usually occur? What does it typically look like on magnetic resonance imaging (MRI) and ultrasound (US)?
BPH usually starts in the transitional zone of the central gland, which is the portion that is most intimate to the urethra. BPH is generally of more heterogeneous signal intensity on T2-weighted MR images than the normal gland and can indent the bladder base. On US, BPH is usually hypoechoic to normal gland.

6. What is the distribution of prostate cancer within the gland?
About 70% of tumors begin in the peripheral gland, and the remainder begin in the central gland.

7. What is the primary role of US and MRI in the evaluation of prostate cancer?
US has low sensitivity for detecting prostate cancer (60% to 70%) and is not used for screening. It is used to guide random biopsies of the gland. MRI also has inadequate sensitivity for screening purposes and is primarily used to stage cancer patients at clinical risk for extracapsular spread of tumor. Accuracy of MRI for staging is 50% to 90%.

8. What is the typical imaging appearance of prostate cancer on transrectal US and MRI?
- *US*: Prostate cancer appears as a hypoechoic mass in 70% of cases. Its appearance in the remaining cases is hyperechoic or of mixed echogenicity.
- *MRI*: Prostate cancer typically is isointense to gland on T1-weighted images and hypointense to the normally high-intensity peripheral zone on T2-weighted images (Fig. 27-2). Central gland malignancy is generally difficult to identify because of the presence of BPH, which distorts normal anatomy.

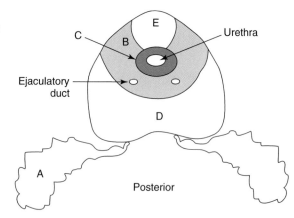

Figure 27-1. Axial line drawing of the prostate and seminal vesicles (*A* = seminal vesicles, *B* = central zone of prostate, *C* = transitional zone of prostate, *D* = peripheral zone of prostate, *E* = fibromuscular stroma of prostate). The right ejaculatory duct connects the seminal vesicle to the urethra.

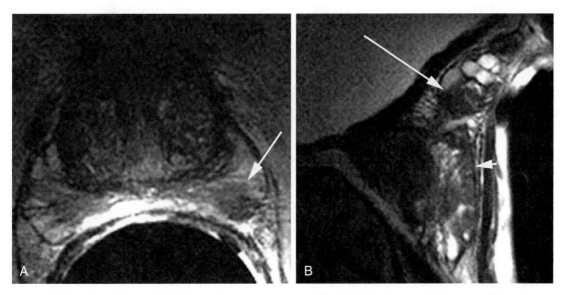

Figure 27-2. Prostate cancer. **A,** Axial T2-weighted MR image. *Arrow* points to the focus of prostate cancer in the normally T2-hyperintense peripheral zone. **B,** T2-weighted sagittal image in another patient shows a low signal tumor in the normally hyperintense seminal vesicles (*long arrow*), representing extracapsular spread of tumor (*short arrow*) and nonsurgical disease. The same patient also had lymphadenopathy and osseous metastases.

9. **When should MRI be performed after biopsy? How is postbiopsy hemorrhage differentiated from tumor in the peripheral zone?**
   MRI should be performed about 3 weeks after biopsy. At this time, less than 50% of patients have residual hemorrhage. Hemorrhage and tumor are distinguished by comparing T1-weighted and T2-weighted images. T1-hyperintense/T2-hypointense areas correspond to postbiopsy hemorrhage. T1-isointense/T2-hypointense areas are more likely to correspond to tumor.

10. **How is prostate cancer staged? How does the cancer stage affect patient management?**
    The American Urological Association stages prostate cancer with the following classification:
    - Stage A: Clinically unapparent
    - Stage B: Tumor confined to prostate
    - Stage C: Tumor extends beyond the capsule (may involve the seminal vesicles)
    - Stage D: Metastatic disease to pelvic or distant nodes, bones, soft tissues, or organs

    Surgery is generally recommended for patients with stage A and B cases. Stage C (extracapsular extension) cases preclude radical prostatectomy in younger patients. Patients with stage D cases are treated with palliative radiation and hormonal treatment.

11. **What signs of nonsurgical (stage C or D) disease can be seen on MRI?**
    Direct extracapsular spread of tumor nodule into periprostatic fat or neurovascular bundle, direct ascent of tumor up the ejaculatory ducts into the seminal vesicles, lymph node involvement (particularly in obturator and pelvic side-wall chains), and osseous metastatic disease can be seen on MRI.

12. **Where does capsular penetration most commonly occur?**
    Capsular penetration most commonly occurs at the prostatic apex (inferiorly). An irregular capsular bulge is more likely than a smooth bulge to reflect capsular penetration.

Key Points: Prostate Cancer

1. Prostate cancer usually occurs in the peripheral zone.
2. Bone metastases are very unlikely with a PSA of less than 10.
3. Extracapsular extension indicates nonsurgical disease. Patients are treated with chemotherapy or hormonal therapy.
4. Prostate cancer (hypointense) may be distinguished from postbiopsy hemorrhage (hyperintense) on T1 sequences. Both are generally hypointense on T2 sequences.

13. What is hematospermia? What causes it?

Hematospermia is blood in the ejaculate. It is usually benign before age 40, when it is commonly due to prostatitis or orchitis. In patients older than 40, benign causes still predominate, but 5% to 10% of cases are related to malignancy. Carcinoma of the bladder and carcinoma of the prostate are most common.

14. Where do the testicular arteries arise?

The testicular arteries supply the testes and arise from the aorta near the level of the renal vessels. The normal testes descend from this level into the scrotum.

15. Describe the normal appearance of the testis and epididymis on US.

Each testis is ovoid, homogeneous in echotexture, and measures approximately 3 × (2 to 4) × (3 to 5) cm. Centrally within each testis is an echogenic linear structure, the mediastinum testis, which is an invagination of the surrounding tunica albuginea (Figs. 27-3 and 27-4). The testicles and epididymides should have symmetric vascularity and echotexture. Each epididymis is located posterolateral to the testis and is either isoechoic or slightly hyperechoic to the testis. The epididymis comprises a head, body, and tail. The epididymal head measures 9 to 12 mm in diameter and is triangle-shaped. The epididymal body and tail are thinner, measuring 2 to 5 mm in diameter.

16. How does the testicle appear on MRI?

T2-weighted images are best for evaluating testicular parenchyma. As on US, testicular tissue is relatively homogeneous and is very T2 hyperintense to nearby soft tissue structures. The surrounding tunica albuginea is well delineated as a low T1, low-T2 signal intensity band surrounding each testicle. The mediastinum testis, as an invagination of the tunica, is also hypointense to testicular parenchyma.

17. What is cryptorchidism? What does a cryptorchid testicle look like?

Cryptorchidism is incomplete descent of a testicle into the scrotum. It occurs in 3% of neonates, but many testicles descend by age 1 (prevalence of 1%). The cryptorchid testis is commonly located in or below the inguinal canal and can be found by physical examination, US, or MRI. In about 10% to 20% of cases, the cryptorchid testis is located intra-abdominally, and MRI is the modality of choice for detecting the testis. On US, the cryptorchid testicle is identified by the presence of its echogenic mediastinum; it is usually small and hypoechoic relative to a normal testicle. On MRI, the cryptorchid testicle is generally smaller than a normal testicle. It is generally T2 hyperintense, similar to a normally descended organ.

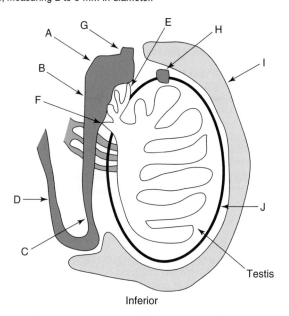

Figure 27-3. Sagittal drawing of the testicle and epididymis (*A* = epididymal head, *B* = epididymal body, *C* = epididymal tail, *D* = vas deferens, *E* = efferent ductules, *F* = rete testis; *G* = appendix epididymis, *H* = appendix testis, *I* = tunica vaginalis, *J* = tunica albuginea).

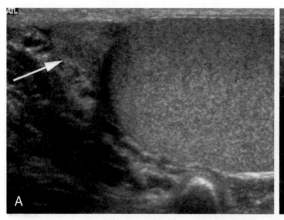
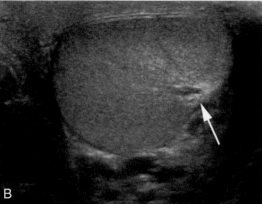

Figure 27-4. A, Sagittal view of epididymis (*arrow*) and superior pole of the testis. **B,** Transverse view of the testis; *arrow* points to the echogenic mediastinum where vessels and ductules enter the testis.

18. What are complications of cryptorchidism?

Cryptorchid testes have an 8 to 30 times increased risk for malignancy, mostly by seminomas. Cryptorchid testes are also more likely to experience torsion. Affected patients also have a higher-than-baseline risk of infertility.

19. What is testicular microlithiasis? Name diseases commonly associated with microlithiasis.

Testicular microlithiasis can be seen on US, but generally is not visible on MRI (Fig. 27-5). Testicular microlithiasis refers to minute calcifications (more than five foci per cross-sectional image) associated with cryptorchidism, Klinefelter syndrome, and pseudohermaphroditism. Although not a premalignant condition, it may be a marker of increased risk for testicular cancer. Yearly US examinations are recommended at some institutions to screen for tumor.

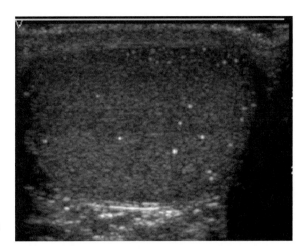

Figure 27-5. US image shows multiple echogenic foci in the testicle, representing testicular microlithiasis.

20. What is the most important question to consider when imaging a palpable scrotal abnormality? Why?

Is there a mass in the testicle? Most intratesticular masses are malignant. Most extratesticular scrotal masses are benign.

21. What is the most common cause of a scrotal mass?

A spermatocele or an epididymal cyst is the most common cause of a scrotal mass. Spermatoceles and epididymal cysts are generally indistinguishable on US: Both appear as anechoic (homogeneously dark) lesions in the epididymis. Epididymal cysts contain simple fluid. Spermatoceles contain spermatozoa. Differentiating epididymal cysts from spermatoceles is rarely of clinical importance.

22. Do cysts occur in the testicle? Is there anything else in the differential diagnosis?

Yes. Cysts have been reported in 10% of testicular US images, more commonly in elderly men, and are typically located near the mediastinum testis. Testicular cysts are benign. Common mimics of testicular cysts include tunica albuginea cysts and tubular ectasia of the retia testes (Fig. 27-6), which result in multiple, tubular cystic structures in the region of the mediastinum testis (usually bilateral and associated with epididymal cysts and history of vasectomy or epididymitis). Other things to consider in the differential diagnosis are a testicular abscess, which should not appear simple and may contain gas, and a cystic tumor, which is differentiated by a thick wall or solid component.

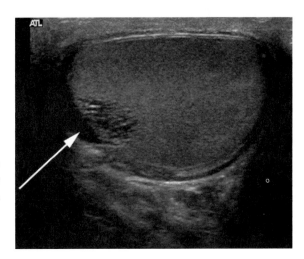

Figure 27-6. US image shows dilation of the rete testis (*arrow*); this is a benign condition.

23. What is the differential diagnosis of a solid testicular mass? Can these be distinguished on US and MRI?

Testicular malignancies are the most common. Less common entities include focal orchitis, hematoma, infarction, and rare benign tumors such as epidermoid inclusion cyst. Most of these entities are not reliably distinguished on US because small tumors may appear avascular on color Doppler. On MRI, hematoma, infarction, and epidermoid do not enhance. Orchitis can be very difficult to differentiate from tumor using either modality. Performing imaging again after successful treatment of infection may be useful.

24. Name the different types of malignant testicular lesions.

- Germ cell tumors include seminoma (which is overall the most common type), endodermal sinus (yolk sac), teratoma, embryonal cell, choriocarcinoma, and mixed germ cell types (second most common type).

- Stromal tumors include Leydig cell and Sertoli cell tumors.
- Metastatic disease is most commonly from lymphoma/leukemia. Prostate, lung, melanoma, colon, and renal cell carcinomas also can metastasize to the testicle.

25. What are the most common types of tumors in young adults (20 to 34 years old), children, and older adults (>50 years old)?
In young adults, seminoma is the most common tumor. In children, teratomas and yolk sac tumors are the most common. In older adults, lymphoma and metastases are more common than primary germ cell tumors. In men older than 50, lymphoma accounts for 25% of testicular tumors, and it is the most common testicular neoplasm in men older than 60.

26. Which category of testicular tumors is most common overall?
Germ cell tumors account for approximately 95% of cases.

27. Germ cell tumors are generally classified according to whether they are seminomatous or nonseminomatous. Why is this distinction important? Describe the general differences between the tumors in these two categories.
Seminoma has a better prognosis, occurs in an older age group (fourth decade), is more sensitive to radiation, and usually appears as a homogeneous hypoechoic intratesticular mass that generally does not invade the tunica albuginea or have cystic components. It does not produce alpha fetoprotein. Any tumor that produces alpha fetoprotein is considered nonseminomatous.

Nonseminomatous germ cell tumors are often of mixed cell type. Relative to seminomas, they have a worse prognosis and are less radiosensitive. Expression of tumor markers depends on constituents. Usually, they are ill-defined inhomogeneous masses, commonly with cystic components, areas of hemorrhage, and calcification or fibrosis. They are more commonly associated with invasion of the tunica albuginea.

28. List the stages of primary testicular tumor.
- Stage I: Confined to scrotum
- Stage II: Involves lymph nodes inferior to the diaphragm
- Stage III: Has metastasized to extra-abdominal nodes
- Stage IV: Extranodal disease

29. Describe the spread of primary testicular tumors.
Primary testicular tumors usually spread along gonadal lymphatics to retroperitoneal lymph nodes, often appearing first at approximately the level of the renal hilum on the left and slightly lower on the right (Fig. 27-7). Inferior iliac and inguinal lymph nodes are usually spared, unless the primary tumor has invaded the scrotal skin or epididymis, or unless there has been prior surgery (e.g., in recurrent disease after orchiectomy). Hematogenous spread generally occurs after lymphatic spread, usually to the lungs.

30. Which germ cell tumor has a tendency for early hematogenous metastases?
Choriocarcinoma often metastasizes to the lung. It is known for its tendency to produce hemorrhagic metastases.

Key Points: Testicular Cancer

1. Testicular cancer is the most common solid neoplasm in men 20 to 40 years old.
2. Germ cell tumors are most the common tumor type overall.
3. The most common testicular neoplasm is seminoma in young men and lymphoma in elderly men.
4. Seminoma has the best prognosis of germ cell tumors and is radiosensitive.
5. Lymphatic spread of testicular cancer is first to retroperitoneal lymph nodes, unless there is invasion of the scrotal skin or prior surgery, in which case pelvic nodes may be involved early.

---

31. What types of testicular tumors are hormonally active? Which of these is most common?
Stromal tumors (Leydig and Sertoli) are hormonally active. Leydig tumor is more common and can produce androgens. Sertoli tumors may produce estrogens. Ten percent of Leydig tumors are malignant.

32. What is the differential diagnosis for multiple intratesticular masses?
- Lymphoma—generally older patients; bilateral in 10% to 20% of cases; involvement of epididymis and spermatic cord favors lymphoma over seminoma, which can otherwise be very similar in appearance

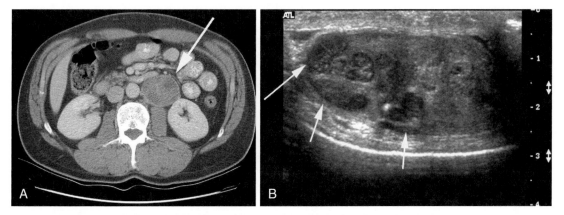

Figure 27-7. A, Axial CT scan shows retroperitoneal lymphadenopathy (*arrow*) near the left renal hilum. **B,** Sagittal US image of the left testicle of the same patient shows multifocal seminoma (*arrows*).

- Leukemia—testes commonly involved, similar in appearance to lymphoma, bilateral or unilateral
- Bilateral seminomas
- Metastases, other than leukemia/lymphoma
- Adrenal rests—benign, bilateral, seen in 8% of patients with congenital adrenal hyperplasia, may regress with therapy
- Leydig cell hyperplasia—often bilateral, commonly seen in Klinefelter syndrome

33. What is an epidermoid inclusion cyst? Is it malignant?
Epidermoid inclusion cyst is (along with simple testicular cyst) one of the few intratesticular entities that is benign. It is a nonvascular, well-circumscribed solid tumor of germ cell origin that consists only of ectodermal elements (in contrast to teratoma, which contains all tissue elements).

34. What does an epidermoid inclusion cyst look like?
Classic epidermoid lesions have a lamellated "onion-skin" appearance on US and MRI (Fig. 27-8). They can also appear as target lesions with a hyperechoic center and a hypoechoic rim, or as rim calcified hypoechoic lesions.

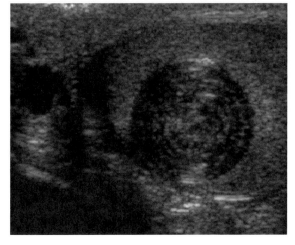

Figure 27-8. US image shows characteristic "onion-skin" appearance of epidermoid inclusion cyst.

35. Name several structures that may herniate through the inguinal canal into the scrotal sac.
Bowel (which can be identified by the presence of gas and peristalsis), mesenteric fat, the peritoneum with ascites, and the urinary bladder all can herniate into the scrotal sac.

36. What is a varicocele, and how is it diagnosed? Is it more common on the left or the right?
A varicocele is a dilated, tortuous vein of the pampiniform plexus, or a vein that is more than 2 mm in diameter located posteriorly near the upper pole of the testes. A varicocele shows little flow on color Doppler at rest and shows increased distention and flow when the patient is upright or performs the Valsalva maneuver. Approximately 85% of these veins are on the left because of compression of the left renal vein by the superior mesenteric artery as it crosses the aorta. Varicoceles occur in 15% of the population and are bilateral 10% of the time.

37. What are complications of a varicocele?
Complications of varicocele include infertility (50% of men presenting with infertility have varicoceles) and pain.

38. Under what circumstances is a varicocele concerning? Why?
Varicoceles are more concerning if they are nondecompressible or right-sided, or if the patient presents with one after age 40. In these cases, cross-sectional imaging is indicated to evaluate for a possible ipsilateral mass obstructing gonadal venous return.

39. What is a hydrocele?
A hydrocele is excess fluid within the tunica vaginalis. On US, a hydrocele typically is hypoechoic with good sound transmission. If complicated by blood (hematocele) or pus (pyocele), it may contain septations or echogenic material.

40. Name the common causes of a hydrocele.
Causes are diverse and include congenital patent processus vaginalis, trauma, surgery, diabetes, neoplasm, epididymo-orchitis, and torsion.

41. What is the clinical differential diagnosis for an acutely painful scrotum? How is this usually evaluated with imaging?
US is used to evaluate the painful scrotum. Epididymitis/orchitis accounts for 75% to 80% of cases of acute scrotal pain. Testicular torsion, or torsion of the testicular appendage, is also an important cause. Strangulated hernia, testicular neoplasm, and trauma can also cause scrotal pain.

42. What are the most common types of testicular torsion? Why does it occur?
Intravaginal torsion is more common and is due to the "bell clapper" deformity. It is present in 10% of men in autopsy series and refers to the complete investment of the testes and epididymis by the tunica vaginalis, which results in incomplete fixation of the testis. The testicle can freely rotate around its vascular pedicle, causing torsion. Intravaginal torsion manifests during the teenage years. Extravaginal torsion, in which the tunica and testes twist at the external ring, occurs in neonates. It is not associated with the bell clapper deformity.

43. What is the key criterion in diagnosing testicular torsion?
Absent or decreased blood flow is the key criterion. It is often stated that compromise of venous flow is more sensitive for detection of torsion than abnormal arterial flow.

44. Why is the sensitivity of US for torsion only about 90%?
At the time of imaging, a testicle may have untwisted or torsion may be incomplete (<360 degrees), and the testicle may have blood flow (Fig. 27-9).

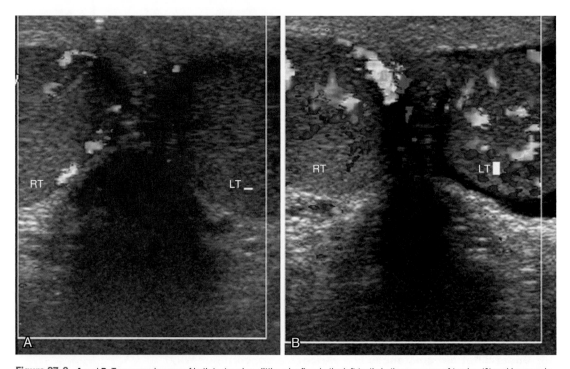

Figure 27-9. A and **B,** Transverse images of both testes show little color flow in the left testis in the presence of torsion (**A**) and hyperemia after detorsion (**B**).

> **Key Points: Testicular Torsion**
>
> 1. A testicular torsion is usually due to the bell clapper deformity in teenagers.
> 2. The diagnosis of testicular torsion is based on the identification of abnormal blood flow, not the gray-scale appearance
> 3. A normal gray-scale appearance (<6 hours) suggests viability.
> 4. Venous flow becomes abnormal before arterial flow.
> 5. False-negative results may be due to detorsion or partial torsion.
> 6. A testicle may be hyperemic after detorsion, simulating orchitis.

45. What is the imaging appearance of acute epididymitis?

The epididymis is enlarged and has increased blood flow. Epididymitis most commonly involves the epididymal head and is often diffuse, but also commonly can involve only the epididymal body and tail, which must be examined. In subtle cases, asymmetry can be a helpful clue to the presence of epididymitis. Accessory findings include hydrocele (simple), pyocele (echogenic), and skin thickening.

46. What are the complications of epididymitis?

Complications include orchitis (diffuse or focal hyperemia and enlargement of the testicle, which may also be relatively hypoechoic, occurs in 20% to 40% of cases), pyocele, scrotal abscess, infarction, chronic epididymitis, and infertility (Fig. 27-10).

47. What is a cause of isolated diffuse hyperemia of the testicle (orchitis without epididymitis)?

Viral causes of orchitis (e.g., mumps) or syphilis causes isolated diffuse hyperemia of the testicle.

48. What else may cause hyperemia of the testicle and epididymis?

Post-torsion luxury perfusion (increased blood flow may result after a time of hypoperfusion) and trauma may cause hyperemia of the testicle and epididymis. The clinical history may help differentiate among possibilities.

49. What are the possible US findings after testicular trauma?

Nonsurgical findings include extratesticular hematoma/hematocele (simple to complex extratesticular fluid collection or cystic mass) or traumatic epididymitis. Findings that indicate surgery include testicular fracture or rupture (look for fracture line in testicle), devascularization, intratesticular hematoma, and disruption of normal contour/tunica albuginea. This is a surgical emergency; if surgery is performed within 72 hours of injury, 90% of fractured testicles can be restored.

50. Describe the normal appearance of the penis on MRI.

The penis is composed of three vascular cylinders. There are two dorsally located corpora cavernosa and the single ventral midline corpus spongiosum. Each cylinder is surrounded by a T2 hypointense fibrous band, the tunica albuginea (Figs. 27-11 and 27-12). All three cylinders tend to be T2 hyperintense to surrounding structures. The cavernosal bodies

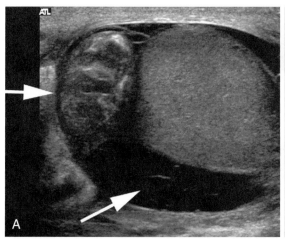 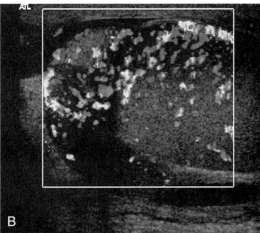

Figure 27-10. A and B, Sagittal images of the right testis in a patient with epididymo-orchitis. An enlarged, inflamed epididymis is represented by the *short arrow,* and a complex hydrocele with septations is represented by the *long arrow.* Note the enlargement, heterogeneity, and hypervascularity of the epididymis and testis.

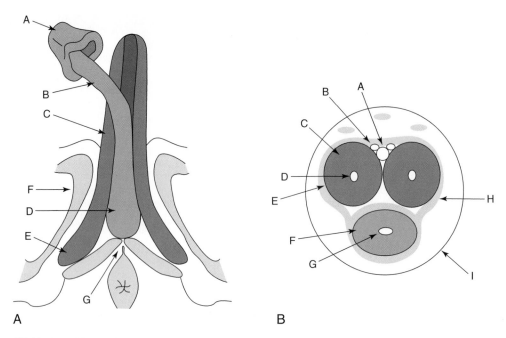

Figure 27-11. **A,** Axial line drawing of the penis (*A* = glans penis, *B* = corpora spongiosum, *C* = right corpus cavernosum, *D* = cavernosal artery, *E* = crus, *F* = ischiopubic ramus, *G* = perineal body). **B,** Coronal line drawing of the penis (*A* = dorsal artery of the penis, *B* = deep dorsal vein [note also the superficial dorsal veins], *C* = right corpus cavernosum, *E* = tunica albuginea, *F* = corpora cavernosa, *G* = urethra, *H* = Buck fascia, *I* = epidermis).

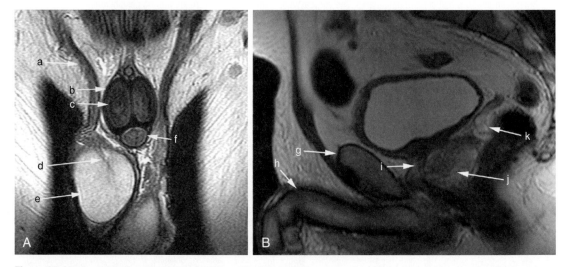

Figure 27-12. Normal penile anatomy. **A,** Coronal T2-weighted MR image (*a* = spermatic cord, *b* = Buck fascia and tunica albuginea, *c* = corpus cavernosum, *d* = central cavernosal artery, *e* = testis, *f* = corpus spongiosum). **B,** T2-weighted image (*g* = symphysis pubis, *h* = corpora cavernosum [again], *i* = urethra, *j* = prostate, *k* = seminal vesicles).

communicate with one another through holes in the intercavernosal septum and should always be isointense to one another. The spongiosum also tends to be relatively T2 hyperintense, but may have different signal from the cavernosa because it is functionally a separate space and may have a different rate of vascular flow within its channels than do the cavernosa. When viewed in cross section, the cavernosa each have a small, medially located T2 hyperintense "dot," which is the cavernosal artery. The flattened T2 dark band seen in the spongiosum is the urethra.

51. Describe the physiologic factors behind erection.

After an appropriate stimulus, vascular resistance decreases, and blood flow through the cavernous arteries increases, resulting in expansion of blood sinusoids in the cavernosa. Expansion of the corpora compresses the draining veins in the nonexpendable tunica albuginea, and penile erection is sustained.

52. What congenital abnormality of the penis is associated with bladder exstrophy?

Epispadias, the absence of the dorsal covering of the penis and ectopic dorsal location of the meatus, is associated with bladder exstrophy. Epispadias also may be associated with a foreshortened penis.

53. The penile meatus is located more ventrally and proximally than expected. What is this congenital malformation called? What is an associated finding?

This congenital malformation is termed *hypospadias*. A dilated utricle, which is a midline cystic structure typically within the prostate, is an associated finding.

54. What is the most common cancer of the penis in an adult? What are the risk factors?

Squamous cell cancer is the most common cancer of the penis, although it still accounts for less than 1% of all genitourinary malignancies in men. Risk factors include infection with human papillomavirus 16 or 18, lack of circumcision (owing to the chronic irritative effect of smegma), and patient age (sixth and seventh decades are the most common). Carcinoma of the penis is much more common in Asia and Africa than in Europe and the Americas.

55. Where is the cancer most commonly located?

Carcinoma of the penis, which is most commonly found in the glans penis, is hypointense to the corpora on both T1 and T2 images.

56. A patient with known prostate or bladder cancer presents with priapism. What must be considered?

A metastasis to the penis may result in abnormal vascular shunting, a high-flow state called *malignant priapism*.

57. What is Cowper duct syringocele? What does it look like on MRI?

Cowper duct syringocele is cystic dilation of the main duct of the bulbourethral glands. It appears as a T2-hyperintense midline structure ventral to the proximal bulbous urethra (in the expected region of the Cowper ducts). It may manifest with vague clinical symptoms, including postvoid dribbling, weak stream, frequency, and hematuria.

58. A patient has a clinical history of painful deviated erections. What disease does the clinician suspect? What should one look for on MRI or US?

Peyronie disease represents inflammation that causes fibrosis of the connective tissue/tunica albuginea surrounding the corpora cavernosa (Fig. 27-13). It may be painful in its inflammatory form, but is often painless in more chronic cases. On MRI, the fibrosis is identified as T1-hypointense and T2-hypointense areas, which may enhance peripherally in association with the tunica albuginea. On US, hyperechoic plaques are identified, which may shadow if calcium is present.

59. Describe the characteristic clinical history or physical examination findings associated with penile fracture. What are the findings on MRI?

Penile fracture occurs secondary to trauma to an erect penis, usually as a consequence of vigorous intercourse. The patient may describe acute onset of pain, rapid detumescence, and purple discoloration/deformity of the penis. Penile fracture is a surgical emergency. On MRI, look for discontinuity of T1-hypointense and T2-hypointense tunica albuginea and associated hematoma.

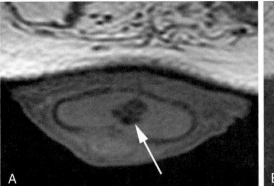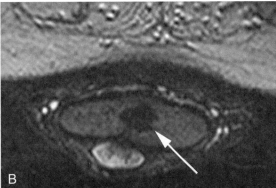

Figure 27-13. Peyronie disease. **A** and **B,** Axial T1-weighted (**A**) and axial T2-weighted (**B**) images show hypointense, densely calcified plaque (*arrows*) along the intercavernosal septum.

60. A patient presents with a history of impotence. What can one look for on US to evaluate for potential causes?

Doppler US can measure arterial flow in cavernosal arteries after administration of a vasodilator (normal peak systolic velocity is >30 cm/s; if velocity is <25 cm/s, arterial disease may be the cause).

BIBLIOGRAPHY

[1] F. Cornud, T. Flam, L. Chauveinc, et al., Extraprostatic spread of clinically localized prostate cancer: factors predictive of pT3 tumor and of positive endorectal MR imaging examination results, Radiology 224 (2002) 203–210.

[2] T.J. Dambro, R.R. Stewart, B.A. Carroll, The scrotum, in: C.M. Rumack, S.R. Wilson, J.W. Charboneau (Eds.), second ed., Diagnostic Ultrasound, 1, St. Louis, Mosby, 1998, pp. 791–821.

[3] V.S. Dogra, R.H. Gottlieb, M. Oka, et al., Sonography of the scrotum, Radiology 227 (2003) 18–36.

[4] N.R. Dunnick, C.M. Sandler, J.H. Newhouse, E.S. Amis Jr., Textbook of Uroradiology, third ed., Lippincott Williams & Wilkins, Philadelphia, 2001, pp. 394–450.

[5] T.C. Noone, R.C. Semelka, R.A. Kubik-Huch, et al., Male pelvis, in: R.C. Semelka (Ed.), Abdominal-Pelvic MRI, Wiley-Liss, New York, 2002, pp. 981–1019.

[6] E.S. Pretorius, E.S. Siegelman, P. Ramchandani, et al., MR imaging of the penis, Radiographics 21 (2001) S283–S299.

INTERVENTIONAL RADIOLOGY

PATIENT SEDATION AND PAIN MANAGEMENT

Charles T. Lau, MD, and
S. William Stavropoulos, MD

CHAPTER 28

1. What is the purpose of sedation and pain management during an interventional radiology procedure?

The purpose is to enable a patient to tolerate a potentially painful procedure yet still maintain satisfactory cardiopulmonary function and the ability to cooperate with verbal commands and tactile stimuli.

2. What is the difference between analgesia and anesthesia?

Analgesia is the relief of pain without alteration of a patient's state of awareness. *Anesthesia* is the state of unconsciousness.

3. What is the difference between anxiolysis and amnesia?

Anxiolysis is the relief of fear or anxiety without alteration of awareness. *Amnesia* is the loss of memory.

4. What capabilities should the patient maintain during conscious sedation?

The patient should:
- Remain responsive and cooperative.
- Maintain spontaneous ventilation.
- Be able to protect the airway.
- Maintain protective reflexes.

5. Describe the levels of patient sedation.

The levels of patient sedation exist along a continuum: light sedation, moderate sedation, deep sedation, and general anesthesia. A patient under light sedation can respond to stimuli and maintains intact airway reflexes. A patient under moderate sedation should maintain spontaneous ventilation and be able to protect the airway. A patient under deep sedation can respond to vigorous stimuli, but may lack airway reflexes. A patient under general anesthesia has no response to stimuli and lacks all protective reflexes.

6. List the details that should be included in the presedation evaluation of a patient.

- Patient medical history
- Previous adverse experience to sedation or anesthesia
- Current medication use and drug allergies
- Time and nature of last oral intake
- History of alcohol or substance abuse
- Focused physical examination including heart, lungs, and airway
- Pertinent clinical laboratory findings

7. How long should a patient typically fast before undergoing conscious sedation?

A patient should not have solid foods for 6 to 8 hours and clear liquids for 2 to 3 hours before undergoing sedation.

8. The physical status of a patient is often quantitated on a 5-point scale, known as the American Society of Anesthesiologists Physical Assessment Status. Describe this scale.

- Class I: Healthy patient
- Class II: Mild to moderate systemic disturbance, well controlled
- Class III: Severe systemic disturbance that limits normal activities
- Class IV: Severe life-threatening illness
- Class V: Moribund, poor chance for survival

9. **Commonly, conscious sedation is administered by the provider (e.g., interventional radiologist) with patient monitoring provided by a qualified nurse. What patient factors should influence a provider to consider consulting an anesthesiologist to administer conscious sedation?**

Patient factor should include:

- ASA classification of III, IV, or V.
- Obesity.
- Pregnancy.
- Mental incapacity.
- Extremes of age.

10. **What patient factors must be monitored during conscious sedation?**

Level of consciousness, ventilation, oxygenation, and blood pressure should be monitored, along with continuous cardiac monitoring.

11. **What equipment must be present when administering conscious sedation to a patient?**

A patient undergoing conscious sedation should be under direct observation until recovery is complete. Equipment needed to monitor oxygenation; blood pressure; and heart rate, rhythm, and waveform should be present. Pharmacologic antagonists and commonly used agents, supplemental oxygen, a defibrillator, and appropriate equipment to establish airway and provide positive-pressure ventilation need to be at hand.

12. **What pharmacologic agents are commonly used for patients undergoing conscious sedation? What is their reversal agent?**

Benzodiazepines are typically used to provide conscious sedation. Common benzodiazepines include midazolam, lorazepam, and diazepam. Flumazenil is used as a reversal agent for benzodiazepines. The effect of flumazenil is usually visible in 2 minutes, with peak effects at 10 minutes. In adults, an initial dose of 1 mg may be needed.

13. **What are the usual effects of benzodiazepines?**

Benzodiazepines produce sedation and amnesia, but do not provide analgesia. Significant adverse effects of benzodiazepines include respiratory and cardiovascular depression. Paradoxic reactions can occur with benzodiazepines and are more common in the elderly.

14. **What pharmacologic agents are commonly used for pain control? What is their reversal agent?**

Opiates are commonly used to provide pain control. Commonly used opiates include fentanyl, morphine, and meperidine. Naloxone is used as a reversal agent for opiates and is typically administered as 0.4-mg intravenous doses (in adults) to a total of 2 mg. The effect of naloxone is usually visible in 2 to 3 minutes; however, its duration of action may be substantially shorter than many long-acting opiates, and repeated dosing may be necessary.

15. **What are the typical effects of opiates?**

Opiates provide systemic analgesia, mild anxiolysis, and mild sedation. Opiates do not induce amnesia.

16. **What pharmacologic agent used for pain control is contraindicated in patients taking a monoamine oxidase (MAO) inhibitor?**

Meperidine administered to patients taking MAO inhibitors can cause various undesirable and potentially lethal side effects and is contraindicated. Side effects include agitation; fever; and seizures progressing in some instances to coma, apnea, and death. The narcotic analgesic of choice for patients taking MAO inhibitors is morphine.

17. **What are the strategies for dealing with a patient who has a known hypersensitivity to iodinated contrast agents?**

Adverse reactions to iodinated contrast agents range from nuisance side effects, such as hives and emesis, to potentially lethal reactions, such as anaphylaxis and laryngeal edema. Patients with a history of even a minor hypersensitivity reaction to contrast agent may be at increased risk for a severe reaction, and special precautions should be exercised when administering contrast agent to these patients. Premedicating the patient with oral steroids and the use of low-osmolar contrast agents may reduce the risk of minor reactions, but there is no proof that this strategy prevents or reduces the risk of lethal contrast agent reactions. Alternative contrast agents, such as gadolinium or CO_2 or both, may be used in patients with a history of severe contrast agent reactions. If an iodinated contrast agent must be used in a patient with a history of bronchospasm, laryngeal edema, or anaphylaxis, it may be wise to have an anesthesiologist standing by.

18. List possible options for the management of an acute vasovagal reaction.

A rapid infusion of normal saline or atropine (0.6 to 1 mg) may be given intravenously.

19. What are the ABCs of patient resuscitation?

Advanced Cardiac Life Support (ACLS) guidelines provide a series of algorithms regarding distressed patients in various clinical settings. The ABCs of resuscitation is a part of these algorithms. Intervention in a patient with an unstable condition should always begin with the establishment of an *A*irway, followed by assessment of *B*reathing (ventilation) and *C*irculation (heart rate and blood pressure).

20. Describe the management of acute hypotension.

Remember your ABCs! During conscious sedation, an overdose of either a benzodiazepine or an opiate may cause respiratory depression that manifests as acute hypotension. Vigorous stimulation (sternal rub) may remedy the situation. If not, pharmacologic reversal may be needed. If hypoxia is not the etiology of the hypotension, evaluation of a patient's heart rate provides a simple algorithm for treating acute hypotension. A vasovagal reaction should be suspected if the patient is bradycardic, and treatment should proceed accordingly. If the patient is tachycardic, one should immediately evaluate for a source of blood loss. A fluid challenge with normal saline may help determine whether a patient has intravascular volume depletion. Pharmacologic intervention with epinephrine, phenylephrine, or dopamine may be indicated if the patient fails to respond to the fluid challenge. A complete algorithm for treating hypotension can be found in the ACLS guidelines.

21. List possible options for the management of an acute hypertensive crisis.

During a procedure, pain and anxiety may precipitate hypertension. A benzodiazepine, such as midazolam (Versed), mixed with an opiate, such as fentanyl, is likely to decrease the blood pressure of an uncomfortable or anxious patient. To treat a patient in true hypertensive crisis further pharmacologic intervention may be needed. Intravenous labetalol, given as a bolus or a constant infusion, often normalizes blood pressure. Hydralazine and nitroprusside are other intravenous agents that may also be useful in this setting.

Key Points: Patient Sedation and Pain Management

1. A patient under moderate sedation should maintain spontaneous ventilation and be able to protect the airway.
2. The following equipment should be present when administering conscious sedation: pharmacologic antagonists, appropriate equipment to establish airway and provide positive-pressure ventilation, supplemental oxygen, and a defibrillator.
3. The medications used to treat an anaphylactic reaction include diphenhydramine, methylprednisolone, and epinephrine.
4. Naloxone is used as a reversal agent for opiates.
5. Flumazenil is used as a reversal agent for benzodiazepines.
6. ACLS guidelines provide complete recommendations for the distressed patient.
7. Evaluation of a patient with an unstable condition should always begin with the ABCs.

---

22. How can acute pulmonary edema be managed?

Pulmonary edema interferes with the ability to oxygenate blood. Therapy consists of securing an airway, providing supplemental oxygen, and administering intravenous furosemide or other agents to induce diuresis.

23. Describe the immediate options for management of an anaphylactic reaction.

An anaphylactic reaction can be rapidly fatal. An airway should be secured immediately, and oxygen should be administered. The mainstay of therapy consists of epinephrine (1:1000), 0.1 to 0.3 mL given subcutaneously every 15 minutes up to 1 mL total. Additional therapy includes saline for pressure support, diphenhydramine (50 mg intravenously), methylprednisolone (50 mg intravenously), and dopamine (5 to 10 µg/kg/min intravenously). Cardiopulmonary resuscitation may be required.

24. Describe the immediate options for management of acute laryngeal edema.

Laryngeal edema may lead to airway obstruction and death. An airway should be established, and oxygen should be administered. Epinephrine (1:1000), 0.1 to 0.3 mL given subcutaneously every 15 minutes up to 1 mL total, should be administered immediately. Additional agents include diphenhydramine (50 mg intravenously) and cimetidine (300 mg by mouth).

25. Describe the immediate options for management of bronchospasm.

The patient should be monitored closely, and oxygen should be administered by nasal cannula or facemask. In severe cases, intubation may be required. Pharmacologic treatment includes epinephrine (1:1000), 0.1 to 0.3 mL given subcutaneously every 15 minutes up to 1 mL total, and aminophylline (4 to 6 mg/kg intravenous loading dose, then 25 mg/min continuous infusion). These agents may be supplemented with inhaled albuterol or metaproterenol.

26. What are possible options for the management of generalized urticaria?

A patient with generalized urticaria can be treated with either diphenhydramine (50 mg intravenously) or cimetidine (300 mg by mouth). Vital signs should be obtained, and the patient should be observed to ensure that a more severe reaction is not evolving. The reaction should be documented in the patient's medical record.

WEBSITE

http://www.emedicine.com/emerg/topic695.htm

BIBLIOGRAPHY

[1] Ray CE, Turner JH, Cothren CG, Moore EE, Smith W, Scatorchia G, et al., Do CT emergency CT scans add value in hemodynamically unstable patients undergoing pelvic embolization?, 2004 Society of Interventional Radiology, 29th Annual Scientific Meeting, Phoenix Arizona.
[2] M. Wojtowycz, Handbook of Interventional Radiology and Angiography, second ed., St. Louis, Mosby, 1995.

CHAPTER 29

EQUIPMENT, TERMS, AND TECHNIQUES IN INTERVENTIONAL RADIOLOGY

Jeffrey A. Solomon, MD, MBA, and
S. William Stavropolous, MD

1. What are the characteristics of a diagnostic catheter?

Catheters may be selected for a specific application based on many characteristics (Fig. 29-1). Although there are numerous catheters, experience and personal preference play a large role in the selection process.

- *Length*: Catheters are available in various lengths, the most common being 65 cm and 100 cm. The appropriate length is based on the access site and desired application. From a femoral approach, a 100-cm-long catheter may be used for a cerebral arteriogram, whereas a 65-cm-long catheter would suffice for a renal arteriogram.
- *Tip configuration*: Tip configuration describes the curve on the leading edge of the catheter. Various curves are available that are designed to select branch vessels that originate at different angles. Common catheter curves include Cobra, Simmons, and Berenstein (see Fig. 29-1).
- *Outer diameter*: Most diagnostic catheters used today are 4 or 5 Fr, meaning that they are less than 2 mm in diameter.
- *Inner diameter*: This describes the inner channel of the catheter. Most catheters are designed to accommodate guidewires that are either 0.035 inch or 0.038 inch in diameter. It is important to match the inner diameter of the catheter with the devices (wire or coil) that are placed through it.
- *Coating*: Some catheters have a hydrophilic coating that becomes very slippery when wet. This may facilitate crossing a stenosis.
- *Stiffness*: Some catheters may contain braided fibers within the shaft. Braiding of polymers increases the stiffness of the catheter. Some clinical applications are better suited to stiffer catheters, whereas others are better served by floppier ones.

2. What is the difference between a Cobra 1 and a Cobra 2 catheter?

A Cobra 1 catheter and a Cobra 2 catheter have the same general shape except that the radius of the secondary curve of the catheter is greater for the Cobra 2 (Fig. 29-2). A Cobra 3 catheter has the same general "Cobra" shape, but the secondary curve is even greater still. The same nomenclature applies to Simmons catheters and others as well.

3. What is a French? What is a gauge?

A *French (Fr)* is a unit of measure of diameter that is often applied to catheters. 1 Fr is equal to one third of a millimeter. A 6-Fr catheter is therefore 2 mm in diameter. A *gauge (G)* is also a unit used to measure diameter and although it can be used to measure catheters, it is frequently used for needles. An approximation used for needles is that the diameter (in inches) is equal to the reciprocal of the gauge. Therefore a 21-gauge needle is about 1/21 of an inch in diameter.

4. What are the two general categories of stents? How do they differ?

Improvements in biomedical engineering and metallurgy have helped expand the clinical applications for noncoronary stents. Although various commercial stents are available, they can be

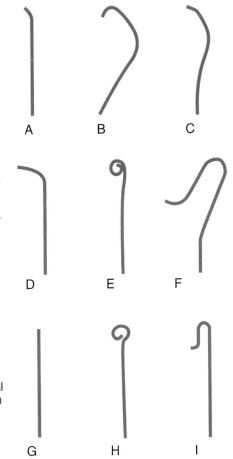

Figure 29-1. Types of catheters. *A* = Berenstein, *B* = Cobra, *C* = H1H, *D* = multipurpose-A, *E* = pigtail, *F* = Simmons, *G* = straight, *H* = tennis racket, *I* = SOS.

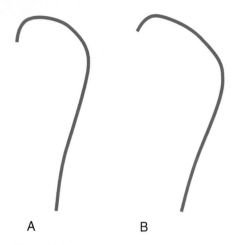

A   B

Figure 29-2. **A** and **B**, The difference between a Cobra 1 and a Cobra 2 catheter: The radius of the secondary curve on the Cobra 1 catheter (**A**) is smaller than the Cobra 2 (**B**), although the overall configuration of the catheters is similar.

classified as either balloon-expandable or self-expanding. The characteristics of each type vary, making one type more suitable for certain clinical applications than the other. There is significant overlap for uses of both types of stent, and user preference plays a role in selection.

5. How is a balloon-expandable stent deployed?

The Palmaz stent is the prototypic balloon-expandable stent. Such stents come packaged either individually or premounted on a balloon. When the balloon is inflated, the stent expands to the diameter of the balloon. As the stent expands, it changes very little in length. The relatively constant size and method of delivery/deployment of this type of stent makes for precise and predictable placement. Balloon-expandable stents are the stent of choice for treating renal artery stenosis. Because they are made of laser-cut stainless steel, these stents may cause significant artifact on magnetic resonance imaging (MRI) examinations. Balloon-expandable stents may be permanently deformed by extrinsic compression and should not be used in situations in which they could be subject to these forces.

6. What two materials are used to make self-expanding stents?

There are two broad categories of self-expanding stents: stents made from woven Elgiloy wires, and stents laser-cut from nitinol tubes. Self-expanding stents exert a continuous outward force and resist deformation, and are preferable to balloon-expandable stents in regions potentially subject to external compressive forces. To ensure full expansion, self-expanding stents are dilated with a balloon of appropriate diameter after deployment.

7. How do woven Elgiloy and nitinol self-expanding stents differ?

- Woven stents, such as Wallstent (Boston Scientific), have several unique characteristics. They are very radiopaque and can be easily seen on fluoroscopy, even in obese patients. The stents are reconstrainable, meaning that they can be almost entirely deployed, recaptured, moved, and then deployed in a different location. The tradeoff is, however, that the length of the stent depends on its fully expanded diameter. These stents may shorten significantly as they expand over time, uncovering a region of pathology. Alternatively, if the stent does not expand to the degree expected, the stent may remain too long. Woven stents are available in large sizes (up to 24 mm in diameter) and are often used to create transjugular intrahepatic portosystemic shunts or to stent large central veins.
- Laser cut self-expanding stents are not reconstrainable. Because the stents are constructed of rings linked together they are subject to significant foreshortening and remain at a relatively stable length regardless of diameter. Nitinol is less radiopaque then Elgiloy, and these stents may be difficult to see, especially in obese patients.

Key Points: Choice of Stent Type

1. Balloon-expandable stents are the stent of choice for renal arteries because they can be placed with greater accuracy.
2. Self-expanding stents are indicated when there may be an extrinsic compressive force acting on the stent.

8. What is nitinol?

Nitinol was developed by the U.S. Navy and stands for nickel titanium alloy. This metal is particularly useful for medical applications because it has thermal memory. This property allows stents to be made at a certain diameter, cooled, and then compressed onto a delivery system. When the stent is deployed at body temperature, the stent attempts to regain its original configuration and diameter. A nitinol stent that is slightly oversized (by approximately 20%) with regard to the vessel exerts an outward force to keep the vessel open as the stent attempts to regain its original diameter.

9. What do the terms *hoop strength* and *radial force* mean?

- *Hoop strength* is a measure of a stent's ability to avoid collapse and withstand the radial compressive forces of a vessel after dilation.

- Chronic outward *radial force* is the force a self-expanding stent exerts on a vessel as it tries to expand to its original diameter. The radial resistive force is the force a self-expanding stent exerts as it resists squeezing by a vessel.

10. What is a sheath?
A sheath is a device that may be placed into a vessel at the site of percutaneous access. Sheaths permit rapid exchanges of guidewires and catheters while maintaining access. Sheaths are sized based on the diameter of the catheter or device that they allow to pass. A 7-Fr sheath accepts devices up to 7 Fr in outer diameter. A 7-Fr sheath is in fact closer to 8 or 9 Fr in diameter.

11. What is a guiding catheter?
A guiding catheter is a special type of catheter that does not taper at its tip to the diameter of the guidewire. This configuration allows the passage of devices of large diameter through the catheter. When used in this manner, a guiding catheter functions similarly to a long sheath. In contrast to sheaths, guiding catheters lack a side-port and hemostatic valve. Guiding catheters are sized based on the outer diameter. A 7-Fr guiding catheter fits through a 7-Fr sheath, but a 7-Fr device does not fit through a 7-Fr guiding catheter. Guiding catheters are available with various tip configurations.

12. What is an up-and-over sheath?
Sometimes called a Balkin sheath, an up-and-over sheath is a U-shaped sheath (Fig. 29-3). It is designed to facilitate interventions in which the arterial access is in one femoral artery, and the lesion to be treated is in the contralateral extremity. A catheter and guidewire are placed into the aorta, and the contralateral iliac artery is selected. The sheath is placed over the wire. The preshaped "U" curve assists passage over the aortic bifurcation. After angioplasty or stenting, arteriography can be performed by injecting contrast agent through the side-arm of the sheath.

13. Explain the Trojan horse technique.
The original balloon-expandable stents came from the manufacturer packaged in a small box. To use the stent, an appropriate balloon was selected, and the stent was hand-crimped onto the balloon by the operator. If not mounted properly, stents had the tendency to slip on the balloon when being advanced across a tight stenosis. The Trojan horse technique minimizes this risk. Instead of pushing the stent across the lesion, the lesion is crossed with a sheath or guiding catheter (Fig. 29-4). The balloon-mounted stent is advanced through the catheter or sheath to the desired location, and then the sheath or catheter is withdrawn to expose the stent in the proper location. In this way, complications related to stent slippage are minimized. This is just one example of how the Trojan horse technique is used. The term applies to the technique in general and can be used to deliver any device in this manner, not just a balloon-expandable stent.

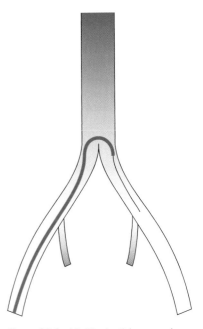

Figure 29-3. A Balkin sheath is commonly used when performing interventions in the contralateral lower extremity. The "up-and-over" design allows diagnostic angiography and interventional procedures to be performed via an access site in the contralateral leg.

14. What are the defining characteristics of guidewires?
Guidewires are available in numerous configurations. The selection of wire type depends on the intended application. Defining characteristics include the following:
- *Length*: Wires are available in lengths from 70 cm to more than 300 cm. Short wires may be used for obtaining vascular access or placing drains. Longer, 300-cm wires are used in catheter exchanges or to perform procedures at a great distance from the access site.
- *Diameter*: The most commonly used wires are 0.035 inch, 0.038 inch, or 0.018 inch in diameter. Wires 0.010 inch are available for special applications, such as cerebral interventions. The size of the wires should be selected based on the catheter used and the intended application.
- *Stiffness*: Wires vary from very floppy to extremely stiff.
- *Coating*: Some wires may have a hydrophilic coating. When wet, these wires become very slippery, and the coating may facilitate the crossing of tight stenoses.

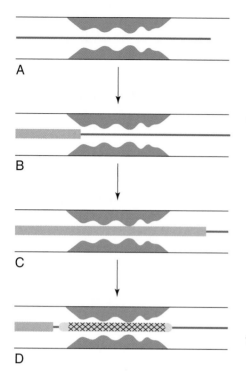

A

B

C

D

Figure 29-4. Trojan horse technique. **A,** The lesion is crossed with a wire. **B,** A sheath or guiding catheter is used to cross the lesion. **C,** A stent is advanced through the sheath or guiding catheter and centered over the lesion. **D,** The guiding catheter or sheath is withdrawn exposing the stent.

- *Tip configuration*: Wires have specialized tips that have been engineered for specific applications. Some wires have preformed angles to assist the selection of vessels. Other wires have floppy or atraumatic tips to prevent vascular injury. Some specialized wires have tips that can be shaped during a procedure to accomplish a specific task.

15. **What is an exchange-length wire? How long does it have to be?**
An exchange-length wire is long enough to perform a catheter exchange without having to withdraw the wire. Most wires are 150 cm long and are paired with catheters that are either 65 or 100 cm long. If a catheter needs to be exchanged over a wire, the wire needs to be at least twice as long as the catheter to make the exchange without having to pull the wire back and risk losing access. This is easy to remember: If a 100-cm-long catheter is advanced all the way into a vessel, a 200-cm wire would be needed to exchange the catheter; 100 cm of the wire would be used before the tip of the wire comes out of the catheter, and another 100 cm of wire is needed so that the catheter can be pulled out without moving the wire.

16. **What is a Cope loop?**
Dr Cope is one of the pioneers of interventional radiology and is credited with some of the field's most ingenious inventions. One of these is the Cope loop, which is a pigtail catheter with a locking mechanism to prevent accidental displacement. A small string runs through the center of the catheter and is fixed to the distal curved end. The other end of the string exits the hub of the catheter. The curl on the catheter is straightened out as it is advanced over a guidewire. After the wire is removed, the string is pulled and tied, which causes the end of the catheter to curl and lock. The fixed diameter of the locked coil prevents migration. To remove the catheter, the hub and string are cut, releasing the distal lock.

17. **What is the origin of the term *stent*?**
The word *stent* derives from the surname of 19th century English dentist Stent. He developed gums and resins used to make models of jaws, and the verb "to stent" came to mean "to hold tissue in place." The term *stent* was later adopted by surgeons to describe a device or material used to prop open a space.

18. **What does it mean to "Dotter" a lesion?**
Dr Charles Dotter was an early pioneer in interventional radiology. Before the availability of angioplasty balloons, he described a technique in which stenoses were treated by passing dilators of successively larger diameter through them.

19. **What is a micropuncture set?**
A micropuncture set is used to obtain vascular access. It contains a 21G, single-wall needle; an 0.018-inch wire, and a dilator. The dilator is tapered to the 0.018-inch wire to allow easy placement. The inner portion of the dilator can be removed along with the wire to allow the dilator to accept a standard 0.035-inch wire. This set can be used as an alternative to double-wall needles. Some prefer this set for gaining access for thrombolysis because it uses the single-wall technique.

20. **What is the difference between the single-wall and the double-wall technique?**
To perform a single-wall technique, only the ventral wall of the vessel is punctured to gain entry to the vessel. A double-wall puncture (Seldinger technique) is performed by puncturing the dorsal and ventral walls of the vessel and subsequently withdrawing the needle. When pulsatile blood is encountered, the tip of the needle is in an intraluminal position, and a guidewire can be placed safely.

21. **What are the advantages and disadvantages of a single-wall puncture?**
The single-wall technique is preferred for bypass grafts and for patients at risk for puncture site hemorrhage, such as patients undergoing thrombolysis. The disadvantage is an increased risk for access site dissection.

22. What is a snare?

A snare is a device that may be used to remove intravascular foreign bodies, such as wires or coils (Fig. 29-5). A snare consists of a wire with a nitinol loop at the end. The plane of the loop is oriented perpendicular to the long axis of the wire. The snare is advanced through a catheter. Under fluoroscopic guidance, the loop is used to engage a free edge of the foreign body. The wire and loop are retracted into the catheter. This locks the foreign body between the snare loop and catheter. The snare, loop, and foreign body are removed in unison.

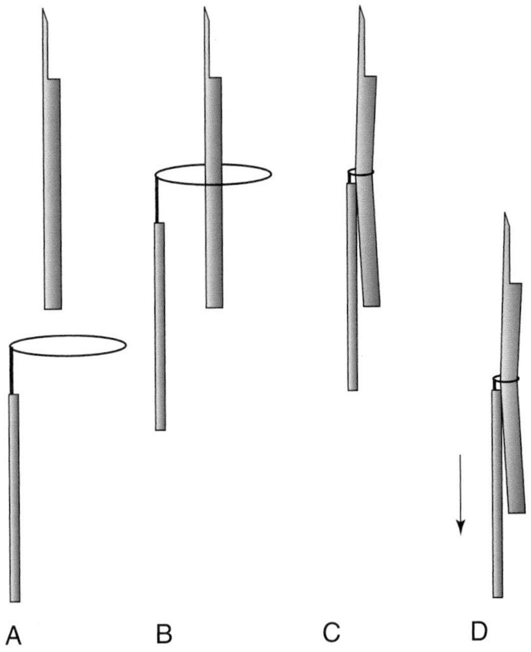

23. What is a reverse curve catheter?

A reverse curve catheter is one in which the tip of the catheter doubles back on itself to form a partial loop (Fig. 29-6). Because of the loop at the end, special maneuvers must often be done to form the loop when the catheter is inside the patient. After the loop is formed, the catheter is pulled down to select a branch vessel. When the tip of the catheter engages the orifice of the vessel, the use of the catheter may be slightly counterintuitive. The presence of the loop at the end of the catheter causes the tip of the catheter to advance distally in the selected vessel if the catheter is pulled out. This is exactly opposite of what happens with a conventional catheter. One must push a reverse curve catheter inward to deselect a branch vessel. Reverse curve catheters may often provide stable access to vessels because of the way they behave. The Simmons catheter is the prototypic reverse curve catheter.

Figure 29-5. Steps used to retrieve a catheter fragment. **A,** A gooseneck snare is deployed in the vessel adjacent to the free end of the fragment. **B,** The free end of the catheter is engaged by the loop of the snare. **C,** The snare is pulled back into its outer catheter to grasp the catheter tightly. **D,** The snare, outer catheter, and catheter fragment are withdrawn in unison.

24. What are the different ways to form a Simmons catheter?

One way is first to place a wire over the aortic bifurcation and then form the catheter by placing the tip over the bifurcation and pushing up. The catheter may also be formed in the thoracic aorta where the diameter is sufficiently large. A technique commonly used at the Hospital of the University of Pennsylvania involves anchoring a suture with a wire in the tip of the catheter. The loop is formed by gently pulling on the string while advancing the catheter.

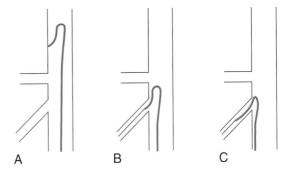

Figure 29-6. Steps in using a reverse curve catheter. **A,** The catheter is formed in the aorta. **B,** The vessel is selected. **C,** As the catheter is pulled out, its tip moves further into the vessel.

25. What is a Waltman loop?

The distal tip of any catheter can be looped back to form a reverse curve catheter. A Waltman loop is the configuration of a standard catheter when the distal end has been formed into a reverse curve loop. The simplest technique to do this involves selection of an aortic branch vessel. The tip is maintained in a constant position as wire and catheter are advanced in unison. This creates a large reverse curve that can stabilize access and facilitate difficult catheterizations.

26. What is a "road map"?

"Road mapping" is an imaging technique present on many modern fluoroscopy units. An arteriogram is performed first. When the road map function is selected, the fluoroscopy monitor displays a static subtracted angiographic image from the prior run. When fluoroscopy is performed, a live subtracted fluoroscopic image is superimposed on the static angiogram. In effect, the vessels are highlighted with everything but the motion of the catheter and guidewire subtracted out. This technique facilitates selection of small or tortuous vessels.

27. How do you select the proper injection rate for an arteriogram?

The easiest way to select the proper rate is to give a test injection of contrast agent by hand to estimate the rate of flow. The injection rate should approximate the intrinsic rate of flow of the vessel. Giving a test injection is always wise to ensure that the catheter is in the appropriate location. Accidental power injection into the subintimal space or a tiny branch vessel may occur if this recommendation is not followed.

> ### Key Point: Injection Rate
>
> 1. The best way to determine the appropriate injection rate for a given vessel is to give a test injection by hand and then to approximate the native rate of flow.

28. What is meant by an injection of "20 for 40"?

One must dictate the rate and volume for a power injected run. The term "20 for 40" means that the injection rate is 20 mL/s for a total volume of 40 mL. This would be a 2-second injection.

29. What is a rate rise?

A rate rise is another way that a power injection can be modified and describes the time in seconds that it takes from the beginning of the injection to reach the desired injection rate. For an injection of "20 for 40" with no rate rise, the velocity of contrast agent in the catheter immediately jumps from 0 to 20 mL/s. No rate rise implies a step function. If a rate rise of 0.6 second is used, it takes 0.6 second for the injection to reach maximum velocity. Rate rises are used to minimize the recoil of the catheter during rapid injections.

30. What is a Hickman catheter?

A Hickman catheter is a device used for long-term intravenous access, most commonly for chemotherapy or total parenteral nutrition. The line is available in single-lumen, double-lumen, or triple-lumen models. It is ideally placed in the internal jugular vein, with the exit site tunneled several centimeters away. The catheter has an antimicrobial cuff on its surface.

31. What is a PermaCath?

PermaCath is a brand name and should not be used to describe the device in general terms. It is a type of tunneled dialysis catheter.

32. What is a Medcomp?

Medcomp is also a brand name and should not be used as a generic reference. It is a brand of nontunneled dialysis catheter.

BIBLIOGRAPHY

[1] S.H. Duda, J. Wiskirchen, G. Tepe, et al., Physical properties of endovascular stents: an experimental comparison, J. Vasc. Interv. Radiol. 11 (2000) 645–654.

INFERIOR VENA CAVA FILTERS

CHAPTER 30

S. William Stavropoulos, MD, and
Jeffrey A. Solomon, MD MBA

1. What is an inferior vena cava (IVC) filter?
An IVC filter is a device inserted percutaneously into the IVC designed to prevent pulmonary emboli (PE) originating from lower extremity deep vein thrombosis (DVT) and to maintain caval patency.

2. What are some common indications for IVC filter placement?
For patients with lower extremity DVT, accepted indications include:
- A contraindication to anticoagulation.
- Recurrent thromboembolic disease despite adequate anticoagulation.
- Significant bleeding complication while undergoing anticoagulation.
- Inability to achieve anticoagulation.

3. List relative indications for IVC filter placement.
- Thromboembolic disease with limited cardiopulmonary reserve
- Poor compliance with anticoagulation therapy
- Chronic PE with pulmonary hypertension
- Prophylaxis in the setting of prolonged immobilization
- Large clot burden or free-floating pelvic/IVC thrombus

4. What is a prophylactic IVC filter?
A prophylactic IVC filter is placed in patients who are at an increased risk for, but do not currently have, DVT or PE. These filters are most commonly placed in patients who face prolonged immobilization. This population primarily consists of trauma patients with long bone or pelvic fractures and neurosurgical patients with transient or permanent motor deficits. Prophylactic filters may also be placed in patients with DVT risk factors before having surgery.

5. What is Virchow triad?
Virchow triad is a basis for understanding the factors that contribute to thrombosis, including:
- A hypercoagulable state, such as caused by malignancy, nephrotic syndrome, or oral contraceptives.
- Vascular stasis resulting from shock, heart failure, venous obstruction, extrinsic compression, or other causes.
- Vascular injury secondary to various causes, such as trauma, inflammation, surgery, or central lines.

6. What are absolute contraindications to IVC filter placement?
Although rare, absolute contraindications are a lack of venous access; complete thrombosis of the IVC; or a severe, uncorrectable coagulopathy.

7. What are relative contraindications to IVC filter placement?
The decision to place a permanent medical device should be made on a case-by-case basis, and only after careful deliberation of the patient's history. One relative contraindication to filter placement is septic emboli or active bacteremia because of the theoretical risk of infectious seeding of the filter. IVC filters are not routinely placed in adolescents or pregnant women. A severe hypercoagulable state or a history of IVC thrombus may preclude filter placement because of the risk of complete IVC thrombosis.

8. How many PE originate from the lower extremities?
Of PE, 75% to 90% originate from the lower extremities. Remaining PE originate from the right atrium and upper extremities and likely account for some of the cases of recurrent PE after IVC filter placement.

9. When would a superior vena cava (SVC) filter be placed?

Filters are rarely placed in the SVC because the small clot burden in the upper extremities is rarely thought to lead to clinically significant PE. SVC filters are indicated in the unique setting of symptomatic PE that can be traced with a high degree of certainty to upper extremity clot.

10. Why is a venacavogram performed before IVC filter placement?

A venacavogram is performed to evaluate the size, anatomy, and patency of the IVC. It is important to know the diameter of the IVC because each filter can be safely placed in vessels up to a certain size. A Greenfield filter can be placed in a cava up to 28 mm in diameter, whereas a Bird's nest filter can be used in an IVC up to 40 mm. Filters can migrate into the heart or pulmonary artery if they are not sized appropriately. Ideally, the tip of the filter should rest in the infrarenal IVC. A venacavogram is helpful in identifying the location of the renal veins and variant anatomy that may affect filter placement. The presence of a nonocclusive clot in the cava may change the approach used to place the filter or its location. A jugular approach may be used when there is a large clot low in the IVC to help prevent pushing the clot centrally. To be effective, a filter needs to be placed above any clot in the IVC; this may warrant suprarenal placement.

11. How is a venacavogram performed before IVC filter placement?

A venacavogram can be performed via access from a jugular or femoral vein or an arm vein. A 5-Fr pigtail catheter with radiopaque markers is recommended so that accurate measurements of the IVC can be taken. The tip of the catheter is placed just above the confluence of the iliac veins, and an injection rate is chosen that causes contrast agent to flow down the left and right common iliac veins. Identifying both iliac veins excludes the existence of a duplicated IVC, a normal anatomic variant that alters filter placement. Patients should perform a Valsalva maneuver to distend the IVC maximally during the contrast agent injection so that the caval diameter can be accurately measured, preventing caval migration. A radiopaque ruler can be placed underneath the patient to be used as a landmark to facilitate accurate filter placement.

12. What do the renal veins look like on a cavogram?

Usually, the renal veins are not opacified by contrast agent injected into the IVC because the opacified blood in the cava flows preferentially back to the right atrium. The location of the renal veins can be determined, however, because unopacified blood from the renal veins mixes with and dilutes opacified blood in the cava. The location of the renal veins can be inferred from inflow defects in the stream of contrast agent in the IVC. If there is doubt about their location, a selective injection of the renal veins may be performed.

13. Can a cavogram be performed if the patient is allergic to iodinated contrast agent or has an elevated creatinine level?

If iodinated contrast agent cannot be used because of an elevated creatinine level or a severe contrast agent allergy, a cavogram can be performed using intravenous CO_2 or gadolinium as an alternative contrast agent. If available, intravascular ultrasound (IVUS) can also be used.

14. What common venous anomalies are seen on a cavogram?

In interpreting a cavogram, one should be familiar with the common venous anomalies, including circumaortic renal vein, retroaortic left renal vein, caval duplication, and left-sided IVC.

15. How common is IVC duplication? What does it look like on a cavogram?

IVC duplication occurs in 0.2% to 0.3% of patients. In a patient with a duplicated IVC, the left common iliac vein does not join with the right common iliac vein, but instead extends cranially to join the left renal vein. Simultaneous injections of the right and left femoral veins reveal two IVCs. The one on the right extends from the right common iliac vein into the right atrium. The one on the left extends from the left common iliac vein and joins with the left renal vein, which empties into the right-sided IVC. If one understands this anatomy, one can understand why refluxing contrast agent down both common iliac veins during the cavogram excludes the presence of a duplicated IVC.

16. What should be done in a patient with duplicated IVC who needs an IVC filter?

Failure to recognize the presence of a duplicated IVC may lead to the placement of a single filter in the right-sided cava. A filter in this position would leave the entire left leg and left pelvis "unprotected" because a clot could bypass the filter by traveling from the leg, up the left-sided cava to the left renal vein, and then to the heart and lung. If the left-sided cava is recognized, a filter could be placed in each cava, or a single suprarenal filter could be placed.

17. What are the characteristics of a left-sided IVC?

Left-sided IVC occurs in 0.2% to 0.5% of patients. This vessel usually crosses to the right side of the abdomen at the level of the left renal vein and suprarenally continues in the position of the normal right-sided cava.

18. What are characteristics of a circumaortic left renal vein? How common are they?
A circumaortic left renal vein is an anatomic variant in which the left renal vein forms a ring around the aorta. It has a prevalence of 1.5% to 8.7%. The anterior segment of the ring connects with the IVC at the expected level of the left renal vein, and the posterior segment connects with the IVC below the insertion of the anterior segment.

19. Where should a filter be placed in a patient with a circumaortic left renal vein?
If unrecognized, a circumaortic left renal vein may provide a collateral pathway for a clot to circumnavigate a filter and embolize to the lungs. If the filter is placed above the posterior segment, a clot may travel up the posterior segment to the anterior segment that is above the filter and then pass on to the lungs. The filter should be placed below the lowest renal vein. This placement ensures that a clot would encounter the filter as it travels centrally.

20. List the IVC filters that are currently approved by the U.S. Food and Drug Administration (FDA).
The following are FDA-approved caval filters: Bird's nest filter, titanium Greenfield filter, stainless steel over-the-wire Greenfield filter, Simon Nitinol filter, Vena Tech LGM filter, Vena Tech LP filter, TrapEase filter, Optease filter, Gunther Tulip filter, and Recovery filter (Fig. 30-1).

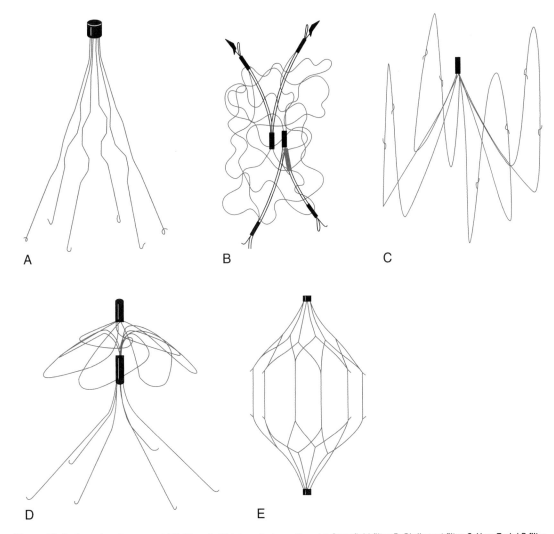

A

B

C

D

E

Figure 30-1. Examples of permanent IVC filters. **A,** Stainless steel over-the-wire Greenfield filter. **B,** Bird's nest filter. **C,** Vena Tech LP filter. **D,** Simon Nitinol filter. **E,** TrapEase filter.

Key Points: IVC Filters

1. IVC filters prevent approximately 97% of symptomatic PE that originate from the lower extremities.
2. A cavogram before IVC filter placement is essential.
3. Retrievable IVC filters may be removed when they are no longer needed.
4. In most cases, IVC filters should be placed below the lowest renal vein when possible.
5. When fishing with a wire in a patient with a filter, be careful! You might actually "catch" something.

---

21. What is a nonpermanent IVC filter?

Nonpermanent IVC filters can be removed. There are two categories of nonpermanent IVC filters: temporary and retrievable filters. A retrievable filter can be left in place permanently or can be removed if it is no longer needed. Currently, three FDA-approved retrievable IVC filters are available in the United States (Fig. 30-2). A temporary IVC filter must be removed at some point and is usually tethered to the skin by a wire or a catheter. There are no FDA-approved temporary IVC filters available in the United States at this time.

22. What patients could benefit from a nonpermanent IVC filter?

Patients who could benefit from a nonpermanent IVC filter include young trauma patients who are expected to recover, preoperative patients who need only short-term protection from PE, pregnant patients, young patients, and patients with a temporary contraindication to anticoagulation.

23. Which of the currently FDA-approved filters can be used as a retrievable filter?

The Gunther Tulip filter, the Recovery filter, and the Optease filter are currently approved by the FDA as permanent and retrievable IVC filters.

24. Can patients with an IVC filter still get PE?

Yes. There are several ways for patients with a filter to get PE. A patient may have had an anatomic variant that was not recognized during filter placement that permitted a clot to bypass the filter. Even in the absence of such variants, a filter would not protect a patient from PE originating in every part of the body. A filter would not offer protection from a clot originating in the upper extremities or right atrium. Similarly, a clot from an ovarian vein that embolizes to the renal vein and then centrally would not be stopped by an infrarenal filter. Small clots may pass through a filter, and large clots may propagate through a filter as pieces break off and embolize centrally. Overall, the rate of recurrent PE in patients with caval filters ranges from 3% to 5%. These rates are based on clinical findings and imaging studies performed in patients to detect symptomatic PE. The rates of asymptomatic PE after IVC filter placement are largely unknown.

25. Where in the IVC should the filter be placed, and why?

It is preferable that the filter be placed immediately below the lowest renal vein. With the apex of the filter sitting just below the renal veins, any clot caught by the filter is subject to high blood flow from the renal veins and may be more likely to lyse. Theoretically, this may help maintain caval patency over the lifetime of the patient. Placement below the renal veins also decreases the risk of renal vein thrombosis if the filter is subject to a large clot burden. Suprarenal

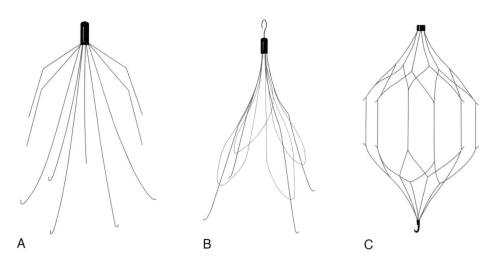

Figure 30-2. Examples of retrievable IVC filters. **A,** Recovery filter. **B,** Gunther Tulip filter. **C,** Optease filter.

IVC filters are relatively safe, but have a theoretical increased risk of renal vein thrombosis and should be reserved for instances in which there is thrombus in the infrarenal IVC.

26. What complications are related to IVC filter placement?

Complications of filter placement can be related to the access site and include hematoma, venous thrombosis, and accidental arterial puncture. Complications related to the device include filter migration, malposition, fracture, infection, IVC perforation, failed deployment, and caval inclusion. IVC filter migration into the right atrium and pulmonary artery has been reported and can be fatal. IVC filters can be dislodged by wires or catheters placed during venous access performed at a later time. A potential complication for house staff may occur during central line placement. If the wire is inserted too far down the IVC in a patient with a filter, it may become entrapped. Attempts to pull the wire out may pull the filter with it and lacerate the cava. If you are placing a central line, and the wire feels like it is "stuck," check the patient's record to see whether he or she has a filter. If the patient has a filter, you may want to call the interventional radiologist who can help remove the wire using fluoroscopic guidance.

27. How often does IVC occlusion occur after IVC filter placement?

IVC occlusion after filter placement can be due to either trapped thrombus in the filter or primary IVC thrombosis. Rates of symptomatic IVC occlusion are 2% to 10% according to reports in the literature.

BIBLIOGRAPHY

[1] M.R. Asch, Initial experience in humans with a new retrievable inferior vena cava filter, Radiology 225 (2002) 835–844.
[2] D.M. Becker, J.T. Philbrick, J.B. Selby, Inferior vena cava filters: indications, safety, effectiveness, Arch. Intern. Med. 152 (1992) 1985.
[3] K.J. Cho, L.J. Greenfield, M.C. Proctor, et al., Evaluation of a new percutaneous stainless steel Greenfield filter, J. Vasc. Interv. Radiol. 8 (1997) 181–187.
[4] D.P. Crochet, O. Stora, D. Ferry, et al., Vena Tech-LGM filter: long-term results of a prospective study, Radiology 216 (1993) 857–860.
[5] G.S. Dorfman, J.J. Cronan, T.B. Tupper, et al., Occult pulmonary embolism: a common occurrence in deep venous thrombosis, AJR Am. J. Roentgenol. 148 (1987) 263–266.
[6] E.J. Ferris, T.C. McCowan, D.K. Carver, et al., Percutaneous inferior vena cava filters: follow-up of seven designs in 320 patients, Radiology 216 (1993) 851–856.
[7] M.L. Friedell, R.J. Goldenkranz, V. Parsonnet, et al., Migration of a Greenfield filter to the pulmonary artery: a case report, J. Vasc. Surg. 3(1986) 929.
[8] P.J. Golueke, W.V. Garrett, J.E. Thompson, et al., Interruption of the inferior vena cava by means of the Greenfield filter: expanding the indications, Surgery 103 (1988) 111–117.
[9] C.J. Grassi, Inferior vena caval filters: analysis of five currently available devices, AJR Am. J. Roentgenol. 156 (1991) 813–821.
[10] M.V. Huisman, H.R. Buller, J.W. ten Cate, et al., Unexpected high prevalence of silent pulmonary embolism in patients with deep venous thrombosis, Chest 95 (1989) 498–502.
[11] A.A. Katsamouris, A.C. Waltman, M.A. Delichatsios, et al., Inferior vena cava filters: in vitro comparison of clot trapping and flow dynamics, Radiology 166 (1988) 361–366.
[12] T.B. Kinney, Update on inferior vena cava filters, J. Vasc. Interv. Radiol. 14 (2003) 425–440.
[13] S.F. Millward, J.I. Marsh, R.A. Peterson, et al., LGM (Vena Tech) vena cava filter: clinical experience in 64 patients, J. Vasc. Interv. Radiol. 2 (1991) 429–433.
[14] C.P. Molgaard, E.K. Yucel, S.C. Geller, et al., Access-site thrombosis after placement of inferior vena cava filters with 12–14 F delivery sheaths, Radiology 185 (1992) 257–261.
[15] J.M. Neuerburg, R.W. Gunther, D. Vorwerk, et al., Results of a multicenter study of the retrievable Tulip vena cava filter: early clinical experience, Cardiovasc. Intervent. Radiol. 20 (1997) 10–16.
[16] F.B. Rogers, S.R. Shackford, J. Wilson, et al., Prophylactic vena cava filter insertion in severely injured trauma patients: indications and preliminary results, J. Trauma 35 (1993) 637–641.
[17] H. Rousseau, P. Perreault, P. Otal, et al., The 6-F Nitinol TrapEase inferior vena cava filter: results of a prospective multicenter trial, J. Vasc. Interv. Radiol. 12 (2001) 299–304.
[18] R. Schutzer, F. Ascher, A. Hingorani, et al., Preliminary results of the new 6F TrapEase inferior vena cava filter, Ann. Vasc. Surg. 17 (2003) 103–106.
[19] S.W. Stavropoulos, M. Itkin, S.O. Trerotola, In vitro study of guide wire entrapment in currently available inferior vena cava filters, J. Vasc. Interv. Radiol. 14 (2003) 905–910.
[20] M.B. Streiff, Vena caval filters: a comprehensive review, Blood 95 (2000) 3669–3677.
[21] K.B. Tobin, S.O. Pais, C.B. Austin, Femoral vein thrombosis following percutaneous placement of the Greenfield filter, Invest. Radiol. 24 (1989) 442–445.
[22] R.J. Winchell, D.B. Hoyt, J.C. Walsh, et al., Risk factors associated with pulmonary embolism despite routine prophylaxis: implications for improved protection, J. Trauma 37 (1994) 600–606.
[23] M.M. Wojtowycz, T. Stoehr, A.B. Crummy, et al., The Bird's Nest inferior vena cava filter: review of a single-center experience, J. Vasc. Interv. Radiol. 8 (1997) 171–179.

AORTIC ANEURYSM STENT GRAFTS

1. What is the basic composition of a stent graft?

A stent graft is composed of a metallic stent structure covered by a medical-grade fabric. The stents are typically made from stainless steel or nitinol (nickel titanium alloy), and the fabric is either Dacron (polyester) or expanded polytetrafluoroethylene (ePTFE). A stent graft comes compressed and loaded in a delivery catheter. Stent graft designs include straight tubes and bifurcated "pant leg" designs to accommodate the iliac branch. Bifurcated designs can either be unibody (one piece) or modular (multiple pieces).

2. What are the prevalence, incidence, demographics, and risk factors for abdominal aortic aneurysms (AAAs)?

The prevalence of AAA in the United States is estimated at 1 million to 1.5 million, and more than 75% of these are asymptomatic. There are more than 200,000 new diagnoses and more than 15,000 rupture deaths annually (13th leading cause of death). The prevalence is higher in older men with risk factors (4.5%) and lower in older women with risk factors (1%). The main risk factors for AAAs include male gender and age older than 65, smoking history, atherosclerosis, hypertension, and family history.

3. What is the natural history of AAA, and when is intervention indicated?

Aneurysms grow over time. Matrix metalloproteinases and their inhibitors result in the loss of aortic wall structural integrity, which leads to AAA formation and expansion. The rate of growth is 1 to 4 mm per year for aneurysms less than 4 cm in diameter, 4 to 5 mm per year for aneurysms 4 to 6 cm, and 7 to 8 mm per year for aneurysms greater than 6 cm. Intervention is typically indicated when the aneurysm reaches 5.5 cm, although many clinicians treat at the 5-cm threshold. The risk of rupture increases as the aneurysm grows: greater than 5 cm = 20% eventual, 4% annual; greater than 6 cm = 40% eventual, 7% annual; greater than 7 cm = 50% eventual, 20% annual. Given that aneurysms grow, studies are ongoing to determine the benefit of earlier intervention when aneurysm diameters are smaller, and patients are relatively healthier.

4. How are most AAAs detected, and what is the role of screening programs?

Symptomatic aneurysms manifest with back, abdominal, buttock, groin, testicular, or leg pain. Most AAAs are asymptomatic, however. AAAs can be easily detected via a simple ultrasound (US) study, which has been shown to be cost-effective in targeted, high-risk patients. If aneurysms rupture, the mortality rate is greater than 85%, and the morbidity rate and cost are significant for patients who survive. Elective repair of aneurysms is associated with low rates of mortality and morbidity, so aneurysmal disease is well suited to screening. Many hospitals and private, mobile screening companies offer aneurysm screening, often in conjunction with screening for other conditions such as peripheral and carotid arterial disease. The U.S. Congress passed the SAAAVE Act (Screen Abdominal Aortic Aneurysms Very Efficiently) in late 2005. Medicare-funded AAA screening is limited to male ever-smokers and to men and women with a positive family history of AAA.

5. In general, when is endovascular aneurysm repair (EVAR) favored over open repair?

EVAR is preferred over operative repair when the surgical operative risk is higher because of comorbidities and older age. Endovascular repair has been shown in studies to have lower short-term rates of death and complications, but the survival curves merge in the long-term. Generally, open repair is preferred for younger, healthier patients, in whom longer term durability is a primary concern. EVAR versus open repair is essentially a matter of proper patient selection based on physiologic and anatomic risk factors, and is often a matter of patient preference for less invasive therapy.

6. Describe briefly the traditional open surgical repair of AAA.

With the patient under general anesthesia, a vascular surgeon makes an incision in the abdominal wall and exposes the aorta and the aneurysm. The incision is either down the center of the abdomen from immediately below the sternum to below the umbilicus or across the abdomen from underneath the left arm across to the center of the abdomen and down to below the umbilicus. Clamps are placed above and below the aneurysm to arrest blood flow; the surgeon then butterflies the aneurysm and removes blood clots and plaque. A surgical tube graft is sewn to the healthy sections of the aorta connecting both ends of the aorta together. The clamps are removed, the wall of the aneurysm is wrapped around the graft, and the incision is closed. Recovery from AAA surgery is typically 7 to 10 days.

7. Name some findings on preprocedure imaging of AAA that would preclude a patient from EVAR.

A major preclusion is proximal neck complexity or lack of a suitable landing zone just below the renal arteries to ensure fixation and seal of the stent graft. A short neck is defined as less than 10 cm from immediately below the renal arteries to the beginning of the aneurysmal zone. An angulated neck is defined as greater than 45 degrees from immediately below the renal arteries to the beginning of the aneurysmal zone. A wide neck is greater than 32 mm. A neck that flares immediately below the renal arteries or an aneurysm that extends into and above the renal arteries (juxtarenal) would also preclude safe landing of a stent graft. Another contraindication is complex iliac arteries. The arteries may be tortuous or calcified, precluding passage of the delivery catheter, or they may be aneurysmal in which case it may be difficult to achieve fixation and seal of the iliac "legs" of a bifurcated stent graft. Lower profile delivery systems, branched and fenestrated grafts, and more flexible and conformable designs are under development to attempt to solve some of these contraindications to EVAR.

8. What is an endoleak? What are the different types of endoleak, and how are they treated?

An endoleak is persistent blood flow into the aneurysmal sac after placement of a stent graft. A type I endoleak results from poor attachment to the vessel wall. It can be caused by poor apposition of the stent graft to the aortic or iliac wall, often owing to tortuosity, angulation, or disease (e.g., thrombus or calcification). Stent graft undersizing and aortic neck dilation are also causes of type I leaks. Type I leaks are typically treated with balloon dilation or the placement of an additional stent graft or balloon-expandable stent. Type II endoleaks are not caused by the graft itself, but rather by retrograde flow into the sac from collateral arterial branches such as lumbar arteries or the inferior mesenteric artery. Type II endoleaks sometimes resolve spontaneously or are monitored to see if they contribute to sac expansion or pressurization. If intervention is indicated, they are treated using coils or embolic glues. Type III endoleaks are caused by modular disconnections of stent graft pieces or by graft or metal fatigue causing tears in the fabric. This type of endoleak was more common in the early days of EVAR, but is now decreasing in incidence because of more durable designs and more overlap of stent graft pieces in the initial procedure. Type IV endoleaks are transgraft endoleaks caused by fabric porosity or microabrasion caused by graft or metal fatigue. Type III and type IV endoleaks are treated by placement of additional stent graft pieces or through open repair.

Key Points: Abdominal Aortic Aneurysm

1. AAA is an asymptomatic but often fatal disease when rupture occurs; AAAs must be detected, monitored, and treated. Intervention is typically indicated when the aneurysm reaches 5.5 cm, although many clinicians treat at the 5-cm threshold. The main risk factors for AAAs include male gender and age older than 65, smoking history, atherosclerosis, hypertension, and family history.
2. There are two primary treatment options for AAAs: EVAR and surgical repair. Endovascular repair is preferred over operative repair when the surgical operative risk is higher because of comorbidities and older age. Open repair is preferred for younger, healthier patients, in whom longer term durability is a primary concern.
3. The advantages of EVAR are that it is less invasive than open surgery, has a lower surgical morbidity and mortality rate, and reduces the length of postoperative hospital stays. EVAR complications include endoleak, continued enlargement or pressurization of the aneurysm sac without endoleak, delayed aneurysm rupture, graft migration, graft limb occlusion, graft infection, stent-graft structural breakdown, and groin or access complications.

---

9. What kind of follow-up imaging do patients treated with EVAR undergo?

Patients require lifelong imaging surveillance to monitor for endoleak, aneurysm expansion, and graft integrity. Imaging follow-up after EVAR is usually performed by periodic contrast-enhanced computed tomography (CT) scans. The typical regimen is a baseline CT study at 1 month, with a follow-up study at 6 months and annually thereafter. To reduce the need for expensive, radiation-exposing serial CT scans, some experts advocate for follow-up via color flow duplex US scanning in the absence of endoleak and no clinical suspicions based on anatomy.

10. What are some of the complications related to EVAR?

Complications of EVAR include endoleak, continued enlargement or pressurization of the aneurysm sac without endoleak, delayed aneurysm rupture, graft migration, graft limb occlusion, graft infection, stent-graft structural breakdown, and groin or access complications.

11. What are the major studies that have looked at the outcomes of EVAR?

The major randomized controlled studies include (1) the Dutch Randomized Endovascular Aneurysm Management (DREAM) trial, (2) the EVAR versus open repair in patients with abdominal aortic aneurysm randomised controlled trial (EVAR trial 1), and (3) the EVAR and outcome in patients unfit for open repair of abdominal aortic aneurysm randomised controlled trial (EVAR trial 2). Major registry data include the European EUROSTAR database, the U.S.-based Lifeline Registry of Endovascular Aneurysm Repair, and the Medicare matched cohort data published in the *New England Journal of Medicine.* Short-term and long-term data from Investigational Device Exemption (IDE) studies from all U.S. Food and Drug Administration (FDA)–approved stent grafts are available at the respective manufacturers' websites.

12. What are the results of the major EVAR studies?

The EVAR 1 trial showed a 3% lower initial mortality for EVAR, with a persistent reduction in aneurysm-related death at 4 years. Improvement in overall late survival was not shown. Similarly, the DREAM trial observed an initial mortality advantage for EVAR, but overall 1-year survival was equivalent in both groups. The EVAR 2 trial did not show a survival advantage of EVAR with respect to nonoperative management, although the design of this trial has been heavily debated. The Medicare matched cohort study concluded that, compared with open repair, endovascular repair of AAA is associated with lower short-term rates of death and complications. The survival advantage was more durable among older patients. In the Lifeline Registry, patients receiving endovascular grafts were older and had more cardiac comorbidities compared with surgical controls (e.g., open repair), but there was no difference in the primary end points of all-cause mortality, AAA death, or aneurysm rupture between the endovascular graft and surgical control groups up to 3 years.

13. What devices are currently commercially available in the United States for EVAR, and how do they differ?

Current FDA-approved devices include the Cook Zenith, the Endologix Powerlink, the Gore Excluder, the Medtronic AneuRx, and the Medtronic Talent. Except for the unibody Powerlink platform, all platforms are modular in design. Each manufacturer offers a slightly different range of widths and lengths, including tapered and flared iliac extensions. The Zenith and the Excluder are equipped with tiny hooks or barbs to aid in fixation of the graft to the aortic wall. Some stent grafts are suprarenal, meaning they have uncovered stent structures that extend across and above the renal arteries. The Zenith and the Talent are suprarenal stent grafts. The AneuRx and the Excluder are infrarenal stent grafts. The Powerlink offers infrarenal and suprarenal aortic cuffs and is the only graft that is designed to "sit" on the iliac bifurcation. All stent grafts are self-expanding, but each has a different delivery catheter and actuator mechanism.

14. What advantages will future generations of stent grafts have over ones that are currently available?

Currently approved stent grafts have catheter delivery profiles ranging from 20 to 24 Fr. New designs currently in clinical trials have profiles ranging from 14 to 18 Fr, which would decrease access complications and significantly improve the ability to treat patients (especially women) with complex and narrow iliac arteries, for which EVAR is currently contraindicated. Patients with complex proximal aortic necks and juxtarenal aneurysms would benefit from branched and fenestrated grafts that permit endovascular repair, while preserving renal patency. More durable fixation methods (e.g., endostapling) and more flexible stent graft designs would expand the applicability of EVAR further.

15. What are advantages of EVAR over traditional surgical repair?

The advantages of EVAR are that it is less invasive than open surgery, has a lower surgical morbidity and mortality rate, and reduces the length of postoperative hospital stays. The disadvantages of EVAR are the initial cost of the devices, the need for lifelong follow-up imaging, and the question of long-term durability.

TRANSARTERIAL CHEMOEMBOLIZATION

16. What is meant by transarterial chemoembolization (TACE)?

TACE is a procedure that involves blocking (embolizing) the blood supply to a tumor and injecting chemotherapeutic drugs directly into the artery that feeds the tumor. A catheter is placed in the femoral artery and used to select the hepatic artery. The catheter in the hepatic artery is used for delivery of the embolic agent and drug delivery. The catheter is removed immediately after treatment.

17. What types of hepatic malignancies can be treated with TACE?

TACE is most often used for liver tumors. The most common tumors treated with chemoembolization are hepatocellular carcinomas (HCC) and metastatic lesions from colon cancer. Other tumors include metastatic hepatic lesions from carcinoid tumors and other neuroendocrine tumors, breast cancer, islet cell tumors of pancreas, ocular melanomas, and sarcomas. Benign tumors such as adenomas can also be treated with chemoembolization.

18. What is a typical mixture used to perform TACE?

There is no standard mixture of chemotherapy drugs or embolic agents that is widely used for TACE.

19. What is the purpose of ethiodized oil (Ethiodol) in the TACE mixture?

Ethiodol is used during TACE because it is selectively retained by tumor cells and is radiopaque and can be seen under fluoroscopy during chemoembolization.

20. What types of patients should be considered candidates for TACE?

TACE is a liver-directed therapy for liver tumors. It works best in HCC when the tumor has not spread to extrahepatic sites. The best therapy for HCC is often liver transplantation. TACE is used to control HCC while the patient is on the transplant list awaiting a liver transplantation. For patients who are not transplant candidates, TACE offers a noncurative treatment for HCC. For metastatic lesions to the liver, TACE is best used when disease outside the liver is well controlled, and the metastatic lesions to the liver represent the biggest threat to the patient's health.

21. How are patients followed after TACE, and when is retreatment indicated?

Patients are generally admitted 1 night in the hospital after TACE. Patients receive a post-TACE CT or magnetic resonance imaging (MRI) examination and are seen in an outpatient interventional radiology clinic 1 month after TACE. Additional clinic visits and imaging with MRI or CT of the liver are done every 3 months to evaluate the success or failure of the procedure. Retreatment can be done and is usually indicated if follow-up imaging shows new masses in the liver or recurrent disease at the site of the treated tumor.

22. What is the typical imaging and work-up required before TACE?

Before TACE, patients are seen in the interventional radiology clinic, and a full history and physical examination are performed. MRI is done within 1 month of the planned TACE. Within 1 week of the procedure, blood work is performed that should include complete blood count, international normalized ration (INR), creatinine levels, and liver function tests.

23. What is postembolization syndrome?

Nearly all patients get postembolization syndrome after TACE. This condition includes low-grade fever, nausea, abdominal pain, and fatigue. It is worst in the first 24 to 48 hours after the procedure and usually resolves 1 week after TACE.

24. What medications are patients typically treated with after TACE?

After TACE, patients are given powerful antibiotics to lessen the chance of infection and intravenous medications to control nausea and pain while they are in the hospital. When they are sent home, patients receive a 5-day course of an oral antibiotic (usually amoxicillin and clavulanate potassium [Augmentin]) and oral medications for nausea and pain.

25. What is the major risk factor for hepatic abscess formation secondary to TACE?

Hepatic abscess is always mentioned as a risk after TACE, but the risk increases greatly if the patient does not have a competent ampulla of Vater. This can occur because of biliary stent placement or because of a biliary bypass procedure that results in resection of the ampulla. Bacteria from the intestines can colonize the biliary tree if the ampulla is not patent. A biliary tree that is colonized with bacteria is at an increased risk for abscess formation after TACE.

26. What tumor markers are used to follow HCC? What about metastatic colon cancer?

For HCC, the most reliable tumor marker is alpha fetoprotein. For colon cancer, the tumor marker commonly used is carcinoembryonic antigen.

27. What laboratory values should be checked when determining candidacy for TACE?

Within 1 week of the procedure, blood work is performed, which should include complete blood count, INR, creatinine, and liver function tests. If the patient has an elevated INR, bilirubin, aspartate aminotransferase, or alanine aminotransferase, this may indicate that the patient has some degree of liver failure. Preexisting liver failure increases the risk of TACE and could be an reason not to perform the procedure.

28. How can the liver tolerate embolization of the hepatic artery without undergoing infarction?

The liver can tolerate TACE because it receives its blood supply from two sources: the hepatic artery and the portal vein. Liver tumors derive most of their blood supply from the hepatic artery. The normal portion of the liver gets most of its blood supply from the portal vein. Before the TACE agents are delivered, an arteriogram is done to confirm patency of the portal vein. If the portal vein is completely occluded, the risk of liver failure and infarction after TACE increases significantly. An occluded portal vein may be reason not to perform TACE.

29. What does one look for on follow-up imaging to evaluate the success of a TACE procedure?

After TACE, MRI or CT of the abdomen and pelvis is done with intravenous contrast agent. The intravenous contrast agent causes the tumors to enhance if they are still viable. If a tumor is successfully treated, it is necrotic and does not enhance after contrast agent administration on CT or MRI. In patients who have elevated tumor markers, a decrease in the tumor marker levels would also be an indication of successful TACE.

30. What is radiofrequency ablation (RFA), and how does it work?

RFA is a technique for generating heat in living tissues through alternating electrical currents. The alternating currents result in agitation of ions and frictional heat, which can result in coagulation necrosis of tissue. This technology has been applied to the treatment of many conditions, including the treatment of liver, kidney, bone, and lung tumors. A metal probe can be placed percutaneously in the tumor using US or CT guidance and is attached to the RF machine. RFA results in tumor death via thermal energy.

31. What characteristics of hepatic lesions are considered treatable by RFA? What are the characteristics of renal lesions treatable by RFA?

RFA is best done when there are three or fewer tumors to treat in the liver or kidney. Liver or kidney tumors 3 cm or smaller in size respond best to RFA. Larger tumors can be treated, but results are not as good.

32. What are the imaging characteristics on MRI and CT of a lesion successfully treated with RFA?

MRI or CT is done with intravenous contrast agent 1 month after RFA to evaluate the success of the treatment. The intravenous contrast agent causes tumors to enhance if they are still viable. If a tumor is successfully treated, it is necrotic and does not enhance after contrast agent administration on CT or MRI.

33. How are patients followed after RFA procedures?

Patients usually have CT or MRI performed 1 month after the procedure and then at 3- to 6-month intervals as determined by the tumor type and institutional protocol.

34. What subset of patients is best treated with RFA of renal lesions?

Currently, RFA is usually reserved for patients who are not surgical candidates because of comorbid medical conditions or renal insufficiency, or who have refused surgical resection of the kidney mass. As more long-term studies of RFA in renal masses are done, more patients may be considered candidates for this therapy.

35. What are complications of RFA?

Complications after RFA include bleeding, infection, injury to the organ being treated, and injury to surrounding organs including bowel.

UTERINE FIBROID EMBOLIZATION

36. What are typical symptoms of uterine fibroids?

Symptoms can be diverse, but may include menorrhagia (abnormal bleeding with menses), dysmenorrhea (painful menses), and bulk symptoms such as pain and pressure. Other symptoms include infertility, urinary urgency and incontinence, and constipation.

37. What clinical work-up is required before undergoing uterine fibroid embolization (UFE)?

Work-up should include a thorough history focusing on the presence of symptoms compatible with uterine fibroids. A physical examination should be performed directed at evaluating the fibroid uterus. Laboratory evaluation should include a Pap smear and endometrial biopsy depending on symptoms, complete blood count, creatinine, and coagulation factors.

38. What imaging is required before UFE?

Cross-sectional imaging is performed before embolization. This can be either US or preferably MRI with contrast agent. The purpose of imaging is to evaluate fibroid size and location and to determine presence of possible adnexal disease that may change the management of the patient. Knowledge of the size and location of fibroids is important because submucosal fibroids are usually associated with bleeding and are at risk for being expelled after embolization. Large intracavitary fibroids may be a relative contraindication because of the risk of infection.

39. How is a patient followed after undergoing UFE?

Patients are followed closely in the immediate postembolization period to help manage pain. Usually MRI is obtained 3 to 6 months after the procedure to ascertain the degree of fibroid infarction and correlate imaging with changes in symptoms.

40. What are the risks associated with UFE?

Aside from the risks that are common to any angiographic procedure, such as bleeding and reaction to contrast agent, complications associated with UFE include infection or infarction of the uterus that might result in hysterectomy, fibroid expulsion, and premature menopause.

41. What are the alternatives to UFE?

Medical management consisting of hormonal therapy exists, but most patients presenting for UFE have already failed this treatment. Myomectomy is an option for patients seeking therapy for infertility. Hysterectomy is an option for patients with fibroids when pregnancy is not a consideration.

42. How do symptoms typically respond to UFE?

There is a success rate of 85% to 90% in controlling bleeding and bulk symptoms. Urinary symptoms may not respond as well.

43. Are there any other indications for UFE other than fibroids?

Uterine embolization can be used to treat bleeding emergencies such as postpartum hemorrhage, uterine atony, and cervical ectopic pregnancy. Uterine embolization may also be used for other conditions such as adenomyosis; however, its success may not be as durable as with the treatment of fibroids.

44. What type of embolic is typically used?

Polyvinyl alcohol particles or trisacryl particles (Embosphere) have been shown to have the best success to date for UFE. Absorbable gelatin sponge (Gelfoam) has been shown to work when treating acute bleeding.

45. Is there a correlation between postprocedure pain and clinical outcomes?

There is no correlation between degree of pain and outcomes. Patients usually return to normal activities in 1 to 2 weeks after UFE.

46. What is a typical analgesia protocol for patients undergoing UFE?

Patients receive ketorolac tromethamine (Toradol), 30 mg intravenously, periprocedure and are managed with fentanyl (Fentora) and midazolam (Versed) during the procedure. Postprocedure, a patient-controlled analgesia pump with morphine or hydromorphone (Dilaudid) along with an oral nonsteroidal anti-inflammatory drug (NSAID) is used to control pain. Some authorities advocate the use of epidurals during hospitalization. Patients are discharged with an oral narcotic, such as oxycodone with acetaminophen and an NSAID, such as ibuprofen.

47. What are the indications for discharge from the hospital after UFE?

Patients may be discharged when they are able to tolerate oral intake, and pain is controlled with oral medications.

48. Describe the vascular anatomy relevant to UFE.

Although anatomic variations exist, the paired uterine arteries are typically the first branch of the anterior division of the internal iliac arteries. Embolization is usually performed with the tip of the catheter in the horizontal segment of the uterine artery that is past the cervical-vaginal branch. The ovarian arteries usually arise from the aorta and can also supply the uterus. This collateral blood supply is a potential cause for poor clinical response to UFE.

49. What is the risk of premature menopause related to UFE?

The risk is low for patients younger than 45 years old, and the risk increases after this age. The rate of premature menopause may be 40% in patients older than 51 years.

50. Is pregnancy possible after UFE?

Yes, however, the incidence of placental location abnormalities, such as placenta previa, may be increased. There may also be a higher rate of miscarriage, but it is uncertain if this is related to a history of UFE or the higher maternal age in this specific patient population.

BIBLIOGRAPHY

[1] L.J. Leurs, J. Buth, P.L. Harris, J.D. Blankensteijn, Impact of study design on outcome after endovascular abdominal aortic aneurysm repair: a comparison between the Randomized Controlled DREAM-trial and the Observational EUROSTAR-registry, Eur. J. Vasc. Endovasc. Surg. 33 (2007) 172–176.

[2] Lifeline Registry of EVAR Publications Committee, Lifeline registry of endovascular aneurysm repair: long-term primary outcome measures, J. Vasc. Surg. 42 (2005) 1–10.

[3] M.L. Schermerhorn, A.J. O'Malley, A. Jhaveri, et al., Endovascular vs. open repair of abdominal aortic aneurysms in the Medicare population, N. Engl. J. Med. 358 (2008) 464–474.

DREAM TRIAL

[1] J.D. Blankensteijn, S.E. de Jong, M. Prinssen, et al., Dutch Randomized Endovascular Aneurysm Management (DREAM) Trial Group: two-year outcomes after conventional or endovascular repair of abdominal aortic aneurysms, N. Engl. J. Med. 352 (2005) 2398–2405.

[2] M. Prinssen, E.L. Verhoeven, J. Buth, et al., Dutch Randomized Endovascular Aneurysm Management (DREAM)Trial Group: a randomized trial comparing conventional and endovascular repair of abdominal aortic aneurysms, N. Engl. J. Med. 351 (2004) 1607–1618.

EVAR TRIAL

[1] E.V.A.R. trial participants, Endovascular aneurysm repair versus open repair in patients with abdominal aortic aneurysm (EVAR trial 1): randomised controlled trial, Lancet 365 (2005) 2179–2186.

[2] E.V.A.R. trial participants, Endovascular aneurysm repair and outcome in patients unfit for open repair of abdominal aortic aneurysm (EVAR trial 2): randomised controlled trial, Lancet 365 (2005) 2187–2192.

[3] R.M. Greenhalgh, L.C. Brown, G.P. Kwong, et al., EVAR trial participants: comparison of endovascular aneurysm repair with open repair in patients with abdominal aortic aneurysm (EVAR trial 1), 30-day operative mortality results: Randomised controlled trial, Lancet 364 (2004) 843–848.

PERIPHERAL VASCULAR DISEASE

Jeffrey A. Solomon, MD, MBA, and
Jeffrey I. Mondschein, MD

CHAPTER 32

1. What is the appropriate landmark for a femoral artery puncture?

Some risks of arteriography can be minimized by properly selecting the puncture site. Above the inguinal canal, the femoral artery (or, more correctly, the external iliac artery) dives posteriorly. Punctures above the inguinal canal may be problematic for several reasons. Because the artery is so deep to the puncture site, manual compression may be difficult, leading to a hematoma or pseudoaneurysm formation. In the event of an access site complication that requires surgical intervention, the surgical approach for puncture above the inguinal ligament is more involved. A puncture that is too low may result in an arteriovenous fistula. The inguinal crease is a landmark that is commonly used for femoral artery puncture. This is a very inaccurate estimate for the location of the inguinal ligament, especially in obese patients. The best landmark is the middle of the medial third of the femoral head identified fluoroscopically (Fig. 32-1).

2. What is Cope's law of vascular access?

"You can't stick a vessel where it isn't." The puncture site should not be where you think the artery might be, but instead where it actually is as determined with palpation or ultrasound (US).

3. If the femoral artery cannot be accessed, what are other options for obtaining access for an arteriogram?

Multiple options for access may exist in any given patient. The appropriate access site depends on the patient's symptoms, intended procedure, prior surgical history, and clinical setting. A brachial approach may be used if a femoral approach is impossible. Other access options include direct puncture of bypass grafts, direct translumbar aortic puncture, and retrograde popliteal access.

4. If a brachial approach must be used, is the right or left arm used?

A left brachial approach is preferred. A catheter placed from the left arm traverses the left vertebral artery orifice, but not that of the left common carotid artery; this may reduce the risk of stroke.

5. What are some complications unique to brachial access?

There is a small risk of stroke associated with brachial access. The arm cannot tolerate large hematomas, and bleeding after removal of a catheter or sheath may result in compartment syndrome. If a hematoma does develop, it must be followed up carefully to ensure that neurovascular compromise does not occur. Surgical evacuation of the hematoma may be required to prevent a neurologic deficit.

6. What is claudication?

Claudication is derived from the Latin verb *claudicare,* which means "to limp." Claudication describes exercise-induced leg pain secondary to peripheral vascular disease (PVD). Patients with claudication typically complain of a burning or aching sensation in the thigh or calf, which starts after a predictable distance and remits with rest. With advanced disease, there may be progression to rest pain, skin ulceration, and tissue loss.

7. What are the risk factors for PAD (Peripheral arterial disease)?

Risk factors for claudication and PAD include hypertension, diabetes, high cholesterol, cigarette smoking, and older age. Claudication is also more likely in individuals who already have atherosclerosis in other arteries, such as the coronary or carotid arteries.

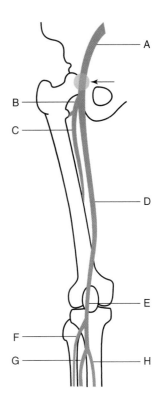

Figure 32-1. Leg arterial vascular anatomy. The *arrow* and *blue circle* indicate the preferred site for percutaneous access to the common femoral artery, over the middle third of the femoral head (A = external iliac artery, B = femoral bifurcation, C = deep femoral artery, D = superficial femoral artery, E = popliteal artery, F = anterior tibial artery, G = peroneal artery, H = posterior tibial artery).

8. Does the location of leg pain suggest the location of arterial stenosis?

Leg pain usually occurs downstream to hemodynamically significant stenoses. Calf pain may result from disease of the superficial femoral artery, whereas thigh or buttock pain may be caused by iliac disease.

9. What is Legs For Life?

Legs For Life is a national screening program initiated by the Society of Interventional Radiology (http://www.sirweb.org/) that is dedicated to improving the cardiovascular health of the community. It is a public education/community wellness program that screens people who may be at risk for PVD and helps them take the next step in resolving the pain they are experiencing. The primary goals of the Legs For Life program are to educate the public, primary care physicians, and medical community; identify patients at risk; and strengthen collaborative relationships among health care professionals who treat this condition.

10. Why is it important to identify patients with claudication?

PVD affects more than 10 million Americans, and its prevalence is increasing. PVD is an important marker for many other serious conditions, including coronary artery disease, cerebrovascular disease, aneurysms, diabetes, and hypertension. Patients with PVD have a fourfold to sixfold increase in cardiovascular mortality compared with age-matched controls. The mortality rate for patients with claudication may be 75% 15 years after diagnosis of PVD. Early diagnosis of claudication gives patients the chance to modify their atherosclerotic risk factors and reduce their risk of coronary and carotid artery disease.

Key Points: Peripheral Vascular Disease

1. Asymptomatic arterial lesions rarely require treatment.
2. Patients rarely die from PVD, but this disease serves as a marker for other, potentially life-threatening processes, such as cerebrovascular disease and coronary artery disease.
3. PVD is underdiagnosed in women.

11. What is the Fontaine classification?

The Fontaine classification is a widely used classification system for lower extremity ischemia. It describes four stages based on signs and symptoms.
- Stage 1 is asymptomatic disease.
- Stage 2a is intermittent claudication when walking more than 200 m.
- Stage 2b is intermittent claudication when walking less than 200 m.
- Stage 3 is rest pain.
- Stage 4 is tissue necrosis or gangrene.

12. What is the Rutherford-Becker classification system?

This is another classification system for chronic lower extremity ischemia. It is popular in the United States and is based on clinical and objective criteria (Table 32-1).

Table 32-1. Rutherford Becker Classification System

GRADE	CATEGORY	CLINICAL DESCRIPTION	OBJECTIVE CRITERIA
0	0	Asymptomatic	Normal treadmill/stress test
1	1	Mild claudication	Complete treadmill test, ankle pressure after exercise <25-50 mm Hg less than blood pressure
	2	Moderate claudication	Between categories 1 and 3
	3	Severe claudication	Cannot complete treadmill test, ankle pressure after exercise <50 mm Hg
2	4	Rest pain	Resting ankle pressure <40 mm Hg, flat or barely pulsatile ankle or metatarsal pulse volume recording
3	5	Minor tissue loss, nonhealing	Resting ankle pressure <60 mm Hg
	6	Major tissue loss, functional foot no longer salvageable	Same as category 5

13. What are the clinical categories of leg ischemia?

The clinical categories of leg ischemia are presented in Table 32-2.

Table 32-2. Clinical Categories of Acute Leg Ischemia						
CATEGORY	DESCRIPTION	CAPILLARY RETURN	MUSCLE WEAKNESS	SENSORY LOSS	ARTERIAL DOPPLER	VENOUS DOPPLER
Viable	Not immediately threatened	Intact	None	None	Audible (ankle pressure >32 mm Hg)	Audible
Threatened	Salvageable if treated promptly	Intact, but slow	Mild, partial	Mild, incomplete	Inaudible	Audible
Irreversible	Major tissue loss, amputation indicated regardless of treatment	Absent (marbling)	Profound paralysis, rigor	Profound, anesthetic	Inaudible	Inaudible

14. What is the ankle-brachial index (ABI)?

The ABI is an essential component used for risk stratification for PVD. The ABI is used to screen for hemodynamically significant disease and to help define its severity. With the patient in the supine position, bilateral brachial blood pressures are obtained. A blood pressure cuff is placed on the calf of each leg, and an ankle systolic pressure is obtained. Determining ankle systolic pressure may require the use of Doppler. The ABI is calculated by dividing the ankle systolic pressure by the highest systolic pressure from either arm.

15. How is the ABI interpreted?

A normal ABI is slightly greater than 1. A significant obstruction to blood flow to the lower extremities reduces the ankle pressure and the ABI. The risk of PVD and symptoms increases as the ABI decreases (Tables 32-3 and 32-4).

Table 32-3. Ankle-Brachial Index (ABI) by Symptoms	
ABI	SYMPTOMS
1-1.10	Normal
0.3-0.9	Claudication
≤0.5	Rest pain
≤0.2	Tissue loss

Table 32-4. Ankle-Brachial Index (ABI) by Risk	
ABI	CATEGORY
≥1	Normal (no/low risk)
0.90-0.99	Borderline (probably normal; no/low risk)
0.70-0.89	Mildly abnormal (low/moderate risk)
0.50-0.69	Abnormal (moderate/high risk)
<0.49	

16. What can cause a falsely elevated ABI?

The ability to determine the systolic blood pressure accurately is predicated by the ability to compress the artery and obstruct blood flow. Diabetes may cause significant calcification of peripheral vessels, making them difficult to compress; this would factiously elevate the observed cuff pressure and the calculated ABI.

17. What is meant by the terms *inflow* and *outflow*?

At least two criteria must be met for an artery to remain patent. There must be sufficient flow of blood into the vessel. With respect to the femoral artery, *inflow vessels* include the aorta, common iliac artery, and external iliac artery. A stenosis of any of these vessels constitutes an inflow lesion. Even with perfect inflow, there also must be flow out of a vessel for it to remain patent. With respect to the femoral artery, the popliteal, peroneal, anterior, and posterior tibial arteries constitute *outflow vessels.*

18. What are the basic steps in performing an angioplasty?

A thorough diagnostic arteriogram is performed first. This is important so that the lesion can be sized, and an appropriate balloon can be selected. The patient is then given heparin. It is important to give heparin before crossing the lesion to prevent thrombosis. The next step involves crossing the lesion with a catheter and guidewire. The lesion is then dilated. After the balloon is removed, an arteriogram is performed with the wire across the lesion to evaluate the result of the angioplasty. It is important to leave the wire in place until the follow-up arteriogram is performed in case a complication, such as a flow-limiting dissection or arterial rupture, occurs.

> **Key Point: Angioplasty**
> 1. Outflow is a key determinant for the long-term patency of angioplasty.

19. What constitutes a technically successful angioplasty?

- Restoration of luminal diameter with less than 32% residual stenosis
- A pressure gradient less than 5 mm Hg across the lesion
- Absence of a flow-limiting dissection or vessel rupture
- Relative reduction in the number and caliber of collateral vessels after a venous angioplasty

20. What are the complications of angioplasty?

The type and incidence of complications vary with the location and morphology of the lesion. Complications include spasm, flow-limited dissection, plaque embolization, vessel rupture, access site trauma, renal dysfunction, contrast allergy, and death.

21. What are the indications for stenting?

Primary indications for stenting include failed angioplasty caused by a flow-limiting dissection or elastic recoil.

22. What constitutes a hemodynamically significant arterial stenosis?

A stenosis is generally considered significant if the luminal diameter is reduced by 50%, and the systolic pressure gradient is greater than 10 mm Hg across the lesion. A lumen that is diminished by 50% would have a corresponding 75% reduction in cross-sectional area, which would likely reduce flow to a clinically significant level. In patients with claudication and lesions that are equivocal based on the aforementioned criteria, provocative testing may be performed. Tolazoline (Priscoline), a potent arterial dilator, is no longer commercially available. One may stimulate arterial dilation with a prolonged inflation of a blood pressure cuff above the systolic pressure. A gradient greater than 20 mm Hg after dilation is considered significant. One should remember to treat the patient and not the arteriographic or pressure findings. The clinical history is also important in deciding whether a lesion is significant. There are few reasons to treat a patient with an entirely asymptomatic lesion.

23. What is the kissing balloon technique?

This technique is most commonly used to perform angioplasty of the common iliac arteries (Fig. 32-2). Often, stenoses of the proximal common iliac arteries are associated with large, eccentric, calcified plaques. Sequential—as opposed to simultaneous—angioplasty may displace the plaque and lead to compromise of the contralateral iliac artery. The kissing technique mitigates this risk through the use of simultaneous angioplasty. This requires bilateral retrograde femoral artery access. The kissing technique may be used for the dilation of complex bifurcation stenosis in other locations as well.

24. What are the basic principles in performing a thrombolysis procedure?

Thrombolysis therapy consists of the delivery of a lytic agent directly into a thrombosed vessel or graft. The catheter is largely responsible for the specificity of the lysis. The immediate goal of the procedure is to lyse an unwanted clot while preventing a systemically lytic state to minimize bleeding complications. The secondary goal of a thrombolysis procedure is to uncover the cause of the thrombosis. Commonly, bypass grafts and native vessels thrombose because of stenoses in inflow vessels, anastomoses, or outflow vessels. Unless the underlying cause for the thrombosis is treated, thrombosis is likely to recur. Less commonly, there are instances in which grafts or vessels thrombose without underlying stenoses. Embolic disease, diminished cardiac output, and noncompliance with anticoagulation therapy are some causes of thrombosis in the absence of an underlying stenosis.

25. In general, how is a thrombolysis procedure performed?

A thorough history and physical examination of the patient are performed. Particular attention should be given to any prior surgeries described in the history. Understanding the patient's vascular anatomy is key for planning access and intervention. Prior arteriograms, if available, should be reviewed. These may also help in the planning of the access site and in determining an appropriate end point to the procedure. A baseline physical examination is essential to monitoring the patient's progress or deterioration during the procedure. After laboratory findings are reviewed and consent has been obtained, a thorough diagnostic arteriogram is performed. The patient is given heparin, and a sheath is placed. The thrombosis is crossed with a wire, and an infusion catheter is placed across the clot. Lytics are infused through the catheter, and the patient is sent to the intensive care unit for monitoring. Every 12 to 24 hours, the patient is brought back to the interventional suite for a follow-up arteriogram. When the clot has resolved, the underlying lesion is treated.

26. What is the guidewire traversal test?

The guidewire traversal test is an attempt to pass a guidewire across a thrombosed vessel before lysis. If the wire can be successfully passed across the occlusion, the clot is more likely to be fresh and lyse. If the guidewire traversal test fails, the occlusion is more likely to be chronic and less responsive to lytics. An end-hole catheter, positioned proximal to the clot, may be used to deliver lytics and soften the clot to facilitate wire traversal. When a wire has been passed, an infusion catheter can be placed. Placement of an infusion catheter within the bulk of the clot helps lend specificity to the lysis procedure and may reduce the overall time required for lysis.

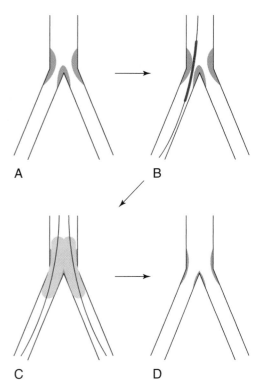

Figure 32-2. Kissing balloon technique. **A,** Bifurcation lesion. **B,** Sequential angioplasty risks occlusion of the unprotected vessel. **C,** Simultaneous angioplasty prevents plaque displacement. **D,** Desired result.

27. List the contraindications to thrombolysis.

- *Absolute*: Active internal bleeding, known intracranial pathology, stroke within the past 6 months, craniotomy in the past 2 months, irreversible limb ischemia, and infected bypass graft
- *Relative*: Uncontrollable hypertension, history of gastrointestinal bleeding, bacterial endocarditis, diabetic retinopathy, coagulopathy, pregnancy, recent major surgery, recent major trauma, and recent cardiopulmonary resuscitation.

In patients with relative contraindications, it is imperative to analyze the potential risk-to-benefit ratio carefully in each case.

28. What is a PVR examination?

PVR stands for *pulse volume recording,* and it is a noninvasive method to evaluate arteries of the lower extremity. A brachial pressure and arterial waveform are obtained as reference standards. The process is repeated at different stations, including the high thigh, low thigh, calf, ankle, and foot. The segmental pressures and waveforms are analyzed to identify the level and severity of possible stenoses. Arterial waveforms provide especially useful information in the setting of calcified vessel. This test is one way that surveillance may be performed after a vascular intervention. It can also be used to plan an intervention in a symptomatic patient.

29. What is Leriche syndrome?

Leriche syndrome comprises chronic, lower extremity ischemia resulting from aortoiliac obstruction that is characterized by intermittent buttock claudication, absent femoral pulses, and sexual impotence (Fig. 32-3).

30. What is an ACT measurement?

ACT stands for *activated clotting time.* It is a clotting test that may be performed in the interventional suite and is commonly used to monitor the effect of heparin. A small sample of whole blood is placed in the testing machine, and a result is available in less than 5 minutes. The reference range varies considerably, but it is usually 70 to

180 seconds. Although it can be obtained quickly, ACT is less precise than partial thromboplastin time and can be affected by a host of factors, including ambient temperature, platelet count, and hemodilution.

31. How are groin pseudoaneurysms managed?

Pseudoaneurysms resulting from femoral artery puncture can be managed in several ways, based on the patient's clinical status and the anatomy of the lesion. The first step is recognizing that the complication has occurred. A postprocedure groin check may reveal a pulsatile mass or ecchymosis. The patient may complain of groin pain. US can be used to diagnose or exclude the injury. If a pseudoaneurysm is found, several options exist. Manual or US-guided compression may cause the pseudoaneurysm to thrombose. Direct thrombin injection can also be performed if the anatomy of the lesion is suitable. Surgical intervention is also an option if other techniques fail.

32. What are the major pathways of collateral circulation to supply the lower extremities in a patient with known aortic occlusion?

A simple way to help remember the collateral supply is to divide it into anterior, middle, and posterior pathways:

- *Anterior*: Subclavian artery through the internal mammary to the superior epigastric artery to the inferior epigastric artery and then into the external iliac artery
- *Middle*: Superior mesenteric to the inferior mesenteric artery via the arc of Riolan and the marginal artery of Drummond to the superior and inferior hemorrhoidal arteries to the internal iliac arteries and then to the external iliac arteries
- *Posterior*: Lumbar arteries to the internal iliac arteries via the retroperitoneal collaterals and then to the external iliac arteries by way of the iliolumbar and circumflex iliac arteries

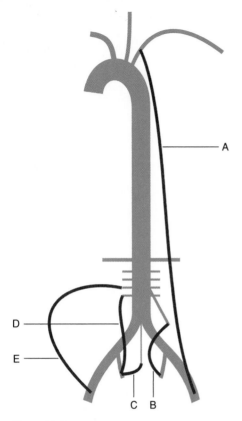

Figure 32-3. Collateral vascular pathways in aortic occlusion. Anterior supply: Left subclavian artery to left external iliac artery, via internal mammary and inferior epigastric arteries (*A*). Middle supply: Inferior mesenteric artery to internal iliac artery (*B*). Posterior supply: Median sacral artery to internal iliac artery (*C*). Lumbar artery to internal iliac artery (*D*). Lumbar artery to external iliac artery (*E*).

WEBSITE

http://www.legsforlife.org

BIBLIOGRAPHY

[1] M.J. Pentecost, H. Michael, G.D. Criqui, et al., Guidelines for peripheral percutaneous transluminal angioplasty of the abdominal aorta and lower extremity vessels: a statement for health professionals from a special writing group of the Councils on Cardiovascular Radiology, Arteriosclerosis, Cardio-Thoracic and Vascular Surgery, Clinical Cardiology, and Epidemiology and Prevention, the American Heart Association, J. Vasc. Interv. Radiol. 14 (2003) 495S–515S.

[2] D. Sacks, C.W. Bakal, P.T. Beatty, et al., Position statement on the use of the ankle brachial index in the evaluation of patients with peripheral vascular disease: a consensus statement developed by the Standards Division of the Society of Interventional Radiology, J. Vasc. Interv. Radiol. 14 (2003) 389S.

EMBOLIZATION TECHNIQUES AND APPLICATIONS

Sara Chen Gavenonis, MD, and
S. William Stavropoulos, MD

CHAPTER 33

1. Describe embolotherapy and some of its indications.

Embolotherapy is temporary or permanent vascular occlusion induced by the intravascular administration of materials via a percutaneous route. Embolization has various clinical applications, including control of bleeding; treatment of vascular malformations; and tumor or organ ablation for curative, palliative, or preoperative purposes.

2. What materials are most commonly used for embolization?

Various embolic materials are commercially available. The most widely used embolic materials are absorbable gelatin sponge (Gelfoam), a temporary agent; metallic coils; and polyvinyl alcohol (PVA) particles. Specific clinical situations may warrant the use of other agents, such as absolute ethanol, synthetic microspheres, or liquid "glues."

3. What is Gelfoam, and how is it used?

Gelfoam is a reabsorbable gelatin that is most widely used in its sheet form. Wedges (1 to 2 mm) of Gelfoam are divided from the larger sheets. The Gelfoam can be injected as "torpedoes" through a catheter placed in a blood vessel, or the Gelfoam can be suspended in a contrast/saline slurry, which can be injected.

4. How does Gelfoam work? When is it used?

Gelfoam causes vascular occlusion by mechanically obstructing vessels, serving as a matrix for thrombus formation, and by causing endothelial inflammation that incites further thrombus formation. Gelfoam is reabsorbed in 5 to 6 weeks, during which time vessel recanalization is anticipated. Clinical situations in which temporary vascular occlusion is preferred include pelvic arterial hemorrhage after trauma, priapism, peripartum hemorrhage, and some cases of upper gastrointestinal (GI) bleeding. The rationale for using Gelfoam in these situations is based on the belief that the use of a temporary agent would minimize the long-term ischemic effect on the end organ.

5. What are metallic coils?

Metallic coils are made of either stainless steel or platinum. Dacron fibers are woven into some coils to promote thrombosis. Coils are available in a wide variety of shapes, sizes, and configurations. Special wires are used to push the coils through catheters that have been placed into the vessel intended to be embolized. Coils occlude vessels by causing mechanical obstruction, inducing clot formation, and provoking an inflammatory reaction.

6. When are coils preferred?

One way to classify embolic materials is based on whether they cause permanent or temporary occlusion. Another way is based on the size (diameter) of the vessel where the occlusion occurs. Coils cause vascular occlusion in vessels that are 1 to 2 mm in diameter and larger. Coils are preferred in clinical situations in which permanent occlusion is intended in vessels of this size. This includes the treatment of arteriovenous fistulas, GI bleeding, aneurysms, endoleaks after endovascular repair of abdominal aortic aneurysms, and traumatic vascular injuries in the proper clinical settings. Coils should not be used if occlusion is desired in vessels smaller than 1 mm, including situations in which the target of the embolization is an organ. When embolizing the uterus or performing chemoembolization of the liver, coils are not used. PVA particles or ethanol can be used to cause microvascular thrombosis, depending on the specific clinical situation.

7. What happens when coils are the wrong size?

Although there is no TV show called "When Coil Embolization Goes Bad," any experienced interventional radiologist can tell a good tale about inappropriately sized coils. When coils are undersized, they can remain mobile after they are pushed out of the catheter and continue to travel with the flow of blood until they embolize to a vessel that is smaller than the diameter of the coil. If this happens while a venous embolization is being performed, the coils travel back toward the right heart and often out the pulmonary artery before lodging in a small vessel. The lungs are also a likely final destination for coils that inadvertently pass through an arteriovenous fistula. When deployed in an artery, coils that are too small can migrate into distal branches or into another vascular distribution. This migration may result in nontarget embolization and decreased efficacy of the intended embolization. Coils that are too large can partially recoil into the parent vessel or cause the catheter to back out of the proper vessel. Retrievable coils are now available and allow optimization of positioning, configuration, and sizing before full deployment.

8. When are PVA particles used?

PVA particles range in size from 50 to 2000 μm. Their mechanism of action is to obstruct vessels physically and incite extensive granulation tissue formation. PVA particles result in permanent occlusion. The size of the particle used is based on the location of desired thrombosis. The smaller the particles are, the more distal the embolization. Particle selection is often based on the experience of the operator. If the particles selected are too small, end-organ ischemia and necrosis may occur. If the particles are too large, collateral vessels may quickly reconstitute blood flow to the target organ, significantly decreasing the efficacy of the procedure. The smallest particles are reserved for tumor embolization or preoperative devascularization of other tissues because they can cause significant tissue ischemia via occlusion down to the capillary level.

9. When performing an embolization procedure, why is it recommended always to place a vascular sheath at the access site?

A vascular sheath assists in catheter exchanges during the procedure. More importantly, the sheath maintains vascular access in the event the embolic agent clogs the delivery catheter, and the catheter needs to be removed.

10. What is postembolization syndrome?

Postembolization syndrome is an expected set of symptoms, including pain, fever, nausea, vomiting, and leukocytosis, that patients may experience after an embolization. The cause is likely secondary to organ ischemia/infarction. Prophylactic antibiotics to prevent superinfection of the ischemic tissue and pain control and antiemetic agents are helpful in treating postembolization syndrome. The syndrome is transient and should resolve within 3 to 5 days after the procedure.

11. How can nontarget embolization be minimized?

Meticulous pre-embolization diagnostic angiography can ensure proper selective catheterization of the desired vessel.

12. When performing an embolization procedure for an upper GI bleed, what information from the endoscopy report is essential?

Because clinically significant upper GI bleeding may be intermittent or too slow to be identified angiographically, arteriograms performed in this setting often display normal results. Empiric embolizations are commonly performed even when arteriograms have normal results. Embolization of an arteriographically "normal" vessel can be performed safely because of the redundant collateral supply to the stomach and duodenum. Ischemic complications of such embolizations are rare unless the patient has a compromised network of collaterals from previous surgery. Before the procedure, it is necessary to know exactly where the patient is bleeding. If the source is duodenal, the gastroduodenal artery is embolized. If the source is gastric, the left gastric artery is embolized.

13. Can a lower GI bleed be treated with empiric embolization?

The colon and small bowel lack the extensive collateral network present in the stomach and duodenum. Empiric embolization of a vascular distribution would cause extensive ischemia and bowel necrosis. The approach to lower GI bleeds is much different. To perform an embolization, the site of bleeding must be identified on the angiogram. Nuclear medicine scans to detect bleeding are often performed before an arteriogram. These scans are noninvasive and can detect intermittent bleeding and hemorrhage that is much slower than that which can be detected on an arteriogram. If the nuclear medicine scan shows negative results, it is of virtually no value to perform an arteriogram. If the nuclear medicine scan shows positive results, and the site of hemorrhage can be identified on the arteriogram, embolization can be attempted.

14. In the setting of pelvic trauma or peripartum hemorrhage in a patient with an unstable condition, is superselective embolization always indicated?

In emergent settings, with a patient with an unstable condition, the goal is efficient hemostasis and stabilization of the patient's condition. Embolization of the entire internal iliac artery, if necessary, can be performed, usually with Gelfoam. The time saved by avoiding further catheterization may be lifesaving. If the patient's condition is stable, selective embolization may be performed to reduce ischemic complications (Fig. 33-1).

15. Name some clinical indications for angiography in patients with pelvic trauma.

The human pelvis represents a very large potential space, often able to accommodate 4 to 5 L of blood. Traumatic diastasis of the symphysis pubis can double the effective potential space of the pelvis. Pelvic bleeding can be difficult to control surgically. Splinting and external fixation are usually performed first to help reduce bleeding. Indications for

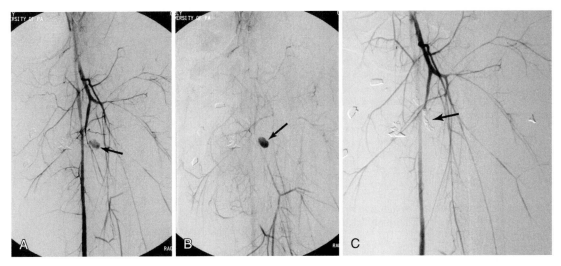

Figure 33-1. A, Digital subtraction angiography (DSA) after a gunshot wound reveals acute hemorrhage from a branch of the left deep femoral artery (*arrow*). **B,** Delayed image from DSA prominently shows the hemorrhage (*arrow*). **C,** DSA after successful coil embolization of the injured artery shows cessation of bleeding (*arrow*).

arteriography include open pelvic fracture, expanding pelvic hematoma, and transfusion requirement greater than 4 U over 24 hours.

16. Is empiric embolization indicated in pelvic trauma?
In the setting of a pelvic fracture, bleeding may be from numerous sources. Venous bleeding is the most common etiology. Bleeding from the periosteal surface of fractured bones is the next most common etiology, followed by arterial hemorrhage. In the setting of an arteriogram with normal results, arterial embolization is not usually performed.

17. In bronchial artery embolization for hemoptysis, vigilance for which vessels is imperative?
Anterior spinal arteries arising from bronchial arteries must be identified to prevent nontarget embolization and subsequent paraplegia. Anterior spinal artery branches that arise from bronchial arteries have a classic "hairpin" appearance, traveling cranially for 1 cm or so before forming a loop and doubling back to travel caudally over the midline of the spine.

18. Why should coils not be used in the bronchial arteries?
Life-threatening hemoptysis is often caused by chronic lung disease, such as sarcoidosis or cystic fibrosis. Because of the chronic nature of the lung disease, hemoptysis is likely to recur. Embolization with coils makes future access to the embolized vascular territory difficult, if not impossible. Particulate agents such as PVA are preferred.

19. Why is it necessary to embolize both sides of a pseudoaneurysm, aneurysm, or arteriovenous fistula?
Significant reconstitution of flow via collaterals can occur and cause recurrence of the lesion. If only the proximal feeding vessel to a pseudoaneurysm is embolized, flow may reverse in the outflow vessel and feed the pseudoaneurysm. Embolizing both sides of a pseudoaneurysm, aneurysm, or arteriovenous fistula is called "embolizing the front and back door of a lesion" and is also sometimes needed when embolizing bleeding vessels.

20. What should always be placed when absolute ethanol is being used for renal artery sclerosis?
An occlusion balloon must always be placed to prevent reflux of absolute ethanol into the aorta. The balloon should also be distal to the origin of the adrenal and gonadal arteries because catecholamine release or gonadal ischemia can result if ethanol is instilled into the respective arteries.

21. How is chemoembolization theorized to work?
Embolization of tumor vessels causes ischemia. This ischemia disables tumor cell membrane ion pumps and exocytosis functions, and increases capillary permeability. As a result, there is increased intracellular accumulation and dwell time of the concomitantly delivered chemotherapeutic agent, leading to increased tumor cell apoptosis.

Key Points: Embolization Techniques and Applications

1. Embolotherapy has various clinical applications, including control of bleeding; elimination of vascular malformations; and tumor or organ ablation for curative, palliative, or preoperative purposes.
2. Postembolization syndrome is a transient and expected set of symptoms, including pain, fever, nausea, vomiting, and leukocytosis, probably secondary to organ ischemia/infarction.
3. Meticulous pre-embolization diagnostic angiography to ensure appropriate selective catheterization of the desired vessel is required to minimize nontarget embolization.
4. Embolization on both sides of a pseudoaneurysm, aneurysm, or arteriovenous fistula is necessary to prevent reconstitution of flow via collaterals, which causes recurrence of the lesion.
5. Gas in the target organ within 3 to 5 days postembolization is thought to arise from tissue necrosis and does not automatically equal infection.

22. What happens when the cystic artery is embolized during hepatic lesion embolization/chemoembolization?

A transient chemical cholecystitis may result. This condition can be self-limited and may resolve with conservative management. Incidental embolization of the cystic artery is believed to contribute to postembolization pain in patients undergoing hepatic chemoembolization.

23. What happens if the left or right gastric artery is embolized during hepatic chemoembolization?

Injecting chemotherapeutic agents directly into the bowel can cause irreversible gastric ischemia and eventual necrosis. Meticulous attention to possible variants in gastric/bowel vascular supply is necessary when performing pre-embolization diagnostic arteriograms.

24. What is the significance of gas in the target organ postembolization?

There is little significance. Gas is often present in the target organ after embolization and, as mentioned earlier, is thought to arise from tissue necrosis. The presence of gas does not always indicate infection. Resorption of the gas may take weeks.

25. What findings suggest that postembolization gas is due to infection?

Beyond 5 days postprocedure, when postembolization syndrome is expected to resolve, persistent fever, elevated serum markers of inflammation (erythrocyte sedimentation rate, C-reactive protein), or a fluid level in the embolized area suggests superinfection of the embolized tissue.

26. When is uterine artery embolization used in a nonemergent setting?

Uterine fibroids causing menorrhagia or pelvic pain can be treated effectively with bilateral uterine artery embolization. Uterine artery embolization can be performed with permanent particles.

BIBLIOGRAPHY

[1] D.M. Coldwell, K.R. Stokes, W.F. Yakes, Embolotherapy: agents, clinical applications, and techniques, Radiographics 14 (1994) 623–643.
[2] M. Gee, M.C. Soulen, Chemoembolization for hepatic metastases, Tech. Vasc. Interv. Radiol. 5 (2002) 132–140.
[3] K.D. Murphy, Embolotherapy, in: D.S. Katz, K.R. Math, S.A. Groskin (Eds.), Radiology Secrets, Hanley & Belfus, Philadelphia, 1998, pp. 502–510.
[4] J.P. Pelage, O. Le Dref, J. Mateo, et al., Life-threatening primary postpartum hemorrhage: treatment with emergency selective arterial embolization, Radiology 208 (1998) 359–362.
[5] R.S. Salem, J.J. Borsa, R.J. Lewandowski, et al., Arterial embolotherapy, in: Proceedings of the Society of Interventional Radiology Workshop, 29th Annual Meeting, 2004, pp. 237–249.
[6] I. Wells, Internal iliac artery embolization in the management of pelvic bleeding, Clin. Radiol. 51 (1996) 825–827.
[7] M. Wojtowycz, Handbook of Interventional Radiology and Angiography, second ed., Mosby, St Louis, 1995, pp. 229–251.

1. **What are the indications for percutaneous transhepatic biliary drainage?**
   Percutaneous biliary drainage is indicated for the treatment of cholangitis or pruritus related to hyperbilirubinemia in the setting of benign or malignant obstructive biliary disease. Biliary drainage may also be performed in the setting of a traumatic bile leak to help divert bile and promote healing of the injured duct. Generally, percutaneous drainage is indicated only if access of the ducts via endoscopic retrograde cholangiopancreatography is impossible.

   > **Key Points: Biliary Drainage**
   > 1. An obstructed, infected biliary system constitutes a medical emergency.
   > 2. Complications from percutaneous biliary drainage can be life-threatening. An endoscopic approach is preferred when possible.

2. **List the causes of benign and malignant biliary obstruction.**
   - Common *benign* causes include bile duct calculi (Fig. 34-1), benign strictures, pancreatitis, and sclerosing cholangitis (Fig. 34-2).
   - Less common *benign* causes include Caroli disease, Mirizzi syndrome, and parasites.
   - Common *malignant* causes include pancreatic cancer (Fig. 34-3), metastatic disease, and cholangiocarcinoma.
   - Less common *malignant* causes include gallbladder carcinoma and ampullary tumors.

3. **What is the most commonly encountered biliary ductal anatomy?**
   The main left bile duct is formed by the union of two horizontally oriented superior and inferior segmental ducts. Right lobe ductal anatomy is more complex and variable. The posterior-inferior and posterior-superior portions of the right hepatic lobe are drained by the right posterior ducts (also known as the right dorsal caudal ducts). The anterior-inferior and anterior-superior portions of the right hepatic lobe are drained by the right anterior ducts (also known as the right ventral cranial ducts). The main right hepatic duct is formed by the union of the right posterior and anterior ducts. The confluence of right and left ducts forms the common hepatic duct, which is joined by the cystic duct (from the gallbladder) to form the common bile duct. The most common biliary ductal anatomy (approximately 60% of the population) consists of a right posterior segment duct that joins the right anterior segment duct to form the main right duct (Fig. 34-4).

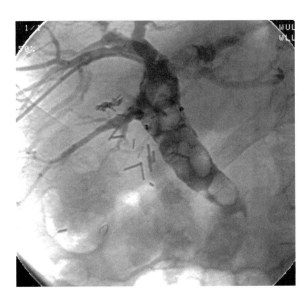

Figure 34-1. Percutaneous transhepatic cholangiogram performed to relieve biliary obstruction shows multiple common bile duct stones, seen as filling defects among the injected intrabiliary contrast material.

4. **Describe the basic steps required to perform diagnostic percutaneous transhepatic cholangiography.**
   Under fluoroscopic guidance, a 21G or 22G needle is passed into the liver through an inferior intercostal or subcostal space at the level of the right mid-axillary line. It is important to verify that the needle does not pass through the pleural space. The needle is withdrawn during injection of contrast agent in an effort to opacify a bile duct that may have been traversed as a result of the needle pass. When a bile duct is identified, injection of contrast agent is continued, and the biliary tree is opacified. A diagnostic cholangiogram is performed with spot images obtained in anteroposterior and multiple bilateral oblique projections.

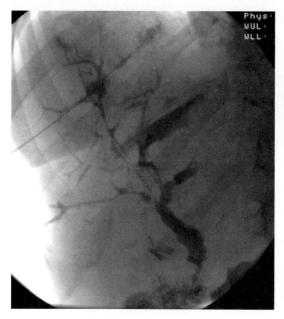

Figure 34-2. Percutaneous transhepatic cholangiogram shows "beading" of intrahepatic biliary ducts, with segments of duct dilation proximal to regions of duct stricture. This stricture-dilation pattern is common in sclerosing cholangitis.

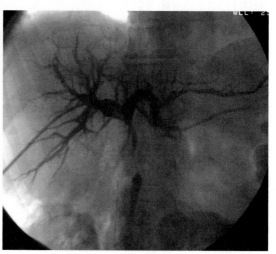

Figure 34-3. Percutaneous transhepatic cholangiogram shows intrahepatic biliary dilation secondary to malignant stricture of the common bile duct. This condition was due to carcinoma of the pancreatic head.

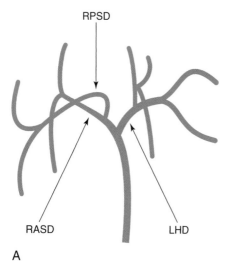

RPSD

RASD   LHD

A

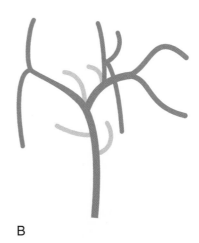

B

Figure 34-4. A, The most common biliary ductal anatomy consists of a right posterior segment duct (RPSD) that joins the right anterior segment duct (RASD) to form the main right duct. LHD = left hepatic duct. **B,** Variant insertions of the RPSD.

5. Describe the basic steps required to perform percutaneous transhepatic biliary drainage.

If indicated by the diagnostic percutaneous transhepatic cholangiogram and clinical symptoms, a wire can be placed via the accessing needle into the biliary tree, followed by tract dilation and biliary drainage catheter placement. This is called the "one-stick" method. If the initial puncture was directed into a central duct, a "two-stick" technique may be used. Central duct punctures are not ideal because the risk of injuring a major hepatic vessel is significant. A second needle may be placed into an appropriate duct that subsequently is dilated and used for access. The ideal access site is an opacified peripheral duct that can be easily accessed under fluoroscopic guidance. Aside from a peripheral location, the duct's path should course through an angle that is gentle enough to allow a catheter to be advanced into the small bowel without extreme angulation. After the second access is obtained, the first needle can be removed. If left-sided biliary drainage is being performed, the needle is passed into the liver from a left subxiphoid approach.

6. **What is the difference between an external biliary drainage catheter and an internal/external biliary drainage catheter?**

External drains end internally within the bile ducts above the site of obstruction. The obstructed biliary tree is decompressed by draining the bile externally into a drainage bag. Internal/external drains cross the site of obstruction and end within the small bowel. Bile may drain internally from the biliary tree through side-holes in the catheter into the small bowel, and the catheter may be capped externally. Internal/external drainage catheters are placed whenever it is possible to cross the site of obstruction because this type of drainage is more physiologic. Internal drainage prevents loss of bile salts and electrolytes and allows the bile to aid in fat metabolism within the bowel. It is important to monitor the volume status and electrolytes of patients draining bile externally. These patients can lose a large volume of fluids rich in electrolytes.

7. **When should an internal/external drain be capped? When should this drain be uncapped?**

After a de novo biliary drainage, catheters are almost always attached to a bag for gravity drainage for a specified time. External drainage helps to decompress the biliary system. A pressurized system may promote bacterial translocation into the hepatic vasculature, resulting in sepsis. Obstructed systems are likely to be pressurized, and this is exacerbated by the contrast agent injected into the ducts during the procedure. Pruritus often resolves faster if drainage is maximized. In the setting of a malignant obstruction, administration of chemotherapeutic agents may be delayed if the serum bilirubin level is excessively elevated. In certain situations, internal and external drainage may accelerate normalization of the serum bilirubin level and allow for the subsequent administration of chemotherapeutic agents.

Patients with drains placed for external drainage can lose a significant amount of fluids and electrolytes. Tubes are commonly capped when possible to allow more physiologic drainage of bile. Usually this occurs when concerns over infection have subsided, and pruritus has resolved. If chemotherapy is planned, tube capping may be delayed until the serum bilirubin level is within an acceptable range.

After a tube has been capped, it should be uncapped because of infectious concerns (fever, bacteremia, sepsis, elevated white blood count), leakage of bile around the catheter, pain, and increasing bilirubin or other liver enzyme levels. After the tube is uncapped, additional tests may be indicated, such as a tube check to determine whether the tube is clogged or malpositioned.

8. **A patient begins to leak bile around an indwelling biliary drain. Why does this happen? What can be done?**

Biliary drains require considerable maintenance after they are placed, and the maintenance often adversely affects the quality of life of patients. Tubes leak for various reasons. Standard biliary tubes consist of a catheter with side-holes and a distal locking loop. For the tube to work properly, the side-holes must be patent and properly positioned. The key to proper positioning is the proper location of the most peripheral side-hole. This hole should be located just inside the biliary duct where access was obtained. If the most peripheral side-hole of the catheter is malpositioned, leakage also occurs. Migration or malposition of the tube so that the hole is outside of the duct and in the parenchymal tract results in bile leaking back along the catheter onto the skin. If the hole is too far in, the bile duct peripheral to the catheter may become obstructed and leak along the course of the catheter. A careful cholangiogram and meticulous tube placement solve these problems. Another common cause of leakage is clogging of the side-holes of the catheter with viscous bile. This situation can be managed with catheter exchange with consideration given to upsizing the tube if the complication occurs frequently.

9. **What are the potential complications associated with percutaneous transhepatic biliary drainage?**

Even in the absence of clinical signs of cholangitis, bile in an obstructed system is often colonized with bacteria. Biliary sepsis, a potentially lethal complication, may occur during or after a cholangiogram or biliary drainage. Antibiotics should be given during a biliary drainage, and patients should be monitored closely for signs of sepsis. Injury to blood vessels adjacent to the bile ducts within the hepatic parenchyma may be associated with pseudoaneurysms, hemorrhage, and hemobilia. Bile leakage and bile peritonitis, and complications related to intraprocedural sedation (respiratory failure and aspiration) may occur. Pneumothorax and reactive or bilious pleural effusions are uncommon complications if care is taken during initial needle placement.

10. **After an initial drainage procedure, what additional management measures may be performed to treat benign biliary obstruction?**

Biliary drainage provides access to the bile ducts that may allow for retrieval of biliary calculi. Balloon dilation of benign ductal strictures with gradual upsizing of drainage catheter diameter may allow for remodeling of the bile duct with eventual relief of obstruction and removal of the drainage catheter. This therapy, when successful, usually takes several months. If unsuccessful, surgical intervention may still be possible, or catheters may be left in place for the long-term.

11. What can be done to manage the treatment of malignant biliary obstruction after initial drainage?

With some tumor types, access to the bile ducts allows for the placement of radioactive isotopes for ductal brachytherapy. If the patient is not a candidate for surgical resection, the drainage catheters may be left in long-term. Sometimes, internal metal stents may be placed across malignant strictures to allow for catheter removal for patient comfort. The decision to place a metallic stent depends on patient prognosis and life expectancy because internal metal stents have limited long-term patency.

12. What does the term *isolated ducts* mean? What is its significance?

In the case of a low obstruction of the common bile duct, the right and left systems still communicate. A right-sided biliary drain can be used to drain the right and the left sides. If the level of obstruction is higher, as might occur with cholangiocarcinoma, this might not be the case, and some ducts may not communicate with others—they are "isolated." This is one reason why it is important to obtain cross-sectional imaging before biliary drainage. If only one ductal system is dilated, this information helps determine the access site (left-sided drainage vs. right-sided drainage). By definition, patients with isolated ducts have a portion of the biliary system that remains undrained if only a single catheter is placed. These patients may require more than one tube to treat infection, pruritus, or hyperbilirubinemia.

13. How does stricture morphology help differentiate between benign and malignant disease?

Benign strictures tend to taper smoothly, with gradual narrowing across their length. Malignant strictures, by contrast, are points of obstruction that end abruptly, sometimes with irregular borders or an appearance of "shouldering."

14. If a histologic diagnosis is required, what methods may be used to obtain a biopsy specimen of the bile ducts?

When access to the bile ducts has been achieved, biopsy of a stricture site may be performed under fluoroscopic guidance. Various devices may be used to obtain tissue samples, including biopsy brushes, forceps, and needles. Often, several samples obtained on different days are required to obtain a diagnosis.

15. When is percutaneous cholecystostomy indicated?

Although cholecystectomy is the preferred therapy for acute cholecystitis, some patients may not be surgical candidates because of their overall clinical status, sepsis, or other comorbid conditions. Percutaneous cholecystostomy combined with broad-spectrum antibiotic coverage is a temporizing measure until the patient's clinical status may be optimized for surgery.

16. Name the basic steps involved in performing percutaneous cholecystostomy.

With ultrasound (US) guidance, the gallbladder is accessed with a needle. A wire is placed, and after tract dilation, a drainage catheter is placed into the gallbladder and allowed to drain externally. A subcostal, transhepatic path to the gallbladder is generally preferred because it may guard against bile leakage into the peritoneal space if the catheter is inadvertently dislodged.

17. What are potential complications associated with percutaneous cholecystostomy?

Complications include hemorrhage, infection, bile peritonitis, and respiratory failure or aspiration related to intraprocedural sedation. Pneumothorax is possible, but relatively rare if a subcostal approach can be used.

18. How long must a percutaneous cholecystostomy catheter remain within the gallbladder before it can be removed?

Although some investigators have shown that catheters may sometimes be safely removed in less time, most believe that the cholecystostomy catheter should stay within the gallbladder for at least 4 to 6 weeks. This allows time for a mature tract to form between the gallbladder and skin surface in an effort to prevent bile leakage into the peritoneal space when the catheter is removed.

19. Should the cholecystostomy catheter be placed to external drainage indefinitely?

In the acute phase, although there is evidence of active inflammation, the catheter should be maintained on external drainage. In the setting of cholecystitis secondary to obstructing biliary calculi, the catheter should be maintained on external drainage. In the setting of acalculous cholecystitis, the catheter may be capped to allow for internal drainage after a cholangiogram is performed to document that there is no evidence of cystic duct obstruction.

20. When is transjugular liver biopsy indicated and preferred over percutaneous liver biopsy?

Because a transjugular liver biopsy specimen is obtained from within a hepatic vein, bleeding complications resulting from transgression of the liver capsule may be avoided. The transjugular procedure is indicated for patients with coagulopathies or platelet deficiency. Platelet dysfunction because of renal failure may also be an indication. In addition, any other issue that may make percutaneous biopsy difficult or risky (e.g., ascites) would be a potential indication for transjugular liver biopsy. Because transjugular biopsy cannot generally be used to obtain tissue from a specific liver lesion, it is used only to obtain a tissue diagnosis for medical (diffuse) liver disease, such as viral hepatitis or transplant rejection.

21. How is transjugular liver biopsy performed?
A hepatic vein (most commonly, the right hepatic vein) is accessed using a transjugular approach (jugular vein to superior vena cava, through right atrium to inferior vena cava, and into right hepatic vein), and a stiff wire is placed. A stiff metal cannula is placed over the wire into the hepatic vein. An 18G or 19G core biopsy needle is placed through the cannula and used to obtain multiple samples of liver tissue. Because the right hepatic vein courses posteriorly through the right lobe, the needle is directed anteriorly to avoid transgression of the liver capsule. Because the middle hepatic vein courses more anteriorly, however, lateral or posterior sampling may be safer with this approach.

22. What are the clinical signs and symptoms associated with portal hypertension?
Esophageal, gastric, mesenteric, and rectal varices may bleed in response to elevated portal pressures; mortality from the initial bleeding episode may be 20% to 60%. Increased intrasinusoidal pressure may result in ascites and hepatic hydrothorax. Hepatic encephalopathy, hepatorenal syndrome with renal dysfunction, and hepatopulmonary syndrome with hypoxemia may also be encountered.

23. How can one indirectly estimate portal venous pressure to confirm the diagnosis of portal hypertension?
Catheterization of a hepatic vein is performed via jugular or femoral vein access. The catheter is advanced until it obstructs a small hepatic vein branch, or a balloon occlusion catheter is inflated within the hepatic vein to obstruct its outflow. The wedged hepatic vein pressure is actually a measure of sinusoidal pressure, but allows for a reasonable indirect estimate of portal pressure. A corrected sinusoidal pressure measurement is obtained by subtracting the measured free hepatic venous pressure from the wedged hepatic venous pressure. Corrected sinusoidal pressure measurements less than or equal to 5 mm Hg are considered normal. Measurements of 6 to 10 mm Hg are compatible with mild portal hypertension, and measurements greater than 10 mm Hg are compatible with more severe portal hypertension.

24. What are the indications for creating a transjugular intrahepatic portosystemic shunt (TIPS)?
The most common indication for TIPS placement is variceal bleeding related to portal hypertension that is refractory to endoscopic therapy (Fig. 34-5). Other indications include refractory ascites or hepatic hydrothorax, Budd-Chiari syndrome, portal hypertensive gastropathy, and hepatorenal or hepatopulmonary syndrome. TIPS placement may be an effective bridge to liver transplantation for patients with end-stage liver disease and manifestations of portal hypertension.

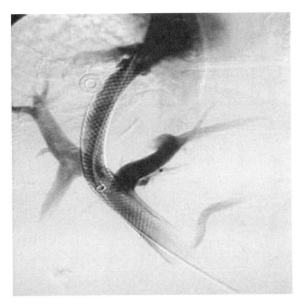

Figure 34-5. TIPS with a stent from the right hepatic vein to the right portal vein.

25. What are the contraindications to TIPS creation?
A pre-TIPS total bilirubin level greater than 3 mg/dL, refractory coagulopathy with an international normalized ratio greater than 1.8, a Child-Pugh score greater than 12, and a serum creatinine level greater than 1.9 mg/dL all have been found to be associated with poor outcomes. TIPS creation that is performed on an emergent basis is also associated with high mortality, and hemodynamic stabilization with transfusions, other medical interventions, and balloon tamponade of gastroesophageal varices are preferred before the TIPS procedure.

26. Describe the steps of the TIPS procedure.
- A hepatic vein, most commonly the right hepatic vein, is accessed via a right internal jugular vein approach. A wedged hepatic venogram may be obtained to opacify the portal vein and map its location.
- A stiff metal cannula is placed, and a needle is passed from the right hepatic vein into the right portal vein under fluoroscopic guidance. Often, several needle passes are required to obtain portal access. The portosystemic pressure gradient measurement is obtained.

- A stiff wire is placed into the portal vein, and dilation of the intrahepatic parenchymal tract is performed with an angioplasty balloon.
- A flexible, self-expanding stent (usually 8 or 10 mm in diameter) is placed from the portal vein to the confluence of the hepatic vein with the inferior vena cava.
- A venogram and repeat portosystemic pressure gradient measurements are obtained.

27. What are the potential complications of TIPS creation?

Complications include hemorrhage, infection, allergic reaction to contrast agent, and respiratory failure or aspiration because of intraprocedural sedation. In addition, because the TIPS causes shunting of portal venous blood away from the liver, the procedure may be complicated by decline in liver function and hepatic encephalopathy.

28. What are the short-term and long-term goals of TIPS creation?

Successful TIPS creation is associated with a final portosystemic pressure gradient measurement of less than 12 mm Hg to prevent variceal bleeding. If the TIPS has been placed to treat refractory ascites, lower pressures may be necessary for success (≤8 mm Hg). If the patient has significant encephalopathy, and treatment with lactulose is insufficient to control symptoms, a reducing stent may be placed into the TIPS to create an intentional increase in the portosystemic pressure gradient. TIPS patency should be monitored at intervals using duplex Doppler US, which allows velocity measurements within the TIPS to be obtained noninvasively. Significant velocity increases from baseline may indicate the presence of TIPS stenosis, which may prompt TIPS venography and revision by balloon dilation or additional stent placement.

BIBLIOGRAPHY

[1] J.M. LaBerge, A.C. Venbrux (Eds.), SCVIR Syllabus: Biliary Interventions, SCVIR, Fairfax, VA, 1995.
[2] N.H. Patel, Z.J. Haskal, R.K. Kerlan (Eds.), SCVIR Syllabus: Portal Hypertension: Diagnosis and Interventions, second ed., SCVIR, Fairfax, VA, 2001.

GENITOURINARY AND GASTROINTESTINAL INTERVENTIONAL RADIOLOGY

Charles T. Lau, MD, and
S. William Stavropoulos, MD

CHAPTER 35

1. List the indications for a percutaneous nephrostomy (PCN) (Fig. 35-1).
- To relieve obstruction in the setting of infection or to preserve renal function
- To assist in the removal of a stone or foreign body
- To divert urine to permit healing of a leak or fistula
- To provide access for ureteral intervention

2. What is the indication for an emergent PCN?
Pyonephrosis (infected urinary obstruction) may rapidly lead to urosepsis and death. It is a urologic emergency, and emergent drainage is indicated.

3. What are important technical factors to consider when performing a PCN?
A PCN is a relatively safe, minimally invasive technique that can be used to treat various conditions efficiently. The safety and efficacy of the procedure are predicated, however, on the following well-established guidelines to help prevent complications. The skin puncture should be sufficiently lateral to the midline; this ensures a relatively straight tract that avoids kinking of the catheter. The needle entry into the kidney should traverse the least vascular plane, and the access obtained should provide a path to all portions of the collecting system. It is also important that organs adjacent to the kidney, such as the colon, are not in the needle path.

4. What is the most common method of visualizing the collecting system for a PCN?
Fluoroscopy is the most common method, but this requires opacification of the collecting system. This can be accomplished by intravenous contrast agent injection with anterograde excretion, if the patient has satisfactory renal function. If the patient has impaired renal function or has a completely obstructed renal collecting system, fluoroscopy may not be a viable option. In these situations, an anterograde pyelogram can be performed via a 22G or 25G needle. An anterograde pyelogram can be performed with iodinated contrast agent or CO_2 gas (Fig. 35-2).

5. What are alternative means other than fluoroscopy of visualizing the collection system for a PCN?
Ultrasound (US) imaging can be used, which eliminates the need for contrast agent opacification of the collecting system. US imaging also can be used to ensure that adjacent organs do not lie along a proposed nephrostomy tract. If the collecting system is not dilated, however, it may be difficult to visualize it with US. Computed tomography (CT) is another option, particularly if the kidney is in an anomalous position.

6. Should access for a PCN be obtained through the renal parenchyma or directly into the renal pelvis?
Puncture of the collecting system should occur through the renal parenchyma because this is the

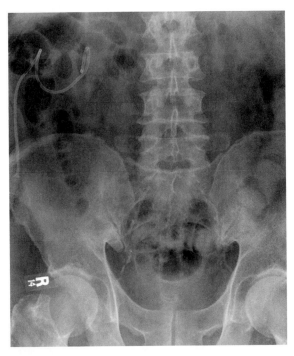

Figure 35-1. PCN tube.

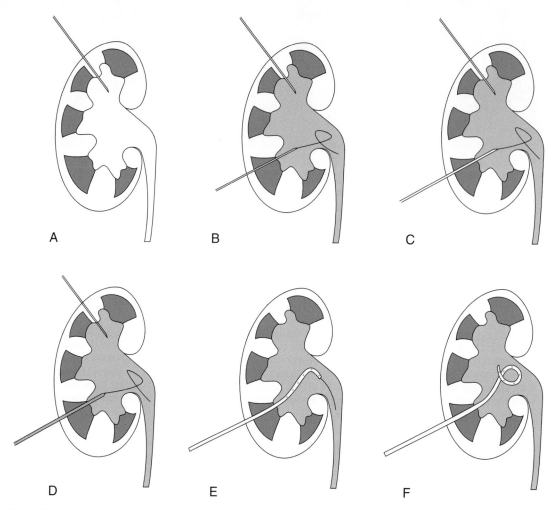

Figure 35-2. Schematic illustration of PCN using the Seldinger technique. **A,** A posterior calyx is punctured with a 22G needle under US guidance. **B,** After performing an anterograde pyelogram through this access point, a second 22G needle is inserted into the opacified collecting system along the expected tract of the nephrostomy catheter. A 0.018-inch wire is advanced through this needle. **C,** Exchange is made for a catheter that allows conversion to a 0.035-inch wire. **D,** Nephrostomy tract is dilated by exchanging successive dilators over the wire.

least vascular plane. Direct access to the pelvis has a higher rate of vascular complications. Puncture through the renal parenchyma also helps to provide support for the catheter, minimize urine leakage, and decrease the chance of catheter displacement.

7. From what approach should a PCN be performed?
A PCN tract should pass through the least vascular region of the kidney to minimize bleeding complications. Renal calyces are arranged in an anterior and posterior row. Between these two rows, in the interpolar kidney, is a relatively avascular plane of renal parenchyma called *Brödel line*. This plane usually lies at 30 to 45 degrees, and the PCN tract should be made along this line.

8. Aside from decreasing the chance of bleeding, what are the other benefits of performing a PCN through Brödel line?
The approach through Brödel line also results in a PCN catheter exiting through skin near the posterior axillary line, so the catheter does not kink and the patient is not uncomfortable lying on it when supine.

9. What imaging modalities can be used to perform a percutaneous drainage of renal or perinephric abscesses?
Percutaneous drainage of renal and perinephric abscesses can be performed with US, CT, or fluoroscopic guidance. US is usually preferred because it provides real-time imaging, which allows for an accurate, safe, and fast procedure.

It is important to place the drainage catheter in the most dependent portion of a large abscess cavity to ensure complete drainage of infected material.

10. **What are possible complications resulting from percutaneous drainage of renal or perinephric abscesses?**
Percutaneous drainage is a safe and effective technique that can be used in the management of an abscess. Complications may still occur, however. When collections adjacent to or within the kidney are being drained, some infected material may intravasate into the vascular system, resulting in bacteremia or sepsis. It is important to administer intravenous antibiotics before and after drain placement. Drains placed within the kidney may accidentally traverse a blood vessel. Bleeding can be inconsequential and resolve spontaneously; may result in hematuria, if bleeding tracks into the collecting system; or may lead to a perinephric hematoma, if the hemorrhage tracks around the kidney. Rarely, adjacent organs may be inadvertently punctured during catheter placement.

11. **When is percutaneous management of urinary tract calculi preferred over extracorporeal shock wave lithotripsy (ESWL)?**
ESWL is the sole therapy used in approximately 90% of patients with symptomatic urinary tract calculi. Percutaneous management is preferred, however, in patients with a large stone burden. Percutaneous management may also be used as an adjunct to ESWL if large stone fragments remain or if obstruction occurs after ESWL.

12. **What is the role of PCN in percutaneous treatment of urinary tract calculi?**
PCN is used to obtain a tract through which the endoscope may access the collecting system. It is important in this situation to create a tract that is straight and permits the endoscope access to all portions of the collecting system.

13. **How are calculi removed during percutaneous treatment of the urinary tract?**
Different devices can be used through the endoscope when access to the collecting system has been obtained. These include various stone baskets, which are three to eight wires arranged in a helical pattern. Forceps may be used to grab individual stones. US and electrohydraulic lithotripters can also be used to pulverize calculi within the collecting system to facilitate removal.

14. **What are indications for ureteral stenting?**
Common indications include urinary tract calculi and benign ureteral stricture. Ureteral stenting is also indicated in patients with extrinsic ureteral obstruction, ureteral trauma, and retroperitoneal fibrosis. In the setting of malignant ureteral obstruction, stenting may be performed if the patient does not have bladder outlet obstruction. Stenting allows the affected kidney to drain, and the patient is able to void. The most commonly used ureteral stents are the double-J stent and nephroureteral stent.

15. **Describe the difference between a double-J ureteral stent and a nephroureteral stent.**
All ureteral stents are made of polyurethane or silicone; metallic stents are not used in ureters. A double-J ureteral stent is completely internal and has a "pigtail" at each end (Fig. 35-3A). Its proximal coil is situated in the renal pelvis, and its distal coil is situated in the urinary bladder. A nephroureteral stent has a "pigtail" at its distal end that is placed in the bladder and another one that is looped in the renal pelvis (Fig. 35-3B). The catheter exits through the skin at the percutaneous access site.

16. **How does a ureteral stent work?**
A ureteral stent is hollow and has multiple side-holes. It drains urine past obstructions from the collecting system into the urinary bladder. Some authorities believe that an element of capillary action augments this process. A ureteral stent also causes passive dilation of the ureter, which may or may not persist after the stent is removed.

17. **What are indications for esophageal stenting?**
Esophageal stenting is most commonly performed in the treatment of dysphagia secondary to cancer ingrowth and bronchoesophageal fistula (Fig. 35-4).

18. **What technical complications are associated with esophageal stenting?**
Even with the most experienced operators, stents may be malpositioned or migrate. Because esophageal malignancies may be friable, stenting may occasionally result in esophageal perforation, a potentially life-threatening complication.

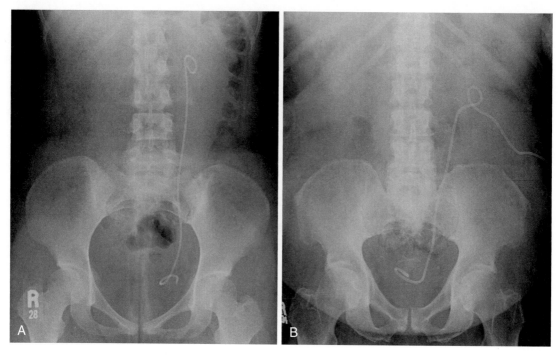

Figure 35-3. **A,** Double-J ureteral stent. **B,** Nephroureteral stent.

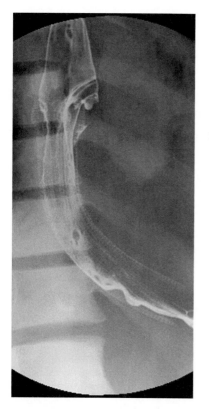

Figure 35-4. Esophageal stent.

19. What factors should be considered when selecting the puncture site for a percutaneous gastrostomy?

The site of the percutaneous gastrostomy should be subcostal and to the left of the midline (Fig. 35-5). The outer third of the rectus abdominis muscle should be avoided because the inferior epigastric artery courses in this region. Fluoroscopy should be performed so that the puncture avoids the colon and small bowel.

20. What is the difference between a G tube, G-J tube, and J tube?

A simple rule to follow in selecting an enteral access site is to use the stomach whenever possible. Direct gastrostomy (G) tubes are safe and easy to use. The stomach performs important digestive functions, and gastric access allows patients to receive bolus feeds. Jejunal access (via jejunostomy [J] tube) necessitates continuous feeds, which are not as well tolerated. The needs of most patients can be met with G tubes.

- A *G tube* is placed directly into the stomach and can be used for feeding or gastric decompression.
- *Gastrojejunostomy tubes* (*G-J tubes*) enter the stomach similar to a G tube, but pass through the stomach and duodenum and terminate in the proximal jejunum (Fig. 35-6). G-J tubes are technically simpler to place than J tubes and are associated with a lower procedural risk (remember, use the stomach, even for access, whenever possible). G-J tubes may have a single port that enters the small bowel. In patients with gastric outlet obstruction, G-J tubes with two ports may be used. One port is used to vent the stomach, and the other is used to administer feeds. In addition, a previously placed G tube can be converted to a G-J tube.
- *J tubes* enter the small bowel directly (Fig. 35-7). They may be used for feedings or for palliative decompression when placed above an obstruction.

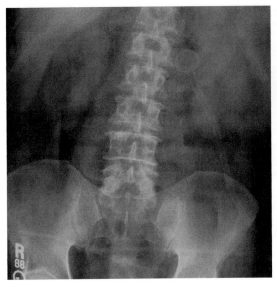

Figure 35-5. Gastrostomy tube.

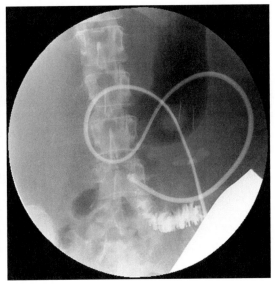

Figure 35-6. Gastrojejunostomy tube.

Key Points: Genitourinary and Gastrointestinal Interventional Radiology

1. Urosepsis is an indication for emergent PCN.
2. A PCN tract should pass through the skin near the posterior axillary line, pass through the renal parenchyma in the relatively avascular plane denoted by the Brödel line, and enter the collecting system.
3. Although ureteral stents successfully drain the collecting system into the bladder and cause passive dilation of the ureter, they are considered a temporary measure and are not curative.
4. Patients with ascites should receive large-volume paracentesis before percutaneous gastrostomy.
5. J tubes and G-J tubes are reserved for patients with known gastroesophageal reflux disease or documented aspiration.

21. When are feeding G tubes not the tube of choice?

Patients may not be candidates for feeding G tubes because of anatomic or functional reasons. Anatomic contraindications include prior gastrectomy or gastric pull-through, colon adhered to the stomach, and ascites. Patients with ascites are at high risk for constantly leaking fluid through the puncture site. Functional reasons include severe reflux with aspiration, gastroparesis, and gastric outlet obstruction. Decompressive G tubes may be indicated in patients with gastric outlet obstruction.

22. When are small bowel feeding tubes indicated?

J tubes and G-J tubes are usually reserved for patients with known severe gastroesophageal reflux disease with the risk of aspiration.

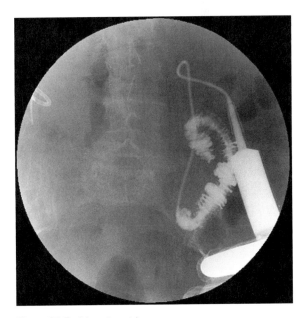

Figure 35-7. Jejunostomy tube.

WEBSITES

http://www.emedicine.com/radio/topic796.htm

http://www.medscape.com/viewarticle/423508_1

http://www.emedicine.com/radio/topic798.htm

BIBLIOGRAPHY

[1] N.R. Dunnick, C.M. Sandler, J.H. Newhouse, E.S. Amis, Textbook of Uroradiology, second ed., Williams & Wilkins, Baltimore, 1997.
[2] M. Wojtowycz, Handbook of Interventional Radiology and Angiography, second ed., Mosby, St. Louis, 1995.

EXTREMITY PLAIN FILMS AND TRAUMA

Woojin Kim, MD

CHAPTER 36

1. How are fractures evaluated with plain films?

At least two views of the fracture site, taken at 90 degrees to each other, must be obtained. Remember, "one view equals no view." The radiographs obtained should include joints immediately above and below the fractured area for evaluation of associated dislocations.

2. Define the following terms: dislocation, subluxation, closed fracture, open fracture, intra-articular fracture, pathologic fracture, and occult fracture.

- *Dislocation* is complete loss of contact between the articular surfaces of a joint. *Subluxation* is a partial loss of congruity between articular surfaces.
- *Closed fracture* has intact skin over the fracture site. If there is communication between the fracture site and the outside environment, it is considered an *open fracture,* regardless of how small the overlying skin defect is.
- *Intra-articular fracture* involves the articular surface of a joint.
- *Pathologic fracture* is a fracture in abnormal bone weakened by a disease process.
- *Occult fracture* is a fracture that is not visible on a plain radiograph.

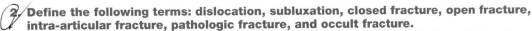

> ### Key Points: Basic Terminology
>
> 1. *Dislocation* is complete loss of contact between the bones of a joint.
> 2. *Subluxation* is partial loss of contact between the bones of a joint.
> 3. *Open fracture* has an open wound that allows communication between the outside environment and the fracture site.
> 4. *Intra-articular fracture* involves the articular surface.
> 5. *Pathologic fracture* is a fracture in an abnormal, diseased bone.

3. What is an avulsion fracture?

An avulsion fracture occurs when a fragment of bone is pulled off at the site of insertion of muscles, ligaments, and tendons.

4. What is a comminuted fracture?

A comminuted fracture is a fracture with more than two fracture fragments.

5. What is an os acromiale?

Os acromiale is an accessory ossification center of the acromion. Although the os acromiale is normally fused in an adult by age 25, it remains unfused in some individuals. It is an important entity to be aware of because it may be misinterpreted as an acromial fracture. In addition, higher prevalence of subacromial impingement and rotator cuff tears have been associated with os acromiale.

6. Describe types I, II, and III acromioclavicular (AC) separation.

As the term suggests, AC separation is widening of the AC joint space because of ligamentous injury.

- *Type I AC separation* is stretching or partial tear of the AC ligament with no displacement seen on a radiograph. One can assess this condition radiographically by obtaining and comparing weight-bearing views of the uninjured shoulder and injured shoulder. This is a stable injury and has excellent prognosis of healing.
- *Type II AC separation* is complete tear of the AC ligament with widening of the AC joint. Most of these injuries heal without surgery.
- *Type III AC separation* is complete disruption of the AC and coracoclavicular ligaments. Abnormal widening of the AC and coracoclavicular joints results. This type of injury requires internal fixation (Fig. 36-1).

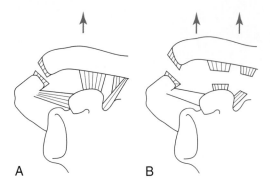

Figure 36-1. A, Type II AC separation. Only the AC ligament is ruptured. **B,** Type III AC separation. There is complete tear of the AC and coracoclavicular ligaments.

7. What is a "Y" view?
A "Y" view is a special radiographic view of the shoulder that shows the head of the humerus sitting between the two projections off the scapula—the acromion and the coracoid process—forming a "Y." This view is helpful in determining the relative position of the humeral head and the glenoid fossa, and aids in the diagnosis of shoulder (glenohumeral) dislocation.

8. What are the radiographic features of anterior shoulder dislocation on an anteroposterior view?
The most common type of shoulder dislocation is anteroinferior. The humeral head is displaced anteromedially and typically rests slightly inferior to the coracoid process. It is also known as *infracoracoid dislocation* or *subcoracoid dislocation*.

9. What are Hill-Sachs fractures and Bankart fractures?
Hill-Sachs fracture and Bankart fracture are complications of anterior shoulder dislocation. Hill-Sachs fracture is a defect in the posterolateral aspect of the humeral head. It occurs when there is contact between this region of the humeral head and the anterior-inferior glenoid rim during anterior dislocation. The Bankart fracture is a fracture of the anterior-inferior glenoid rim secondary to this trauma.

10. What is pseudosubluxation of the humerus?
With pseudosubluxation of the humerus, there is inferior displacement of the humeral head with widening of the glenohumeral space. This entity is usually caused by hemarthrosis or lipohemarthrosis after trauma to the shoulder. As the term suggests, this is not true dislocation of the glenohumeral joint.

11. What are the "posterior fat pad" sign and the "sail" sign in the elbow?
The "posterior fat pad" and "sail" signs indicate the presence of an intra-articular elbow fracture. Fat is normally present between the synovium and capsule of the elbow joint, which is normally not radiographically visible, with the exception of an occasional normal anterior fat pad that may be seen as a small lucency immediately adjacent to the anterior cortex of the distal humerus. With intra-articular fracture, subsequent hemarthrosis distends the synovium and causes displacement of this fat. The posterior fat pad becomes visible as a radiolucency, and the anterior fat pad is lifted away from the bone as a triangular radiolucency, causing it to resemble a sail.

12. Describe Monteggia fracture and its associated finding.
Monteggia fracture is a fracture of the proximal ulna with radial head subluxation or dislocation. This fracture-dislocation was originally described by Monteggia in 1814. It is important to remember to look for the associated radial head dislocation or subluxation when you see a proximal ulnar fracture because failure to do so would result in radial head necrosis.

13. Describe Galeazzi fracture and its associated finding.
Galeazzi fracture is a fracture of the distal radius with associated distal radioulnar dislocation/subluxation. Galeazzi described this fracture in 1935.

14. Name all eight carpal bones.
A well-known mnemonic used for memorizing all the carpal bones is the following (proximal row from radial to ulnar direction and then distal row from radial to ulnar direction): "*s*ome *l*overs *t*ry *p*ositions *t*hat *t*hey *c*annot *h*andle," which stands for *s*caphoid, *l*unate, *t*riquetrum, *p*isiform, *t*rapezium, *t*rapezoid, *c*apitate, and *h*amate. The following tip can help you remember the respective positions of trapezium and trapezoid: trapezium is associated with the thumb.

15. Which carpal bone gets fractured the most often?
The scaphoid is the carpal bone that is fractured the most often. Fracture of the scaphoid should be suspected when there is tenderness of the anatomic snuff box. Scaphoid fractures can be difficult to visualize on plain radiographs. The blood supply to the scaphoid enters from the waist (middle third) and distal pole by the scaphoid branches of the radial artery. As result, blood flows proximally from the distal pole. When this is disrupted by a fracture, avascular necrosis of the proximal fracture fragment occurs and can be seen as sclerosis.

16. What is the "Terry Thomas" sign?

Scapholunate dissociation results from ligamentous disruption between the scaphoid and lunate. This is manifested by widening of the space between the scaphoid and lunate on the anteroposterior view of the wrist and is known as the "TerryThomas" sign. Terry Thomas (1911-1990) was a gap-toothed British comic actor.

17. Define dorsal intercalated segmental instability (DISI) and volar intercalated segmental instability (VISI).

DISI and VISI describe carpal instability based on the tilt of lunate on the lateral radiograph of the wrist. With DISI, the lunate tilts dorsally. With VISI, the lunate tilts in a volar direction (Fig. 36-2).

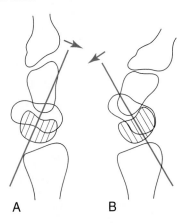

A   B

Figure 36-2. **A,** DISI. Note the dorsal tilt of the lunate (indicated by the vertical lines). **B,** VISI. Conversely, there is volar tilt of the lunate.

18. Match the following fractures with the radiographic images in Fig. 36-3:

Barton
Baseball (mallet) finger
Bennett
Boxer
Colles
Smith
Triquetral

19. Which is more common, anterior or posterior dislocation of the hip?

Posterior hip dislocation is more common. It is manifested by superior displacement of the femoral head. In anterior hip dislocation, the femoral head is displaced anteriorly and medially.

20. What is a bipartite patella?

Bipartite patella is another normal anatomic variant that one should not misinterpret as being a fracture of the patella. It is a secondary ossification center that is seen in the upper outer quadrant of the patella. It is usually bilateral and has a smooth and sclerotic cortical border.

21. What is a Segond fracture, and what is its clinical implication?

Segond fracture is an avulsion fracture of the proximal lateral tibia at the site of attachment of the lateral ligament. The fracture fragment may be very small. Although it may not look so terrible on a radiograph, it is commonly associated with anterior cruciate ligament tear and meniscal injury.

22. What is a tibial plafond fracture?

A tibial plafond fracture is an intra-articular fracture of the distal tibia caused by impaction of the talus and is often comminuted.

23. Match the following fractures with their radiographic images in Fig. 36-4:

Freiberg
Jones
Maisonneuve
Segond

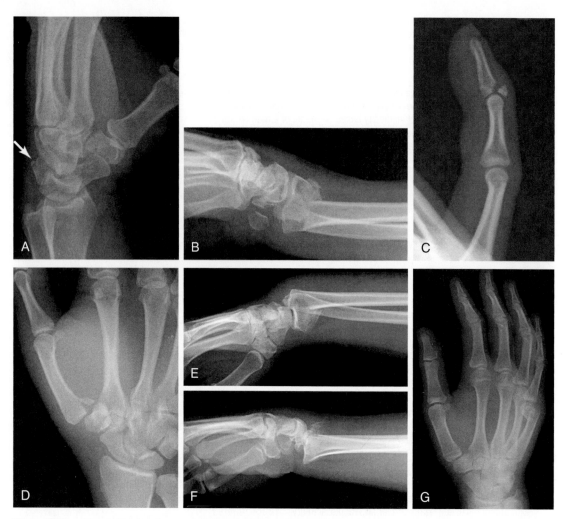

Figure 36-3. **A,** Triquetral fracture. Dorsal avulsion fracture (*arrow*) is seen best on the lateral view. **B,** Colles fracture. Nonarticular distal radial fracture with dorsal displacement of the distal fracture fragment. **C,** Mallet finger. Avulsion fracture of base of the distal phalanx at the extensor digitorum tendon insertion site. **D,** Bennett fracture. Intra-articular fracture-dislocation of base of the first metacarpal. **E,** Smith fracture. Nonarticular distal radial fracture with volar displacement of the distal fracture fragment. **F,** Barton fracture. Intra-articular oblique fracture of dorsal aspect of the distal radius. **G,** Boxer's fracture. Transverse fracture of the distal fifth metacarpal.

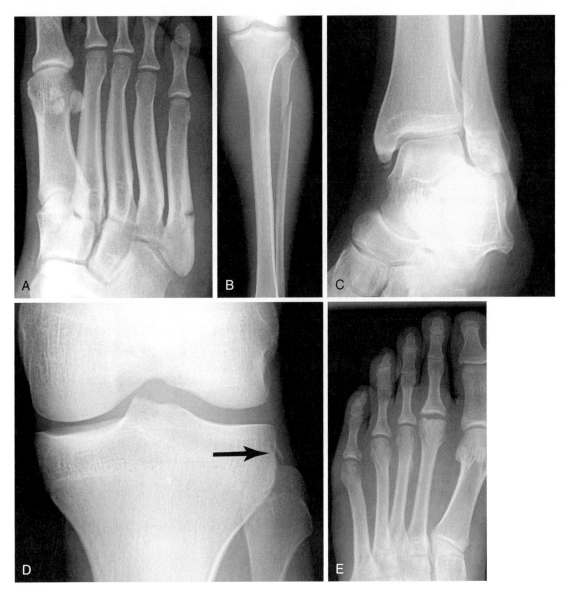

Figure 36-4. A, Jones fracture. Transverse fracture of base of the fifth metatarsal. **B** and **C,** Maisonneuve fracture. Tear of interosseous membrane and fracture of the upper third of fibula (**B**) with associated medial malleolus fracture (**C**). **D,** Segond fracture. Small cortical avulsion fracture (*arrow*) of the proximal lateral tibia. **E,** Freiberg infraction is osteonecrosis of the second or third metatarsal head from subchondral fatigue fracture.

BIBLIOGRAPHY

[1] J.H. Harris, W.H. Harris, The Radiology of Emergency Medicine, Lippincott Williams & Wilkins, Philadelphia, 2000.
[2] T.B. Hunter, L.F. Peltier, P.J. Lund, Radiologic history exhibit: musculoskeletal eponyms: who are those guys? Radiographics 20 (2000) 819–836.
[3] R.J. Schultz, The Language of Fractures, second ed., Williams & Wilkins, Baltimore, 1990.

PLAIN FILM EXAMINATION OF SPINAL TRAUMA

Woojin Kim, MD

1. Describe a standard cervical spine radiograph examination.

A standard cervical spine radiograph study includes anteroposterior, lateral, and open-mouth odontoid views. Occasionally, bilateral oblique views may be obtained for evaluation of the neural foramina and facet joints. In a trauma setting, computed tomography (CT) is the preferred modality of choice because of higher sensitivity in detecting acute abnormalities.

2. Describe how to interpret a lateral cervical spine film.

- Count the vertebral bodies. All seven cervical vertebral bodies and C7-T1 should be visualized. If not, either a swimmer's view or CT can be obtained.
- Evaluate the thickness of prevertebral soft tissue. It should be less than 5 mm anterior to C1-C3. From C4-C7, its thickness should not exceed 20 mm.
- Assess four parallel lines for alignment. From anterior to posterior, these lines are anterior vertebral, posterior vertebral, spinolaminar, and posterior spinous (Fig. 37-1).
- Examine the atlantoaxial interval, which is the distance between the posterior aspect of the anterior arch of C1 and the anterior aspect of the odontoid process of C2 (axis). This space should not exceed 3 mm in adults and 5 mm in children. This interval should remain constant with flexion and extension in adults. Widening of this space indicates disruption of the transverse atlantal ligament.
- Compare the intervertebral disc spaces for widening or narrowing.

Key Points: How to Interpret Cervical Spine Radiographs

1. Count vertebral bodies.
2. Evaluate prevertebral soft tissue.
3. Assess alignment.
4. Examine the atlantoaxial interval.
5. Compare the intervertebral disc spaces for widening or narrowing.

---

3. What is a swimmer's view?

A swimmer's view is obtained when the lower cervical vertebrae cannot be seen on the lateral view, usually because of a patient's inability to cooperate or a large shoulder girdle obscuring the view. This view is obtained by having the patient, in the supine position, raise his or her arm over the head while lowering the other arm.

4. Describe Jefferson fracture and its mechanism of injury.

Jefferson fracture is an unstable burst fracture involving the ring of C1 with lateral displacement of lateral masses and disruption of the transverse ligament. This fracture is associated with axial load injuries.

5. Describe three different types of odontoid process (also known as *dens*) fractures.

- *Type I* fracture involves the superior tip of the odontoid process. It is extremely rare, and some authorities even argue over its existence.
- *Type II* is the most common and is characterized by a fracture through the base of the odontoid process. In contrast to the other two types, this fracture is considered mechanically unstable.
- *Type III* fracture involves the body of C2.

6. What is os odontoideum?

Os odontoideum describes separation of the dens from the body of C2. It appears as a well-circumscribed ossicle with a smooth, thin cortex that is separated from the adjacent dens by a radiolucent gap. It was originally thought that this entity represented failure of fusion of the secondary ossification center with the remaining dens. Such a congenital anomaly is now known as *persistent ossiculum terminale,* however, and appears as a small ossicle at the tip of the dens. Most authorities now agree that os odontoideum is more likely an acquired post-traumatic abnormality.

Regardless, this entity can be differentiated from an acute odontoid fracture by the presence of a sclerotic cortical margin and occasional hypertrophy of the anterior arch of axis. Os odontoideum can cause atlantoaxial instability. Some studies have shown increased frequency of this entity in patients with Down syndrome.

7. What is a hangman's fracture?
Hangman's fracture can be seen after a motor vehicle accident in which the chin strikes the dashboard. It is a hyperextension injury with bilateral fracture of the pars interarticularis. This type of fracture can be subtle on radiography and be easily overlooked (Fig. 37-2).

8. What is a flexion teardrop fracture? What is its prognostic significance?
A flexion teardrop fracture is a severe hyperflexion injury of the cervical spine that results in anterior compression fracture of the vertebral body and disruption of the posterior ligament. Because of severe kyphotic angulation of the cervical spinal cord at this level, there is usually associated anterior cervical cord syndrome. The teardrop component is seen as a fracture fragment off the anterior-inferior corner of the involved vertebral body (Fig. 37-3). Flexion teardrop fractures are the most severe and unstable spinal fractures. In 1956, Schneider described this fracture as a "teardrop" fracture-dislocation because it reminded him of the tear from a patient after he conveyed the seriousness of the injury.

9. What is a clay shoveler's fracture?
A clay shoveler's fracture is a fracture of the spinous process, often seen in the lower cervical spine (Fig. 37-4). In the 1930s, numerous men worked as clay shovelers in Australia. This injury occurred as result of hyperflexion when the worker attempted to throw a shovel full of clay with the shovel stuck in the clay. Currently, this fracture occurs as result of football and power-lifting injuries.

10. What is the difference between unilateral and bilateral interfacetal dislocations?
Unilateral interfacetal dislocation (also known as *unilateral locked facet injury*) is a rotational injury of the cervical spine that results in unilateral facet joint dislocation with associated posterior ligamentous tear. Bilateral interfacetal dislocation (also known as *bilateral locked facet injury*) results from extreme hyperflexion, causing anterior dislocation of both facet joints. This is a serious injury that is commonly associated with spinal cord damage.

11. What is the "hamburger" sign?
The "hamburger" sign refers to the appearance of a dislocated facet joint on axial CT images where there is uncovering of the articular facet. The superior facet of the level below normally constitutes the top bun of the hamburger, the facet joint itself constitutes the meat patty, and the inferior articular facet of the level above constitutes the bottom bun. When there is facet dislocation, there is loss of the "hamburger" sign, where the meat patty is exposed without the top bun, also known as the "naked facet" sign.

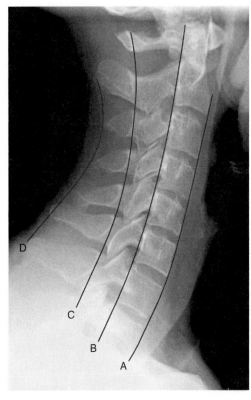

Figure 37-1. Normal lateral view of the cervical spine. Cervical vertebrae to C7-T1 can be visualized. Four parallel lines used for assessment of alignment are drawn: *A,* anterior vertebral; *B,* posterior vertebral; *C,* spinolaminar; and *D,* posterior spinous process.

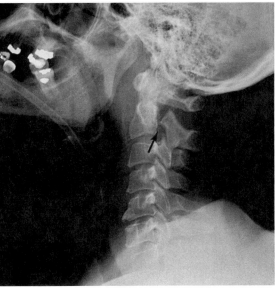

Figure 37-2. Lateral plain film radiograph of a hangman's fracture. Note the disruption of the spinolaminar line (*arrow*).

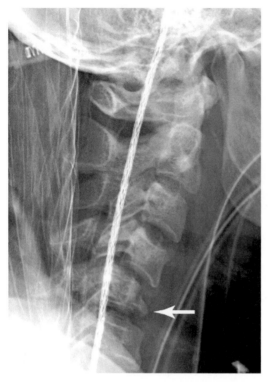

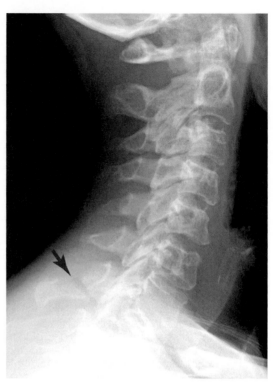

Figure 37-3. Flexion teardrop fracture. There is focal kyphosis at C5 with posterior displacement of the vertebral body and a teardrop fracture fragment (*arrow*).

Figure 37-4. Clay shoveler's fracture. There is a minimally displaced fracture of the posterior spinous process of C7 (*arrow*).

12. What is the difference between compression and burst fractures?

Compression fractures are caused by anterior flexion. There is anterior wedging of the affected vertebral body, with the middle vertebral column remaining intact. Because only the anterior vertebral column is affected, this fracture is usually stable. Burst fractures are caused by axial loading injuries. The fracture lines extend through the anterior and posterior cortices of the vertebral body. The posterior displacement of fracture fragments can cause spinal cord injury, and these fractures are considered unstable.

13. What is a Chance fracture?

There is horizontal splitting of the posterior elements extending anteriorly to involve the vertebral body or intervertebral disc space or both. It is often associated with tearing of the posterior ligament complex. It is also called a seat belt fracture after acute hyperflexion. Presence of this fracture should alert the clinician to the existence of significant intra-abdominal injury.

14. What is a "Scotty dog"?

On the oblique view of the lumbar spine, an outline of what looks like a dog can be seen. The parts of the dog are as follows: the transverse process constitutes the nose; the pedicle, the eye; the superior articular facet, the ear; the pars interarticularis, the neck; the inferior articular facet, the front leg; the lamina, the body; the contralateral superior articular facet, the tail; and the contralateral inferior articular facet, the hind leg (Fig. 37-5).

15. What is spondylolysis?

Spondylolysis is a defect or fracture of the pars interarticularis. On the "Scotty dog" view, it is seen as a band of radiolucency through the "neck," similar to a collar. L5 is most commonly involved.

16. Describe spondylolisthesis and its grading method.

When spondylolysis involves bilateral pars interarticularis, it is commonly associated with a condition called *spondylolisthesis,* which is anterior translation of the involved vertebral body with respect to its inferior adjacent vertebral body. It is graded I through IV, based on the degree of anterior displacement. If it is displaced anteriorly less than 25% of the vertebral body's anteroposterior dimension, it is considered to be grade I. Displacements of 25% to 50%, 50% to 75%, and greater than 75% constitute grades II, III, and IV. Its etiology can be congenital, traumatic, degenerative, or pathologic, such as from Paget disease or osteogenesis imperfecta.

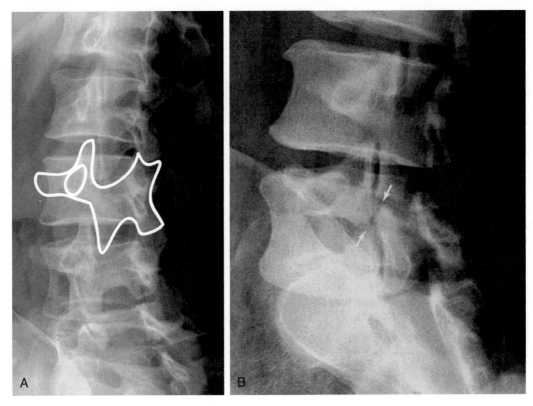

Figure 37-5. A, "Scotty dog" (see question 14). **B,** Fracture of pars interarticularis, the "neck" of the "Scotty dog."

BIBLIOGRAPHY

[1] J.H. Harris, W.H. Harris, The Radiology of Emergency Medicine, Lippincott Williams & Wilkins, Philadelphia, 2000.
[2] T.B. Hunter, L.F. Peltier, P.J. Lund, Radiologic history exhibit: musculoskeletal eponyms: who are those guys? Radiographics 20 (2000) 819–836.
[3] R.J. Schultz, The Language of Fractures, second ed., Williams & Wilkins, Baltimore, 1990.

CHAPTER 38

NONTRAUMATIC SPINE PLAIN FILMS AND DEGENERATIVE DISEASE

Christopher J. Yoo, MD, and
Neil Roach, MD

1. Define *scoliosis*, and name the most common cause.
Scoliosis refers to lateral curvature of the spine in the coronal plane; kyphosis and lordosis refer to anterior and posterior curvature in the sagittal plane. In most cases, the cause of scoliosis is idiopathic.

2. Describe the three subgroups of idiopathic scoliosis.
- *Infantile idiopathic scoliosis* is typically detected before 4 years of age and is more common in boys. Of cases diagnosed in the first year of life, 92% resolve spontaneously.
- *Juvenile idiopathic scoliosis* is diagnosed in children 4 to 10 years old, and is seen predominantly in boys before age 6 and predominantly in girls between ages 7 and 10. Only 7% of cases resolve spontaneously.
- *Adolescent idiopathic scoliosis* is diagnosed between age 10 and skeletal maturity and is the most common type of idiopathic scoliosis. There is a heavy predominance in girls.

3. Although idiopathic scoliosis is the most common type of scoliosis, what other etiologic factors should be considered before making this diagnosis?
Other etiologic factors can be grouped as shown in Table 38-1.

4. What is a limbus vertebra?
A limbus vertebra is an abnormality of the anterior-inferior or anterior-superior corner of a vertebral body secondary to an unfused ring apophysis of the end plate. It appears as a corticated ossicle, usually triangular in shape and separated from the rest of the vertebral body by herniated disc material. It is unknown whether this abnormality is congenital or traumatic in nature (Fig. 38-1).

5. What is a butterfly vertebra, hemivertebra, and block vertebra?
These are congenital vertebral anomalies. The vertebral bodies form initially from two chondral centers, side by side, which eventually fuse to form a single body. If one chondral center fails to form, a hemivertebra results. If the chondral centers fail to fuse in the midline, and there is hypoplasia centrally, a butterfly vertebra results (Fig. 38-2A). If there is nonsegmentation of these centers from the chondral centers above or below, a block vertebra may result (Fig. 38-2B). These congenital anomalies can result in premature degenerative disease or structural abnormalities, such as congenital scoliosis and kyphosis. These anomalies should also alert the radiologist to the possibility of other anomalies in the VACTERL complex (vertebral, anorectal, cardiac, tracheal, esophageal, rectal, and limb anomalies).

6. List important descriptors when reporting scoliosis.
The following descriptors are important: location and direction of the curvature, Cobb angle, rotational component, whether it is fixed (structural) versus not fixed (nonstructural), presence of congenital anomaly or neoplasm, and Risser stage.

Table 38-1. Etiologic Factors to Consider before Making the Diagnosis of Idiopathic Scoliosis

CATEGORY	EXAMPLES
Congenital*	Block vertebra, hemivertebra, vertebral bar
Neuromuscular	Cerebral palsy, muscular dystrophy, spinal cord injury
Developmental	Skeletal dysplasia, neurofibromatosis
Neoplasm*	Osteoid osteoma, osteoblastoma
Trauma and other	Trauma, postradiation

*Particularly in otherwise healthy patients, effort should be focused on excluding congenital vertebral segmentation, fusion anomalies, and neoplasm.

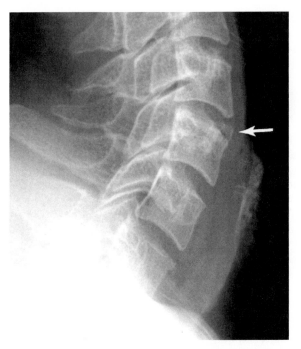

Figure 38-1. Lateral plain film examination of the neck shows a triangular-shaped, well-corticated ossicle at the superior end plate of C5 (*arrow*). This is a limbus vertebra.

7. How is the Cobb angle measured?
One of two methods is used, depending on the severity of the scoliosis. Visually determine the highest vertebra at the beginning and the lowest vertebra at the end of the curvature. Draw a line parallel to the superior end plate of the top vertebral body and a line parallel to the inferior end plate of the lower vertebral body. The angle at the intersection of these two lines is the Cobb angle. If the scoliosis is mild, the intersection of the two lines would be far away. Draw lines perpendicular to the previously described lines, and measure the Cobb angle at their intersection. Use whichever method is convenient because they result in the same angle measurement (Fig. 38-3).

8. What is the Risser classification, and why is it significant in scoliosis?
The Risser classification is a gross measure of skeletal maturity as determined by the amount of ossification of the iliac apophysis. The apophyseal ossification begins laterally and progresses medially with increasing skeletal maturity. The Risser classification is significant in scoliosis because the likelihood of progression is high in low Risser stages (e.g., skeletal immaturity) and decreases when the patient reaches skeletal maturity (Fig. 38-4).

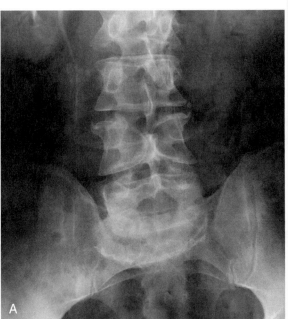

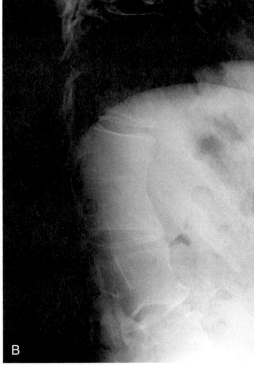

Figure 38-2. A, Frontal radiograph of the lumbar spine shows a butterfly vertebral body segment at L4. **B,** Lateral radiograph of the thoracolumbar junction shows nonsegmented block vertebrae.

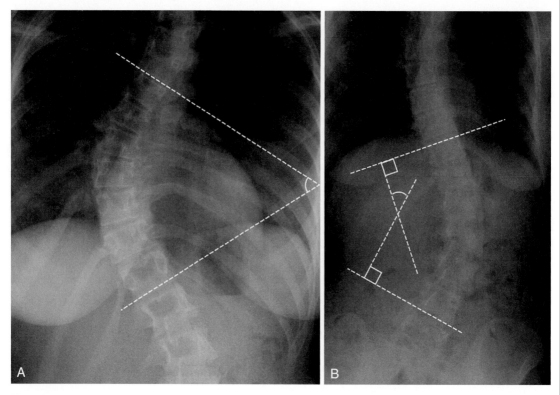

Figure 38-3. **A** and **B,** Frontal radiographs of patients with scoliosis show methods for measuring the Cobb angle in moderate (**A**) and mild (**B**) scoliosis.

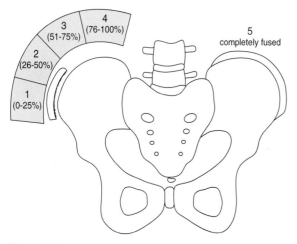

Figure 38-4. Risser stages for determining skeletal maturity through evaluation of degree of ossification of the iliac apophysis.

9. List the radiographic signs of degenerative disc disease.
- Disc space narrowing
- Osteophyte formation
- End-plate sclerosis
- Schmorl nodes
- Vacuum disc phenomenon
- Facet osteoarthritis
- Neural foraminal narrowing
- Uncovertebral joint hypertrophy in the cervical spine

10. What is a Schmorl node?
A Schmorl node is a herniation of intervertebral disc material through the vertebral end plate, resulting in a lucent area at the end plate with surrounding sclerosis on radiographs and computed tomography (CT) and possibly surrounding edema on magnetic resonance imaging (MRI) (Fig. 38-5).

11. What is the best way to image degenerative disc disease?
MRI is now the modality of choice for anatomic accuracy in imaging degenerative disc disease and its effects on the spinal canal and neural foramina.

12. What are Modic changes of the vertebral end plates?
These are MRI findings of the marrow adjacent to the vertebral end plates associated with degenerative disc disease in the lumbar spine.
- *Modic type I* change refers to a marrow edema–like pattern that histopathologically correlates with subchondral vascularized fibrous tissue with end-plate fissures and is seen as low signal on T1-weighted images and high signal on T2-weighted images relative to normal marrow signal.

- *Modic type II* change refers to a fatty marrow change seen as increased signal on T1-weighted images and as isointense or increased signal on T2-weighted images relative to normal marrow signal.
- *Modic type III* change refers to subchondral sclerosis, which is seen as low signal on T1-weighted and T2-weighted images.

13. What terms are used to describe the different types of disc extension beyond the vertebral body margin?
The spectrum includes disc bulge, protrusion, extrusion, and sequestration (Fig. 38-6).
- *Disc bulge* is diffuse enlargement of the intervertebral disc, which is usually symmetric or slightly eccentric to one side and results from laxity or stretching of the anulus fibrosus.
- *Disc protrusion* is an area of more focal disc extension beyond the boundaries of the remainder of the disc, but still contained within the anulus fibrosus. The neck of the protrusion is the widest portion of the abnormality.
- *Disc extrusion* is a focal disc extension in which the neck is narrower than the extruded portion of the disc and indicates extrusion through an annular fissure. Extrusions often extend superiorly or inferiorly, along the long axis of the spinal canal.
- *Disc sequestrum* is a free fragment of the intervertebral disc, which has extruded through the annulus and separated from the remainder of the disc to lie within the extradural space.

14. Other than degenerative disc pathology, what other factors commonly contribute to neural foraminal narrowing and central canal stenosis?
Facet osteoarthritis, which can result in sclerosis and subsequent enlargement of the facet joint complex, and ligamentum flavum hypertrophy contribute to narrowing. Spondylolisthesis can also contribute, particularly if it is secondary to degenerative disease, rather than spondylolysis. In the cervical spine, osteophytes along the posterior margins of the vertebral end plates and uncovertebral hypertrophy, in addition to the previously mentioned factors, can contribute to narrowing.

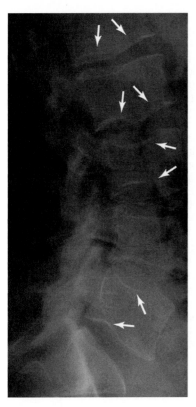

Figure 38-5. Lateral radiograph of the lumbar spine shows multiple degenerative end-plate Schmorl's nodes (*arrows*).

Key Points: Terminology of Degenerative Disc Pathology

1. *Disc bulge:* Diffuse, symmetric extension of the disc beyond the end plate.
2. *Disc protrusion:* More focal extension of the disc. It may be central, left/right paracentral, or left/right lateral. The "neck" is wider than the more distal portion.
3. *Disc extrusion:* Herniation of a portion of the disc. The "neck" is the narrowest part. The extrusion often extends superiorly or inferiorly along the long axis of the spinal canal.
4. *Disc sequestrum:* Free disc fragment in the epidural space that has lost its connection to the disc.

---

15. What nerve root exits the C3-C4 neural foramen; C7-T1; T3-T4; L3-L4?
In the cervical spine, C1 exits between the occiput and C1, whereas C8 exits at C7-T1. The cervical nerve roots exit above the pedicles of the same-numbered vertebral body (i.e., the C4 nerve root exits through the C3-C4 foramen). Because there are eight cervical roots, the relationship switches at the cervicothoracic junction, and in the thoracic and lumbar spine, the nerve root exits below the pedicle of the same-numbered vertebral body (i.e., T3 exits though the T3-T4 foramen, and L3 exits through the L3-L4 foramen).

Key Points: C8 Nerve Root

1. C8 is a nerve root without a vertebral body. It exits between C7 and T1.
2. As a result of C8 exiting between C7 and T1, cervical nerve roots exit above the pedicles of the same-numbered body.
3. As a result of C8 exiting between C7 and T1, thoracic and lumbar nerve roots exit below the pedicles of the same-numbered body.

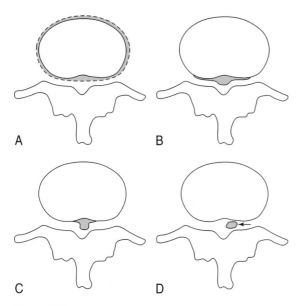

A   B

C   D

Figure 38-6. Illustrations of terms used to describe extension of the intervertebral disc beyond the margin of the vertebral body. **A,** A *disc bulge* is diffuse and symmetric. **B,** A *disc protrusion* (in this case, a central disc protrusion) has focality, and the neck is the widest part of the abnormality. **C,** An *extrusion* also has focality, but the neck is the narrowest part. **D,** A *disc sequestrum* has lost all connection to the disc and lies in the epidural space.

16. What nerve root may be compressed by a right posterior disc protrusion at L3-L4?

On a sagittal T1-weighted MR image of the lumbar spine, the nerve root exits the foramen just below the pedicle of the upper vertebral body (i.e., L3 root exits just below the L3 pedicle, which happens to be above the level of the intervertebral disc space). A posterior disc bulge at L3-L4 would not impinge the L3 root because it has already exited unless the disc protrusion is large or extends craniad in the neural foramen. Instead, the right L4 nerve root is descending slightly lateral to the cauda equina, in the lateral recess, toward the L4-L5 neural foramen and can be impinged by a right posterior disc protrusion.

17. What is failed back syndrome? What is the best way to evaluate affected patients?

After spine surgery, 5% to 40% of patients have persistent symptoms, and this is referred to as failed back syndrome. Approximately 10% of these patients undergo another operation. Causes of failed back syndrome include residual or recurrent disc herniation; residual central canal, foraminal, or lateral recess stenosis; formation of scar tissue in the surgical bed; instability; arachnoiditis; surgical error (operating on the wrong level); and surgical complications, including infection, hematoma, and cerebrospinal fluid leak. The best method for evaluating these patients is with MRI, with and without intravenous gadolinium enhancement, which can help distinguish recurrent disc pathology versus postoperative fibrosis, two common causes of the syndrome.

18. What is spondylolisthesis? Name the two major causes.

Spondylolisthesis is displacement of one vertebral body with respect to the vertebral body below. Anterolisthesis is more common than retrolisthesis. The most common causes are spondylolysis and degenerative facet arthrosis.

19. What is the "inverted Napoleon hat" sign?

This is a radiographic sign seen on the anteroposterior view of the lateral spine or pelvis and can be due to spondylolisthesis of L5 on S1. The anterior-inferior vertebral margin and transverse processes have the appearance of Napoleon's hat turned upside down (Fig. 38-7).

20. What is OPLL?

OPLL stands for *ossification of the posterior longitudinal ligament* and typically involves the cervical spine. OPLL appears as a longitudinal bony ridge parallel and adjacent to the posterior vertebral margins. It is more common among individuals of Japanese descent and occurs in 50% of patients with DISH (see question 21).

21. What is DISH?

DISH stands for *diffuse idiopathic skeletal hyperostosis* (also known as *Forestier disease*). DISH has many manifestations throughout the body,

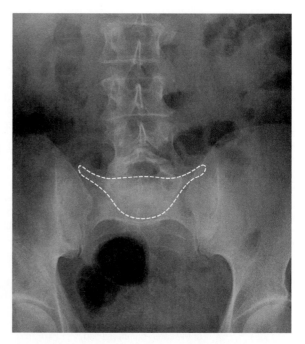

Figure 38-7. The "inverted Napoleon hat" sign, which can indicate anterolisthesis of L5 on S1 as depicted on an anteroposterior view of the lumbar spine.

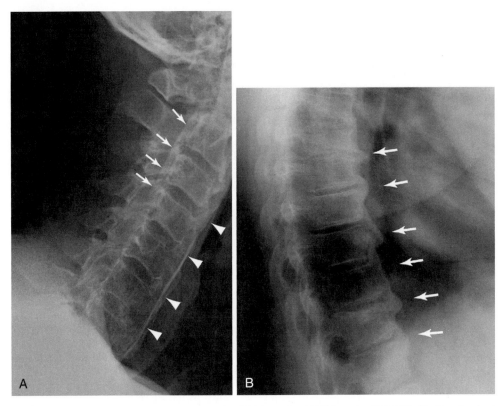

Figure 38-8. A, Lateral view of the cervical spine. The patient has OPLL (*arrows*) and DISH (*arrowheads*). **B,** DISH of the thoracic spine (*arrows*).

including calcification and ossification of ligamentous and tendinous insertion sites, particularly involving the pelvis and patella (known as "whiskering"); enthesophyte formation on the calcaneus and olecranon processes; and para-articular osteophyte formation, particularly around the hip joints. Its most common manifestation is in the spine, however, where it is associated with calcification and ossification of the anterior longitudinal ligament and large bridging osteophytes anteriorly and laterally, sometimes interrupted by linear lucencies owing to herniation of intervertebral disc material. OPLL can occur in DISH as well (Fig. 38-8).

22. What are three radiographic criteria for the diagnosis of DISH?
Criteria are (1) flowing ossification over at least four contiguous vertebrae, (2) minimal loss of disc height relative to ossification formation, and (3) absence of bony ankylosis and sacroiliac joint disease.

23. What is the difference between an osteophyte and a syndesmophyte?
- *Osteophyte* formation begins at the site of Sharpey fibers attachment between the anulus fibrosus and the anterior margin of the vertebral body just above or below the end-plate margin. Osteophytes typically begin by growing outward. An osteophyte eventually grows and meets an osteophyte on the other side of the disc space and may be called a *bridging osteophyte*.
- *Syndesmophytes* are ossifications of the anulus fibrosus and are more vertically oriented, attaching right at the end-plate margin. DISH in the spine is ossification of the anterior longitudinal ligament and, similar to an osteophyte, is also seen originating away from the end-plate margin.

24. What is Scheuermann disease?
Scheuermann disease is an osteochondrosis of the thoracic spine, which occurs in adolescents typically 13 to 17 years old. It is characterized by vertebral end-plate sclerosis, multiple Schmorl nodes, anterior wedging, and resultant kyphosis. Radiographic criteria for diagnosis require three contiguous abnormal vertebrae with at least 5 degrees of anterior wedge deformity.

25. What is the radiographic appearance of Kümmell disease?
The radiographic appearance shows compression fracture of the vertebral body with intraosseous vacuum phenomenon. This is believed to represent osteonecrosis of the vertebral body with secondary fracture.

BIBLIOGRAPHY

[1] D. Resnick, Degenerative disease of the spine, in: D. Resnick (Ed.), Bone and Joint Imaging, second ed., Saunders, Philadelphia, 1996, pp. 355–377.
[2] D. Resnick, Diffuse idiopathic skeletal hyperostosis (DISH), in: D. Resnick (Ed.), Bone and Joint Imaging, second ed., Saunders, Philadelphia, 1996, pp. 378–387.
[3] D.W. Stoller, S.S. Hu, J.A. Kaiser, The spine, in: D.W. Stoller (Ed.), Magnetic Resonance Imaging in Orthopaedics and Sports Medicine, second ed., Lippincott Williams & Wilkins, Philadelphia, 1997, pp. 1059–1162.

OSTEOPOROSIS

Neil Roach, MD

1. **What is osteoporosis? How does it differ from osteomalacia and osteopenia?**
   - *Osteoporosis* is characterized by low bone mass and microarchitectural deterioration of bone tissue, leading to increased bone fragility and an increased risk of fracture. The bone has normal mineralization and histologic characteristics.
   - *Osteomalacia* is characterized by incomplete mineralization of normal osteoid tissue. Osteomalacia in a growing child is also known as *rickets*.
   - *Osteopenia* is a descriptive term for decreased calcification or density of bone. Osteopenia if not due to a particular cause, pathophysiology, or disease.

2. **What are potential causes for generalized osteoporosis?**
   Arthritis may be either primary or secondary. Any patient who presents with osteoporosis should be evaluated for secondary causes before being diagnosed with primary osteoporosis. Causes of primary osteoporosis include involutional osteoporosis, juvenile osteoporosis, and idiopathic osteoporosis (premenopausal women or middle-aged men). Secondary osteoporosis has a wide differential diagnosis, including:
   - Endocrine diseases (e.g., hypogonadism, ovarian agenesis, hyperadrenocorticism, hyperthyroidism, hyperparathyroidism, diabetes mellitus, and acromegaly)
   - Gastrointestinal diseases (e.g., subtotal gastrectomy, malabsorption syndromes, chronic obstructive jaundice, primary biliary cirrhosis, severe malnutrition, and anorexia nervosa)
   - Bone marrow disorders (e.g., multiple myeloma, systemic mastocytosis, and disseminated carcinoma)
   - Connective tissue diseases (e.g., osteogenesis imperfecta, homocystinuria, Ehlers-Danlos syndrome, and Marfan syndrome)
   - Miscellaneous causes (e.g., immobilization, chronic obstructive pulmonary disease, chronic alcoholism, long-term heparin therapy, and rheumatoid arthritis)

3. **What are some causes for regional or localized osteoporosis?**
   A focal area of bone loss can be highly localized (also known as a *lytic lesion*). Metastasis, multiple myeloma, and osteomyelitis are the most common causes of lytic lesions. Larger areas of bone loss, usually without violation of cortical bone, may be caused by a stroke or immobility of an extremity. Another cause for regional osteoporosis is reflex sympathetic dystrophy syndrome, or Sudeck atrophy. Reflex sympathetic dystrophy is a multifactorial disorder. The underlying cause is typically trauma, followed by regional or localized osteoporosis.

4. **In what demographic groups is generalized osteoporosis most prevalent?**
   Bone loss starts to occur in men and women around 35 years old. Women have a greater rate of bone loss. Whites and Asians are more likely to develop osteoporosis than blacks. A white or Asian woman has the greatest risk of developing osteoporosis.

5. **Are conventional radiographs sensitive enough to diagnose osteoporosis?**
   No. A large percentage (30% to 40%) of bone must be lost to appreciate a change on radiographic examination. There is also marked intrareader and inter-reader variability for this diagnosis on radiographs.

6. **What radiographic features are useful in diagnosing osteoporosis?**
   Decreased bone density, prominence of vertebral body end plates, and cortical thinning can be seen with osteoporosis, but are subjective. Accentuation of trabecular stress lines from resorption of secondary trabecula is another radiographic sign of osteoporosis; this is best appreciated around the femoral neck.

7. **Is computed tomography (CT) more sensitive than conventional radiographs for evaluating bone mineral density (BMD)?**
   Yes. Quantitative CT can be performed using software that is added to a standard CT scanner to measure BMD. Other methods of assessment based on relative absorption of x-rays using a less expensive scanner are preferred.

8. What are other quantitative methods of measuring BMD?

Single-photon absorptiometry and dual-photon absorptiometry were the early techniques for measuring BMD. Both used radioactive sources to produce photons. These units have essentially been replaced with dual x-ray absorptiometry (DXA) units. DXA uses the same principles as dual-photon absorptiometry except that the radionuclide source is replaced with an x-ray tube. Two distinct energy x-ray beams are used (usually 70 kVp and 140 kVp). DXA is the examination of choice for the diagnosis and follow-up of osteoporosis.

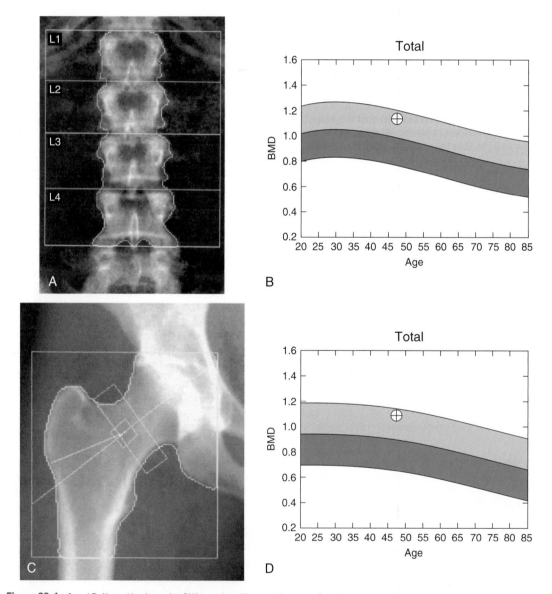

Figure 39-1. A and **B,** Normal lumbar spine DXA scan in a 47-year-old woman. **C** and **D,** Normal right hip DXA scan in the same patient.

9. What are the units of measurement of BMD?

BMD is measured in grams divided by area: g/cm^2. Technically, it is not a density (weight/volume) being measured, but a weight divided by area.

10. What sites of the skeleton are routinely assessed on a DXA scan?

The lumbar spine, from L1 or L2 to L4, and the proximal femur (regions of interest are the femoral neck, trochanteric region, and Ward triangle) are routinely assessed on a DXA scan. Ward triangle is a site at the proximal femur where bone mineral loss is thought to occur first (Figs. 39-1 and 39-2).

11. How can large osteophytes and sclerotic changes in a patient with lumbar degenerative disease affect bone densitometry assessment?

On an anteroposterior evaluation of the lumbar spine, the osteophytes and other degenerative changes in the vertebrae and posterior elements can cause pseudoelevation of the BMD. This pseudoelevation can result in the BMD of an osteoporotic patient appearing falsely normal. This is one reason that BMD measurements are routinely obtained in two separate locations.

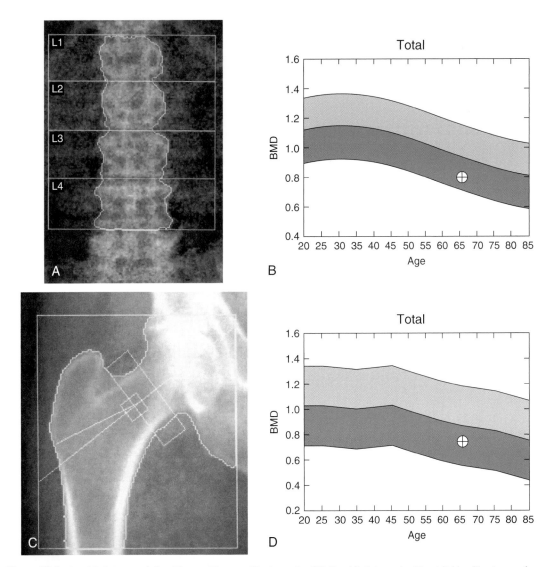

Figure 39-2. A and **B,** Osteoporosis in a 65-year-old woman. The *t* score is −2.9. **C** and **D,** Osteopenia of the right hip with a *t* score of −1.8 in the same patient.

12. What are the World Health Organization criteria for the diagnoses of normal BMD, osteopenia, and osteoporosis?

- Normal is a BMD within 1 SD of the young adult reference mean.
- Osteopenia is a BMD 1 to 2.5 SD below the young adult reference mean.
- Osteoporosis is a BMD more than 2.5 SD below the young adult reference mean.

13. What are *t* and *z* scores?

- The *t* score is the number of standard deviations above or below the young adult mean. The young adult mean is the expected normal value for the patient compared with others of the same sex and ethnicity in a reference population the manufacturer builds into the DXA software. It is approximately what the patient should have had at his or her peak bone density at about age 20.
- The *z* score is the number of standard deviations of the patient's bone density above or below the values expected for the patient's age. By comparing the patient's BMD with the expected BMD for his or her age, the *z* score can help classify the type of osteoporosis. Primary osteoporosis is age-related osteoporosis in which no secondary causes are found.

BIBLIOGRAPHY

[1] National Osteoporosis Foundation, Physicians Resource Manual on Osteoporosis: A Decision-making Guide, second ed., National Osteoporosis Foundation, Washington, DC, 1991.

[2] World Health Organization, Assessment of fracture risk and its application to screening for postmenopausal osteoporosis: report of a WHO study group, WHO Technical Report Series 843 (1994) 1–129.

CHAPTER 40

OSTEOARTHRITIS AND INFLAMMATORY ARTHRITIS

Joseph R. Perno, MD, PhD, and
Neil Roach, MD

1. What imaging modality is best for diagnosis and follow-up of arthritic diseases?
Plain films are the mainstay for arthritis imaging. They are easy to obtain and give high-resolution information about cortical bone changes such as erosions, joint space narrowing, and osteophytes. The sensitivity of plain radiographs to detect early changes of rheumatoid arthritis (RA) is limited, however. Magnetic resonance imaging (MRI) has been shown to be sensitive to early changes, such as marrow edema, erosions, and synovial inflammation.

2. What is the difference between an inflammatory arthritis and a degenerative arthritis?
Inflammatory arthritides are diseases of the synovium, which subsequently produce erosive changes of the adjacent bones. Examples of inflammatory arthritis include RA and psoriatic arthritis. Degenerative arthritis/osteoarthritis is secondary to articular cartilage damage from repetitive microtrauma that occurs throughout life, although multiple other factors, such as heredity, nutrition, metabolic factors, preexisting articular disease, and body habitus, may contribute to development of the radiographic features of osteoarthritis, which include osseous proliferation, joint space narrowing, and subchondral sclerosis.

3. Which joints are most often affected in RA?
RA has a predilection for the carpal/ tarsal, carpometacarpal/tarsometatarsal, metacarpophalangeal/metatarsophalangeal, and proximal interphalangeal joints (Fig. 40-1). In adults, the distal interphalangeal joints rarely are affected. Joint involvement tends to be bilateral, but not always symmetric. Generally, the metacarpophalangeal and the metatarsophalangeal joints are affected first.

4. What portion of the spine does RA most commonly affect?
In the cervical spine, RA commonly causes atlantoaxial (C1 to C2) subluxation because of laxity of the transverse ligament and pannus formation. Other disease entities may affect this region of the cervical spine, including gout, calcium pyrophosphate dihydrate (CPPD) crystal deposition disease, and hydroxyapatite deposition disease. Some of these other disease processes may cause erosions of the dens, atlantoaxial subluxation, and radiopaque calcifications.

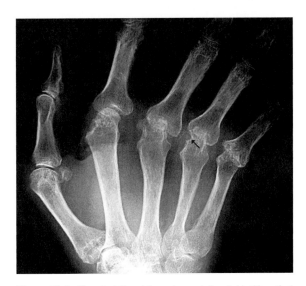

Figure 40-1. Ulnar deviation of the metacarpals is noted in this patient with RA. There is a typical marginal erosion of the metacarpal head (*arrow*).

5. Can RA affect nonarticular structures?
Yes. Retrocalcaneal bursitis is common and is detected when the retrocalcaneal fat at the posterior-superior aspect of the calcaneus is obscured by edema. It is often accompanied by bone erosion.

6. How do inflammatory arthritides affect cartilage?
Inflammatory arthritides are a chronic synovitis, eroding bone that is "unprotected" by cartilage. These changes are noted first at the margins of joints, where cartilage is thinnest. Cartilage is also eroded by the joint inflammation, but tends to erode in an even and uniform manner.

7. What finding, which is common in osteoarthritis, is virtually never seen with RA?

The presence of significant osteophytes (productive bone changes) is not consistent with the diagnosis of RA. A joint that has been destroyed by RA may then develop osteoarthritis, however, owing to cartilage loss.

8. What additional joint findings are seen with RA?

Subluxations and malalignments at the metacarpophalangeal and metatarsophalangeal joints are typical. The subluxations tend to deviate the phalanges in the ulnar direction (see Fig. 40-1).

9. Where are the swan neck and boutonnière deformities located?

The chronic inflammatory changes of RA in the joints of the fingers produce retraction of the tendons. The *swan neck deformity* is caused by hyperextension of the proximal interphalangeal joint with simultaneous flexion of the distal interphalangeal joint. If you try this manipulation on yourself, you will recognize the reason for the name. The *boutonnière (or buttonhole) deformity* is caused by hyperextension of the distal interphalangeal joint with simultaneous flexion of the proximal interphalangeal joint.

10. When can RA be confused with other arthritides?

Severe erosions of the subchondral bone may develop late in RA after the cartilage is destroyed and may give an appearance similar to erosive osteoarthritis.

11. What joints are typically affected by osteoarthritis?

Osteoarthritis most often affects the proximal and distal interphalangeal joints of the hands and the major weight-bearing joints—the hips and the knees. In addition, the carpal joints at the base of the thumb are commonly affected (trapeziometacarpal and scaphotrapeziotrapezoidal joints). The most commonly affected joint in the foot is the first metatarsophalangeal joint. Any joint damaged by trauma that results in an irregular articular surface can become prematurely arthritic.

12. Where are Heberden and Bouchard nodes located?

- *Heberden nodes* are osseous outcroppings involving the distal interphalangeal joints.
- *Bouchard nodes* involve the proximal interphalangeal joints.

Bouchard and Heberden nodes are physical examination signs of hand osteoarthritis.

13. Which joints are rarely involved in primary osteoarthritis?

Involvement of the radiocarpal, pan-carpal, and metacarpophalangeal joints is rare in osteoarthritis, but is common in RA and psoriatic arthritis.

14. What are the hallmarks of osteoarthritic change in a joint?

Erosive arthritides have uniform cartilage loss, whereas degenerative osteoarthritis results in segmental cartilage loss. In small joints, such as joints in the fingers, the loss may seem to be uniform. The layer of bone just beneath the cartilage is called the *subchondral bone*. When exposed to increased stress, this layer becomes sclerotic. As this process continues, the cartilage and the underlying bone can become eroded, producing cystlike pockets in the bone, called *geodes*. At the edge of a joint where the cartilage is thinnest, exposed bone becomes hypertrophic, resulting in irregular or pointed outcroppings of bone, called *osteophytes*.

15. What is erosive osteoarthritis?

Erosive osteoarthritis is a form of osteoarthritis that is sometimes called *inflammatory osteoarthritis* (Fig. 40-2). Although the joint distribution is the

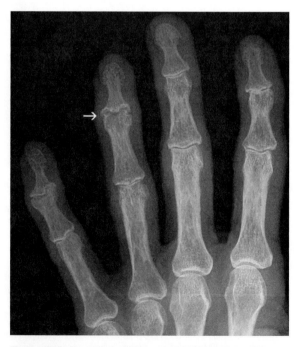

Figure 40-2. Erosive osteoarthritis involving the distal interphalangeal joints, with a combination of productive and erosive changes. Note the classic "gull wing" deformity of the distal interphalangeal joint (*arrow*).

same as in typical osteoarthritis, the erosive changes are more severe, and there is soft tissue swelling, which may give a similar appearance to RA or psoriatic arthritis. These changes involve the subchondral cortex in the main portion of the joint, however, rather than the peripheral "bare areas." Ultimately, the phalangeal joints may become fused.

16. Name the seronegative spondyloarthropathies.

Seronegativity refers to the absence of rheumatoid factor in blood tests of patients who present with inflammatory arthritis. This group of diseases includes psoriatic arthritis, reactive arthritis (Reiter syndrome), ankylosing spondylitis (AS), and enteropathic arthritis (associated with inflammatory bowel diseases such as Crohn disease and ulcerative colitis).

17. What mnemonic can be used to remember the triad of symptoms seen with reactive arthritis (also known as Reiter syndrome)?

"Can't see (uveitis), can't pee (urethritis), can't bend your knee (arthritis)."

18. What are the different presentations of psoriatic arthritis?

Psoriatic arthritis tends to involve the terminal interphalangeal joints of both hands; this is in contrast to RA, which more commonly involves more proximal joints in the hands and wrists. A second presentation pattern of psoriatic arthritis may involve multiple joints of a single hand. The third pattern involves only the joints of a single ray. The appearance is a combination of erosive and productive bony changes. The erosive changes occur at the peripheral bare areas, similar to RA. Psoriatic arthritis also has productive bone formation adjacent to the joint, however, typically in an exuberant and irregular manner. Although the clinical symptoms of psoriatic arthritis develop in 30% to 40% of patients with psoriasis, psoriatic arthritis usually does not occur concomitantly with the dermatologic diagnosis and may take 10 years or longer to manifest. It has been estimated, however, that 10% to 15% of patients have musculoskeletal complaints as the first manifestations of psoriasis.

19. What is the "pencil-in-cup" deformity?

The advanced erosive changes seen in psoriatic arthritis can produce a pointed appearance of the proximal phalanx that then pushes into the base of the more distal phalanx and deforms it to look like a cup.

20. Does AS have a specific pattern of joint involvement?

AS preferentially involves the sacroiliac joints and lumbar spine, and then may advance craniad to involve the thoracic and cervical spine. *Ankylosis* refers to the bony fusion of the opposing surfaces, which results in sclerosis and loss of the normal sacroiliac joint cartilage space (Fig. 40-3). Focal cortical irregularities at the anterior margin of the superior and inferior discovertebral junctions are considered early and significant features of AS seen on conventional radiographs and have been termed *Romanus lesion*. The MRI correlate has been described and is termed the "MRI corner" sign. Healing of the Romanus lesion leads to sclerosis at the end-plate corners and has been termed the "shiny corner" sign.

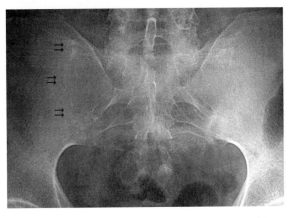

Figure 40-3. AS causes fusion of the sacroiliac joint. When this joint fuses, the normally dark-appearing cartilage becomes replaced by bone matrix (*double arrows*).

21. What does the term *bamboo spine* describe?

AS produces syndesmophytes, which are osseous bridges of the intervertebral disc spaces along Sharpey fibers in the anulus fibrosus. Combined with fusion of the facet joints and ossification of the longitudinal spinal ligaments, the appearance is similar to that of a stick of bamboo.

22. What is the radiologic appearance of gout?

Gout classically involves the first metatarsophalangeal joint. Other joints of the hand and foot can also be affected, however. Although more than one joint may be involved, it does not tend to be symmetric as other inflammatory arthritides can be. The classic appearance of a gout erosion is termed the *overhanging margin,* with a rim of eroded cortex hanging over a soft tissue density called a *tophus.* Tophi are soft tissue deposits of monosodium urate crystals that may occur anywhere, particularly in the dorsal aspect of the foot and the extensor aspect of the elbow.

23. What is pseudogout?

Pseudogout is not a radiographic diagnosis; it refers to a goutlike clinical syndrome with acute attacks of intermittent pain.

24. What are the differences between pyrophosphate arthropathy and CPPD crystal deposition disease?

CPPD crystal deposition disease is a specific term for a disorder characterized by the exclusive presence of CPPD crystals in and around joints. *Pyrophosphate arthropathy* describes a pattern of joint damage that is secondary to CPPD crystal deposition disease. Although the radiographic changes of pyrophosphate arthropathy may be similar to osteoarthritis (osteophytosis, subchondral sclerosis, and joint space narrowing), there is a tendency to develop prominent subchondral cystic changes and decreased osteophytosis (as seen in osteoarthritis), and it tends to involve non–weight-bearing joint spaces, such as the shoulder, patellofemoral, and radiocarpal joints. It also tends to be symmetric. In the hand, CPDD crystal deposition disease tends to involve the metacarpophalangeal joints, particularly the second and third, but spares the interphalangeal joints. The subchondral bone becomes involved by multiple cystlike lucencies that can eventually lead to collapse of the articular surface (scapholunate advanced collapse wrist).

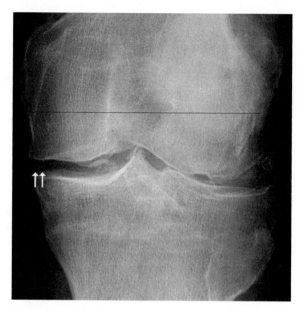

Figure 40-4. CPDD with calcium crystal deposition in the meniscus (*double arrows*). This is called chondrocalcinosis.

Calcium pyrophosphate crystals tend to deposit within fibrocartilage. The menisci of the knee, triangular fibrocartilage of the wrist, labra of the acetabulum and glenoid, symphysis pubis, and anulus fibrosus of the intervertebral disc are common sites. These cartilage calcifications are termed *chondrocalcinosis* (Fig. 40-4). These deposits may also affect the hyaline cartilage, which becomes a more specific radiologic marker for the disease. Soft tissue calcification is also common in tendons, bursae, and synovium.

Key Points: Differentiating Arthritis on Hand Radiograph

1. Symmetric erosive change of the metacarpophalangeal and proximal interphalangeal joints of both hands, periarticular osteopenia, and symmetric joint space loss suggest RA.
2. Extensive productive osteophyte changes of the distal interphalangeal joints, with less severe changes of the proximal interphalangeal and metacarpophalangeal joints, or a thickened "sausage-digit," suggests psoriatic arthritis.
3. Osteophyte production and joint space narrowing without marginal erosions of the distal interphalangeal and proximal interphalangeal joints, with little or no involvement of the metacarpophalangeal joints, suggests degenerative joint disease.
4. A soft tissue mass with an overhanging rim of bone, adjacent to a joint space, suggests gout. Gout also tends to preserve the joint space and the mineralization of the bone.
5. Calcifications within the soft tissues of the fingertips, resorption of the cortex of the finger tufts, or both suggest scleroderma or polymyositis.

BIBLIOGRAPHY

[1] A. Brower, Arthritis in Black and White, Saunders, Philadelphia, 1988.
[2] J.M. Farrant, P.J. O'Connor, A.J. Grainger, Advanced imaging in rheumatoid arthritis, part 1: synovitis, Skeletal Radiol. 36 (2007) 269–279.
[3] A. Feydy, F. Lioté, R. Carlier, et al., Cervical spine and crystal-associated diseases: imaging findings, Eur. Radiol. 16 (2006) 459–468.
[4] C.A. Helms, Fundamentals of Skeletal Radiology, second ed., Saunders, Philadelphia, 1995.
[5] N.R. Kim, J.Y. Choi, S.H. Hong, et al., "MR corner sign": value for predicting presence of ankylosing spondylitis, AJR Am. J. Roentgenol. 191 (2008) 124–128.
[6] J.A. Jacobson, G. Girish, Y. Jiang, B.J. Sabb, Radiographic evaluation of arthritis: degenerative joint disease and variations, Radiology 248 (2008) 737–747.
[7] C.C. Peterson, M.L. Silbiger, Reiter's syndrome and psoriatic arthritis: their roentgen spectra and some interesting similarities, AJR Am. J. Roentgenol. 100 (1967) 860–871.
[8] L.S. Steinbach, D. Resnick, Calcium pyrophosphate dihydrate crystal deposition disease revisited, Radiology 200 (1996) 1–9.
[9] J.M. Taveras, J.T. Ferrucci, Radiology: Diagnosis, Imaging, Intervention, 2002 ed. on CD-ROM, Lippincott Williams & Wilkins, Philadelphia, 2002.

OSTEOMYELITIS

Joseph R. Perno, MD, PhD,
Andrew Gordon, MD, and
Neil Roach, MD

CHAPTER 41

1. What are the initial plain film findings in osteomyelitis?

Soft tissue swelling and blurred fascial planes are the initial findings. As the infection ensues, osteopenia, periosteal reactions, and a permeative process of bone destruction may be seen.

2. What is meant by periosteal reaction? Does it occur only in osteomyelitis?

Periosteal reactions have been described radiographically in two broad categories: solid and interrupted. *Solid reactions* may be defined as a single layer of new bone greater than 1 mm in thickness of uniform density. This type of periosteal reaction indicates a benign process. Processes that produce solid periosteal reactions include osteomyelitis, hemorrhage, vascular disease such as venous stasis, pulmonary hypertrophic osteoarthropathy, and osteoid osteoma. Periosteal reactions are not specific for the diagnosis of osteomyelitis.

Interrupted reactions are not uniform with varying radiographic patterns. These patterns are concerning for malignancy. Because this pattern represents an aggressive process with rapid bone turnover, interrupted periosteal reactions are inherently unstable and can change their radiographic appearance in weeks to days. Common appearances include lamellated (also known as "onion-skin"), which is parallel to bone cortex, and "sunburst," which is perpendicular to bone cortex.

3. How long does it take before the initial skeletal findings of osteomyelitis are seen on a plain film?

Radiographically evident bone changes often take at least 7 to 14 days to develop. Skeletal lesions appear as enlarging ill-defined radiolucencies in the infected bone. Periosteal reaction is common (Fig. 41-1).

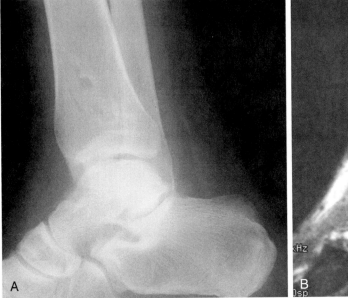
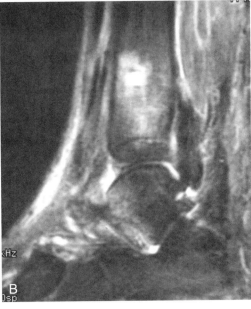

Figure 41-1. Acute osteomyelitis of the distal tibia in a teenager bitten by a dog approximately 1 week earlier. **A,** Lateral radiograph of the ankle shows an ill-defined lucency in the metaphysis of the distal tibia. **B,** On a sagittal STIR MR image of the ankle, there is increased signal intensity in the marrow of the distal tibia, most focal at the site corresponding to the abnormality seen on the plain film. High-signal edema is also noted in the anterior soft tissues because of associated cellulitis. STIR images can be thought of as equivalent to fat-saturated T2-weighted images.

4. Define sequestrum, involucrum, cloaca, and sinus tract.

- A *sequestrum* is a fragment of necrotic bone that is separate from the living parent bone. A sequestrum may be resorbed, be discharged through a sinus tract, or persist as a focus of infection (Fig. 41-2).
- An *involucrum* is a layer of healthy bone that has formed around the dead bone. It may merge with the parent bone or become perforated with tracts through which pus can escape.
- A *cloaca* is an opening in the involucrum through which granulation tissue and the sequestra may be discharged.
- A *sinus tract* is a channel extending from the bone to the skin surface that is lined with granulation tissue.

5. What is Brodie abscess?

Brodie abscess is a bone abscess found characteristically in subacute pyogenic osteomyelitis, but which also may be identified in chronic osteomyelitis. Brodie abscess typically occurs near the ends of tubular bones, is especially common in children, and may be single or multiple. The wall of the abscess is lined by granulation tissue surrounded by dense bone. On radiographs, Brodie abscess appears as a well-defined circular or elliptic radiolucency with adjacent sclerosis. When located in the metaphysis of children, it may connect with the growth plate through an identifiable channel (Fig. 41-3).

6. Name the two imaging modalities that may be used to diagnose acute osteomyelitis if plain films show negative or equivocal results.

Magnetic resonance imaging (MRI) and three-phase bone scan may be used to diagnose acute osteomyelitis.

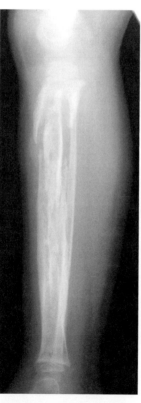

Figure 41-2. Sequestrum. Lateral radiograph of the tibia and fibula in a child with chronic osteomyelitis shows a long segment of bone in the medullary canal of the tibia, separate from the parent bone. This finding is in keeping with a devascularized sequestrum. There has been marked resorption and cortical destruction of the tibia, indicated by radiolucency surrounding the sequestrum.

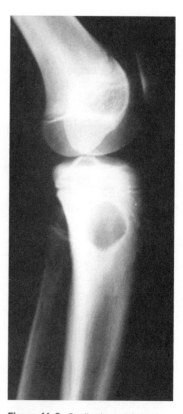

Figure 41-3. Brodie abscess. Lateral radiograph of the knee of a child shows a well-defined circular lucency with a sclerotic border in the proximal metaphysis of the tibia. This is the typical appearance of a Brodie abscess of subacute osteomyelitis.

7. What is the appearance of acute osteomyelitis on MRI?

Because inflammation causes edema to replace marrow fat, a focus of osteomyelitis shows low to intermediate signal intensity on T1-weighted MR images and high signal intensity on fat-saturated T2-weighted and short-tau inversion recovery (STIR) images (see Fig. 41-1).

Intravenous gadolinium-based contrast agents may be administered when performing MRI for the purpose of diagnosing osteomyelitis. Gadolinium is useful in differentiating an abscess from bone marrow edema in the marrow space or in differentiating a soft tissue abscess from surrounding cellulitis or phlegmon. An abscess exhibits a thick, enhancing wall without central enhancement. Detection of sinus tracts and sequestra is also improved after gadolinium administration. Bone marrow enhancement is nonspecific; it may be seen in infected bone and in noninfected regions of reactive marrow hyperemia. MRI contrast enhancement is useful to differentiate cellulitis from edema. Cellulitis shows enhancement, whereas soft tissue edema usually does not.

8. Are the MRI findings of osteomyelitis specific?

The MRI findings for osteomyelitis are not specific. Bone contusion, occult fracture, neuropathic joint, and neoplastic processes may show marrow signal intensity changes similar to those seen in osteomyelitis. Correlation with clinical history and laboratory values is important for proper image interpretation.

> **Key Points: Osteomyelitis**
> 1. Plain film radiography, MRI, and nuclear medicine studies have roles in the imaging diagnosis of osteomyelitis.
> 2. The knee and hip are the most commonly infected joints of infants and children. The knee is the most common joint infected in adults.

9. Diabetic patients are at increased risk of osteomyelitis, in particular in their feet. Is there a best imaging test for evaluation?

Initial evaluation should be performed with plain film radiography. As indicated in question 2, the plain film findings are insensitive to the detection of osteomyelitis and may take 7 to 14 days to develop. Nuclear medicine and MRI are good imaging modalities for further evaluation. A three-phase nuclear medicine scan in the peripheral skeleton of adults shows a sensitivity and specificity of approximately 95%. In the setting of previous trauma, orthopedic hardware, or a neuropathic joint, bone scintigraphy is less useful, and positron emission tomography (PET) imaging may be helpful. Collins et al evaluated the MRI findings of pedal osteomyelitis (all patients had a tissue diagnosis of osteomyelitis) based on geographic medullary signal loss on T1-weighted images with concordant signal abnormality (increased) with fat-suppressed T2-weighted and T1-weighted postcontrast images, and were able to identify osteomyelitis versus reactive marrow edema correctly in 100% of the patients.

10. List the three classes of radiotracers used predominantly to diagnose osteomyelitis.

- *Technetium (Tc)-99m diphosphonates* (most commonly methylene diphosphate [MDP]). Tc-99m MDP is the radiotracer used in three-phase bone scans and is typically all that is required for diagnosing uncomplicated osteomyelitis.
- *Gallium-67 citrate.* Gallium may be used in combination with Tc-99m MDP bone scans in more complicated cases. Gallium activity greater than Tc-99m MDP suggests infection.
- *Autologous leukocytes* labeled with indium-111 or Tc-99m hexamethyl-propyleneamine oxime (HMPAO). Radiolabeled autologous leukocytes are also used in combination with Tc-99m MDP bone scans in a similar fashion to gallium.

11. Name the three phases of a three-phase bone scan, and describe the timing of each.

The three phases are angiographic (blood flow) phase, blood pool phase, and delayed phase. During the angiographic phase, serial images are obtained every 5 seconds for the first minute after injection of the radiotracer. During the blood pool phase, an image is obtained approximately 5 minutes after injection. Images are obtained 2 to 3 hours later for the delayed phase.

12. How can the diagnosis of osteomyelitis be differentiated from cellulitis on a three-phase bone scan?

Cellulitis and osteomyelitis show high soft tissue uptake of the radiotracer in the blood flow and blood pool phases. Differentiation between the two types of infection occurs in the delayed phase. In cellulitis, there is mild, diffuse bone uptake on delayed images. In osteomyelitis, there is focal, intense radiotracer uptake of the infected bone.

13. List the four main routes through which osteomyelitis (and septic arthritis) may be acquired.

- Hematogenous spread of infection from the bloodstream
- Spread of infection from adjacent soft tissues
- Direct inoculation (e.g., penetrating trauma)
- Postoperative infection (a postoperative infection may result from hematogenous spread, spread from contiguous tissues, or direct implantation)

14. Which organism is accountable for most cases of hematogenous osteomyelitis and septic arthritis?

Staphylococcus aureus account for most cases of hematogenous osteomyelitis and septic arthritis.

15. Which disease is associated with an increased incidence of *Salmonella* osteomyelitis?

Sickle cell disease is associated with an increased incidence of *Salmonella* osteomyelitis.

16. How does the vascular anatomy of tubular bones affect the location of infection in infants, children, and adults?

Until about 1 year of age, a fetal vascular pattern may be present in tubular bones. Some vessels at the surface of the metaphysis penetrate the preexisting physeal plate and extend into the epiphysis. These transphyseal vessels allow a pathway for the spread of infection. In addition to infection at the metaphysis, epiphyseal and articular infection may occur in infants.

After about 1 year of age, there is obliteration of the transphyseal vessels. The physeal plate serves as a barrier keeping the metaphyseal and epiphyseal blood supplies completely separate; hematogenous osteomyelitis arising in the metaphysis cannot extend into the epiphysis. The terminal metaphyseal vessels turn acutely at the growth plate to join large sinusoidal veins, where the blood flow is slow and turbulent. The frequency of metaphyseal osteomyelitis in children is due to this combination of venous stasis and the barrier formed by the growth plate. When the growth plate closes in the mature skeleton, vascular communications between the metaphysis and epiphysis become re-established, and infection may localize from the metaphysis to the epiphyseal subchondral bone. Involvement of the joint may complicate epiphyseal infection.

17. What are the plain film findings of chronic sclerosing osteomyelitis?

The chronic phase of osteomyelitis, termed *chronic sclerosing osteomyelitis,* is characterized by thickened trabecula and thick, wavy periosteal new bone with resultant radiodensity and contour abnormalities of the affected bone (Fig. 41-4).

18. Is malignancy a potential complication of osteomyelitis?

Yes. Epidermoid carcinoma arises in 0.5% of patients with chronic osteomyelitis and draining sinus tracts. The latent period is usually 20 to 30 years. Radiographically, progressive destruction of the bone may suggest the diagnosis. Other secondary neoplasms arising in chronic osteomyelitis have also been described.

19. Describe the plain film and MRI findings in septic arthritis.

Septic arthritis is the infection of a joint and should always be considered when there is monarticular inflammatory arthritis. Widening of the joint space is initially seen secondary to joint effusion. There may also be regional soft tissue swelling and periarticular osteopenia secondary to hyperemia. Later, cartilage destruction results in concentric joint space narrowing, and an inflamed pannus results in osseous erosions. Bone ankylosis and destruction can occur in the late stages of disease. The poorly defined osseous destruction is most characteristic (Fig. 41-5).

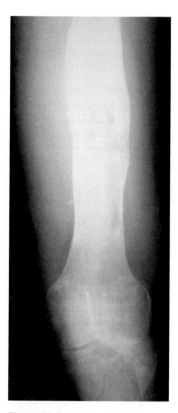

Figure 41-4. Chronic sclerosing osteomyelitis of the femur. The femoral shaft is markedly sclerotic (dense). Thick, wavy periosteal reaction on the medial and lateral aspects of the femur causes the bone to have an abnormal contour. The thick periosteal new bone is the involucrum.

MRI may be used as an adjunct to joint aspiration in the diagnosis of septic arthritis. The MRI findings of septic arthritis are not specific, however, and are the same as in any inflammatory arthritis. Initially, the joint effusion and synovitis are characterized by low intra-articular signal intensity on T1-weighted images and high signal intensity on T2-weighted and STIR images. After gadolinium is administered, the synovium enhances, but the joint fluid does not. There may be low to intermediate T1 signal and high T2 signal in the adjacent soft tissues and bone marrow because of sympathetic hyperemia with edema or spread of infection outside of the joint. Later, bone erosions appear as marginal subchondral defects that are low signal on T1-weighted images and high signal on T2-weighted images (Fig. 41-6).

20. Name the joints most commonly infected in infants and children, adults, and intravenous drug abusers.

- *Infants and children*: The knee and hip are most commonly infected.
- *Adults*: The knee is most commonly infected.
- *Intravenous drug abusers*: The sacroiliac, sternoclavicular, and acromioclavicular are most commonly infected (also, although it is not a joint, the spine is commonly infected in cases of osteomyelitis in intravenous drug abusers).

21. How is a definitive diagnosis of septic arthritis made in a child?

Radiographic findings of septic arthritis are nonspecific. Plain films should be obtained first, however, to exclude other potential causes for an irritable hip in a child, such as Perthes disease or occult fracture. Although MRI has a role in the evaluation of suspected septic arthritis, aspiration of the joint is mandatory to establish the diagnosis so that the appropriate antibiotic therapy may be started in a timely manner. The joint may be aspirated under ultrasound or fluoroscopic guidance.

22. List the differential diagnoses for unilateral sacroiliac joint disease.

- Infection
- Psoriatic arthritis
- Reiter syndrome
- Degenerative joint disease
- Gout

See Fig. 41-7.

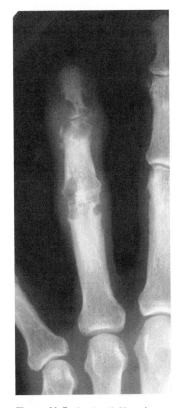

Figure 41-5. Septic arthritis and osteomyelitis involving the fourth finger. Extensive intra-articular and periarticular erosions are seen to involve the proximal and distal interphalangeal joints of the fourth digit. There is marked concentric narrowing of the proximal interphalangeal joint because of cartilage destruction. Soft tissue swelling is evident overlying both joints. Ill-defined radiolucency of the head of the middle phalanx is suggestive of a component of osteomyelitis.

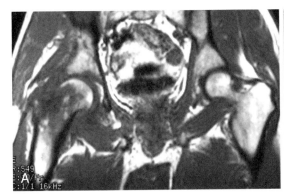
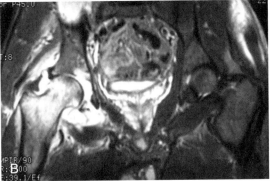

Figure 41-6. Septic arthritis of the right hip on MRI. **A** and **B,** Coronal T1-weighted (**A**) and coronal STIR (**B**) images of the hips show decreased T1 and increased STIR signal within a distended right hip joint, indicating joint effusion and synovitis. There is abnormal signal in the proximal right femur and in the regional hip musculature because of reactive edema. The left hip is normal.

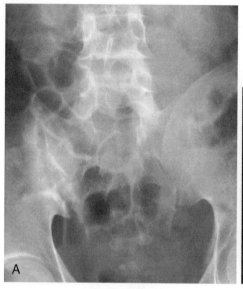
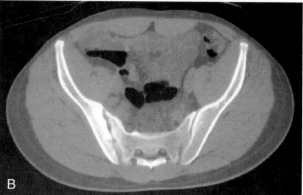

Figure 41-7. Unilateral sacroiliitis. **A** and **B,** Plain film (**A**) and computed tomography (CT) scan (**B**) of the pelvis show erosions with reactive sclerosis at the right sacroiliac joint. The left sacroiliac joint is normal. Although a few processes can manifest as unilateral sacroiliitis, in the appropriate clinical setting, these findings suggest septic arthritis. CT is often helpful in evaluating complicated joints such as those at the pelvis.

23. Describe the radiographic findings of infectious spondylitis (infection of the spine).
Hematogenous spread of infection to the spine initially results in involvement of the anterior subchondral vertebral body and quickly spreads to the adjacent intervertebral disc. The initial findings on radiography are a decrease in the height of the vertebral body with loss of the normal definition of the end plate. Destruction of the vertebral body ensues. Spread of infection through the intervertebral disc results in involvement of the adjacent vertebra. Involvement of two contiguous vertebral bodies and the intervening disc is seen in most patients. After many weeks, reactive sclerosis occurs in the involved vertebra. Soft tissue extension may occur and appears as a displaced psoas shadow in the lumbar spine, a paraspinal mass in the thoracic spine, or prevertebral soft tissue swelling in the cervical spine.

24. Can infection of the intervertebral disc (discitis) occur without involvement of the adjacent vertebral bodies?
Yes. In children and young adults 20 to 30 years old, the intervertebral discs remain significantly vascular, and hematogenous spread of infection may occur directly to the disc tissue. The clinical manifestations of discitis are usually mild, and an organism cannot always be identified. Infection of an intervertebral disc may also occur via direct contamination during invasive diagnostic or therapeutic procedures.

25. How does infectious spondylitis appear on MRI?
Patients are usually first imaged with MRI after the infection has spread through a disc and involves two contiguous vertebral bodies. The MRI findings consist of a triad of (1) low signal intensity of the involved vertebral body marrow on T1-weighted images, (2) enhancement of the marrow and possible intervertebral disc enhancement after the administration of gadolinium, and (3) high signal of the disc on T2-weighted and STIR images. A decreased disc height and destruction of the cortical end plate may also be seen. An epidural, subligamentous, or paraspinal abscess or phlegmon may be present. Differentiation of abscess from phlegmon requires intravenous gadolinium; a phlegmon enhances diffusely, whereas an abscess shows low signal intensity on T1-weighted images with peripheral rim enhancement. Both exhibit high signal intensity on T2-weighted images (Fig. 41-8).

26. What is the Phemister triad?
Phemister triad refers to the classic radiographic findings of tuberculous arthritis: (1) periarticular osteoporosis, (2) peripherally located osseous erosions, and (3) gradual narrowing of the joint space. Preservation of the joint space is the hallmark of tuberculous arthritis and helps to distinguish it from the rapid joint destruction of pyogenic (bacterial) arthritis. Monarticular disease is the rule in tuberculous arthritis. Most joint infections arise secondary to contiguous spread of tuberculous osteomyelitis. Diagnosis of tuberculous arthritis is often delayed and requires synovial fluid and tissue for culture and histopathology.

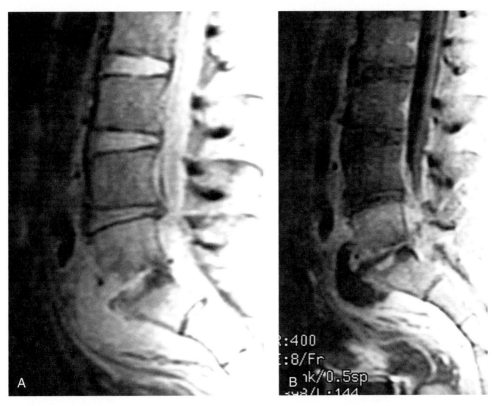

Figure 41-8. Infectious spondylitis. **A,** Sagittal T2-weighted MR image of the lumbar spine shows marked disc space narrowing at L5-S1. High signal is present in what is remaining of the intervertebral disc. There are erosions of the end plates of L5 and S1, and abnormal signal in both vertebral bodies. A paraspinal mass is noted anteriorly at this level. **B,** Sagittal T1-weighted image after the administration of intravenous gadolinium shows enhancement of the involved vertebral bodies. The paraspinal mass remains low in signal intensity with mild peripheral rim enhancement, indicating a paraspinal abscess (as opposed to phlegmon).

27. What is Pott disease?

Pott disease is the eponym of tuberculous spondylitis. The vertebra is affected in 25% to 60% of cases of osseous tuberculosis. The first lumbar vertebral body is most commonly infected, although involvement of more than one vertebral body is typical. Infection may spread to contiguous vertebral bodies or skip multiple levels; it commonly spreads beneath the anterior longitudinal ligament (and, less commonly, the posterior longitudinal ligament). Tuberculous spondylitis characteristically involves the anterior portion of the vertebral body. Destruction and anterior collapse of the vertebral body may result in deformity and an angular kyphosis (gibbous deformity). Epidural or paraspinal abscesses are common and often travel long distances from their site of origin before perforating into a viscus or the body surface. Paraspinal masses out of proportion to the spondylitis may be seen on radiographs. A calcified psoas abscess favors tuberculous over pyogenic spondylitis. Another differentiation point is that tuberculous spondylitis is not as rapidly progressive as pyogenic disease.

28. What plain film findings suggest an infection of a metallic prosthesis?

It is typically impossible to differentiate an infected prosthesis from a loosened, uninfected prosthesis with plain radiographs alone. Both show prominent lucency at the bone-cement interface. A radiolucent zone of 2 mm should suggest loosening or infection, especially if it has increased in size from a prior radiograph.

29. What is a ring sequestrum?

A ring sequestrum indicates infection around a pin tract. A central radiolucent region created by the pin is surrounded by a ring of bone, which is surrounded by an area of osteolysis owing to infection. Pin tract infections are particularly common after percutaneous placement.

Bibliography

[1] M.S. Collins, M.M. Schaar, D.E. Wenger, J.N. Mandrekar, T1-weighted MRI characteristics of pedal osteomyelitis, AJR. Am. J. Roentgenol. 185 (2005) 386–393.

[2] J. Edeiken, New bone production and periosteal reaction, in: J. Edeiken (Ed.), Roentgen Diagnosis of Disease of Bone, vol. 1, Williams & Wilkins, Baltimore, 1981, pp. 11–29.

[3] P.A. Kaplan, C.A. Helms, R. Dussault, et al., Musculoskeletal infections, in: P.A. Kaplan, C.A. Helms, R. Dussault, et al., (Eds.), Musculoskeletal MRI, Saunders, Philadelphia, 2001, pp. 101–116.

[4] T.J. Leach, Imaging of infectious arthritis, Semin. Musculoskelet. Radiol. 7 (2003) 137–142.

[5] C. Love, M.B. Tomas, G.G. Tronco, C.J. Palestro, FDG PET of infection and inflammation, Radiographics 25 (2005) 1357–1368.

[6] D. Resnick, G. Niwayama, Osteomyelitis, septic arthritis, and soft tissue infection: mechanisms and situations, in: D. Resnick (Ed.), Diagnosis of Bone and Joint Disorders, third ed., Saunders, Philadelphia, 1995.

[7] B. Sammak, M. Abd El Bagi, M. Al Shahed, et al., Osteomyelitis: a review of currently used imaging techniques, Eur. Radiol. 9 (1999) 894–900.

[8] D.S. Schauwecker, The scintigraphic diagnosis of osteomyelitis, AJR. Am. J. Roentgenol. 158 (1992) 9–18.

[9] A. Stabler, M.F. Reiser, Imaging of spinal infection, Radiol. Clin. North Am. 39 (2001) 115–135.

[10] J. Tehranzadeh, E. Wong, F. Wang, M. Sadighpour, Imaging of osteomyelitis in the mature skeleton, Radiol. Clin. North Am. 39 (2001) 223–250.

CHAPTER 42

BONE TUMORS

Judy S. Blebea, MD

1. What radiographic features should be considered when evaluating a suspected bone tumor?

When evaluating a suspected bone tumor, morphologic features, periosteal reaction, location in a bone (epiphysis, metaphysis, diaphysis), distribution within the skeleton (axial vs. appendicular), presence of tumor matrix, and soft tissue mass should be considered. Morphologic features to consider are the pattern of bone destruction and the size, shape, margins, and zone of transition of the lesion. A lesion with a sharp border suggests a nonaggressive or benign lesion, whereas a poorly defined margin, especially one associated with cortical destruction, favors malignancy. Periosteal reaction reflects the rate of growth of the underlying lesion. Slow-growing lesions may produce a laminated periosteal reaction with uniform, wavy layers. Malignant lesions that grow in spurts can produce an "onion-skin" pattern, whereas aggressive lesions with rapid growth are associated with a "sunburst" or "hair-on-end" periosteal reaction. Codman triangle is the uplifting of the periosteum in a triangular configuration and can be seen with benign and malignant lesions.

2. How do cartilage tumor matrix and neoplastic bone matrix differ?

Cartilage matrix is typically ringlike, flocculent, or flecklike—in the shape of rings and arcs—whereas neoplastic bone matrix is typically cloudlike, amorphous, or ivory-like. The detection of tumor matrix can be helpful in recognizing the etiologic factor of the underlying lesion—that is, whether it is osseous or cartilaginous in origin.

Key Points: Plain Radiographic Features to Assess for Bone Tumors

1. Morphologic features and pattern of bone destruction, zone of transition
2. Periosteal reaction
3. Location in the bone and distribution in the skeleton
4. Presence of tumor matrix
5. Presence of a soft tissue mass

---

3. Which imaging study is most useful in arriving at an accurate differential diagnosis for a bone tumor?

Plain radiography is the first step in detecting and diagnosing a bone tumor. Plain films should also be obtained initially, even with suspected soft tissue tumors, to identify possible underlying bone involvement or the presence of calcifications.

4. What is the role of magnetic resonance imaging (MRI) and computed tomography (CT) in the evaluation of musculoskeletal tumors?

MRI is the most important diagnostic test for local staging and preoperative planning of primary bone and soft tissue tumors. It is also useful for monitoring the response to chemotherapy or radiation therapy and detecting postoperative tumor recurrence. CT may be helpful in the detection of tumor matrix and the location of the nidus in a suspected osteoid osteoma. CT is also used for percutaneous image-guided biopsy of bone tumors.

5. What are some tumor features evaluated with MRI? Can MRI be used to distinguish between benign and malignant tumors?

The tumor location, extent, and relationship to the neurovascular bundle and the presence of skip lesions and joint involvement are important features that are assessed with MRI and help to determine the stage of the tumor and to plan a surgical approach. Although MRI may help in the assessment of the aggressiveness of a lesion and in the recognition of certain "pathognomonic" lesions, it cannot be used to distinguish reliably between benign and malignant tumors, and is generally nonspecific in determining tumor cell type. Biopsy of the lesion is often required.

6. **What is the role of intravenous gadolinium contrast enhancement in MRI of musculoskeletal tumors?**

There is some controversy about the need for intravenous contrast enhancement during pretherapy MRI for a patient with a suspected musculoskeletal tumor. Contrast enhancement may be used to help distinguish tumor margins and assess tumor vascularity. Its use may also help distinguish malignant viable tissue from inflammatory changes and necrosis for preoperative biopsy planning. For a follow-up or post-therapy MRI evaluation, contrast enhancement can be helpful to assess the patient's response to chemotherapy, to determine the presence of a fluid collection postoperatively, and to detect tumor recurrence.

7. **What is the staging system adopted by the Musculoskeletal Tumor Society, and what three features form the basis of this staging system?**

The Musculoskeletal Tumor Society has adopted the Enneking staging system. Grade, local extent, and presence of metastases are the three features assessed with this system.

8. **Which primary bone tumors tend to involve the epiphysis most commonly?**

Chondroblastoma and giant cell tumors tend to involve the epiphysis most commonly. Chondroblastoma is a benign lesion that is typically well defined and located in the epiphysis. Although benign, chondroblastomas can be locally invasive and metastasize to the lungs. A giant cell tumor usually arises in the metaphyseal region and extends to involve the epiphysis. Giant cell tumors are eccentrically located lesions with a nonsclerotic zone of transition that typically occurs after closure of the growth plate (Fig. 42-1). A clear cell chondrosarcoma may also occur in the epiphyseal region.

9. **What is the difference between a nonossifying fibroma and a fibrous cortical defect?**

Both entities are benign, usually asymptomatic, well-defined cortical-based lesions with sclerotic borders seen in the metaphysis or diametaphysis of long bones, and are identical in their histology. They differ only in size. Fibrous cortical defects are smaller (<2 cm), whereas nonossifying fibromas are larger (>2 cm); both are usually detected incidentally on radiographs in children and often subsequently heal with sclerosis.

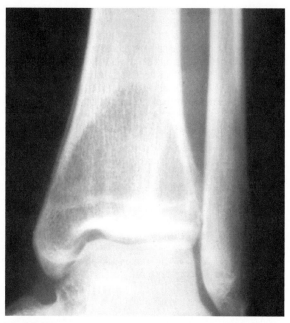

Figure 42-1. Plain film anteroposterior radiograph of the ankle shows a geographic lesion that extends to the epiphyseal region in the distal tibia. In this patient with closed growth plates, the most likely diagnosis is giant cell tumor.

Key Points: Primary Bone Tumors in the Epiphyseal Region

1. Chondroblastoma
2. Giant cell tumor
3. Clear cell chondrosarcoma

---

10. **What is the most common malignant tumor involving the skeleton?**

Metastases are the most common malignant skeletal tumors.

11. **What is the most common primary malignant bone tumor in adults?**

Multiple myeloma represents approximately 1% of all malignant diseases and about 10% to 15% of hematologic malignancies. The excessive proliferation of abnormal plasma cells can result in the formation of a single lesion (plasmacytoma) or multiple lesions (multiple myeloma).

12. If the diagnosis of multiple myeloma is suspected, what radiographic evaluation should be performed?

A skeletal survey is usually obtained. Approximately 75% of patients with multiple myeloma have positive radiographic findings with "punched-out" osteolytic lesions that have discrete margins and uniform size. Multiple compression fractures can also be seen. MRI is very sensitive for detecting the presence of marrow lesions and may help in determining tumor extent.

13. What are the most common primary neoplasms that metastasize to bone?

A few primary tumors account for most metastatic bone lesions. Cancers most likely to metastasize to bone include prostate, breast, kidney, thyroid, and lung, and are remembered by the mnemonic *PB (lead) KetTLe*. Other primary tumors that can metastasize to bone include colon, rectum, stomach, and bladder. The axial skeleton is seeded more than the appendicular skeleton because of the presence of red bone marrow. It is rare to have bone metastases below the elbow or knee. Lytic bone metastases must have destroyed 30% to 50% of the bone to be seen on radiographs. Nuclear medicine bone scans are more sensitive than radiographs for the detection of metastatic bone disease.

14. Which tumors can give rise to lytic, expansile, "blown-out" metastases of bone?

Bone metastases from renal cell carcinoma and thyroid cancer can show this pattern. Bone metastases from malignant melanoma may be expansile as well.

15. What is the second most common primary bone tumor after multiple myeloma?

Osteosarcoma is the second most common primary bone tumor after multiple myeloma (Fig. 42-2). About 75% of osteosarcoma lesions occur around the knee and typically arise in the metaphyseal region. The peak incidence is in the second and third decades, and there is a smaller second peak in patients older than 50 years; this later peak has more pelvic and craniofacial involvement. Osteosarcoma can develop after radiation exposure, with an average latent period of 11 years.

16. Which type of tumor can manifest with bone pain, swelling, tenderness, fever, and increased sedimentation rate, mimicking an infection?

Ewing sarcoma is a malignant round cell tumor with a predilection for the long bones and pelvis. Plain films may show a permeative or moth-eaten pattern of bone destruction with an onion-skin type of periosteal reaction and an associated soft tissue mass.

17. Where do sarcomas most commonly metastasize?

Sarcomas tend to undergo hematogenous spread, with pulmonary metastases being the most common.

18. What is the most common benign skeletal neoplasm?

Osteochondroma is the most common benign skeletal neoplasm (Fig. 42-3). This lesion accounts for 20% to 50% of benign bone tumors and 10% to 15% of all bone tumors. Osteochondromas occur most commonly in the first 2 decades of life, arise from the metaphysis pointing away from the joint, and can be either flattened (sessile) or stalklike. There is usually cessation of growth of the osteochondroma after closure of the growth plate. Osteochondromas can occur after radiation therapy in children and may present with pain because of mechanical irritation or fracture.

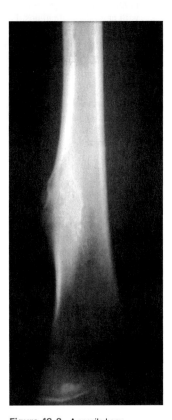

Figure 42-3. A sessile bony protuberance is noted arising from the femur on this plain film radiograph; this represents an osteochondroma. Osteochondromas are the most common benign skeletal neoplasm.

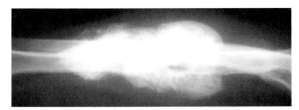

Figure 42-2. Plain film radiograph shows exuberant bone formation in this osteosarcoma.

19. Which clinical and radiographic features suggest malignant degeneration of an osteochondroma?

Features suggesting malignant degeneration include pain, growth after closure of the growth plate, bony destruction, thickened cartilage cap, and soft tissue mass. The risk of malignant transformation of a solitary osteochondroma is approximately 1%, whereas the risk of hereditary multiple osteochondromatosis is much higher and may be 25% to 30%. A sessile lesion is more likely to degenerate, usually undergoing malignant transformation to a chondrosarcoma (Fig. 42-4).

20. What is the most common benign bone tumor of the hand? Where else may these lesions occur, and what are the features of malignant transformation?

An enchondroma is the most common benign bone tumor of the hand. Small, peripheral enchondromas of the hand are usually well-defined lytic lesions that are typically benign, but may be detected as a result of pathologic fracture. Solitary enchondromas can also occur in the long bones and are usually oval in shape with central calcifications (Fig. 42-5). Features suggestive of malignant degeneration include an enlarging painful lesion with progressive destruction of the chondroid matrix and an expansile soft tissue mass.

21. Which primary bone tumor has the characteristic history of pain at night that is relieved by aspirin?

Osteoid osteoma is a primary bone tumor that has a characteristic history of pain at night that is relieved by aspirin. The classic radiographic appearance of this lesion is a round or oval lucent lesion, which represents the nidus, that typically measures less than 1 cm and is surrounded by a zone of bone sclerosis with cortical thickening.

22. What is fibrous dysplasia?

Fibrous dysplasia is a developmental anomaly of bone that usually manifests as a solitary lesion with focal bone expansion, cortical thinning or thickening, and a "ground-glass" appearance. Patients with these lesions may be asymptomatic or present with pathologic fracture. Polyostotic fibrous dysplasia with associated endocrine dysfunction that is usually manifested as precocious female sexual development is known as McCune-Albright syndrome.

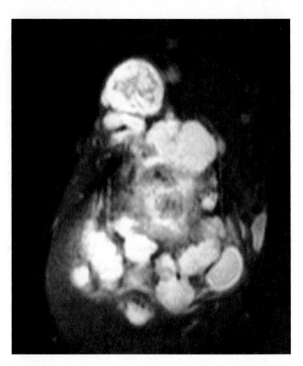

Figure 42-4. Axial T2-weighted MR image permits the evaluation of the extent of this biopsy-proven chondrosarcoma. This image is helpful for staging and preoperative planning.

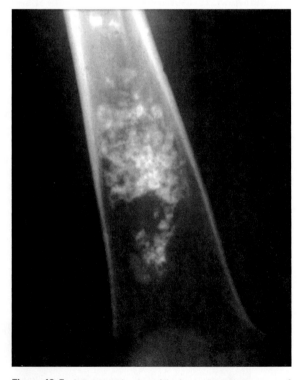

Figure 42-5. Anteroposterior view of the femur shows the presence of cartilage matrix, which is typically ringlike, flocculent, or flecklike, in this patient with an enchondroma.

> **Key Points: Imaging of Bone Tumors**
> 1. Order a plain film first.
> 2. Use MRI for staging and preoperative planning.
> 3. Use CT for image-guided biopsy and detection of the nidus of an osteoid osteoma or pulmonary metastases.
> 4. Use MRI for follow-up to detect response to therapy or tumor recurrence.

23. Which of the following has an increased incidence of skeletal malignancy: high-dose radiation therapy, bone infarction, Paget disease, or chronic osteomyelitis?

All of these entities have an increased incidence of skeletal malignancy; osteosarcoma and fibrosarcoma are the most common forms of malignant degeneration.

24. What is a bone island?

A bone island, or *enostosis,* is a benign lesion that appears radiographically as an oval or round sclerotic focus that may have radiating bone spicules from the center of the lesion. Bone islands are typically asymptomatic, are incidentally discovered, and usually do not show increased radiotracer uptake on a nuclear medicine bone scan.

25. What is the most common location for a skeletal hemangioma?

The most common site of involvement is the spine, particularly the thoracic segment. Most vertebral hemangiomas are small and asymptomatic, with a coarse, vertical trabecular pattern or corduroy appearance in the vertebral body on plain films or CT.

BIBLIOGRAPHY

[1] A. Greenspan, Differential Diagnosis of Tumors and Tumor-like Lesions of Bones and Joints, Lippincott Williams & Wilkins, Philadelphia, 1998.
[2] T. Rand, P. Ritschl, S. Trattnig, et al., Imaging of Bone and Soft Tissue Tumors, Springer Verlag, New York, 2001.
[3] D. Resnick, Diagnosis of Bone and Joint Disorders, fourth ed., Saunders, Philadelphia, 2002.

CHAPTER 43

SHOULDER MRI

Neil Roach, MD

1. What magnetic resonance imaging (MRI) planes are used for evaluating the shoulder?

Because the scapula is attached to the chest wall at approximately 45 degrees, oblique sagittal and oblique coronal planes are used to evaluate the shoulder. Axial images are also obtained.

2. Name the four muscles of the rotator cuff.

The supraspinatus, infraspinatus, and teres minor attach to the greater tuberosity of the humeral head. The subscapularis tendon attaches to the lesser tuberosity.

3. What is impingement syndrome?

This condition is caused by entrapment of the supraspinatus tendon, biceps tendon, and subacromial-subdeltoid bursa between the humeral head and coracoacromial arch. It is thought that 95% of rotator cuff tears are related to chronic impingement. The diagnosis of impingement is made clinically.

4. In what age group do rotator cuff tears most commonly occur?

Rotator cuff tears are rare in healthy individuals younger than 40 years old. Impingement syndrome is a chronic process, beginning at about age 25 years, that causes degeneration of the rotator cuff tendons. Rotator cuff tears can be seen in pitchers and weightlifters before age 40 years.

5. What is the typical MRI appearance of a rotator cuff tear?

Increased T2 signal (fluid) is seen within the tendon (Fig. 43-1). Normal tendons have low signal intensity on all pulse sequences.

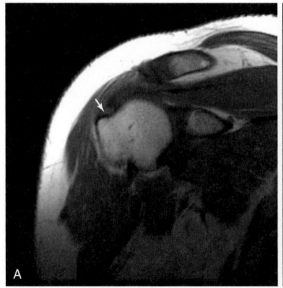
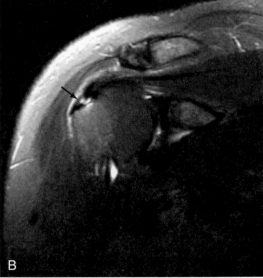

Figure 43-1. A and **B,** Oblique coronal proton density (**A**) and fat-suppressed T2-weighted (**B**) images of the right shoulder at the anterior leading edge of the supraspinatus tendon. A small focal tear (*arrow*) is seen where the supraspinatus tendon (which should be dark) inserts on the greater tuberosity. On T2, fluid is seen in the region of the tear.

6. Which tendon of the rotator cuff is most commonly torn?

The supraspinatus is most commonly torn. Most tears occur in the critical zone of the tendon, which is a relatively hypovascular area of the tendon that is approximately 1 to 2 cm proximal to the insertion of the supraspinatus tendon on the greater tuberosity.

7. What MRI features indicate that a rotator cuff tear is chronic?

A high-riding humeral head in close proximity to the undersurface of the acromion indicates a chronic rotator cuff tear. This can be seen on radiographs or MRI. Atrophy of muscles can be seen on MRI. This is appreciated by fatty infiltration on T1-weighted images and decreased muscle bulk.

8. What are Hill-Sachs and Bankart deformities?

Both of these deformities are secondary to anterior dislocations. The Hill-Sachs lesion is an impaction fracture of the posterolateral aspect of the humeral head and is seen best on axial images above the coracoid process. The Bankart lesion is defined as an injury to the anterior-inferior glenoid and can be an osseous or nonosseous abnormality. Bankart lesions are also best appreciated on axial images (Fig. 43-2).

9. What other shoulder abnormalities can be diagnosed on routine shoulder MRI?

Fractures, biceps tendon tears or dislocations, glenohumeral and acromioclavicular osteoarthritis, glenoid labral tears, joint effusion, osteonecrosis, and osteomyelitis all can be diagnosed on routine shoulder MRI.

Key Points: Shoulder MRI

1. Three primary diseases can be seen on MRI of the shoulder: osteoarthritis, rotator cuff tears, and abnormal structures related to the clinical diagnosis of instability.
2. Radiographs should be obtained before MR images. Many times, rotator cuff tears can be diagnosed by the narrowing of the distance between the undersurface of the acromion and humeral head.

---

10. What is a SLAP lesion?

SLAP stands for superior labrum anterior and posterior. A SLAP lesion is a type of glenoid labral tear that extends anteriorly and posteriorly. It is usually seen in athletes who throw or after shoulder trauma. Subtle SLAP lesions may be difficult to diagnose on routine MRI. Magnetic resonance arthrography (MRA) increases the sensitivity for detecting these abnormalities.

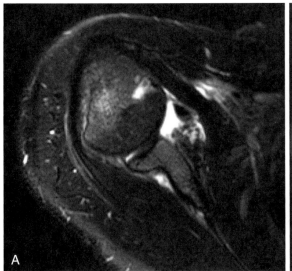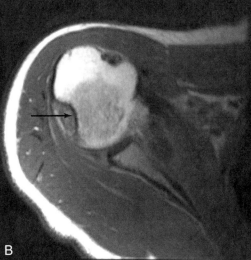

Figure 43-2. A, Axial fat-suppressed T2-weighted image shows an osseous defect in the anterior-inferior aspect of the glenoid, a Bankart lesion. **B,** Axial proton density image shows a defect in the posterior-lateral aspect of the humeral head (*arrow*), representing a Hill-Sachs deformity resulting from prior anterior-inferior humeral dislocation.

11. Which is better for the detection of calcific tendinitis, radiographs or MRI?

Calcific tendinitis is a type of tendon pathology seen around the shoulder. It is formally known as *calcium hydroxyapatite deposition disease*. The shoulder is the most common site of involvement. On MRI, the nodular calcium deposits show low signal intensity on all pulse sequences. The involved rotator cuff tendons may show focal thickening related to the calcified nodules. It can be difficult to appreciate calcific tendinitis on MRI, but this diagnosis can be clearly seen on radiographs.

12. What is meant by glenohumeral instability?

Patients in whom the humeral head slips or subluxates out of the glenoid are said to have instability during activities. Orthopedic surgeons describe instability by direction: anterior, posterior, or multidirectional. Instability can also be characterized as traumatic or atraumatic. *Anatomic instability* refers to subluxation or dislocation of the humeral head. *Functional instability* refers to pain, clicking, or locking of the shoulder. The most common glenohumeral instability is anterior instability from a previous dislocation.

BIBLIOGRAPHY

[1] J. Beltran, D.H. Kim, MR imaging of shoulder instability injuries in the athlete, Magn. Reson. Imaging Clin. N. Am. 11 (2003) 221–238.

[2] J.F. Feller, et al., Magnetic resonance imaging of the shoulder: review, Semin. Roentgenol. 30 (1995) 224–240.

[3] P.A. Kaplan, R. Dussault, M.W. Anderson, N.M. Major, Musculoskeletal MRI, Saunders, Philadelphia, 2001, pp. 175–176.

[4] M. Rafii, et al., Rotator cuff lesions: Signal patterns at MR imaging, Radiology 177 (1990) 817–823.

MRI OF THE ELBOW AND WRIST

Christopher J. Yoo, MD, and
Neil Roach, MD

CHAPTER 44

1. Name the bones and articulations of the elbow.

The elbow joint involves the radius and ulna of the forearm and the humerus of the upper arm. There are three articulations: the radiocapitellar, ulnar trochlear, and proximal radioulnar.

2. Name the muscles that cross or surround the elbow joint.

These muscles are the biceps, brachialis, triceps, brachioradialis, extensor tendons, flexor tendons, anconeus, pronator teres, and supinator.

3. Name the labeled structures on the MR images in Fig. 44-1.

See figure legend for answers.

4. Describe the anatomy of the medial and lateral collateral ligament complexes.

The medial collateral ligament complex consists of three bundles: anterior, posterior, and transverse. The anterior is the most important stabilizer against valgus strain. The lateral collateral ligament complex also consists of three components: the radial collateral ligament, annular ligament, and lateral ulnar collateral ligament (LUCL). The annular ligament encircles the radial head and attaches to the anterior and posterior margins of the radial notch of the ulna. The LUCL arises from the lateral epicondyle, courses posterior to the radial head, and inserts on the lateral aspect of the ulna onto the supinator crest (Table 44-1).

5. What pattern of injury is seen with a valgus injury? Whom does it most commonly affect?

Athletes who throw develop these injuries, which arise from repeated valgus stress and injury. Valgus-type injuries can include the following, even though not all components would be seen because there is a spectrum of severity of injury: medial collateral ligament strain/tear, common flexor tendon/muscle strain/tear, medial epicondyle edema, medial heterotopic ossification, lateral bony impaction injury of the radius and capitellum, and ulnar neuropathy.

6. What is the LUCL? Explain its significance in instability of the elbow joint.

The LUCL is a component of the lateral collateral ligament complex, as previously described, originating from the lateral epicondyle and coursing posterior to the radial head to insert on the lateral aspect of the ulna at the supinator crest. Disruption or laxity of the LUCL results in an entity called *posterolateral rotatory instability,* which is the most common form of chronic elbow instability.

Key Points: MRI Signs of Tendon Injury

1. Tendon enlargement
2. Increased intrinsic signal intensity on T1-weighted, proton density–weighted, and T2-weighted images
3. Fluid and edema surrounding the tendon
4. Disruption of the tendon fibers

---

7. What are golfer's elbow and tennis elbow? Which is more common?

Golfer's elbow and *tennis elbow* are lay terms for medial and lateral epicondylitis. They do not represent inflammation of the epicondyle itself, but rather are injuries of the tendons and muscles, including tendinopathy; partial and complete tendon tears; muscle strain; muscle tear; and, in young patients, perhaps bony avulsion or delayed physeal closure. Lateral epicondylitis (tennis elbow) is more common.

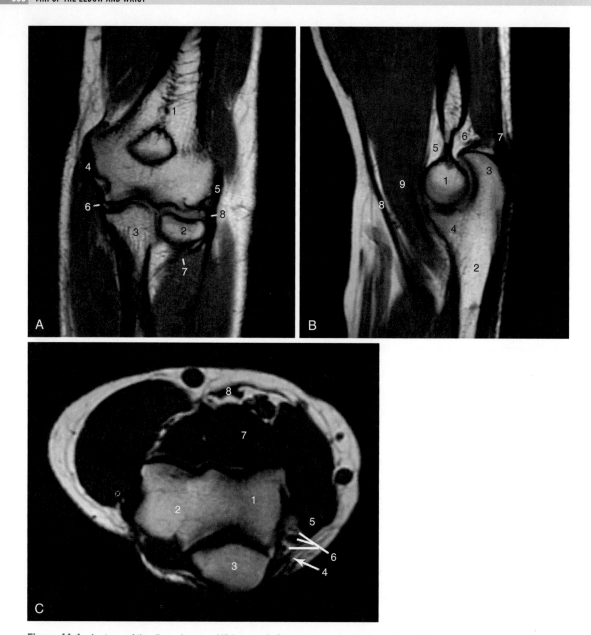

Figure 44-1. Anatomy of the elbow shown on MR images. **A,** Coronal proton density image through the posterior aspect of the radial head (*1* = humerus, *2* = radial head, *3* = ulna, *4* = common flexor tendon, *5* = common extensor tendon, *6* = medial collateral ligament, *7* = lateral ulnar collateral ligament, *8* = radial collateral ligament). **B,** Sagittal proton density image through the ulnar trochlear articulation (*1* = trochlea, *2* = ulna, *3* = olecranon, *4* = coronoid process, *5* = anterior fat pad in the coronoid fossa, *6* = posterior fat pad in the olecranon fossa, *7* = triceps, *8* = biceps tendon, *9* = brachialis). **C,** Axial T1-weighted image at the level of the distal humeral epiphysis (*1* = trochlea, *2* = capitellum, *3* = ulna, *4* = cubital tunnel retinaculum, *5* = flexor carpi ulnaris, *6* = ulnar nerve, artery, and vein in the cubital tunnel, *7* = brachialis, *8* = biceps tendon).

8. What muscle groups do medial and lateral epicondylitis involve?

The common flexor tendon and associated muscles are involved in medial epicondylitis, and the common extensor tendon and associated muscles are involved in lateral epicondylitis (Fig. 44-2).

9. What causes the anterior and posterior fat pad signs in conventional radiographs? What is the significance of these signs?

The anterior fat pad in the coronoid fossa and the posterior fat pad in the olecranon fossa can be displaced by a joint effusion. Elevation of the anterior fat pad has been called the "anterior sail" sign. Visualization of either a posterior fat

Table 44-1. Anatomy of the Medial Collateral Ligament (MCL) and Lateral Collateral Ligament (LCL) Complexes

	ORIGIN	INSERTION
MCL Complex		
Anterior bundle	Medial epicondyle	Medial aspect of coronoid
Posterior bundle	Medial epicondyle	Medial aspect of olecranon
Transverse bundle	Medial aspect of coronoid	Medial aspect of olecranon
LCL Complex		
Radial collateral ligament	Lateral epicondyle	Annular ligament
Annular ligament	Anterior margin of radial notch	Posterior margin of radial notch
Lateral ulnar collateral ligament	Lateral epicondyle	Supinator crest of lateral ulna

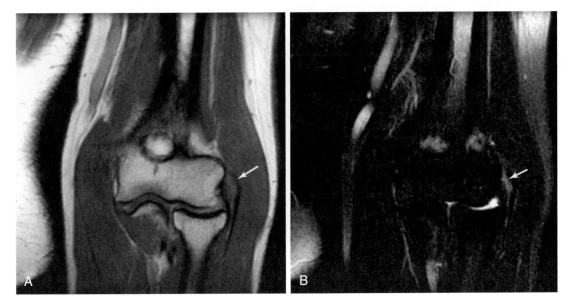

Figure 44-2. Common extensor tendinopathy/tennis elbow. **A,** Coronal T1-weighted image shows thickening and increased intermediate signal in the common extensor tendon insertion (*arrow*). **B,** Coronal T2-weighted image with fat saturation shows increased high signal intensity in common extensor tendon insertion (*arrow*). The tendon is intact, and no full-thickness tear is seen. Compare with Fig. 44-1A.

pad sign or an anterior sail sign may indicate the presence of a joint effusion or hemarthrosis (Fig. 44-3). In the setting of elbow trauma, these signs are highly suggestive for the presence of a fracture, whether or not a fracture is visualized radiographically.

10. **What role does MRI play in the evaluation of patients with anterior and posterior fat pad signs?**
MRI can be used to diagnose fractures when the sail sign or posterior fat pad sign is present but the fracture is radiographically occult, and can detect associated tendon or ligament injury.

11. **Which patients most commonly present with biceps tendon rupture? Describe the MRI appearance of complete rupture.**
Biceps rupture usually involves the dominant arm and is most commonly seen in men, especially weightlifters or workers who perform heavy lifting. The MRI appearance of complete rupture is easily recognized because there is complete disruption of the biceps tendon near the insertion with proximal retraction of the tendon, which often has a wavy appearance (Fig. 44-4). Fluid or hemorrhage usually fills the cubital fossa and surrounds the ruptured tendon.

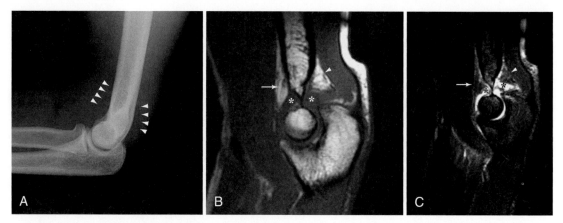

Figure 44-3. A, Lateral plain radiograph of the elbow shows elevation of the anterior fat pad, the "anterior sail sign," and elevation of the posterior fat pad. **B,** Sagittal T1-weighted image through the ulnar trochlear articulation shows high signal intensity anterior (*arrow*) and posterior (*arrowhead*) fat pads displaced by intermediate signal intensity joint fluid (*asterisks*). **C,** Sagittal T2-weighted image with fat saturation in the same plane shows the high signal intensity joint fluid (*asterisks*) displacing the anterior (*arrow*) and posterior (*arrowhead*) fat pads, which now appear dark as a result of fat saturation.

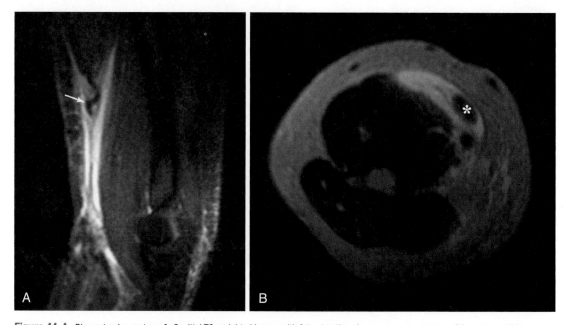

Figure 44-4. Biceps tendon rupture. **A,** Sagittal T2-weighted image with fat saturation shows wavy appearance of the retracted biceps tendon (*arrow*), with extensive edema around the tendon and in the cubital fossa. **B,** Axial T2-weighted image through the distal humeral metaphysis shows the retracted tendon (*asterisk*) with surrounding edema.

12. What are the boundaries and contents of the cubital tunnel?

The cubital tunnel contains the ulnar nerve and the recurrent ulnar artery and vein. The floor of the tunnel comprises the elbow capsule and medial collateral ligament, and the roof consists of the cubital tunnel retinaculum proximally and the flexor carpi ulnaris distally (see Fig. 44-2C).

13. The presence of which anomalous muscle is a rare cause of symptoms related to the cubital tunnel?

The anconeus epitrochlearis, when present, can cause static compression of the ulnar nerve within the confines of the cubital tunnel, resulting in ulnar neuropathy. The anconeus epitrochlearis sits just deep to the cubital retinaculum.

Key Points: Tunnel Neuropathies
1. *Cubital tunnel*: Medial elbow, ulnar neuropathy
2. *Carpal tunnel*: Volar wrist, median neuropathy
3. *Guyon canal*: Volar wrist, ulnar neuropathy

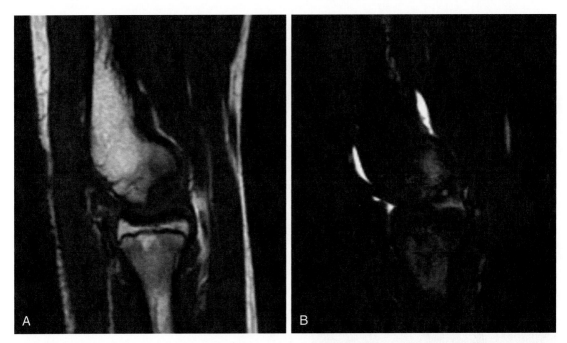

Figure 44-5. Osteochondritis dissecans of the capitellum. **A,** Sagittal T1-weighted image through the radiocapitellar articulation shows a large osteochondral defect and adjacent low signal intensity marrow that represents marrow edema. **B,** Sagittal T2-weighted image with fat saturation at the same level shows the same osteochondral defect with surrounding marrow edema and edema within the osteochondral fragment.

14. What is Panner disease?

Panner disease is an osteochondrosis/avascular necrosis (AVN) of the capitellum, similar to Legg-Calvé-Perthes disease of the femoral epiphysis. On plain radiographs, one may see sclerosis and deformity of the capitellum. On MRI, Panner disease manifests as low marrow signal on T1-weighted images and variable signal on T2-weighted or short-tau inversion recovery (STIR) images, progressing from high to low with more advanced disease.

15. Where does the pseudodefect of the capitellum occur compared with osteochondritis dissecans in the capitellum?

Osteochondritis dissecans typically occurs anteriorly, whereas the pseudodefect is seen posterolaterally. The pseudodefect is actually the normal appearance of the capitellum on sagittal images (Fig. 44-5).

16. What is the differential diagnosis for olecranon bursitis? Describe its appearance on MRI.

The differential diagnosis includes acute or repetitive trauma, gout, rheumatoid arthritis, calcium pyrophosphate deposition disease, hydroxyapatite deposition disease, dialysis, and infection. On MRI, olecranon bursitis typically appears as simple or complex fluid enlarging the bursa, often with surrounding edema in the soft tissues or bone or both, depending on the etiologic factors.

17. Name the labeled structures in Fig. 44-6.

See figure legend for answers.

18. What is the role of MRI in evaluation of scaphoid fractures?

MRI has much higher sensitivity for scaphoid fractures and, more importantly, can be used to diagnose early AVN of the proximal fracture fragment. MRI is useful to assess the viability and probability of successful union of the fracture fragments, helping direct treatment options. In radiographically occult fractures, a low T1-signal and T2-signal intensity fracture line may be seen with surrounding edema on MRI.

19. What is the appearance of AVN of the proximal pole?

In the presence of AVN, the proximal fracture fragment appears as low signal intensity on T1-weighted images and heterogeneously high to low signal intensity on T2-weighted images. Uniformly low T2-signal intensity and lack of enhancement of the proximal fracture fragment on postgadolinium MRI suggest the lack of blood supply and poor prognosis for healing (Fig. 44-7).

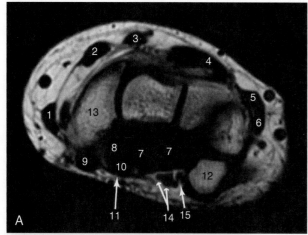

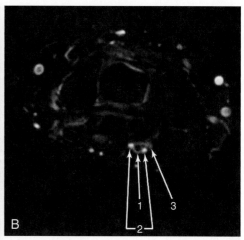

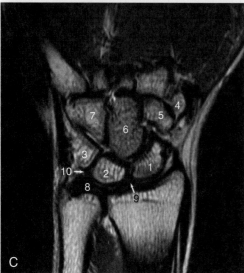

Figure 44-6. A, Axial T1-weighted image through the wrist at the level of the pisiform (*1* = abductor pollicis longus, extensor pollicis brevis, *2* = extensor carpi radialis brevis, extensor carpi radialis longus, *3* = extensor pollicis longus, *4* = extensor digitorum, extensor tendon insertion, *5* = extensor digiti minimi, *6* = extensor carpi ulnaris, *7* = flexor digitorum superficialis and profundus tendons, *8* = flexor pollicis longus tendon, *9* = flexor carpi radialis longus tendon outside the carpal tunnel, *10* = median nerve, *11* = flexor retinaculum, *12* = pisiform, *13* = scaphoid, *14* = ulnar artery and veins in Guyon canal, *15* = ulnar nerve in Guyon canal). **B,** Axial T2-weighted image with fat saturation at the same level as in **A** (*1* = ulnar artery, *2* = ulnar veins, *3* = ulnar nerve, *4* = median nerve). **C,** Coronal gradient-echo image (*1* = scaphoid, *2* = lunate, *3* = triquetrum, *4* = trapezium, *5* = trapezoid, *6* = capitate, *7* = hamate, *8* = triangular fibrocartilage, *9* = scapholunate ligament, *10* = lunatotriquetral ligament).

20. Define negative, neutral, and positive variance. Which of these is related to Kienböck malacia?

Ulnar variance refers to the length of the ulna in relationship to the radius at the distal radioulnar joint. If the ulna is longer than the radius as determined by straight lines drawn along the distal articular surfaces, this is termed *positive ulnar variance*. If the ulna is more than 2 mm shorter than the radius, this is termed *negative ulnar variance*. All other cases are termed *neutral ulnar variance*. Negative ulnar variance is associated with increased incidence of Kienböck disease (AVN of the lunate), which is thought to be due to altered compressive forces at the radiolunate articulation secondary to decreased load bearing at the triquetral–triangular fibrocartilage–ulnar axis.

21. Name the contents of the carpal tunnel. What are classic signs and symptoms of carpal tunnel syndrome (CTS)?

The carpal tunnel contains the median nerve and tendons of the flexor digitorum superficialis and profundus and the tendon of the flexor pollicis longus. Classic signs and symptoms of CTS include paresthesia in the median nerve sensory distribution (the first three digits and the radial aspect of the fourth digit) that may be worse at night, thenar atrophy, and positive Phalen and Tinel tests.

22. Describe the MRI appearance of CTS.

The MRI appearance of CTS includes flattening and edema of the median nerve in the carpal tunnel, enlargement of the nerve proximal to the tunnel, and volar bowing of the retinaculum. The etiologic factor can sometimes be seen on MRI, including flexor tenosynovitis, trauma, infection, and mass (ganglion cyst, lipoma, neuroma, fibrolipomatous hamartoma).

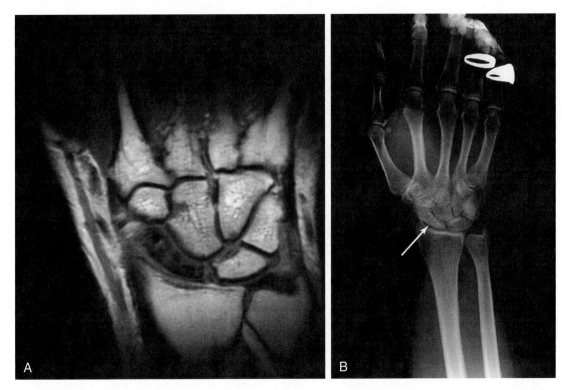

Figure 44-7. AVN of the scaphoid after fracture. **A,** Coronal proton density–weighted image shows irregular shape and abnormal low signal intensity of the scaphoid. **B,** Anteroposterior radiograph of the wrist shows irregular shape and abnormal sclerosis of the scaphoid (*arrow*).

23. What is the role of MRI in CTS?

Currently, MRI is not commonly used as a primary diagnostic tool for CTS because it is costly and neither sensitive nor specific enough. It may be helpful when electromyography is equivocal or when an atypical etiologic factor is being considered. MRI is useful in evaluating for a cause of recurrent symptoms in postoperative patients who have undergone surgical release (Fig. 44-8A and B).

24. What are the two most common causes of recurrent symptoms in patients who have had surgical release of the carpal tunnel?

The two most common causes are an incomplete release, meaning failure to divide the flexor retinaculum completely, and scar formation joining the surgically divided retinaculum, resulting in a closed canal (Fig. 44-8C and D).

25. What are the boundaries and contents of Guyon canal?

Guyon canal is a triangular space on axial images located superficial to the carpal tunnel on the ulnar aspect of the wrist and contains the ulnar nerve, artery, and vein. The flexor retinaculum is the floor. The radial surface of the pisiform is the ulnar margin. A superficial fascial layer is the roof (see Fig. 44-6A).

26. What situations can cause neuropathy related to Guyon canal?

Acute or chronic trauma, mass, anomalous muscle, or inflammation related to infection or arthritis can cause ulnar nerve entrapment within the canal.

27. What is de Quervain tenosynovitis? Describe its MRI appearance.

de Quervain tenosynovitis is tenosynovitis of the first extensor compartment involving the abductor pollicis longus and extensor pollicis brevis. The tendons may be enlarged with increased intrinsic signal, and there should be fluid surrounding the tendons within the tendon sheaths (Fig. 44-9).

28. What ligament is injured in gamekeeper's thumb or skier's thumb?

The ulnar collateral ligament of the first metacarpal joint is injured with forced adduction or hyperadduction of the first digit, often seen in skiers gripping ski poles during a fall, but also seen in other contact sports. Historically, this

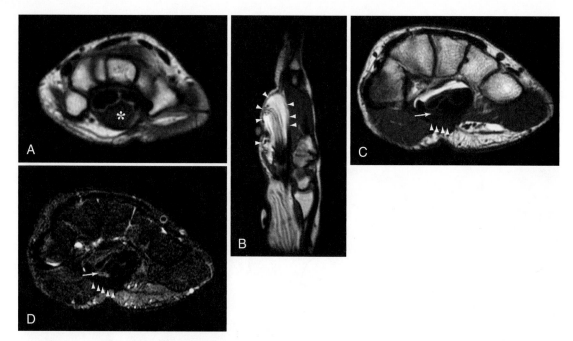

Figure 44-8. **A,** Axial T1-weighted image through the carpal tunnel shows marked enlargement of the median nerve (*asterisk*) within the carpal tunnel secondary to a fibrolipomatous hamartoma. **B,** Sagittal T1-weighted image through the carpal tunnel shows a mixed soft tissue and fatty mass (*arrowheads*) enlarging the median nerve. **C** and **D,** Axial T1-weighted (**C**) and fat-saturated T2-weighted (**D**) images after carpal tunnel release in a patient with recurrent symptoms of CTS. Images show low T1 and T2 signal intensity fibrosis and scarring of the flexor retinaculum (*arrows*) with flattening and increased signal of the median nerve (*arrowheads*).

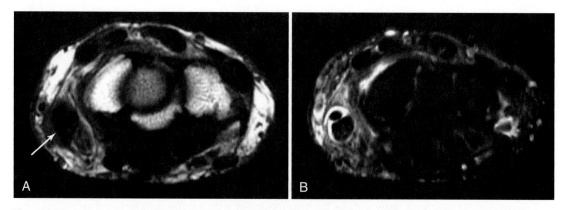

Figure 44-9. **A** and **B,** Axial T1-weighted (**A**) and fat-saturated T2-weighted (**B**) images in the proximal wrist show enlargement and increased T1 and T2 signal intensity within the first extensor compartment (*arrow*) involving the abductor pollicis longus and extensor pollicis brevis tendons with surrounding fluid within the tendon sheath, in keeping with de Quervain tenosynovitis.

injury was seen in European gamekeepers who would grip a small animal's neck, similar to a ski pole, and break the neck using an adduction motion, which would cause chronic repetitive strain on the ulnar collateral ligament (Fig. 44-10).

29. What is a Stener lesion? Describe its significance.

A Stener lesion is characterized by displacement of the avulsed ulnar collateral ligament such that the adductor pollicis aponeurosis is interposed between the avulsed ligament and its insertion, effectively precluding healing. This lesion requires surgical repair to prevent chronic instability.

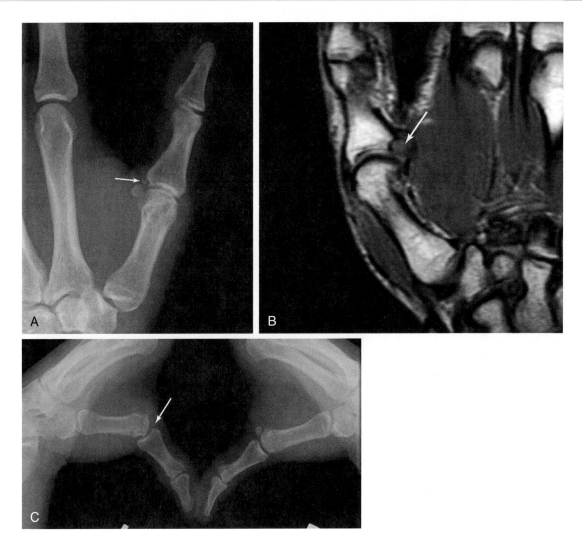

Figure 44-10. Gamekeeper's thumb. **A,** Plain radiograph of the first digit shows a small, bony, ossific density adjacent to the ulnar aspect of the base of the proximal phalanx (*arrow*), representing an avulsion fracture involving the ulnar collateral ligament of the first metacarpophalangeal joint. **B,** Coronal T1-weighted image shows thickening and disruption of the ulnar collateral ligament of the first metacarpophalangeal joint (*arrow*). The avulsed fracture fragment is not seen here. **C,** Stress image of the same patient reveals hyperabduction at the first metacarpophalangeal joint, indicating ligamentous laxity of the affected side (*arrow*).

Key Points: Other Important Clinical Entities

1. Kienböck malacia (negative ulnar variance)
2. Ulnar abutment syndrome (positive ulnar variance)
3. Medial epicondylitis (wrist flexors and common flexor tendon)
4. Lateral epicondylitis (wrist extensors and common extensor tendon)

---

30. What is the most commonly injured intrinsic ligament of the wrist? With what form of instability is this injury associated?

The scapholunate ligament is injured more commonly than the lunatotriquetral ligament. Injury to the scapholunate predisposes the patient to dorsal intercalated segment instability, whereas injury to the lunatotriquetral ligament is associated with volar intercalated segment instability.

31. Describe typical patients who experience traumatic versus degenerative tears of the triangular fibrocartilage.

Typically younger patients have traumatic tears of the triangular fibrocartilage, whereas older patients and patients with positive ulnar variance and ulnar abutment syndrome more commonly develop degenerative tears.

32. What mass in the wrist has been called the "King James lesion"? Where does it most commonly occur?

A ganglion cyst has been called the "King James lesion." This facetious term was derived from the sometimes used "treatment" for this lesion, which consisted of putting the hand on a hard flat surface and slamming it with a King James version of the Bible. Ganglion cysts most commonly occur on the dorsum of the wrist near the scapholunate ligament, but can occur anywhere. The typical patient a young adult, more commonly a woman.

BIBLIOGRAPHY

[1] T.H. Berquist, Nerve compression syndromes, in: T.H. Berquist (Ed.), MRI of the Hand and Wrist, Lippincott Williams & Wilkins, Philadelphia, 2003, pp. 163–178.

[2] C.B. Chung, H.J. Kim, Sports injuries of the elbow, Magn. Reson. Imaging Clin. North. Am. 11 (2003) 239–253.

[3] L. Desharnais, P.A. Kaplan, R.G. Dussault, MR imaging of ligamentous abnormalities of the elbow, Magn. Reson. Imaging Clin. North. Am. 5 (1997) 515–528.

[4] R.C. Fritz, MR imaging of osteochondral and articular lesions, Magn. Reson. Imaging Clin. North. Am. 5 (1997) 579–602.

[5] R.C. Fritz, D.W. Stoller, The elbow, in: D.W. Stoller (Ed.), Magnetic Resonance Imaging in Orthopaedics and Sports Medicine, second ed., Lippincott Williams & Wilkins, Philadelphia, 1997, pp. 743–849.

[6] C.P. Ho, Magnetic resonance imaging of tendon injuries in the elbow, Magn. Reson. Imaging Clin. North. Am. 5 (1997) 529–543.

[7] Z.S. Rosenberg, J. Bencardino, J. Beltran, MR features of nerve disorders at the elbow, Magn. Reson. Imaging Clin. North. Am. 5 (1997) 545–565.

MRI OF THE HIP

Gregory Goodworth, MD, and
Neil Roach, MD

CHAPTER 45

1. What is the first radiologic examination for the evaluation of hip pain?
Plain radiography is the first-choice imaging modality for the evaluation of hip pain. Plain radiographs are inexpensive, easy to obtain, and can often delineate the etiology of hip pain.

2. When should magnetic resonance imaging (MRI) of the hip be performed?
Hip MRI is the modality of choice for symptomatic patients whose conditions cannot be diagnosed after evaluation of plain films. Common indications include osteonecrosis, trauma with radiographically occult fractures, stress and insufficiency fractures, labral tears, musculoskeletal neoplasms, septic arthritis and osteomyelitis of the hip, transient osteoporosis, and bone marrow edema.

3. Which modality is best for the evaluation of suspected osteoarthritis (degenerative changes) of the hip?
Plain radiographs are best for the evaluation of suspected osteoarthritis of the hip.

4. Does an MRI examination of the hip usually include one or both hips?
Both hips are usually included in an MRI examination of the hip. Even if a patient has a complaint of unilateral hip pain, both hips should be examined when a bilateral disease process is suspected, such as osteonecrosis in a patient on long-term steroid therapy. Because most hip MRI examinations are for fracture, tumor, or osteonecrosis, it is often useful to image the entire pelvis to search for other lesions. A unilateral protocol is used to evaluate patients with unilateral hip pain without suspicion of contralateral disease, such as a trauma patient with clinical suspicion of an occult fracture. If very high-resolution images are required, the unilateral protocol allows for a smaller field of view and higher resolution.

5. Is intravenous contrast agent helpful for an MRI evaluation of the hip?
Intravenous contrast agent is only very rarely helpful. Intravenous contrast agent may aid in the guidance of percutaneous biopsy by helping to distinguish viable tumor from cystic or necrotic tumor. Enhanced images may also help localize a soft tissue abscess and guide surgical drainage. Contrast imaging may help assess tissue viability in tumors or osteonecrosis.

6. What is avascular necrosis of the hip?
Osteonecrosis, previously referred to as avascular necrosis or aseptic necrosis, is a process of subchondral bone necrosis secondary to diminished or disrupted blood supply. The pathologic condition is very similar to that of a bone infarct; however, the articular location of hip avascular necrosis makes it clinically more critical than most bone infarcts.

7. What is the natural history of osteonecrosis? Why is the articular location so critical?
Compromised blood supply leads to infarct of the subchondral bone beneath the articular surface of the femoral head. The weight-bearing surface eventually collapses and fragments, disturbing joint mechanics and resulting in severe osteoarthritic changes of the hip. The risk of developing osteonecrosis is greatly influenced by the type of fracture. A nondisplaced fracture carries a low risk, approximately 10%, of developing osteonecrosis. A displaced femoral neck fracture may carry a risk of 80%, depending on vascular anatomy.

8. What is the blood supply to the femoral head?
The femoral head is predominantly nourished by a variable combination of the medial femoral circumflex artery and the ligamentum teres artery, which travels with the round ligament. Hip dislocations may tear the ligamentum teres artery, whereas femoral neck fractures may tear the medial femoral circumflex artery and its branches (Fig. 45-1).

9. Is osteonecrosis a unilateral or bilateral process?
It depends on the etiologic factor. Unilateral osteonecrosis is usually secondary to traumatic disruption of the blood supply to the femoral head and is often a sequela of hip dislocation or femoral neck fracture. Bilateral osteonecrosis is usually nontraumatic in etiology.

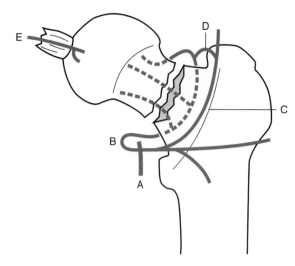

Figure 45-1. Arterial anatomy of femoral head and neck (*A* = deep femoral artery, *B* = medial femoral circumflex artery, *C* = lateral circumflex femoral artery, *D* = anastomosis of medial and lateral circumflex femoral arteries, *E* = artery of round ligament of the femoral head).

10. Which is more common, unilateral or bilateral osteonecrosis?
Bilateral disease accounts for approximately 50% to 80% of cases. The most common cause in the United States is steroid therapy.

11. What is an idiopathic cause of osteonecrosis in children?
Also known as Legg-Calvé-Perthes disease or coxa plana, Perthes disease usually affects children 3 to 12 years old and results from an inadequate blood supply to the femoral head. In most cases (87%), only one hip joint is affected. Most children with Perthes disease eventually recover, but it can take 2 to 5 years for the femoral head to regenerate. Treatments are available to encourage the femoral head to grow into a functional shape.

12. How is MRI useful in the treatment of osteonecrosis?
MRI is useful in the treatment of osteonecrosis because it enables early detection. MRI is the most sensitive modality for detection of early osteonecrosis, before femoral head cortical collapse. Early detection allows for possible joint-sparing therapies such as steroid reduction, supportive therapies such as non–weight-bearing, and core decompression. Small lesions that involve less than 25% of the weight-bearing portion of the femoral head have a better chance of responding to therapy without progression to femoral head collapse. Large areas of osteonecrosis do not respond to minimally invasive therapies such as core decompression. It is generally believed that if more than 50% of the articular surface is involved, the prognosis is poor, with eventual collapse and fragmentation of the femoral head, requiring total hip arthroplasty.

13. What are the MRI characteristics of osteonecrosis?
MRI characteristics are variable with heterogeneous signal characteristics. On fat-saturated T2-weighted images or short tau inversion recovery (STIR) images, 80% of patients may have the characteristic "double line" within the femoral head marrow (Fig. 45-2). This sign is composed of concentric rings with an inner low signal intensity ring surrounded by a high signal intensity outer ring. The irregular, inner low signal intensity line demarcates the peripheral aspect, or reactive interface, of the necrotic segment. This is paralleled by a high signal intensity line of marrow edema.

14. What are radiographically occult hip fractures?
Radiographically occult hip fractures are fractures that are not evident on plain radiographs. Examples include nondisplaced traumatic fractures, stress fractures, and insufficiency fractures. MRI is a very useful modality for detecting these fractures.

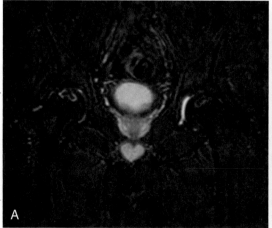
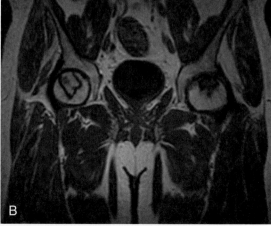

Figure 45-2. A and **B**, STIR (**A**) and T1-weighted (**B**) images of avascular necrosis of both femoral heads.

15. Why is MRI a useful modality for the detection of radiographically occult hip fractures?

MRI has very high sensitivity. Traumatic fractures can be nondisplaced sometimes and often impossible to identify on plain films. As soon as a fracture occurs, there is associated edema, however, which produces an immediate change in the bone marrow signal intensity (increased on fat-saturated T2-weighted or STIR images) that is easily seen on MRI (Fig. 45-3). Fractures are hypointense to marrow on T1-weighted images. Additionally, subtle cortical fracture lines, which may not be evident on plain radiographs for days or weeks until there is visible evidence of healing, may be easily seen on MRI.

16. What are the MRI signal characteristics of an acute fracture?

Fracture lines are low signal intensity on all pulse sequences. The edema associated with a fracture shows low signal intensity on T1-weighted images and high signal intensity on T2-weighted and STIR sequences. Traumatic fractures can sometimes be nondisplaced and are often impossible to identify on plain films. MRI is very sensitive for the identification of a nondisplaced fracture. Usually a fracture line is visible, but occasionally only diffuse edema without a fracture line is present.

17. There is clinical suspicion of an occult fracture related to trauma, but plain radiography displays normal results, and MRI reveals only diffuse edema without any sign of a dark fracture line. Does this scenario exclude a fracture?

No. These findings may represent a bone contusion, which is a microfracture of cancellous bone with associated edema and hemorrhage. On MRI, bone contusions often manifest as a speckled area in cancellous bone with low T1 signal intensity and high T2 signal intensity. The absence of cortical involvement not only explains the lack of a visible pathologic condition on plain radiography, but also highlights why MRI is far superior to computed tomography (CT) for diagnosis of occult fractures. Unless there is cortical disruption, CT may not show the fracture, especially the microfractures of a bone contusion, whereas MRI shows these changes. Contusions within the subchondral portion of the femoral head may lead to subsequent bone resorption and rapid development of osteoarthritis.

18. How many types of stress fractures are there?

There are two types of stress fracture: fatigue and insufficiency. Fatigue fractures are commonly referred to as stress fractures. A fatigue stress fracture results from repeated stress on a normal bone. An insufficiency fracture occurs in abnormal bone that has been weakened by decreased mineralization and fractures under stress of routine or normal activity.

19. In the hip, where do stress fractures usually occur?

Stress fractures usually occur in the transcervical neck. Stress fractures rarely involve the intertrochanteric region. Stress fractures in the femoral neck are not often seen on plain film because 67% may involve only cancellous bone, rather than cortical bone. Fracture in the femoral neck usually can be classified into one of two types: tension or compression. Tension stress fractures are usually perpendicular to the line of force transmission in the femoral neck, usually originate at the superior surface of the neck, and have increased risk of displacement. Compression stress fractures have radiologic changes of callus formation on the inferior femoral neck without apparent cortical disruption.

20. How are stress fractures of the hip usually treated?

Tension stress fractures are unstable and often require surgical stabilization. Treatment of compression stress fractures is usually nonsurgical with conservative measures of rest and protective weight bearing.

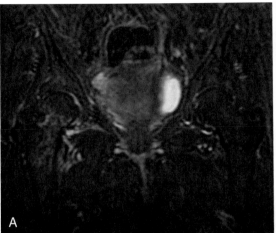 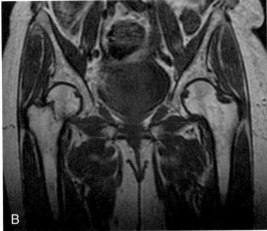

Figure 45-3. **A** and **B**, STIR (**A**) and T1-weighted (**B**) images of occult right hip fracture. The fracture line is hypointense to bone marrow on T1-weighted image and shows surrounding edema, which is hyperintense on STIR image.

Key Points: MRI of the Hip

1. Plain films are the first-choice modality for identification of hip fracture, but MRI shows nondisplaced fractures and microfractures not visible on plain film.
2. The most common cause of hip osteonecrosis in the United States is steroid therapy.

21. When a stress fracture or other occult fracture of the hip is diagnosed, which modality is best for follow-up?

Plain radiographs are best for follow-up. Routine plain films may be used to detect any changes or displacement of the fracture. A displaced femoral neck stress fracture in a young adult is a surgical emergency that requires open reduction and internal fixation.

22. Which individuals are prone to fatigue stress fracture?

Young, active individuals such as endurance athletes, ballet dancers, and military recruits are prone to fatigue stress fracture. Development of a stress fracture is often associated with initiation of a new activity or increased frequency or intensity of a routine athletic activity.

23. Who is most prone to insufficiency stress fracture?

A person prone to osteoporosis, such as a woman or elderly adult, or a patient with metabolic bone disease is most prone to insufficiency stress fracture. In elderly adults, a fall is often thought to be the cause of an acute femoral fracture; however, the fall actually may have resulted from displacement of a long-standing insufficiency fracture. It is thought that the displacement of an insufficiency fracture of the femoral neck may lead to a fall as the hip loses its stability. There is no radiographic difference between a completed insufficiency fracture and an acute, traumatic femoral fracture.

24. Does diffuse marrow edema without a fracture line always indicate a bone contusion or microfracture?

No. Often, the extensive edema related to subchondral contusions or occult fractures, which do not exhibit a fracture line, may lead to their misdiagnosis as osteonecrosis or transient osteoporosis of the hip.

25. What is transient osteoporosis of the hip?

Transient osteoporosis of the hip is most common in women in the later stages of pregnancy, although it may also occur in older men (50 to 70 years old). It manifests as sudden onset of pain that is increased with weight bearing. The cause is unknown, but it generally resolves in 6 to 12 months with supportive therapy. On MRI, transient osteoporosis of the hip is depicted as a marked increase in marrow signal on STIR images and decrease of marrow signal on T1-weighted images, reflecting the presence of marrow edema (Fig. 45-4).

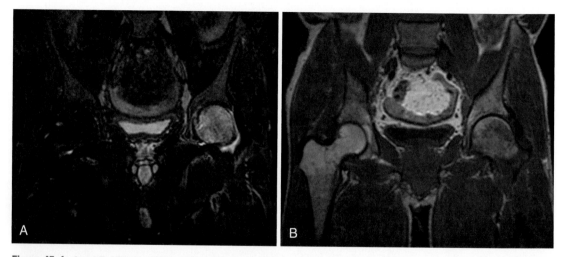

Figure 45-4. **A** and **B**, STIR (**A**) and T1-weighted (**B**) images of transient osteoporosis of the left hip. The bone edema is hyperintense to normal marrow on STIR image and hypointense on T1-weighted image.

MRI OF THE KNEE

Conor P. Shortt, MBBCh, MSc, and
Hanna M. Zafar, MD, MHS

1. What sequences should be included in a standard magnetic resonance imaging (MRI) knee protocol?

Sequences should include sagittal proton density–weighted (non–fat-saturated), and fat-saturated T2-weighted sequences in sagittal, coronal, and axial planes. A non–fat-saturated T1-weighted sequence (preferably in the coronal plane) is also recommended.

2. What structures in the knee are best evaluated in each plane?

- *Sagittal*: Anterior cruciate ligament (ACL)and posterior cruciate ligament (PCL), medial and lateral menisci, medial and lateral compartment cartilage, patellofemoral cartilage, and extensor mechanism
- *Coronal*: Medial and lateral collateral ligaments, medial and lateral menisci, and medial and lateral compartment cartilage
- *Axial*: Patella, patellar retinacula, patellofemoral cartilage, and Baker cysts

3. Identify the following labeled normal structures of the knee on Figs. 46-1 through 46-4.

A. ACL (Fig. 46-1)
B. PCL (Fig. 46-1)
C. Medial collateral ligament (Fig. 46-1)
D. Medial patellar retinaculum (Fig. 46-2)
E. Vastus medialis muscle (Fig. 46-2)
F. ACL (Fig. 46-3)
G. PCL (Fig. 46-3)
H. Patellar tendon (Fig. 46-3)
I. Quadriceps tendon (Fig. 46-3)
J. Anterior horn of lateral meniscus (Fig. 46-4)
K. Posterior horn of lateral meniscus (Fig. 46-4)
L. Popliteal tendon (Fig. 46-4)

4. What is a Baker (popliteal) cyst, where is it located, and what is its significance?

A Baker or popliteal cyst is a bursa that extends from the knee joint posteriorly between the tendons of the semimembranosus and medial head of gastrocnemius (Fig. 46-5). The presence of a Baker cyst suggests a chronic or recurrent knee joint effusion and should prompt a search for intra-articular pathology, particularly meniscal tears or cartilage defects.

5. What tendons compose the pes anserinus?

Remember "SGT": *s*emitendinosus, *g*racilis, and sar*t*orius. These tendons insert on the medial tibia approximately 5 cm distal to the knee joint line and are associated with a bursa, which can become inflamed. The semimembranosus–tibial collateral bursa is a separate entity.

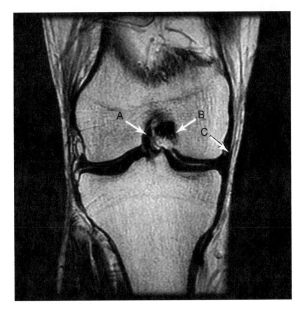

Figure 46-1. Coronal T1-weighted image.

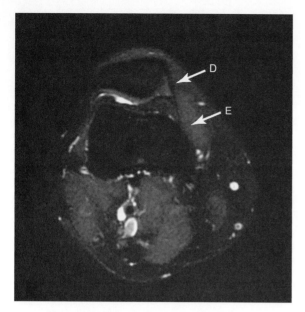

Figure 46-2. Axial fat-saturated T2-weighted image.

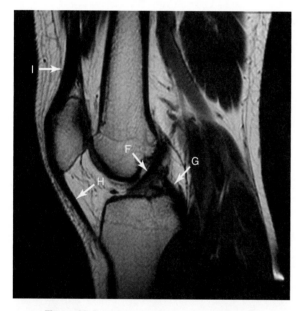

Figure 46-3. Sagittal proton density–weighted image.

6. Describe the clinical presentation of meniscal injury. Which portions of the menisci are more likely to be involved in injury?

The clinical presentation of a patient with a meniscal tear is pain and locking of the knee. The posterior horn of the medial meniscus is the primary weight-bearing surface and is more likely to be injured than the anterior horn of the medial meniscus. Peripheral meniscal tears occur at the more vascular zone of the meniscus, are more likely to heal, and often do not require surgery when they occur in isolation. The anterior horn of the lateral meniscus is the most common site for false-positive diagnoses of meniscal tear, where the normal anterior transverse meniscal ligament may simulate a tear.

7. What is the appearance of a normal meniscus and a torn meniscus on MRI?

The medial and lateral menisci are crescent-shaped structures that lie at the medial and lateral aspects of the superior articular surface of the tibia. They are composed mainly of fibrocartilage and show low signal intensity on all pulse sequences. On sagittal images, the menisci appear as bow tie–shaped structures.

8. What are the criteria for diagnosis of meniscal tear on MRI?

A meniscal tear is diagnosed by two major criteria:

- Increased signal intensity within the meniscus that extends to the articular surface on at least two contiguous slices (Fig. 46-6)
- Abnormal meniscal morphology

9. What common meniscal variant is associated with tears of the lateral meniscus, and what is the appearance on MRI?

Discoid meniscus is a common variant occurring in 3% of the population that appears as morphologic enlargement of the meniscus (Fig. 46-7). Patients usually present with clicking of the knee on extension and flexion. This entity is best diagnosed on coronal imaging and not sagittal views, which may vary in technique. On a coronal MR image taken through the mid–femoral condyle level, a meniscus that extends centrally beyond the mid-point of the femoral condyle should be called a discoid meniscus.

10. How can traumatic meniscal tears be differentiated from degenerative meniscal tears?

Traumatic tears are more likely to be oriented vertically, whereas degenerative tears are more likely to be oriented horizontally.

11. What is a bucket-handle tear? Describe the findings on MRI.

A bucket-handle tear is a subtype of a traumatic tear that constitutes 10% of all meniscal tears. MRI usually shows the following: (1) absence of the inner body segment, resembling a bow tie, known as the "absent bow tie sign," and (2) identification of a displaced meniscal fragment, which is often located in the intercondylar notch on coronal images, simulating a second PCL—the "double PCL" sign.

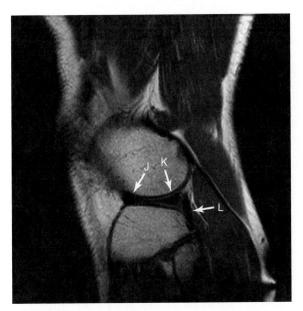

Figure 46-4. Sagittal proton density–weighted image.

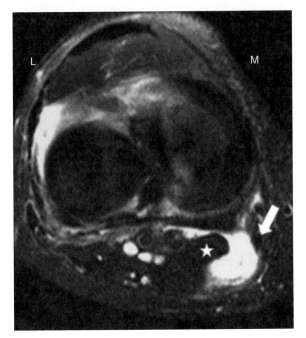

Figure 46-5. Baker cyst. Axial fat-saturated T2-weighted sequence through the level of the menisci. A Baker cyst is seen extending between the tendons of the semimembranosus (*arrow*) and medial head of gastrocnemius tendons (*asterisk*). Note also the normally larger surface area of the medial meniscus compared with the lateral. M = medial; L = lateral.

12. What are the sensitivity and specificity of MRI in the detection of meniscal tears?
MRI has a sensitivity of approximately 88% and a specificity of 94% for detection of meniscal tears. Proton density–weighted sequences are more sensitive than fat-saturated T2-weighted sequences, but less specific.

13. What are meniscal cysts, and what is their significance?
Meniscal (or parameniscal) cysts are due to extrusion of meniscal fluid after a meniscal tear. Typically, they arise within the meniscus or in the parameniscal soft tissues at the meniscocapsular junction. MRI is more sensitive than either physical examination or arthroscopy in the diagnosis of meniscal cysts. On MRI, these cysts have high signal intensity on T2-weighted images. They indicate a meniscal tear, even if a tear is not seen on imaging.

14. What are the points of attachment for the cruciate ligaments?
ACL arises on the medial surface of the lateral femoral condyle at the intercondylar notch and attaches on the anterior portion of the intercondylar eminence of the tibia. PCL arises from the lateral surface of the medial femoral condyle within the intercondylar notch and attaches at the posterior surface of the intercondylar eminence.

15. Which is more commonly injured, ACL or PCL?
ACL is much more commonly injured than PCL.

16. What is the MRI appearance of a torn ACL?
Direct MRI signs of ACL tear include the following:

- Visible disruption of the ligament
- Irregular or wavy contour
- Focal signal abnormality within the ligamentous substance
- "Empty notch" sign on coronal images (absence of ACL in its expected location)
- Anterior tibial spine avulsion

Indirect MRI signs of ACL tear include the following:

- Characteristic pivot-shift bone bruise pattern
- Deep lateral sulcus sign at the site of impaction injury at the anterior aspect of the lateral femoral condyle
- Segond fracture
- Anterior drawer sign (anterior translation of tibia relative to femur by >5 mm) (Figs. 46-8 and 46-9)

17. What are the sensitivity and specificity of MRI for the detection of complete ACL and PCL tears?
MRI has an approximate sensitivity of 94% and a specificity of 94% for complete ACL tears and a sensitivity of 91% and a specificity of 99% for complete PCL tears.

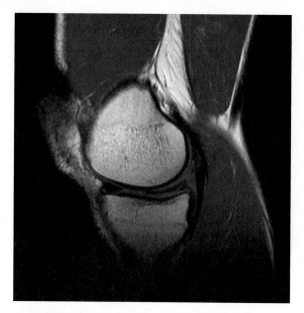

Figure 46-6. Medial meniscal tear. Sagittal proton density–weighted image of the lateral aspect of the knee shows linear high signal intensity within the posterior horn of the medial meniscus. This increased signal extends to the inferior articular surface. Its vertical/oblique orientation is most consistent with a traumatic etiology.

18. What are the components of the medial collateral ligament and lateral collateral ligament complex?

- The medial collateral ligament comprises the deep layer, which includes the medial meniscofemoral and meniscotibial ligaments, and the superficial layer (usually understood as the main medial collateral ligament), which is the tibial collateral ligament.
- The lateral collateral ligament complex (anterior to posterior) comprises the iliotibial band, fibular collateral ligament, and biceps femoris tendon.

19. What structures are important stabilizers at the posterolateral corner of the knee, and why are they important?

The important posterolateral stabilizers are the lateral collateral ligament complex (iliotibial band, fibular collateral ligament, and biceps femoris tendon), popliteus muscle and tendon, lateral head of gastrocnemius tendon, and other ligaments including the arcuate/fabellofibular and popliteofibular ligaments.

High-grade injury to the posterolateral corner, if left untreated, is associated with a poor outcome. If MRI findings of posterolateral injury are detected, the referring clinician should be informed as soon as possible, and clinical correlation should be undertaken for signs of instability.

Key Points: MRI of the Knee

1. Abnormal signal within a meniscus is insufficient to diagnose meniscal tear on MRI. Abnormal meniscal signal intensity must extend to the meniscal surface on two contiguous slices to be called meniscal tear on MRI.
2. Diagnosis of ACL tear should prompt a search for commonly associated injuries, including medial collateral ligament injury, medial meniscal tear, Segond fracture, and bone contusions.
3. Findings of posterolateral corner injury on MRI should be relayed to the referring clinician as soon as possible because untreated high-grade injuries have a poor prognosis.

---

20. What is O'Donoghue's "unhappy triad"?

O'Donoghue's "unhappy triad" is a common football and skiing injury that occurs as a result of valgus stress and twisting motion during weight bearing. Classically, medial collateral ligament injury, ACL tear, and medial meniscal tear result.

21. What is the grading system for medial collateral ligament injury?

See Table 46-1. Medial collateral ligament tears without other injury rarely require surgery.

22. List the signs of lateral patellar dislocation.

- Reciprocal bone bruising at anterolateral aspect of the lateral femoral condyle and medial aspect of the medial patellar facet
- Patellofemoral cartilage injury
- Injury to the medial patellar retinaculum or medial patellofemoral ligament or both
- Knee joint effusion

The presence of a shallow patellar notch may predispose patients to this injury (Fig. 46-10).

23. What is jumper's knee?

Jumper's knee, also known as *patellar tendinitis,* is an overuse syndrome that classically occurs in young athletes who kick, jump, and run. These actions place stress on the patellofemoral joint with intrasubstance degeneration and partial tearing of

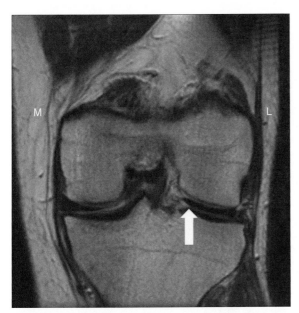

Figure 46-7. Discoid lateral meniscus. Coronal T1-weighted sequence through mid–femoral condyle level shows a lateral meniscus that extends centrally beyond the mid-point of the lateral femoral condyle (*arrow*), representing a discoid lateral meniscus. Note how the normal medial meniscus does not extend beyond the mid-point of the medial femoral condyle. M = medial; L = lateral.

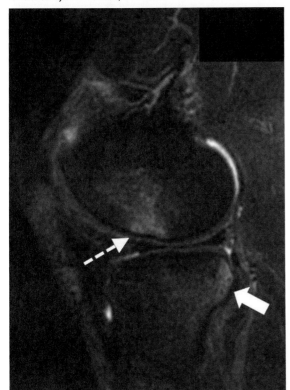

Figure 46-8. Pivot-shift bone bruise pattern. Sagittal fat-saturated T2-weighted sequence shows bone edema (high signal) at the anterior aspect of the lateral femoral condyle (*dashed arrow*) and at the posterolateral tibial plateau (*solid arrow*) indicating reciprocal bone bruise at the site of pivot-shift mechanism of injury during anterior translation of the tibia with respect to the femur. This is one of the most helpful indirect signs of ACL tear.

the tendon. Patellar tendinitis is characterized on MRI by proximal patellar tendon thickening and edema (increased signal on fluid-sensitive sequences). In more severe cases, there is concomitant edema in Hoffa fat and at the inferior pole of patella.

24. What is meant by the term *osteochondral lesion*?

An osteochondral lesion describes an articular surface defect involving separation of the cartilage and a portion of the underlying bone from the remainder of the bone. It encompasses etiologies that may overlap, including traumatic osteochondral fractures, osteochondral lesions associated with insufficiency fractures, and osteochondritis dissecans (OCD).

25. What is OCD?

OCD refers to a chronic separation of subchondral bone and overlying cartilage, which may have been initially precipitated by trauma. OCD most commonly occurs in individuals 10 to 20 years old, particularly in males, and has a predilection for the lateral aspect of the medial femoral condyle.

26. Why is OCD graded?

The management of OCD is contingent on determining fragment stability, with most unstable lesions requiring operative management.

27. How is OCD graded?

MRI signs of an unstable fragment in an adult include one or more of the following findings on fluid-sensitive sequences (T2 or short-tau inversion recovery [STIR]):

- Presence of surrounding high T2 signal intensity rim
- Cysts surrounding an OCD lesion
- High T2 signal intensity fracture line extending through the articular cartilage overlying an OCD lesion
- Fluid-filled osteochondral defect

In juvenile OCD, signs of instability require stricter criteria.

28. Describe the MRI appearances of subchondral insufficiency fracture of the knee.

Spontaneous osteonecrosis of the knee is now considered a subchondral insufficiency fracture. It usually manifests in adults in the sixth or seventh decade as acute onset of pain without inciting trauma and often involves the medial femoral condyle. In the early stages, MRI shows subchondral edema on fluid-sensitive sequences, which may progress to articular surface flattening and subchondral osteonecrosis (low signal). In the later stages of the condition, bone marrow edema decreases as cartilage loss and other changes of osteoarthritis develop.

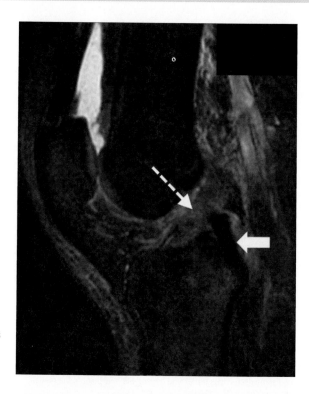

Figure 46-9. Complete ACL tear. Sagittal fat-saturated T2-weighted sequence in the same patient as in Fig. 46-8 shows absence of the ACL at its proximal and mid portion representing complete tear (*dashed arrow*). Note the normal homogeneous low signal of the distal portion of the PCL (*solid arrow*).

Table 46-1. Grading System for Medial Collateral Ligament Injury

Grade I (sprain)	Edema around intact ligament
Grade II (partial tear)	Edema within ligament with or without fiber disruption not involving entire medial collateral ligament at a given level
Grade III (complete tear)	Complete disruption of ligament

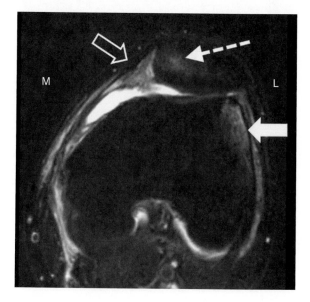

Figure 46-10. Transient lateral patellar dislocation. Axial fat-saturated T2-weighted image through the patella shows reciprocal bone bruising (high signal) at the anterolateral aspect of the lateral femoral condyle (*solid arrow*) and medial patellar facet (*dashed arrow*) from recent transient lateral patellar dislocation. The medial retinaculum (*open arrow*) is thickened with surrounding edema, representing partial tear. M = medial; L = lateral.

BIBLIOGRAPHY

[1] R. Mansour, M. Kausik, E. McNally, MRI of knee joint injury, Semin. Musculoskelet. Radiol. 10 (2006) 328–344.
[2] W.B. Morrison, T.G. Sanders, Problem Solving in Musculoskeletal Radiology, Mosby, Philadelphia, 2008, pp. 565–652.
[3] T.L. Pope, H.L. Bloem, J. Beltran, et al., Imaging of the Musculoskeletal System, Saunders, Philadelphia, 2008, pp. 537–689.

MRI OF THE FOOT AND ANKLE

Neil Roach, MD

CHAPTER 47

1. What are the four compartments around the ankle, and what do they contain?

The four compartments are medial, lateral, anterior, and posterior. The compartmental organization is helpful in thinking of tendon anatomy.

- The *medial compartment* contains (anterior to posterior) the posterior *t*ibialis tendon (PTT), flexor *d*igitorum longus (FDL) tendon, and flexor *h*allucis longus (FHL) tendon: "Tom, Dan, and Harry." (The "an" in Dan refers to the posterior tibial artery and nerve.)
- The *lateral compartment* contains the peroneal brevis and longus.
- The *anterior compartment* contains (medial to lateral) the extensor *t*ibialis tendon, extensor *h*allucis longus tendon, and extensor *d*igitorum longus tendon: "Tom, Harry, and Dick."
- The *posterior compartment* contains the Achilles tendon.

2. What is the most commonly injured ankle tendon?

The Achilles tendon is most commonly injured. It usually tears 3 to 5 cm superior to its calcaneal insertion, where the blood supply of the tendon is poorest. Tears may also occur at the musculotendinous (usually the lateral gastrocnemius) junction, but this is much less common. Tears occur least commonly at the calcaneal insertion secondary to injury or ill-fitting shoes. Normal tendon signal is very low on T1-weighted and T2-weighted MR images. The morphologic features of the tendon should be evaluated on sagittal and axial images, with the anterior surface of the normal tendon flat or concave on axial images.

3. Describe the magnetic resonance imaging (MRI) appearance of Achilles tendon tears.

Achilles abnormalities on MRI tend to cover a progressive sequence of disorders:

- *Peritendinitis*: The Achilles tendon does not have a sheath; only peritendinitis, not synovitis, can occur. Peritendinitis is seen as infiltrative changes in the fat surrounding the tendon.
- *Tendonopathy*: Any internal tendon signal is indicative of tendonopathy.
- *Chronic tendonopathy*: Chronic tendonopathy is visualized on MRI as an enlarged and abnormally shaped tendon.
- *Interstitial tears*: Interstitial tears are depicted on MRI as longitudinally oriented internal signal changes first seen on T1-weighted images. As these tears become more severe, T2-weighted images are abnormal also.
- *Partial tears*: Partial tears are horizontally oriented signal abnormalities.
- *Complete tears*: Complete Achilles disruption with retraction of the torn ends is similar in appearance to the end of a mop.

4. Which of the flexor or medial tendons is most commonly torn?

The PTT is the most common of the medial tendons to tear. These tears most often occur in middle-aged women. PTT disruption results in "adult-onset" flat foot. PTT tears usually occur near the tendon insertion site and are associated with accessory navicular or a cornuate navicular bones. Normally, the PTT is twice the size as the FDL or FHL tendon. One must suspect a PTT tear if there is tenosynovitis or if the tendon is greatly enlarged. Comparing the size of the PTT with the FDL or FHL tendon can be useful.

5. Name the three ligaments that form the lateral collateral ligament.

The anterior talofibular, calcaneofibular, and posterior talofibular ligaments form the lateral collateral ligament.

6. Which of these three ligaments tends to tear first?

The anterior talofibular ligament is the most commonly injured ligament. The calcaneofibular ligament is the next most commonly injured ligament. The posterior talofibular ligament is easily identified on coronal MR images, but is rarely injured.

7. Which bones form the hindfoot, midfoot, and forefoot?

- The *hindfoot* comprises the calcaneus and talus.
- The *midfoot* comprises the navicular, the three cuneiform bones, and the cuboid.
- The *forefoot* comprises the metatarsals and phalanges.

8. What are the articulations of the subtalar joint?

- The *posterior facet* is the largest and the "true" subtalar joint.
- The *middle facet* is formed by the sustentaculum tali (of the calcaneus) and the anterior talus. It has a flat joint surface.
- The *anterior facet* (vestigial) may be independent of or contiguous with the middle facet and has a rounded surface.

9. Describe the tarsal canal and the sinus tarsi.

The tarsal canal and sinus tarsi form the boundary between the posterior subtalar joint and the anteriorly located talocalcaneal navicular joint. The tarsal canal and sinus extend from posteromedial to anterolateral. The tarsal canal extends to the medial aspect of the foot, posterior to the sustentaculum tali. The canal widens to form the sinus tarsi, which is cone-shaped and opens laterally. The sinus tarsi contains fat, blood vessels, and the interosseous and cervical ligaments and branches of the tibial nerve.

10. Which ligament around the ankle is least likely to tear?

The medially located deltoid ligament is very strong and uncommonly tears. Eversion injuries, rather than ligament tears, usually cause avulsion fractures of the medial malleolus. The deltoid is composed of four ligaments—two superficial and two deep.

11. What are the three plantar compartments, and why are they important?

The plantar compartments of the foot are important for the evaluation of infection and tumor extent. The three plantar compartments are separated by fascial planes.

- The *medial compartment (first ray)* contains the abductor hallucis muscle, the flexor hallucis brevis muscle, the tendon of the flexor hallucis longus muscle, the medial plantar nerve and vessels, and the first metatarsal bone.
- The *central compartment (second, third, and fourth rays)* contains the flexor digitorum brevis muscle, the quadratus plantae, the four plantar lumbricales muscles, the tendon of the flexor digitorum longus muscle, a portion of the tendon of the flexor hallucis longus muscle, and the lateral plantar nerve and vessels. The central compartment also contains the second, third, and fourth metatarsals. The thick, longitudinally oriented plantar aponeurosis forms the floor of the central compartment. This compartment is important because it communicates with the calf and can serve as a pathway for spread of infection.
- The *lateral compartment (fifth ray)* contains the fifth metatarsal and the abductor digiti minimi and flexor digitorum minimi brevis muscles.

12. What is tarsal coalition?

Tarsal coalition is fusion of one or more intertarsal joints. The fusion can be osseous, fibrocartilaginous, or fibro-osseous. Patients usually present in adolescence with a spastic flatfoot. It can be bilateral in 20% to 25% of cases. Hereditary forms exist. Calcaneonavicular fusion is the most common type based on plain film experience. Computed tomography (CT) and MRI show that talocalcaneal fusion may be more common. Secondary signs of tarsal coalition include talar beaking and a ball-and-socket ankle joint. MRI diagnosis of an osseous coalition, shown by continuity of the bone marrow, is straightforward (Fig. 47-1). Fibrocartilaginous or fibro-osseous coalitions require evaluation of articular surfaces for irregularities and for low signal fibrous tissue bands that are more difficult to appreciate.

13. What are common sites for stress fractures of the foot?

Calcaneal and metatarsal stress fractures are the most common stress fractures in the foot. On T1-weighted images, the edema and hemorrhage of the fracture appear as bands of low signal traversing the normally high signal bone marrow. Fat-suppressed T2-weighted or short tau inversion recovery (STIR) images show areas of increased signal intensity in the region of the fracture (Fig. 47-2).

14. Which part of the dome of the talus is typically injured in repetitive trauma? What part of the talar dome is typically involved if there is a single bad traumatic event?

Osteochondral injuries are most common in adolescents and in males. If the injury is caused by repetitive injury, the medial talar dome is usually affected. If the injury is caused by a single bad traumatic event, the lateral talar dome is usually involved.

15. MRI and magnetic resonance arthrography of the ankle may be useful in evaluating the different types of osteochondral injuries. How are osteochondral injuries classified?

- *Stable*: Ill-defined rim of high T2 signal is present around the lesion, but the cartilage is intact.
- *Loose in situ*: The cartilage is injured.
- *Partially loose*: Incomplete but well-defined ring of high T2 signal is present around the lesion.
- *Loose complete*: Well-defined ring of signal surrounds the fragment or a cyst associated with the lesion or both.
- *Free*: Intra-articular body has an empty crater.

16. Describe characteristics used to differentiate between osteomyelitis and neuropathic arthropathy?

The distinction between neuropathic joint arthropathy and osteomyelitis is based on distribution of disease, the association with an ulcer, and the MRI signal characteristics of the bone marrow. Neuropathic arthropathy usually affects the Lisfranc, metatarsophalangeal, and subtalar joints. Osteomyelitis can affect any bone, but it is usually associated with contiguous spread from an ulcer and abnormal adjacent soft tissues. STIR sequences are very sensitive to edema in bones, whether the edema is due to osteomyelitis or to neuropathic/osteoarthritic changes. Because bone edema is not specific for bone infection, STIR images may lead to false-positive diagnoses of osteomyelitis, and the finding of bone edema must be interpreted in light of other MRI findings. Postgadolinium images are also helpful in evaluating edema versus cellulitis.

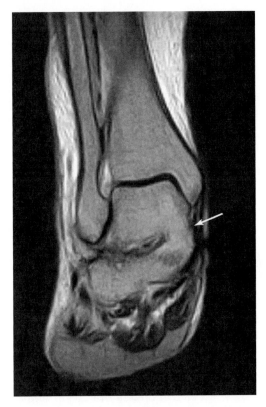

Figure 47-1. Coronal T1-weighted image of the ankle shows an osseous calcaneal-talar coalition (*arrow*) at the level of the middle facet of the subtalar joint.

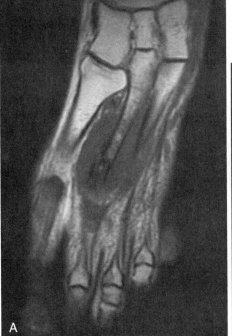

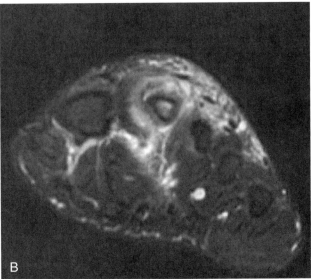

Figure 47-2. A, T1-weighted axial image of the forefoot shows a stress fracture of the second metatarsal. **B,** Coronal fat-suppressed T2-weighted image outlines the soft tissue and bone marrow edema from the stress fracture in **A.**

17. What MRI findings are related to plantar fasciitis?

Plantar fasciitis is seen as increased T2 signal adjacent to the proximal insertion of the plantar fascia with or without a plantar enthesophyte. The fascia may be thickened. Refractory cases can show bone marrow edema adjacent to the plantar fascia insertion on the calcaneus (Fig. 47-3).

18. What is plantar fibromatosis?

Patients present with pain on weight bearing and have palpable nodular thickening along the course of the plantar fascia. Plantar fibromatosis can be bilateral in 10% to 40% of patients and may occur in any age group; males are affected twice as often as females. On T1-weighted images, the lesion can be hypointense or isointense to muscle. On T2-weighted images, the lesion may be hypointense or slightly hyperintense. These lesions enhance intensely with gadolinium and are usually bright on STIR images.

19. What are Morton neuromas?

Morton neuromas are small, focal masses of fibrosis and do not represent a true neuroma involving the plantar digital nerves. They occur most commonly between the third and fourth metatarsals and can be bilateral in 25% of cases. Women 25 to 50 years old are the most likely to be affected. T1-weighted and T2-weighted images show low signal intensity secondary to fibrosis.

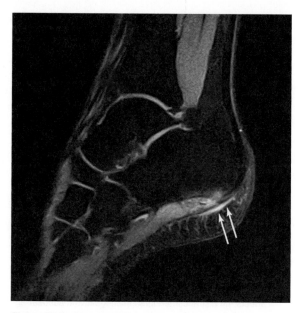

Figure 47-3. Sagittal STIR image of the ankle shows soft tissue and bone marrow edema in a patient with plantar fasciitis (*arrows*).

20. What characterizes the tarsal tunnel?

The tarsal tunnel is located on the medial side of the ankle. It begins superiorly at the medial malleolus and extends inferiorly to the navicular bone. The lateral side of the tunnel is formed by the calcaneus, including the sustentaculum tali, and the talus. The flexor retinaculum forms the medial wall, and the abductor hallucis muscle forms the floor of the tunnel. The posterior tibial nerve and its divisions—the posterior tibial artery and vein and the PTT, FDL tendon, and FHL tendon—are within the tunnel.

21. What is tarsal tunnel syndrome?

Patients with tarsal tunnel syndrome usually present with pain and paresthesia along the distribution of the posterior tibial nerve and its branches. Patients typically complain of pain and burning on the plantar aspect of the foot. Half of cases are idiopathic, with the remainder secondary to scarring, osseous deformities, soft tissue masses, or varicose veins.

22. What is sinus tarsi syndrome, and what does it look like on MRI?

In sinus tarsi syndrome, there is loss of the normal fat within the sinus tarsi. In acute or subacute cases, there is low T1 signal and high T2 signal secondary to inflammation. In chronic cases, there is low T1 and T2 signal secondary to fibrosis. Patients complain of weakness and instability in the ankle with palpable tenderness over the sinus tarsi. Most cases are idiopathic, but some patients have a history of ankle inversion injury. Other causes of sinus tarsi include inflammatory conditions, such as rheumatoid arthritis or gout, and ganglion cysts.

23. Of the bones of the foot and ankle, which is the most likely to develop avascular necrosis? What is the typical cause of this?

The talus is the most likely to develop avascular necrosis related to fracture of the neck of the talus and loss of the blood supply to the dome. Avascular necrosis eventually leads to deformity and collapse of the dome.

Key Points: MRI of the Foot and Ankle

1. Tendon tears are generally related to a progressive sequence of disorders.
2. MRI can commonly detect fractures in the foot and ankle that are not appreciated on radiographs or CT scans.
3. The deltoid ligament practically never tears. Avulsion fractures of the medial malleolus generally occur before deltoid ligament tears.
4. Tarsal coalitions are usually seen in children and adolescents.

BIBLIOGRAPHY

[1] J. Beltran, D.S. Campanini, C. Knight, M. McCalla, The diabetic foot: magnetic resonance imaging evaluation, Skeletal. Radiol. 19 (1990) 37–41.

[2] Y. Cheung, Z.S. Rosenberg, T. Magee, L. Chinitz, Normal anatomy and pathologic conditions of ankle tendons: current imaging techniques, Radiographics 12 (1992) 429–444.

[3] P.A. Kaplan, R. Dussault, M.W. Anderson, N.M. Major, Musculoskeletal MRI, Saunders, Philadelphia, 2001.

[4] M.A. Klein, A.M. Spreitzer, MR imaging of the tarsal sinus and canal: normal anatomy, pathologic findings, and features of the sinus tarsi syndrome, Radiology 186 (1993) 233–240.

[5] R.J. Wechsler, M.E. Schweitzer, D.M. Deely, et al., Tarsal coalition: depiction and characterization with CT and MR imaging, Radiology 193 (1994) 447–452.

VIII
NEURORADIOLOGY

BRAIN: ANATOMY, TRAUMA, AND TUMORS

Ann K. Kim, MD, Gul Moonis, MD, and
Laurie A. Loevner, MD

CHAPTER 48

1. **Identify the parts of the brain labeled *1* through *6* in Fig. 48-1.**
   See figure legend for answers.

2. **What are the two primary imaging modalities used to image the brain?**
   The two major noninvasive cross-sectional imaging modalities used in neuroimaging are computed tomography (CT) and magnetic resonance imaging (MRI). Catheter angiography is reserved for the detection of intracranial vascular processes, such as aneurysms and intracranial vasculitis. Myelography involves the injection of contrast material into the subarachnoid space by lumbar puncture, allowing visualization of the spinal cord and nerve roots, which are seen as "filling defects" within the contrast-opacified cerebrospinal fluid (CSF). Myelography (usually followed by postmyelography CT) is reserved for patients with contraindications to MRI (e.g., patients with pacemakers or severe claustrophobia), patients with surgical hardware (pedicle screws), patients with equivocal MRI findings, and obese patients who exceed weight limits for MRI scanners.

3. **What are the clinical indications for obtaining CT and MRI of the brain?**
   A CT scan is a good initial screening examination for evaluating the brain for the presence of abnormalities. It is the primary imaging modality for assessing for acute intracranial hemorrhage, subarachnoid hemorrhage (SAH), mass effect, hydrocephalus, and stroke. The greater tissue contrast of MRI and its multiplanar capabilities make MRI the imaging modality of choice, however, for the assessment of a large spectrum of pathologic processes, including, but not limited to, metastatic disease, primary glial neoplasms, neurodegenerative disorders, and inflammatory and infectious processes. MRI is less sensitive than CT for the detection of SAH and calcification. In many instances, CT and MRI have complementary roles in the evaluation of pathologic conditions (especially lesions at the skull base and lesions involving the calvaria).

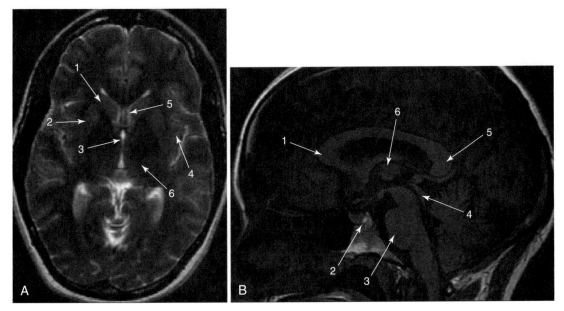

Figure 48-1. **A,** Axial T2-weighted MR image of the brain at the level of the basal ganglia (*1*, caudate head; *2*, putamen; *3*, third ventricle; *4*, insular cortex; *5*, septum pellucidum; *6*, thalamus). **B,** Sagittal T1-weighted image of the brain at midline (*1*, anterior genu of the corpus callosum; *2*, posterior lobe of the pituitary gland ["pituitary bright spot"]; *3*, pons; *4*, tectal plate; *5*, splenium of the corpus callosum; *6*, mass intermedia).

4. What are contraindications for performing MRI of the brain?

Contraindications include implanted electronic devices, such as pacemakers, neurostimulator devices, non–MRI-compatible vascular clips, ferromagnetic metallic implants, and foreign bodies in the eye. Severe claustrophobia is a relative contraindication, and, if necessary, most patients with this condition can successfully undergo MRI with sedation. MRI cannot be performed on individuals who have a metallic intracranial aneurysm clip. Most aneurysm clips used after 1995 are made of titanium and are MRI-compatible.

5. Define the terms *intra-axial* and *extra-axial,* which are commonly used to localize intracranial pathologic conditions.

An *intra-axial* abnormality arises from the brain parenchyma. An *extra-axial* lesion is one that arises outside of the brain substance and may be pial, dural, subdural, epidural, or intraventricular in origin. The most common extra-axial mass is a meningioma. In adults, the most common solitary intra-axial masses are primary brain tumors and metastatic disease. An intra-axial mass lesion expands the brain, results in gyral swelling, or results in effacement of the cerebral sulci. Imaging features that identify a mass as extra-axial include inward buckling of the gray and white matter, the presence of a cleft (which may be CSF, dura, or small vessels) separating the extra-axial mass from the brain, and the presence of remodeling of the adjacent osseous calvaria (Fig. 48-2).

6. What is nephrogenic systemic fibrosis (NSF), and who is at risk for developing this complication?

NSF is a rare systemic syndrome that involves fibrosis of the skin, muscles, joints, eyes, and internal organs. It is a disease process seen in patients with severe renal dysfunction and patients with renal dysfunction awaiting liver transplants (concomitant liver failure). At the time of this writing, no known cases of NSF have been seen in patients with normal renal function. There is an accepted association of the administration of the MRI contrast agent gadodiamide (Omniscan) with the development of NSF in patients with renal failure. Gadolinium-based contrast agents are metabolized entirely through the renal system; gadolinium agents have a prolonged half-life in renal failure patients. Metabolic by-products may result in the formation of free Gd^{3+}, which is very toxic. Not all patients with renal failure who received gadodiamide developed NSF, however, so other factors are present that contribute to its development. Increased incidence of NSF was seen in patients when there was a delay of greater than 2 days between administration of contrast agent and receiving dialysis. Research in this area is ongoing.

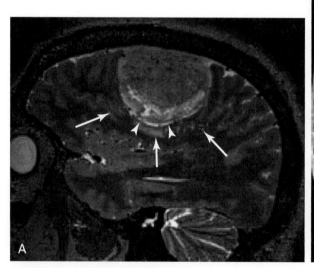
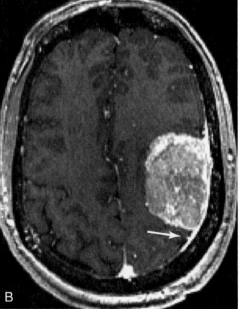

Figure 48-2. A, Intracranial meningioma. Sagittal T2-weighted MR image shows large meningioma in the left frontotemporal region that is isointense to gray matter. Note the inward buckling of the gray and white matter (*arrows*) and the CSF cleft (*arrowheads*), indicating its extra-axial site of origin. **B,** Axial T1-weighted contrast-enhanced image shows homogeneous enhancement of this mass with a dural tail (*arrow*), characteristic of a meningioma.

7. Is gadodiamide the only MRI contrast agent available?

No. There are five U.S. Food and Drug Administration(FDA)–approved gadolinium-containing MRI contrast agents: gadodiamide (Omniscan), gadoversetamide (OptiMARK), gadopentetate dimeglumine (Magnevist), gadobenate dimeglumine (MultiHance), and gadoteridol (ProHance). NSF has been reported only with Omniscan as of this writing. The FDA is actively investigating potential associations with all gadolinium-containing contrast agents. It is imperative for one to be familiar with the specific institution's guidelines on the administration of MRI contrast agents in patients with renal insufficiency.

8. What is the imaging modality of choice for imaging acute head trauma?

The imaging modality of choice for imaging acute head trauma is an unenhanced brain CT scan. CT is readily available and is a fast, accurate method for detecting acute intracranial hemorrhage. On CT, acute hemorrhage is hyperdense to brain and may display mass effect. Emergency physicians and neurosurgeons want to know the exact cause of clinical symptoms in a trauma patient. Specifically, the most significant concern is whether there is a treatable lesion. CT plays a primary role in evaluating the extent of trauma and in determining the appropriate management. It is sensitive in distinguishing brain contusions from extra-axial hematomas (subdural and epidural). CT is also excellent for detecting depressed facial and calvarial fractures. When diffuse axonal shear injury is suspected, MRI is more sensitive and can be obtained when the patient is clinically able to tolerate this examination.

9. How does one differentiate a subdural hematoma from an epidural hematoma?

An epidural hematoma is usually caused by an arterial injury (most commonly, the middle meningeal artery is injured as a result of a fracture of the temporal bone through which it courses) (Fig. 48-3A). An epidural hematoma is extra-axial, runs between the periosteum of the inner table of the skull and the dura, and is confined by the lateral sutures (especially the coronal sutures) where the dura inserts. As a result, an epidural hematoma is usually lenticular in shape. In contrast, a subdural hematoma is usually caused by injury to the bridging cortical veins (Fig. 48-3B). A subdural hematoma runs between the dura and the pia-arachnoid meninges on the surface of the brain and is not confined by the lateral sutures. As a result, subdural hematomas are usually crescentic in shape. In the midline, the dural reflection is attached to the falx cerebri, however. Subdural hematomas (in contrast to epidural hematomas) do not cross the midline, but rather track in the interhemispheric fissure. Subdural hematomas are commonly seen in patients with closed head trauma; elderly patients with minor head trauma; and patients with rapid decompression of hydrocephalus and extra-axial hematomas, where abrupt changes in intracranial pressure make the bridging cortical veins vulnerable.

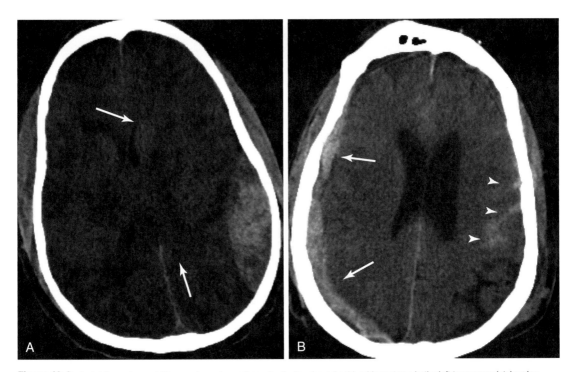

Figure 48-3. **A,** Axial unenhanced CT scan shows hyperdense, lenticular-shaped epidural hematoma in the left temporoparietal region. Note the mass effect on the adjacent left lateral ventricle that is effaced (*arrows*). **B,** Axial unenhanced CT scan shows right hemispheric subdural hematoma (*arrows*) that crosses the coronal and lambdoid sutures. Note the hyperdensity in the sulci of the left cerebral hemisphere, consistent with acute SAH (*arrowheads*).

Key Points: Epidural Hemorrhage

1. This is an arterial injury, usually the middle meningeal artery.
2. It is associated with temporal bone or other skull fractures.
3. It has a biconvex, lenticular shape; blood is contained by dural sutures.
4. This is a surgical emergency.

Key Points: Subdural Hemorrhage

1. This is a venous injury to bridging cortical veins.
2. Skull fracture may not be present.
3. It is usually crescentic in shape and not contained by sutures; it does not cross falx or tentorium.
4. This is found in trauma patients, older patients, and child abuse victims.

10. What is the CT appearance of traumatic SAH?

SAH appears as hyperdensity in the subarachnoid spaces. The subarachnoid spaces are identified by their serpentine appearance, dipping in between the gyri of the brain (see Fig. 48-3B). SAH in the setting of trauma usually indicates the presence of superficial cortical contusions.

Key Points: Subarachnoid Hemorrhage

1. Blood is in subarachnoid spaces; hyperdensity is in CSF spaces.
2. Aneurysm rupture or post-traumatic superficial cortical contusions are the cause.
3. Vasospasm several days afterward may lead to secondary infarction.

11. What is the Glasgow Coma Scale? How is it used?

The Glasgow Coma Scale was devised to provide a uniform approach to clinical assessment of trauma patients with acute head trauma. To measure level of awareness and responsiveness, the scale assigns numeric values (1 to 5) to each of the following: eye opening, best motor response, and best verbal response. Scores of 13 to 15 correspond to mild closed head injury; 9 to 12, to moderate head injury; and 8 or less to severe brain injury. The Glasgow Coma Scale does not correlate with survival outcome in cases of severe head trauma with coma.

12. What are the advantages and drawbacks of MRI in assessing a trauma patient?

The availability and speed of CT and its high sensitivity in detecting treatable lesions make it the imaging modality of choice for the initial assessment of trauma patients with head injury. MRI is more sensitive in distinguishing between the different ages of hemorrhage (hyperacute, acute, subacute, and chronic), in detecting shear injury (diffuse axonal injury), and in detecting injury in the posterior fossa and the undersurfaces of the frontal and temporal lobes. MRI is less sensitive than CT in detecting intracranial air and fractures. In addition, logistic difficulties occur in performing MRI on trauma patients: MRI times are significantly longer, performing MRI in patients on ventilators and other monitoring devices can be very cumbersome, and the location of most MRI scanners is outside of the emergency department. Although the fluid-attenuated inversion recovery (FLAIR) sequence on MRI can be as sensitive or more sensitive than CT in detecting subarachnoid hemorrhage, it is less specific, and the difficulty in quickly obtaining MRI in the acute trauma setting still renders CT the study of choice in assessing a trauma patient.

13. Define penetrating injury to the brain, and identify common causes.

Penetrating injuries result in brain "lacerations," and they are most commonly associated with bullets, stab wounds, and depressed or dislodged bone fragments. There is risk of injury to all vital structures traversed by the penetrating object. The most important of these are the brain and vascular structures (arteries and veins/dural venous sinuses).

14. **What are the five patterns of brain herniation and herniation syndromes?**

The brain is in a confined compartment (the skull) and is compartmentalized further by inelastic dural attachments (falx cerebri, falx cerebelli, and tentorium). Brain swelling, or mass lesions when large enough, forces brain from one compartment into another. If untreated, this herniation can result in further brain damage and vascular injury. Five patterns of brain herniation are as follows:

- Inferior tonsillar/cerebellar
- Superior vermian (upward)
- Temporal lobe
- Subfalcine
- Central transtentorial

Mass effect, especially in the posterior fossa, may also result in acute, obstructive hydrocephalus.

15. **What is the imaging manifestation of a brain contusion?**

Contusions are parenchymal bruises of the brain with associated petechial hemorrhage usually related to direct trauma to the head. The most common locations are the inferior, anterior, and lateral surfaces of the frontal and temporal lobes, owing to direct impact of the brain against the rough edges of the inner table of the skull along the floor of the anterior cranial fossa, the sphenoid wing, and the petrous ridges. On CT, hemorrhagic contusions appear as focal areas of hyperdensity (blood) with surrounding hypodensity (edema) in characteristic anatomic locations of the brain. On T2-weighted MR images, acute hemorrhagic contusions are hypointense (dark) with surrounding high-intensity (bright) edema. On gradient-echo susceptibility images, these lesions are detected with increased sensitivity as areas of signal drop-out (hypointensity, or "dark").

16. **What are the imaging manifestations of diffuse axonal injury?**

Diffuse axonal injury is commonly associated with coma, immediate cognitive decline, and poor outcome in patients with significant closed head injury. The stress induced by rotational acceleration/deceleration movement of the head causes differential motion to occur between the neuronal body and axon, which is the area of greatest density difference in the brain. This motion causes axon disruption and formation of retraction balls. The sites most commonly involved include the body and splenium of the corpus callosum, brainstem, superior cerebellar peduncle, internal capsule, and gray-white junction of the cerebrum. On CT, diffuse axonal injury may not be initially detected. On follow-up MRI, rounded or elliptic T2 hyperintense foci are seen in characteristic locations, and they are commonly hemorrhagic.

17. **Primary brain tumors in adults usually arise from what cell line?**

Most primary intra-axial tumors of the brain arise from the supporting microglial cells. Gliomas account for 35% to 45% of all intracranial tumors. Glioblastoma multiforme accounts for 35% of gliomas and has a very poor prognosis, with survival rates commonly less than 1 year. Astrocytomas, ependymomas, medulloblastomas, and oligodendrogliomas are other, more commonly encountered primary brain tumors.

18. **What is the most common benign extra-axial tumor in adults?**

The prototypic extra-axial tumor in adults is meningioma. This tumor commonly affects middle-aged women and arises from the arachnoid of the meninges. The most common locations are the parasagittal dura of the falx, the cerebral convexities, the sphenoid wing, the olfactory groove, and the planum sphenoidale. Other locations include the tuberculum sella and orbit, the cerebellopontine angle, and the cavernous sinus. On unenhanced CT, most meningiomas are slightly hyperdense compared with normal brain tissue, with calcifications present in approximately 20%. There may be associated osseous hyperostosis involving the adjacent bone. On MRI, meningiomas are isointense to slightly hyperintense relative to gray matter on T2-weighted images. Meningiomas enhance intensely and homogeneously (see Fig. 48-2). A CSF cleft between the mass and the brain is often present, identifying its extra-axial location. Although the presence of a dural tail is typical of a meningioma, it may not be seen in 30% of cases (see Fig. 48-2B).

19. **What are the most common neoplasms arising in the corpus callosum?**

The corpus callosum is the largest white matter tract, and it connects the two cerebral hemispheres in the midline. The most common tumors that affect the corpus callosum are glioblastoma multiforme and lymphoma. The extension of a neoplasm from one hemisphere to the other via the corpus callosum produces the so-called butterfly pattern (Fig. 48-4). Other non-neoplastic white matter diseases that commonly involve the corpus callosum include demyelinating disease (especially multiple sclerosis) and trauma (diffuse axonal injury).

20. **What are the most common systemic neoplasms to metastasize to the brain?**

Breast cancer, carcinoma of the lung, and melanoma most commonly spread hematogenously to the brain. Hemorrhagic brain metastases are common with melanoma, choriocarcinoma, thyroid cancer, and renal cell carcinoma; however, because breast and lung cancer are so much more common, it is more likely that a hemorrhagic metastasis is related to

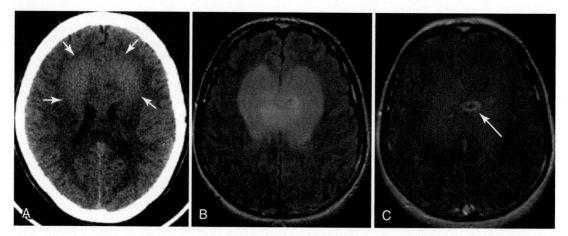

Figure 48-4. Glioblastoma multiforme. **A,** Axial unenhanced CT scan shows ill-defined hyperdense mass in both frontal lobes (*arrows*), crossing the corpus callosum in a pattern characteristic of a "butterfly" glioma. **B,** Axial FLAIR MR image shows the mass is hyperintense (bright) relative to brain. **C,** Axial T1-weighted postcontrast image shows diffuse faint enhancement with a central area of necrosis (*arrow*).

one of these latter cancers. Calcified metastases may be seen with mucinous adenocarcinomas (lung, colon, stomach, ovary, and breast) and bone cancers (osteosarcoma and chondrosarcoma).

21. What are the most common primary brain tumors that calcify?
Oligodendroglioma, ependymoma, astrocytoma, craniopharyngioma, and ganglioglioma are primary central nervous system tumors that most commonly calcify.

22. What is the imaging appearance of leptomeningeal carcinomatosis or subarachnoid seeding? What are the most common tumors producing it in adults?
Subarachnoid seeding or leptomeningeal tumor is characterized by tiny nodules of tumor implanted on the surface of the brain or spinal cord or both. There is "sugar-coating" of the subarachnoid spaces. T1-weighted MRI with contrast enhancement is best at showing this nodular enhancement, particularly in the basilar cisterns, over the cerebral convexities, and along the cranial nerves (Fig. 48-5). Communicating hydrocephalus may result from obstruction of the arachnoid villi.

23. What are the most common tumors producing subarachnoid seeding in adults?
Many primary central nervous system tumors seed the subarachnoid spaces (e.g., glioblastoma multiforme, oligodendroglioma, ependymoma). Metastatic systemic tumors that commonly spread to the CSF or leptomeninges include breast and lung carcinoma, melanoma, and hematologic malignancies (lymphoma and leukemia).

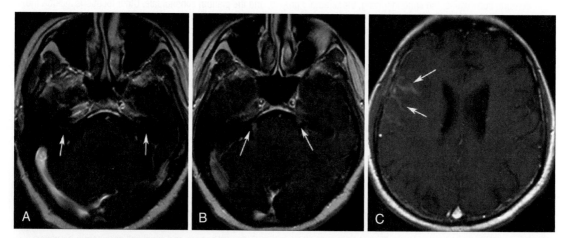

Figure 48-5. Leptomeningeal spread of lymphoma. **A-C,** Axial T1-weighted postcontrast MR images show abnormal enhancement of bilateral internal auditory canals (*arrows* in **A**), bilateral fifth cranial nerves (*arrows* in **B**), and subarachnoid spaces of the right frontal lobe (*arrows* in **C**).

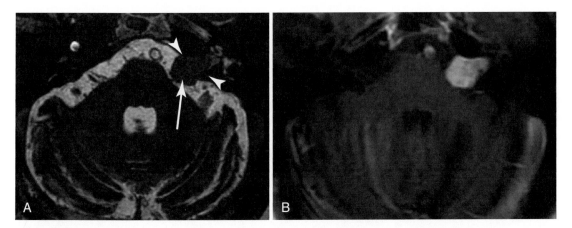

Figure 48-6. Vestibular schwannoma. **A,** Axial high-resolution T2-weighted MR image shows hypointense mass (*arrow*) in the left cerebellopontine angle extending into the internal auditory canal and expanding the porus acusticus (*arrowheads*). **B,** Axial T1-weighted postcontrast image shows characteristic enhancement of the mass.

24. Why would a mass appear hyperdense on unenhanced CT scan of the head?

Masses may be hyperdense because of the presence of acute blood, calcification, dense cellularity (lymphoma, meningioma, medulloblastoma, and germinoma), or proteinaceous material.

25. What is the most common tumor in the cerebellopontine angle cistern?

Most tumors in the cerebellopontine angle cistern are vestibular schwannomas (75%), followed by meningiomas (10%) and epidermoid tumors (5%). Uncommon neoplasms that may involve the cerebellopontine angle include metastatic disease, facial nerve schwannoma, exophytic brainstem glioma, and hemangioma. Non-neoplastic lesions that may occur include aneurysms arising from the vertebrobasilar arteries, arachnoid cysts, and lipomas. On imaging, small vestibular schwannomas are usually isolated to the internal auditory canal (IAC), isointense to brain parenchyma, and homogeneously enhanced. Contrast-enhanced MRI is commonly necessary to detect them. Larger tumors are usually heterogeneous because of the development of cystic or necrotic areas (or both), and they cause expansion of the porus acusticus (the opening of the IAC) (Fig. 48-6). Of vestibular schwannomas, 85% involve the IAC. In contrast, meningiomas rarely involve the IAC (5%), they usually enhance homogeneously, and there is usually associated dural enhancement. It is important for the radiologist to try to distinguish schwannoma from meningioma because this information can affect the surgical approach in resecting these lesions.

26. What is the most common clinical presentation of a vestibular schwannoma?

The most common clinical presentation of a vestibular schwannoma is unilateral sensorineural hearing loss. Adults with unilateral sensorineural hearing loss should be evaluated with enhanced MRI. Conductive hearing loss is usually evaluated with temporal bone CT to assess for an abnormality of the ossicles and middle ear. In children, temporal bone CT is commonly the first imaging modality used to assess sensorineural and conductive hearing loss because the sensorineural hearing loss in pediatric patients is often related to congenital malformations easily detected on CT.

27. Define transtentorial herniation.

To understand this, one must appreciate important central anatomy. The medial temporal lobes (uncus, hippocampus) overhang the tentorium; the brainstem passes through the tentorial hiatus; the posterior cerebral arteries course around the brainstem and medial to the temporal lobes; and the third cranial nerves originate from the midbrain, crossing the interpeduncular cistern below the posterior cerebral arteries and medial to the medial lobes. Transtentorial herniation is caused by a mass effect with a vector force that is directed inferiorly and medially. The temporal lobe shifts over the tentorium, resulting in compression of the third nerve (leading to ipsilateral papillary dilation), posterior cerebral arteries, and midbrain. Compression of the contralateral cerebral peduncle against the tentorium produces ipsilateral motor weakness, referred to as the "Kernohan-Woltman notch" phenomenon (false localizing sign).

28. What is the most common posterior fossa/infratentorial mass in adults?

The most common infratentorial neoplasm in adults is a metastasis. A metastasis appears as a well-defined, enhancing mass at the gray-white junction and may have surrounding vasogenic edema. The most common primary posterior fossa tumor in adults is a hemangioblastoma. The typical imaging findings of hemangioblastoma are a cystic mass with an enhancing mural nodule (Fig. 48-7). The mural nodule is highly vascular. Solidly enhancing hemangioblastomas can also be seen, however. Multiple hemangioblastomas are associated with von Hippel-Lindau disease.

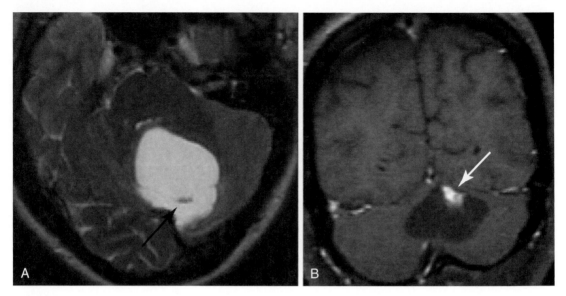

Figure 48-7. Hemangioblastoma. **A,** Axial T1-weighted MR image shows T2 hyperintense, cystic, midline cerebellar mass with a small mural nodule (*arrow*). There is mass effect on the fourth ventricle. **B,** Coronal T1-weighted postcontrast image shows that the mural nodule is intensely enhancing (*arrow*).

29. What are the three parts of the anterior lobe of the pituitary gland?

The pituitary gland is composed of two physiologically and anatomically distinct lobes—anterior and posterior. The anterior lobe, or adenohypophysis, represents 75% of the volume of the gland and is divided into the pars tuberalis, pars intermedia, and the pars distalis. The posterior lobe, or neurohypophysis, is composed of the posterior pituitary lobe, the infundibular stalk, and median eminence of the hypothalamus. Microadenomas are the most common intrasellar neoplasm in adults. Microadenomas are defined as neoplasms that are 10 mm or smaller. They are hypointense relative to the pituitary gland on unenhanced and enhanced T1-weighted MRI (Fig. 48-8A). Autopsy series indicate that small, incidental lesions of the pituitary gland are common. Clinical correlation is crucial so that insignificant lesions (e.g., cysts) are not treated. In about 75% of cases, microadenomas have associated hormonal abnormalities.

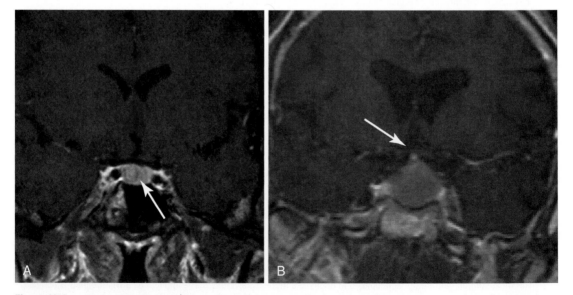

Figure 48-8. **A,** Pituitary microadenoma. Enhanced coronal T1-weighted MR image through the sella turcica shows a small, round lesion in the right lateral aspect of the pituitary gland (*arrow*). **B,** Pituitary macroadenoma. Coronal enhanced T1-weighted image shows large mass centered within the pituitary sella and extending into the suprasellar space. Despite its large size, the mass is not compressing the optic chiasm (*arrow*).

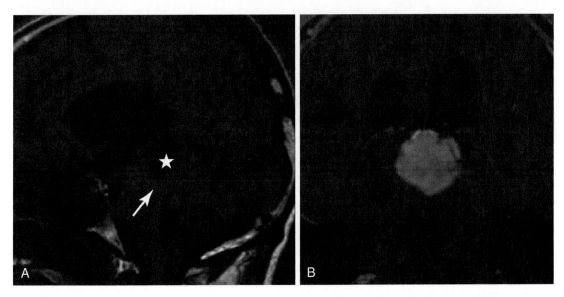

Figure 48-9. Pineoblastoma. **A,** Sagittal T1-weighted MR image shows mass in the region of the pineal gland (*asterisk*) that compresses the tectum (*arrow*). **B,** Enhanced coronal T1-weighted image shows intense enhancement of the mass.

Macroadenomas are larger than 10 mm, enlarge the sella turcica, and commonly spread outside of the sella into the suprasellar cistern or cavernous sinus. As a result, patients with macroadenomas often present with visual symptoms (classically, bitemporal hemianopsia) related to compression of the optic chiasm and prechiasmatic optic nerves (Fig. 48-8B), headache, and other cranial nerve palsies.

30. Name newer imaging techniques that help diagnose brain tumors.

These techniques include magnetic resonance spectroscopy, perfusion MRI, and diffusion MRI. Functional MRI is used for preoperative localization of eloquent brain cortex before surgery.

31. Pineal region masses are associated with what visual disturbance?

The clinical manifestations of pineal region masses depend on their size and location near critical anatomic structures—the aqueduct of Sylvius, the tectal plate, and the vein of Galen/internal cerebral veins. Pineal region masses may cause paresis of upward gaze (Parinaud syndrome) because of compression of the tectal plate or obstructive hydrocephalus because of compression of the aqueduct. Pineal region tumors are categorized into tumors of germ cell origin (60%) and tumors of pineal cell origin. Most of these tumors arise from germ cells, are seen in male patients, and are germinomas. Intrinsic pineal cell tumors (pineocytoma and pineoblastomas) are seen in male and female patients equally. CSF seeding is common. Because pineal tumors are commonly hypercellular, they appear hyperdense on unenhanced CT, and they are intermediate in signal intensity on T1-weighted and T2-weighted MRI (Fig. 48-9).

BIBLIOGRAPHY

[1] S.J. Nelson, T.R. McKnight, R.G. Henry, Characterization of untreated gliomas by magnetic resonance spectroscopic imaging, Neuroimaging Clin. N. Am. 12 (2002) 599–613.
[2] P.E. Ricci, Imaging of adult brain tumors, Neuroimaging Clin. N. Am. 9 (1999) 651–669.
[3] J.G. Smirniotopoulos, The new WHO classification of brain tumors, Neuroimaging Clin. N. Am. 9 (1999) 595–613.
[4] C.D. Wiginton, B. Kelly, A. Oto, et al., Gadolinium-based contrast exposure, nephrogenic systemic fibrosis, and gadolinium detection in tissue, AJR. Am. J. Roentgenol. 190 (2008) 1060–1068.

CHAPTER 49

BRAIN: INFLAMMATORY, INFECTIOUS, AND VASCULAR DISEASES

Gul Moonis, MD, and
Laurie A. Loevner, MD

1. How is multiple sclerosis (MS) diagnosed?

MS is the most common of the acquired demyelinating disorders. The disease has a characteristic relapsing-remitting course and usually manifests between the third and fifth decades of life with a female predominance. On magnetic resonance imaging (MRI), the demyelinating lesions of MS are ovoid and hyperintense (bright) on T2-weighted images and occur predominantly in the white matter, especially in the periventricular location (usually perpendicular to the ventricular surface) (Fig. 49-1). The corpus callosum, white matter around the temporal horns of the lateral ventricles, and middle cerebellar peduncles are other favored locations of MS plaques. There may be enhancement of the plaques (ringlike or solid) that denotes active disease. Occasionally, MS plaques can be large and masslike (tumefactive MS), in which case differentiation from a tumor may be difficult.

2. What is the differential diagnosis of MS based on imaging findings?

The diagnosis of MS is a clinical one (neurologic symptoms spaced over time and in multiple distributions), with supporting radiologic findings. The diagnosis cannot be made on imaging findings alone because other inflammatory and vascular processes can manifest with similar imaging findings. White matter lesions similar to MS can be seen with a spectrum of inflammatory conditions, including Lyme disease, sarcoidosis, and vasculitis.

3. What are the causes of intracranial abscesses?

Infectious agents gain access to the central nervous system (CNS) by direct spread from a contiguous focus of infection, such as sinusitis, otitis media, mastoiditis, orbital cellulitis, or dental infection. Infection from these locations may also spread to the intracranial compartment by retrograde venous reflux. Hematogenous spread of infection can also occur from a distant nidus of infection, such as the lung. Polymicrobial infection is common with brain abscesses. Four stages have been described in abscess evolution: early cerebritis, late cerebritis, early capsule formation, and late capsule formation. A mature abscess is characterized by a "ring-enhancing" lesion on cross-sectional imaging.

4. What is the imaging differential diagnosis of a ring-enhancing lesion in the brain?

The following disease processes can have an imaging presentation identical to brain abscess: metastatic disease, primary CNS glioma, resolving hematoma, and demyelinating disease. Interpreting the radiologic findings in conjunction with the clinical history is usually helpful in differentiating among these possible etiologies.

5. What advanced MRI techniques may be useful in distinguishing brain abscess from neoplasm?

Differentiating a subclinical brain abscess from cystic or necrotic tumor with conventional

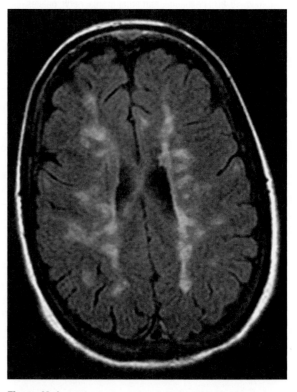

Figure 49-1. MS in a young patient. Axial fluid-attenuated inversion recovery (FLAIR) MR image shows numerous ovoid, periventricular lesions characteristic of MS plaques. These are oriented along the perivascular spaces, and the appearance has been referred to as "Dawson's fingers."

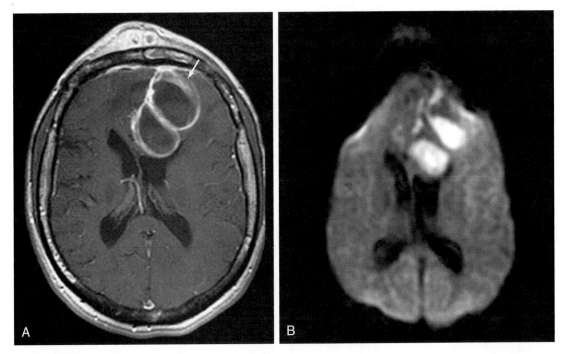

Figure 49-2. A, Frontal lobe abscess secondary to frontal sinusitis. Axial contrast-enhanced T1-weighted MR image shows two ring-enhancing lesions in the left frontal lobe (*arrow*) and enhancing soft tissue within and anterior to the frontal sinus. **B,** On the corresponding diffusion-weighted image, there is restricted diffusion (high signal intensity) within these lesions that is compatible with abscesses.

computed tomography (CT) or MRI can be difficult. ¹H magnetic resonance spectroscopy and diffusion-weighted MRI can be useful in this regard (Fig. 49-2). Typically, on diffusion-weighted MRI, an abscess is hyperintense (bright).

6. **What anatomic location in the brain is preferentially involved by herpes simplex encephalitis?**

   In adults, type 1 herpes simplex virus is responsible for fulminant, necrotizing encephalitis. The virus preferentially involves the temporal lobes, but involvement of the frontal lobes (especially the cingulate gyrus) is common. Often, there is bilateral temporal lobe involvement, although this is usually asymmetric. On MRI, there is T2-weighted hyperintensity in the temporal and frontal lobes with enhancement (Fig. 49-3). Clinically, the patient presents with acute confusion, disorientation, or seizures progressing to stupor and coma. Most cases are a result of reactivation of dormant virus in the trigeminal ganglion. There is commonly asymmetric temporal lobe involvement. Hemorrhage in the affected area is common.

7. **What is the differential diagnosis of an intracranial mass in a patient with human immunodeficiency virus (HIV) infection?**

   It is crucial to determine whether the cause of HIV-related brain mass is neoplastic or infectious because these entities are managed differently. Among infectious etiologies, toxoplasmosis and brain abscesses secondary to fungal or bacterial etiologies have to be considered. The major neoplastic consideration is primary CNS lymphoma. Toxoplasmosis is the leading cause of focal CNS disease in acquired immunodeficiency syndrome (AIDS) and results from infection by the intracellular parasite *Toxoplasma gondii*. It is usually caused by reactivation of old CNS lesions or by hematogenous spread of a previously acquired infection. On imaging, single or multiple ring-enhancing lesions in the white matter or basal ganglia or both with mass effect may be observed. A single lesion favors the diagnosis of lymphoma over toxoplasmosis (Fig. 49-4). Occasionally, progressive multifocal leukoencephalopathy, a demyelinating disease caused by a viral infection, may result in ring-enhancing lesions. Progressive multifocal leukoencephalopathy is caused by a virus that infects the oligodendrocytes in immunocompromised patients.

8. **What is a stroke?**

   A stroke occurs when the blood supply to a vascular territory of the brain is suddenly interrupted (ischemic stroke), or when a blood vessel in the brain ruptures, spilling blood into the spaces surrounding the brain cells (hemorrhagic stroke). Ischemic stroke is the more common form, responsible for approximately 80% of vascular accidents. In adults, these blockages are usually associated with two conditions: atherosclerosis-related occlusion of vessels (60%) and cardiac embolism (20%).

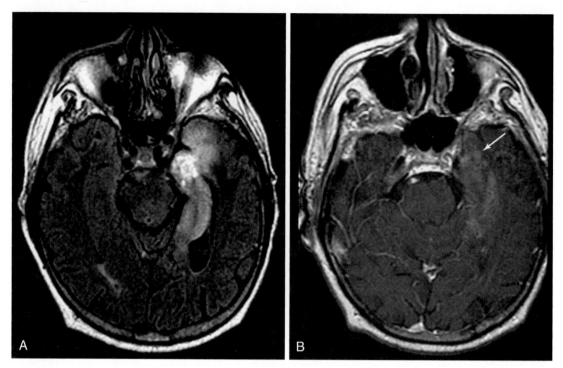

Figure 49-3. A, Herpes simplex encephalitis. Axial FLAIR MR image shows abnormal T2 hyperintensity in the left medial temporal lobe involving gray and white matter. **B,** Axial enhanced T1-weighted MR image shows mild patchy enhancement (*arrow*) that is consistent with cerebritis.

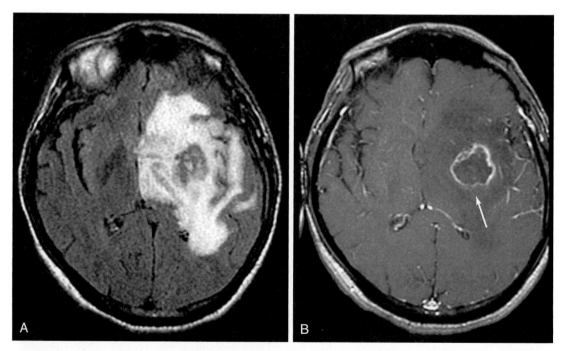

Figure 49-4. A, Toxoplasmosis in an HIV-positive patient. Axial FLAIR MR image shows extensive signal abnormality involving the left basal ganglia and adjacent frontal and temporal lobes with mass effect. **B,** Axial enhanced T1-weighted MR image at the same axial level as **A** shows a rim-enhancing lesion in the center of the left basal ganglia (*arrow*) with extensive surrounding edema and midline shift from left to right.

9. **What are the common causes of stroke that one must consider in children and young adults?**

Only 3% of cerebral infarctions occur in patients younger than 40 years old. The most common causes of stroke in young patients are cardiac disease, hematologic diseases (hypercoagulable states), and vascular dissection (from trauma or disease of the vessel wall). Other causes include CNS vasculitis, fibromuscular dysplasia, and venous sinus thrombosis.

10. **What are the imaging manifestations of ischemic stroke in the acute stage?**

Commonly, in the acute setting, a CT scan of the head may be normal. The earliest signs (≤6 hours) of an acute infarct on CT are loss of the gray-white differentiation with obscuration of the lateral lentiform nucleus. There may be a high density noted in the proximal middle cerebral artery, representing acute thrombus or calcified embolus; this is referred to as the "hyperdense artery" sign (Fig. 49-5A). Within 12 to 24 hours, there is low density in the appropriate vascular distribution, with increasing mass effect. Mass effect peaks between 3 and 5 days. Findings of acute ischemia are detected earlier on MRI. With the use of diffusion-weighted imaging, acute ischemic changes can be seen within minutes of onset of the ictus. High signal intensity is noted within the involved vascular territory on T2-weighted images, with characteristic restricted diffusion (also hyperintense) on diffusion-weighted images (Fig. 49-5B and C). Swelling of the involved cortex and arterial enhancement are noted early in the time course.

11. **How can one differentiate acute from chronic stroke on imaging?**

Chronic stroke is manifested by encephalomalacic change in the involved vascular territory with accompanying dilation of the sulci and cisterns. There is also ex vacuo dilation of the ipsilateral ventricle. There is absence of mass effect. If it is difficult to distinguish the age of a stroke on CT, MRI that includes a diffusion-weighted sequence can be invaluable.

12. **What are watershed infarctions?**

Also known as "border zone infarcts," watershed infarctions occur in the vascular watersheds (the distalmost arterial territory with connection between the major arterial branches). In severe hypotension or shock, the systemic blood pressure is insufficient to pump arterial blood to the end arteries. In the cerebrum, not enough blood gets to the "watershed zones" between the anterior and middle cerebral arteries or the middle and posterior cerebral artery territories, and in those areas infarcts are likely to develop. Some other causes of cerebral watershed infarcts include heart failure, decreased systemic perfusion pressure, and low blood pressure in the setting of a high-grade stenosis of a major artery (internal carotid) supplying the brain.

13. **What are lacunar infarctions?**

Lacunar infarctions are small infarcts caused by occlusion or disease of the perforating arteries (arteriolar lipohyalinosis). Initially, these are slightly hypodense on CT. By 4 weeks, sharply circumscribed, cystic lesions develop. These lesions are most commonly seen in the deep gray matter (basal ganglia, thalami), brainstem, internal capsule, and corona radiata. These small infarctions are usually 1 cm or smaller.

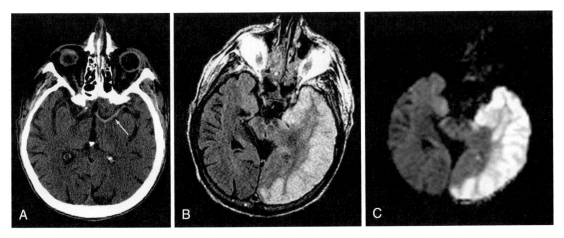

Figure 49-5. Hyperdense middle cerebral artery consistent with acute thrombus or calcified embolus. **A,** Axial unenhanced CT scan of the head shows hyperdensity in the left middle cerebral artery (*arrow*) that is compatible with acute thrombus. **B** and **C,** Corresponding axial FLAIR and diffusion-weighted MR images shows diffuse hyperintensity involving gray and white matter in the left middle cerebral artery territory, which is characteristic of stroke. The hyperintensity on the diffusion-weighted image represents restricted diffusion, which is compatible with acute ischemia.

14. What are the risk factors for venous sinus thrombosis and venous infarction?

Venous sinus thrombosis is associated with many systemic conditions, including acute dehydration, hypercoagulable states, chemotherapeutic agents (L-asparaginase), sinusitis and mastoiditis, hematologic malignancies, pregnancy, and trauma. Unenhanced CT reveals the presence of high density and enlargement of the dural venous sinuses. The "empty delta" sign, which refers to enhancement around the clot in a dural venous sinus, may also be present (Fig. 49-6A). The diagnosis of venous thrombosis is improved significantly with MRI. On unenhanced T1-weighted images, high signal intensity clot is noted within the venous sinuses (Fig. 49-6B). There may be associated venous infarction. Venous infarctions have a high rate of hemorrhagic transformation compared with arterial infarctions.

15. What is the most common cause of nontraumatic subarachnoid hemorrhage (SAH)?

An aneurysm rupture is the most common cause of nontraumatic SAH. An aneurysm is a focal dilation of an artery, most commonly encountered at branching points in the intracranial vasculature. Aneurysms are usually due to a congenital weakness in the media and elastica of the arterial wall, but can be acquired in the setting of trauma or mycotic infections. The approximate relative frequency of aneurysm formation in the intracranial vasculature is as follows: anterior communicating artery (30%), distal internal carotid artery and posterior communicating artery (30%), middle cerebral artery (25% to 30%), and the posterior vertebral-basilar circulation (10% to 15%). Multiple aneurysms are seen in approximately 15% of cases. There is increased incidence of intracranial aneurysms in patients with polycystic kidney disease, Marfan syndrome, and fibromuscular dysplasia (and other rarer entities, including moyamoya disease, Ehlers-Danlos syndrome, and Takayasu arteritis).

16. What is the work-up of a patient presenting with SAH?

If the patient presents with the classic history of "the worst headache of my life," a CT scan should be obtained to look for SAH. If the results of the CT scan are negative, but there is high clinical suspicion for SAH, a lumbar puncture should be performed to look for red blood cells or xanthochromia or both in the cerebrospinal fluid (CSF). If CSF analysis is positive for subarachnoid blood, a diagnostic conventional catheter angiogram is the next step to find the aneurysm, providing an anatomic road map for the neurosurgeon. Increasingly, CT angiography is being used rather than conventional catheter angiography for aneurysm detection.

17. If multiple aneurysms are seen on catheter angiography in a patient with SAH, which one most likely bled?

If multiple aneurysms are identified, greater suspicion falls on the aneurysm that is the largest in size, on the aneurysm with a lobulated contour (nipple sign), or on the aneurysm closest to the largest clot on CT. Extravasation of contrast agent from the aneurysm is rarely seen, but is diagnostic.

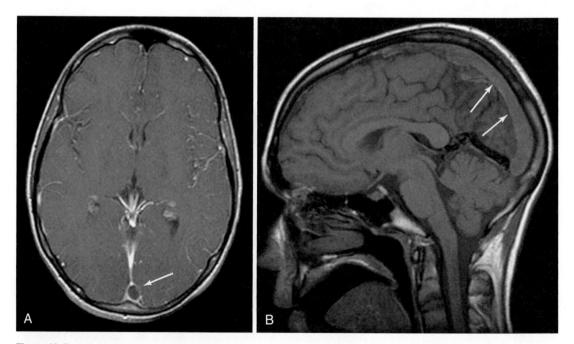

Figure 49-6. A, Venous sinus thrombosis. Axial contrast-enhanced T1-weighted MR image shows acute clot in the superior sagittal sinus. Note the characteristic "empty delta" sign (*arrow*) that represents nonenhancing clot within the superior sagittal sinus. **B,** Sagittal unenhanced T1-weighted MR image taken in the midline shows relative high signal intensity in the superior sagittal sinus (*arrows*), which is consistent with acute thrombosis.

18. What are common locations for hypertensive intraparenchymal hemorrhages?

In adults who present with nontraumatic intraparenchymal hemorrhage in the brain, hypertension is the most common etiologic factor. The arteries in the brain injured by chronic hypertension typically are the perforating arteries, which supply the basal ganglia, thalami, and pons (Fig. 49-7). Other areas that may also be affected by hypertensive bleeds include the centrum semiovale and, occasionally, the cerebellum.

19. What is amyloid angiopathy?

Amyloid angiopathy results from deposition of amyloid in the media and adventitia of small and medium-sized vessels of the superficial layers of the cortex and leptomeninges. Amyloid deposition increases with age. Pathologically, there is loss of elasticity and increased fragility of the vessels that cause hemorrhages that are usually lobar and most often in the frontal and parietal lobes. These parenchymal hemorrhages may be associated with subdural hemorrhage and SAH. The usual course is multiple hemorrhagic incidents spaced over time.

20. Review the MRI signal characteristics of intracranial hemorrhage.

See Table 49-1.

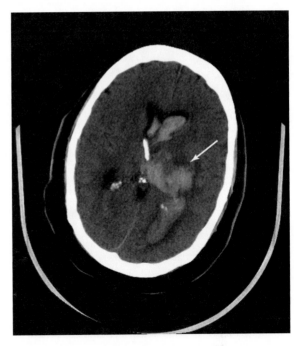

Figure 49-7. Left thalamic hypertensive hemorrhage. Axial unenhanced CT scan of the head shows a large focus of hemorrhage centered in the left thalamus (*arrow*) with extension into the ventricular system and hydrocephalus.

21. What are the imaging features of cerebral hypoxia/anoxia?

Hypoxia refers to a lack of oxygen supply to the cerebral hemispheres. Hypoxia can have a multifactorial etiology, including drowning, asphyxiation from smoke inhalation, severe hypotension, strangulation, perinatal hypoxic insult, cardiac arrest, and carbon monoxide poisoning. On MRI, there is increased T2 signal in the perirolandic and occipital cortex and the basal ganglia (Fig. 49-8). The watershed zones between major vascular territories and the hippocampi are also prone to hypoxic-ischemic damage. Layers three, four, and five of the cortex are sensitive to global hypoxia-ischemia and may become necrotic and hemorrhagic (laminar necrosis).

Table 49-1. MRI Signal Characteristics of Intracranial Hemorrhage

	AGE	T1-WEIGHTED	T2-WEIGHTED
Hyperacute	Hours old, mainly oxyhemoglobin with surrounding edema	Hypointense	Hyperintense
Acute	Days old, mainly deoxyhemoglobin with surrounding edema	Hypointense	Hypointense, surrounded by hyperintense margin
Subacute	Weeks old, mainly methemoglobin	Hyperintense	Hypointense, early subacute with predominantly intracellular methemoglobin
			Hyperintense, late subacute with predominantly extracellular methemoglobin
Chronic	Years old, hemosiderin slit or hemosiderin margin surrounding fluid cavity	Hypointense	Hypointense slit or hypointense margin surrounding hyperintense fluid cavity

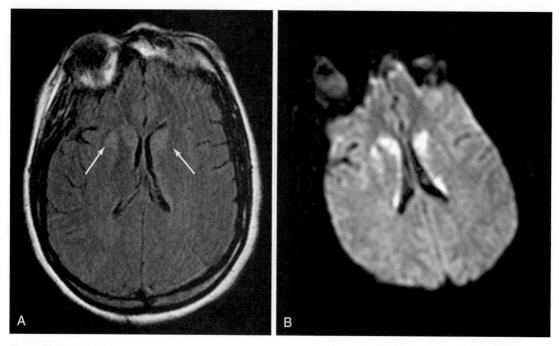

Figure 49-8. Hypoxic injury in a patient who was found in respiratory arrest. **A** and **B,** Axial FLAIR (**A**) and diffusion-weighted (**B**) MR images show abnormal hyperintensity in the bilateral caudate heads and the right putamen (*arrows* on **A**). The diffusion hyperintensity is consistent with acute hypoxic-ischemic injury.

BIBLIOGRAPHY

[1] S. Falcone, M.J. Post, Encephalitis, cerebritis, and brain abscess: pathophysiology and imaging findings, Neuroimaging Clin. North. Am. 10 (2000) 333–353.
[2] M.F. Gaskill-Shipley, Routine CT evaluation of acute stroke, Neuroimaging Clin. North. Am. 9 (1999) 411–422.
[3] S.K. Lee, K.G. Brugge, Cerebral venous thrombosis in adults: the role of imaging evaluation and management, Neuroimaging Clin. North. Am. 13 (2003) 139–152.
[4] T. Yoshiura, O. Wu, A.G. Sorensen, Advanced MR techniques: diffusion MR imaging, perfusion MR imaging, and spectroscopy, Neuroimaging Clin. North. Am. 9 (1999) 439–453.

Linda J. Bagley, MD, and
Laurie A. Loevner, MD

1. **Identify parts of the spine labeled in Fig. 50-1.**
   See the figure legend for the answers.

2. **What imaging modalities are most often used in the evaluation of spine pathology?**
   Radiographs (plain films), computed tomography (CT), magnetic resonance imaging (MRI), myelography, discography, magnetic resonance angiography (MRA), and conventional angiography have roles in spinal imaging.

3. **Describe the strengths, weaknesses, and most appropriate uses of CT in spinal imaging.**
   Radiographs (plain films) are often the initial imaging study of the spine. Pathologic conditions of the osseous spine, including fractures, degenerative changes, tumors, infections, and congenital anomalies (including transitional vertebrae), may be detected with radiographs. Multidetector CT provides superior evaluation, however, of the bony anatomy and pathologic conditions. Images may be acquired rapidly and reconstructed at narrow intervals (≤1 mm) with edge-enhancing algorithms. Multiplanar, three-dimensional images can subsequently be created. In the setting of acute spinal trauma, CT has been shown to be more time efficient and significantly more sensitive than plain radiographs for fracture detection. CT, in contrast to radiography, also allows excellent evaluation of retropulsed bone into the spinal canal. As a result, CT is often used to image traumatic and nontraumatic osseous spinal pathologic conditions. A major drawback of CT is its limited contrast resolution of the soft tissues within the spinal canal, including the spinal cord, nerve roots, epidural compartment, and subdural compartment. A higher radiation dose is also associated with CT scanning compared with plain radiography.

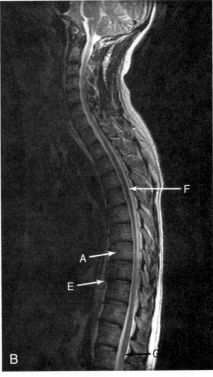

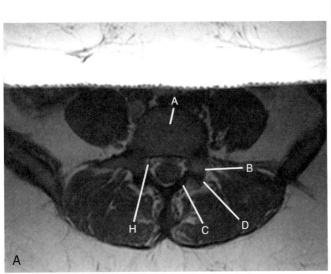

Figure 50-1. A, Axial T1-weighted MR image of normal vertebra. **B,** Sagittal T2-weighted MR image of the spine. (*A,* vertebral body; *B,* pedicle; *C,* lamina; *D,* facet joint; *E,* disc; *F,* spinal cord; *G,* conus medullaris; *H,* nerve root.)

4. Describe the strengths and drawbacks of MRI.

MRI provides the best and most direct evaluation of the contents within the spinal canal, including the spinal cord, nerve roots, and epidural and subdural compartments. MRI also provides the most detailed evaluation of the soft tissues, including the intervertebral discs, ligaments, and musculature. Optimal resolution is obtained at high field strengths using phased array surface coils. Numerous safety concerns arise, however, with the use of MRI. Many implantable devices, such as pacemakers, are not MRI-compatible, and patients must be appropriately screened. Ferromagnetic objects may become projectiles within the magnetic field and injure patients or health care providers. When MRI is performed in critically ill patients, MRI-compatible ventilators and monitoring devices must be used. When patients with spinal cord injuries are imaged, spinal precautions must be maintained, and fixation devices must be MRI-compatible. MRI of patients with prior spinal surgery is often of limited diagnostic value because of artifacts arising from metallic hardware. MRI is also time-consuming and requires patient cooperation (remaining motionless) to obtain high-quality studies.

5. In patients with contraindications to MRI, what radiologic study can be used to assess the contents within the spinal canal?

In patients with suspected spinal cord or nerve root compression who cannot be evaluated with MRI, myelography is an alternative, although invasive, technique that may be used to evaluate the spinal canal contents. Myelography is performed most often in patients with contraindications to MRI or nondiagnostic MRI studies. Nonionic contrast material is instilled into the subarachnoid space of the spinal canal, typically via lumbar puncture. Risks of this procedure are low, but include headache, allergic reaction to contrast agent, infection, hematoma, neural damage, and seizure. The contrast material in the subarachnoid space outlines the spinal cord and nerve roots. Impressions on the contrast column and displacement of neural structures are findings indicative of a pathologic condition (Fig. 50-2). Myelography is often complemented with cross-sectional CT scanning, performed after the myelogram is obtained to distinguish the anatomy and pathologic condition better in the spinal canal.

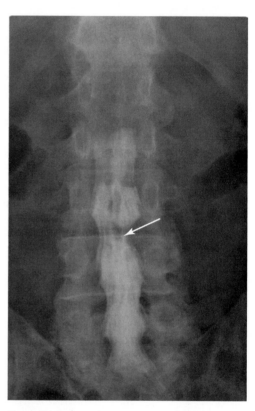

Figure 50-2. Anteroposterior plain film from lumbar myelogram shows extradural impression on the thecal sac at L3-L4 (*arrow*) with decreased opacification of the L3 nerve root sleeve.

6. What is discography, and when is it used?

Discography involves the injection of contrast material into the nucleus of the intervertebral disc, usually followed by CT scanning of the injected disc. This test is usually performed in patients with multilevel disc disease or axial back pain, or both, in an attempt to reproduce the patient's symptoms and identify the "culprit" disc. Patterns of contrast diffusion may suggest annular degeneration or fissures or both, but imaging findings must be correlated with patient symptoms (Fig. 50-3).

7. What is the primary role of catheter angiography of the spine?

Conventional spinal catheter angiography is primarily used for the detection, characterization, and possible endovascular treatment of spinal vascular malformations.

Key Points: Spine Imaging Modalities

1. Spine plain films are used to evaluate for fractures, degenerative changes, and alignment.
2. CT is used to evaluate for osseous pathologic conditions, especially fractures.
3. MRI is the best modality for imaging the spinal cord, bone marrow, and epidural and subdural spaces.
4. Myelography is reserved largely for symptomatic patients who cannot undergo MRI examination.
5. Spinal catheter angiography is used primarily for spinal vascular malformations.

8. What is spinal dysraphia?

Spinal anomalies with incomplete midline closure of mesenchymal, osseous, and neural structures are grouped under the term *spinal dysraphia*. Most defects occur in the lumbosacral region.

9. Differentiate open and occult forms of spinal dysraphia.

Myeloceles and myelomeningoceles are two types of open spinal dysraphia. Neural tissue (the neural placode, with or without associated meninges) protrudes through the spinal canal and soft tissue defects. Associated abnormalities include Chiari II malformation, hydrocephalus, syringohydromyelia, spinal lipomas, dermoid and epidermoid inclusion cysts, agenesis of the corpus callosum, diastematomyelia, and abnormal spinal curvature. In the occult form of dysraphia, the defects are covered by skin, and no neural tissue is exposed. Occult dysraphias include meningoceles, dorsal dermal sinuses (epithelial-lined tubes connecting the spinal cord and the skin), and fat-containing lesions (lipomyelomeningoceles, filum terminale lipomas, and intradural lipomas). Midline cutaneous stigmata (dimples, nevi, and hairy patches) are often present.

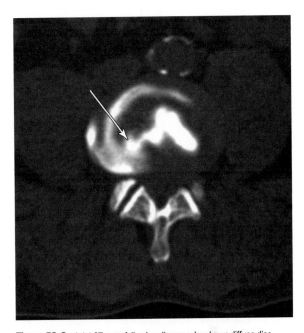

Figure 50-3. Axial CT scan following discography shows diffuse disc bulge with right lateral disc herniation. Contrast material extends to the outer annular fibers at the 7 o'clock position (*arrow*), indicative of a radial tear.

10. What are the clinical findings and imaging features of a tethered spinal cord?

The conus medullaris normally terminates at approximately the L1-L2 level. With a tethered spinal cord/thick filum terminale syndrome, the conus medullaris is identified at L2 or below, and the filum terminale is greater than 2 mm in thickness (Fig. 50-4). Associated anomalies (lipomas, diastematomyelia, and myelomeningoceles) are common. Patients typically present in childhood or young adulthood with pain, dysesthesias, bowel or bladder dysfunction, spasticity, or kyphoscoliosis.

11. List and describe caudal spinal anomalies.

Caudal spinal anomalies are malformations of the distal spine, spinal cord, and meninges associated with disorders of the hindgut, kidneys, urinary bladder, and genitalia. Caudal spinal anomalies include the following:

- *Caudal regression syndrome*: Varying degrees of lumbosacral agenesis with renal and anogenital anomalies and possible fusion of the lower extremities (Fig. 50-5).
- *Terminal myelocystocele*: Cystic dilation of the distal spinal cord, which is tethered, associated with partial sacral agenesis or spina bifida.
- *Anterior sacral meningocele*: Cerebrospinal fluid–filled sac that protrudes into the pelvis anterior to the sacrum.
- *Occult intrasacral meningocele*: Mild dural developmental anomaly with associated remodeling of the sacrum.
- *Sacrococcygeal teratoma*: Most common presacral mass in children; contains tissue from all three germ layers (endoderm, mesoderm, and ectoderm), and is often cystic and solid.

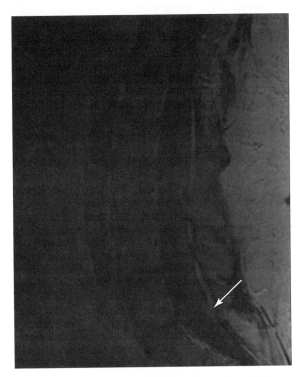

Figure 50-4. Sagittal T1-weighted MR image shows abnormally low position of the termination of the spinal cord with tethering of the filum terminale at L5-S1 (*arrow*).

12. What are the split notochord syndromes?

Persistent midline adhesions between endoderm and ectoderm can result in splitting of the notochord. With this split, paired hemicords (diastematomyelia) may result. Persistent endodermal-ectodermal adhesions or communications may produce dorsal enteric fistulas and neuroenteric cysts.

- *Diastematomyelia* predominantly occurs in female patients. In 85% of cases, the split occurs between T9 and S1. The cord is split by a fibrous, osseous, or osteocartilaginous septum, and the hemicords may or may not share a dural sac. Associated neurologic and orthopedic anomalies are common (Fig. 50-6).
- *Dorsal enteric fistulas* are very rare and extend from the mesenteric surface of the gut through the prevertebral tissues, vertebrae, and spinal cord to the dorsal skin surface.
- *Neuroenteric cysts* are most often intradural, extramedullary cystic masses in the thoracic region. Vertebral anomalies are seen in less than half of the cases.

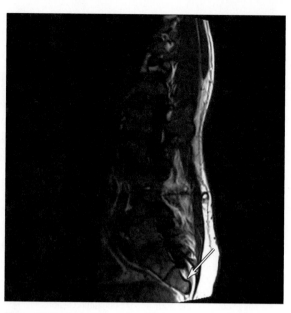

Figure 50-5. Sagittal T1-weighted MR image shows multiple spinal anomalies including partial agenesis of the sacrum (*arrow*).

13. What is the most common disorder of the spine affecting adults?

Degenerative changes in the spine generally begin to appear in adolescence and are often asymptomatic. Degenerative changes occur within the discs; vertebrae; joints; and soft tissues, including the ligaments. Although many degenerative changes are asymptomatic, more than 10 million adults seek medical care, and more than 200,000 operations are performed for back pain each year in the United States.

14. Discuss the MRI findings of degenerative disease affecting the spine.

Degenerative changes within the disc may initially manifest as decreased signal intensity within the disc on T2-weighted MR images, secondary to

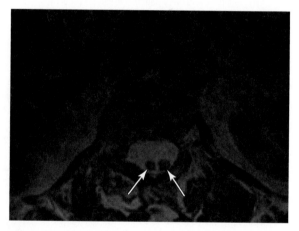

Figure 50-6. Axial T2-weighted MR image shows two spinal cords within the thecal sac (*arrows*).

decreased water content and increased fibrocartilaginous tissue. Discs may lose height. Annular fissures may occur. Diffuse disc bulges, focal disc protrusions, and free disc fragments may be seen. The advantage of MRI over plain film radiographs is that the relationship between the degenerative disc and the contents (neural tissue) within the spinal canal can be seen (Fig. 50-7).

Osseous degeneration may take the form of osteophytes, end-plate changes that include stages of edema, fatty replacement, and eventually sclerosis, which are readily distinguished with MRI. Facet and uncovertebral joint degenerative change may manifest with osteophytes, synovial proliferation, or synovial cyst formation. The ligamentum flavum may hypertrophy, and epidural lipomatosis may contribute to spinal stenosis. Degenerative changes may combine to produce central canal, lateral recess, or foraminal stenosis with possible resultant spinal cord or nerve root compression.

15. What are the most common lumbar and cervical spine levels to be affected by degenerative disease?

Approximately 90% of lumbar disc extensions beyond the vertebral body end plate occur at L4-L5 or L5-S1, with approximately 7% occurring at L3-L4 and 3% at L1-L2 and L2-L3. Most cervical disc extensions beyond the end plate (90%) occur at C5-C6 or C6-C7. Although spondylotic changes are common in the thoracic spine, thoracic disc extensions beyond the end plate are seen less commonly than cervical or lumbar disc abnormalities.

16. What is the natural history of most disc extensions beyond the vertebral body end plate?

Most discogenic disease is asymptomatic. In one study, 64% of normal volunteers showed some abnormality of the lumbar spine on MRI. Symptoms related to most disc abnormalities improve with conservative therapy (i.e., bed rest, anti-inflammatory and pain medication); 90% decrease in size, and clinical symptoms improve in 75% of cases.

17. Define Baastrup disease.

Baastrup disease is apparent enlargement and flattening of the spinous process, particularly in the lumbar spine, which may be secondary to excessive lordosis resulting in close contact of the spinous processes and subsequent sclerosis of the spinous processes and degeneration of the interspinous ligaments. Pain and tenderness may result. Baastrup disease is seen well on radiographs or MRI (Fig. 50-8).

18. How can residual and recurrent disc abnormalities be differentiated from scar tissue?

Scar and granulation tissue and residual and recurrent disc abnormalities often appear as soft tissue adjacent to the disc space, within the lateral recess, and within the neural foramen. This soft tissue may be inseparable from the nerve roots. Contrast-enhanced CT and unenhanced MRI are approximately 80% accurate in differentiating these entities. Contrast-enhanced MRI is the most reliable modality for this task, however, with reported accuracy of approximately 95%. Disc abnormalities are typically of lower signal intensity than scar material on T2-weighted images. Scar and granulation tissue enhance with gadolinium administration; disc material generally does not enhance. Residual and recurrent disc abnormalities and scar tissue sometimes may coexist. In a postoperative patient, enhancement may commonly be seen (and is not indicative of a pathologic condition) in the disc space, vertebral end plates, paraspinal soft tissues, and joints, and within nerve roots that were previously compressed.

19. What is arachnoiditis?

The term *arachnoiditis* refers to inflammation of the nerve roots of the cauda equina with adhesion of the nerve roots to each other or to the thecal sac, or both. Patients may present with nonspecific back pain or paresthesias or both. The key imaging features of this diagnosis are abnormal morphologic features and distribution of nerve roots, which may or may not enhance. Three imaging patterns have been described. The nerve roots may be centrally clumped, appearing as a "pseudocord" within the thecal sac. Alternatively, the nerve roots may be adherent to the periphery of the thecal sac—the "empty sac" appearance. Uncommonly, the nerve roots may clump together to form a large, mildly enhancing mass, which fills the thecal sac.

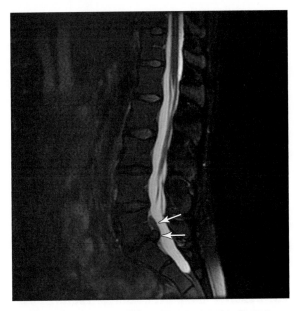

Figure 50-7. Sagittal T2-weighted MR image shows very large disc herniation at L5-S1 extending superiorly behind the L5 vertebral body (*arrows*).

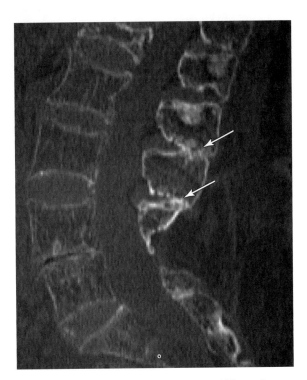

Figure 50-8. Baastrup disease. Sagittal reformatted CT scan shows enlargement and flattening of the spinous processes. Because of the close contact of the spinous processes, there is bony sclerosis (*arrows*).

20. Review the epidemiologic factors of spinal trauma.

Approximately 30,000 injuries to the spinal column occur in the United States each year. Most injuries are secondary to blunt trauma, and penetrating trauma accounts for approximately 10% to 20% of cases. Roughly 2% to 3% of victims of blunt trauma are affected, with a higher incidence of spinal injuries seen in patients with significant craniofacial trauma. Approximately 40% to 50% of spinal injuries produce a neurologic deficit—often severe and sometimes fatal. Survival is inversely correlated with patient age. Mortality during initial hospitalization is approximately 10%. Because most patients with spinal trauma are young, the costs of lifetime care and rehabilitation are extremely high, often exceeding $1 million per individual.

21. What are the appropriate indications for obtaining imaging of the spine in the setting of blunt trauma?

Pain, neurologic deficit, distracting injuries, altered consciousness (owing to head injury, intoxication, or pharmaceutical intervention), and high-risk mechanism of injury have been shown to be appropriate clinical indications for spinal imaging. The NEXUS and C-spine RULE studies have validated the clinical clearance of approximately 10% to 15% of all trauma patients.

22. Name the most common mechanisms of cervical spine injury.

Hyperflexion, hyperextension, and vertical compression (axial loading) are the most common mechanisms of cervical spine injury.

23. Describe the most common fractures associated with each of the mechanisms of injury in question 22.

- Hyperflexion may cause compression fractures, flexion-teardrop fractures, and spinous process fractures. When associated with posterior ligamentous injury, subluxations and bilateral facet dislocations may result. When hyperflexion occurs with rotation, this mechanism may result in unilateral facet dislocations.
- Hyperextension injuries include extension-teardrop fractures, fractures of the atlas, hangman's fractures (through the pars interarticularis of C2), laminar fractures, and fracture-dislocations. When hyperextension occurs with rotation, pillar fractures and pedicle-laminar separation may result.
- Vertical compression or axial loading injuries (when force is transmitted through the top of the skull through the occipital condyles and vertebral column) result in burst fractures of the vertebral bodies. In the cervical spine, burst fracture of the atlas (C1) is most common (Fig. 50-9).
- Lateral flexion usually occurs in conjunction with vertical compression. Isolated lateral flexion is the typical mechanism of injury resulting in isolated fractures of the uncovertebral joint of the cervical spine.
- Some injuries, such as odontoid fractures and atlanto-occipital dislocations, result from complex, often combined forces.

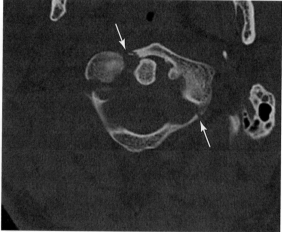

Figure 50-9. Axial CT scan shows fractures (*arrows*) of anterior and posterior rings of C1 with rotational deformity manifest by an asymmetric atlantodental interval.

24. What is the role of MRI in spinal trauma?

Fractures of the spine are best evaluated with thin-section CT with coronal and sagittal reformatted images. Spinal cord injuries and other traumatic sequelae within the spinal canal (e.g., subdural hematoma) are best evaluated with MRI and should be suspected when there are focal neurologic deficits, or when neurologic symptoms are disproportionate to the findings detected on plain films and CT scans. Cord contusions are generally manifested as hyperintense, intramedullary lesions on T2-weighted MR images. The cord may be expanded. The presence of hemorrhage within a contusion is associated with a worse prognosis and may alter the signal intensity characteristics of the lesion. MRI may also characterize many compressive lesions, such as epidural and subdural hematomas, disc abnormalities, and osteophytes.

25. What additional structures may be injured in association with cervical spinal trauma that may not be detected on radiographs or CT scans?

It is always important to consider ligamentous and arterial (especially vertebral artery) injuries in patients with significant trauma to the cervical spine. If there is subluxation or dislocation involving the cervical spine on

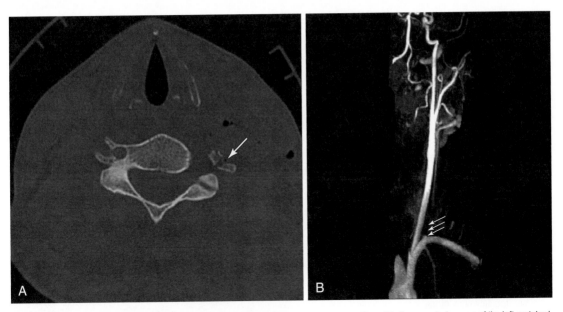

Figure 50-10. A, Axial CT scan shows comminuted fractures of left transverse process adjacent to the expected course of the left vertebral artery (foramen transversarium) (*arrow*) with extensive soft tissue swelling and subcutaneous emphysema in the left neck. **B,** Gadolinium-enhanced three-dimensional MRA of the cervical vasculature shows no flow in the proximal left vertebral artery (*arrows*) secondary to dissection.

plain film radiographs or CT, ligamentous injury must be present. In the absence of subluxation/dislocation, ligamentous injuries may be inapparent, however. Special MRI sequences such as fat-saturated T2-weighted images usually detect ligamentous injury, including frank disruption or edema or both. MRI and MRA may be used to evaluate for associated vascular injuries (dissections, occlusions, pseudoaneurysms) that may accompany spinal trauma (Fig. 50-10). In particular, cervical spine fractures involving a transverse process or the foramen transversarium (the osseous canal where the cervical portion of the vertebral artery lives), or both, are at higher risk of vertebral artery injury.

26. Name the most common sites of infection in the spine.
Infections may occur within the vertebra (most commonly the vertebral body [*osteomyelitis*]), within the disc space (*discitis*), within the epidural space (*abscess*), in the meninges (*meningitis*), and in the paraspinal soft tissues.

27. What patient populations are particularly prone to the development of infectious spondylodiscitis?
Infectious spondylodiscitis most commonly occurs in elderly patients and diabetic patients, and in men more often than women. Other groups particularly susceptible to this disorder include intravenous drug abusers, dialysis patients, alcoholics, and immunocompromised individuals.

28. What is the most common infectious agent responsible for spondylodiscitis?
The infecting organism may be bacterial, fungal, or parasitic. The most common cause of discitis is *Staphylococcus aureus*.

29. What is the typical clinical presentation of discitis?
Patients may present with back pain, fever, focal neurologic deficits, elevated white blood cell count, and elevated erythrocyte sedimentation rate.

30. What are the typical imaging findings of spondylodiscitis on plain film radiographs and CT?
On radiographs and CT, end-plate irregularity/destruction, and demineralization may be apparent (Fig. 50-11). The disc space may be narrowed. These findings commonly occur in the later stages of infection, however. Spondylodiscitis may be detected earlier with MRI. The finding of increased signal intensity within the intervertebral disc on T2-weighted images in the appropriate clinical setting should raise suspicion. Loss of disc height with end-plate irregularity or destruction and abnormal signal intensity in the vertebral bone

consistent with edema or osteomyelitis can be late imaging findings. Paravertebral soft tissue swelling or fluid collections and abscesses may be present. Typically, enhancement is seen within the marrow and disc space. Epidural phlegmons may show solid enhancement, and the presence of peripheral or "rim" enhancement is usually indicative of abscess formation.

31. Describe the imaging appearance of spondylodiscitis caused by atypical organisms, such as tuberculosis.

With granulomatous infections, such as tuberculosis, and fungal infections, there may be relative sparing of the disc space and end plates until late in the infection. Earlier involvement of the vertebral bodies is common. Tuberculosis is typically associated with anterior subligamentous involvement, resulting in infection of multiple, contiguous levels of the spine.

32. List noninfectious disorders that can have imaging findings similar to infectious spondylodiscitis.

* Degenerative disease or instability
* Neuropathic arthropathy
* Dialysis-related arthropathy (amyloid deposition)
* Postoperative changes
* Richter syndrome (lymphomatous transformation of chronic lymphocytic leukemia)

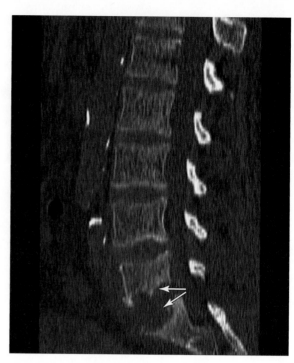

Figure 50-11. Sagittal reformatted CT scan of lumbar spine shows extensive end-plate destruction with sclerosis at L5-S1 (*arrows*).

33. What is the most common inflammatory disorder that affects the spinal cord?

Multiple sclerosis is the most common inflammatory disorder that affects the spinal cord. Patients typically have symptoms of numbness, weakness, or urinary incontinence that wax and wane. Other inflammatory conditions that involve the spinal cord include systemic lupus erythematosus, acute disseminated encephalomyelitis and other autoimmune disorders, sarcoidosis, and infections such as syphilis and HIV. Various other viral, bacterial, fungal, and parasitic organisms can infect the spinal cord.

34. What are the classic imaging findings of multiple sclerosis that affect the spinal cord?

The imaging findings of inflammatory disorders are often nonspecific. All of these processes produce intramedullary lesions that are hyperintense on T2-weighted images (Fig. 50-12). These lesions sometimes enhance and may be associated with cord expansion. More specific diagnoses are often made through correlation of imaging findings with clinical and laboratory data.

The spinal cord is commonly involved in patients with multiple sclerosis. The lesions of multiple sclerosis are often ill-defined, multiple, and located in the dorsolateral white matter of the cord (they are commonly small, but some lesions may extend over several spinal segments). In the active phase of demyelination, the plaques may expand the cord and typically enhance. Chronic lesions lead to focal or generalized cord atrophy.

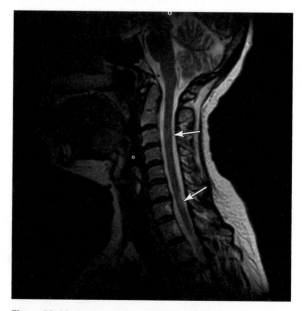

Figure 50-12. Sagittal T2-weighted MR image reveals foci of hyperintensity within the cervical cord (at C3 and at C6-C7) secondary to demyelinating disease (*arrows*).

The imaging findings of Behçet syndrome are similar to multiple sclerosis. With autoimmune diseases—including systemic lupus erythematosus, viral infection, postviral and postvaccination syndromes (including acute disseminated encephalomyelitis), and paraneoplastic disorders—focal cord signal abnormality, sometimes associated with cord expansion and enhancement, is often present.

35. What is the typical MRI appearance of sarcoidosis? How can its appearance, combined with the clinical history, distinguish it from other inflammatory disorders?

The typical MRI appearance of sarcoidosis is extensive leptomeningeal enhancement on the surface of the spinal cord. In sarcoidosis, a long segment of the cord may be expanded with abnormal signal intensity. With sarcoid, in contrast to many of the other inflammatory conditions, there typically is pronounced enhancement of the leptomeninges on the surface of the cord. Foci of intramedullary enhancement may also be present.

36. What is the typical time course for the development of radiation myelitis after irradiation for treatment of tumor?

Radiation myelitis generally manifests within 6 months to 3 years after treatment. It occurs within the treatment portal, and the marrow of the vertebrae within the port typically is fatty replaced. On MRI, the cord usually has T2-weighted hyperintensity, is expanded, and may enhance.

37. What portion of the spinal cord is typically involved with syphilis?

Syphilis has a predilection for the dorsal columns of the spinal cord. With syphilitic infection, enhancement may be seen along the pial surface of the cord and nerve roots. Vasculitis may accompany the infection and lead to cord infarctions. Vacuolar myelopathy occurs in approximately 15% to 30% of patients with AIDS and more commonly affects the posterolateral cord. Pathologically, vacuoles and lipid-laden macrophages are seen in the white matter.

38. Name the two most common vascular disorders of the spinal cord.

The two most common vascular disorders of the spinal cord are spinal cord infarcts and vascular malformations.

39. What is the arterial vascular supply to the spinal cord?

The anterior spinal artery is the main arterial supply to the spinal cord. Additional supply is through paired posterior spinal arteries. The anterior spinal artery is located in the midline. In the cervical and upper thoracic cord, contributions to the anterior spinal artery are from the vertebral, cervical, and superior intercostal arteries. A small component of supply to the mid-thoracic cord arises from the mid-thoracic intercostal arteries. The predominant contribution to the anterior spinal artery in the lower thoracic and lumbar regions (otherwise known as the artery of Adamkiewicz) most often arises from thoracic intercostal or lumbar arteries, usually on the left (Fig. 50-13).

40. What are the typical clinical characteristics and imaging findings of spinal cord infarcts?

Spinal cord infarcts most often occur in elderly patients with atherosclerotic vascular disease. Patients undergoing thoracoabdominal aneurysm repair are particularly at risk. Lower thoracic intercostal or upper lumbar arteries are often sacrificed with aneurysm repair procedures, jeopardizing the artery of Adamkiewicz. Patients experience sudden onset of paraplegia, often associated with pain. On MRI, signal abnormality is seen within the central gray matter (Fig. 50-14).

41. List the four types of spinal vascular malformations, and describe their clinical and imaging characteristics.

* *Dural arteriovenous malformations* are the most common of the spinal vascular anomalies seen in adults. They typically affect middle-aged and older men, who present with chronic, progressive motor and sensory deficits, usually in the lower extremities.

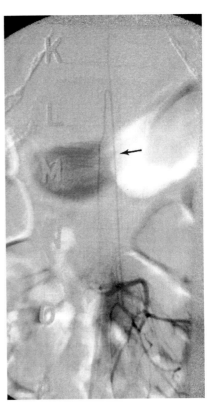

Figure 50-13. Anteroposterior plain film radiograph from a spinal angiogram shows anterior spinal artery (*arrow*) making its classic "hairpin" turn.

Bowel, bladder, and sexual dysfunction also often occur. These are acquired lesions, most often occurring in the lower thoracic and upper lumbar spine. Arterial supply is from the dural arteries. MRI is notable for diffuse enlargement and signal abnormality within the cord, generally involving the conus. Large vessels, representing dilated veins, are seen within the thecal sac. Enhancement may be present within the cord. The diagnosis is confirmed with spinal angiography. Treatment consists of embolization or surgery or both.

- *Arteriovenous malformations* are seen in younger patients (often teenagers) and often occur acutely secondary to intramedullary or subarachnoid hemorrhage. The arteriovenous malformation nidus is located within or on the surface of the cord and is supplied by the anterior or posterior spinal arteries. In the juvenile variant, the nidus also involves the vertebral column.
- *Arteriovenous fistulas* are uncommon. They are direct intradural fistulous connections from the anterior or posterior spinal arteries to the pial veins. These lesions typically occur in the thoracic and lumbar regions. Patients with these lesions may have a slowly progressive myelopathy or radiculopathy or may present with subarachnoid hemorrhage. These lesions usually manifest in the second to fourth decades.

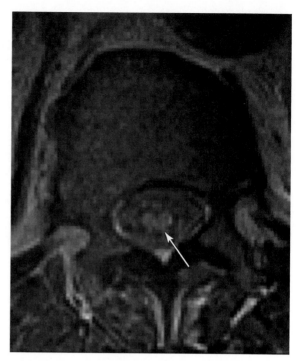

Figure 50-14. Axial T2-weighted MR image shows central hyperintensity of the spinal cord caused by infarct (*arrow*).

- *Cavernomas* may occur anywhere in the spinal cord. They may manifest at any age, chronically or acutely (secondary to hemorrhage). Back pain is often reported. On imaging studies, they are often well-demarcated intramedullary lesions with a surrounding hemosiderin ring (hypointense on T2-weighted MR images). Surrounding signal abnormality owing to edema or gliosis may be present, and these lesions may be calcified. Symptomatic lesions are treated with surgical excision.

42. How are spinal tumors classified anatomically?
- Extradural
- Intradural-extramedullary
- Intramedullary

Key Points: Classification of Tumors and Other Lesions within the Spinal Canal

1. *Extradural* (outside the thecal sac)—disc pathology, metastasis, epidural abscess, hematoma, bone abnormality
2. *Intradural-extramedullary* (inside the thecal sac but outside the cord)—nerve sheath tumor (neurofibroma, schwannoma), meningioma, metastases, lipoma, arachnoid cyst
3. *Intramedullary* (inside the cord)—tumors (astrocytoma, ependymoma, hemangioblastoma), multiple sclerosis, cord infarct, arteriovenous malformation, syrinx

---

43. What is the most common epidural spinal tumor in adults?
Metastases are the most common neoplasms involving the epidural space. Epidural involvement is usually related to direct extension from an adjacent vertebral bone metastasis, although involvement of the epidural space in the absence of bone involvement on imaging can occur (most often with lymphoma, leukemia, Ewing sarcoma, breast cancer, and lung carcinoma). On radiographs and CT, metastases may appear as lytic or sclerotic lesions. Pathologic compression fractures may result. Typically, metastases show increased uptake of radiotracer on bone scintigraphy. MRI is the most sensitive modality for the detection of osseous metastases, which appear as foci of signal abnormality within the marrow space, typically hypointense on T1-weighted images and hyperintense on fat-suppressed T2-weighted images with variable enhancement characteristics. MRI optimizes detection of spinal cord or nerve root compression (Fig. 50-15).

44. What is the most common benign osseous lesion involving the spine?

Usually an incidental finding, hemangiomas are benign, present in approximately 11% of patients, and typically have a characteristic appearance on MRI. They are typically markedly hyperintense on T2-weighted images, and because they contain internal fat, they are also hyperintense on T1-weighted images.

45. What is the differential diagnosis for an intradural-extramedullary tumor?

The most common intradural-extramedullary tumors are benign and include meningiomas and neural neoplasms (neurofibromas and schwannomas). Meningiomas most commonly occur in the mid-thoracic region and are much more common in women than in men. Nerve sheath tumors typically enhance avidly and extend along or envelop a nerve root. These tumors may have intradural and extradural components. These tumors are often slow-growing, and bony remodeling, neural foraminal expansion, and vertebral body scalloping are common secondary imaging findings.

46. What neoplasms are associated with leptomeningeal seeding of tumor?

Leptomeningeal metastatic disease may occur with primary central nervous system neoplasms and with systemic malignancies. Medulloblastoma, ependymoma, glioblastoma multiforme, and other high-grade astrocytomas are the primary central nervous system tumors that have been most often associated with leptomeningeal seeding. This phenomenon may also occur, however, with choroid plexus tumors, other glial tumors (including pilocytic astrocytomas), germ cell tumors, retinoblastomas, and primary spinal tumors.

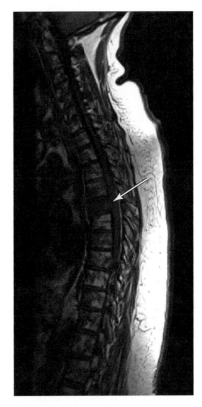

Figure 50-15. Sagittal T1-weighted MR image of the cervical and thoracic spine shows heterogeneous marrow signal intensity with prominent replacement of an upper thoracic vertebral body, and a pathologic compression fracture with resultant compromise of the spinal canal (*arrow*).

Systemic tumors, including lymphoma, may directly invade the subarachnoid space or may disseminate via lymphatic or hematogenous means. On MRI, leptomeningeal tumor often produces enhancement along the surface of the spinal cord that may be nodular and diffuse and is most prominent along the lumbar nerve roots and cauda equina. There may be associated edema (T2-weighted hyperintensity) within the spinal cord. Imaging of the brain may be notable for communicating hydrocephalus. Adequate cerebrospinal fluid sampling (up to three high-volume lumbar punctures) remains more sensitive than imaging for the detection of leptomeningeal disease.

47. List the most common intramedullary spinal tumors.

- Ependymoma
- Astrocytoma
- Hemangioblastoma
- Metastasis

48. Describe the distinguishing clinical and imaging features of intramedullary spinal tumors.

- *Ependymomas* occur in all age groups and are slightly more common in men. Ependymoma is the most common primary tumor of the lower spinal cord, conus medullaris, and filum terminale. Imaging findings include bony remodeling (spinal canal expansion, vertebral body scalloping, or pedicle erosion), spinal cord expansion, centrally located mass within the conus or filum, and heterogeneous signal intensity and enhancement—often with hemorrhage or hypercellularity.
- *Astrocytomas* most often occur in the thoracic cord in young adults and children. On MRI, the spinal cord is typically expanded with decreased T1-weighted and increased T2-weighted signal intensity. These tumors are most often eccentric in location and enhance. Cysts may be seen within or adjacent to the lesions.
- *Hemangioblastomas* are the third most common of the primary intramedullary tumors, but account for less than 5% of such tumors. These tumors are commonly seen in patients with von Hippel-Lindau disease. Hemangioblastomas are most often single, are located in the thoracic region, enhance avidly, and are commonly associated with cysts. Because these tumors are often vascular, enlarged vessels may be seen within the spinal canal. Although most are intramedullary, hemangioblastomas may also be intradural-extramedullary or extradural in location (Fig. 50-16).

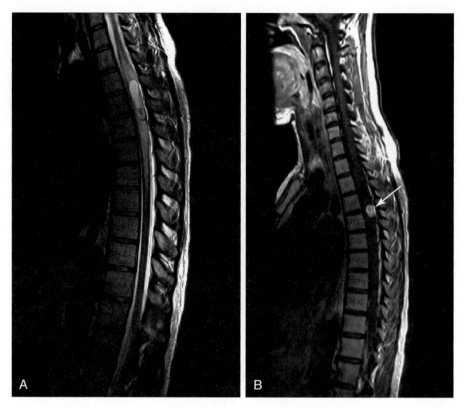

Figure 50-16. A, Hemangioblastoma. Sagittal T2-weighted MR image reveals long area of signal abnormality and expansion within the upper thoracic cord. **B,** Gadolinium-enhanced T1-weighted image of thoracic spine shows a nodule of enhancement (*arrow*) with associated cyst and edema.

- *Intramedullary metastases* are less common and are typically found in patients with widespread metastatic disease. The most common primary tumor to metastasize to the spinal cord is carcinoma of the lung. Cord metastases may also be seen with breast carcinoma, melanoma, lymphoma, colon carcinoma, and renal cell carcinoma.

BIBLIOGRAPHY

[1] L.F. Czervionke, V.M. Haughton, Degenerative disease of the spine, in: S.W. Atlas (Ed.), Magnetic Resonance Imaging of the Brain and Spine, third ed., Lippincott Williams & Wilkins, Philadelphia, 2002, pp. 1633–1714.
[2] A.E. Flanders, S.E. Croul, Spinal trauma, in: S.W. Atlas (Ed.), Magnetic Resonance Imaging of the Brain and Spine, third ed., Lippincott Williams & Wilkins, Philadelphia, 2002, pp. 1769–1824.
[3] J.H. Harris, S.E. Mervis, Mechanistic classification of acute cervical spine injuries, in: J.H. Harris, S.E. Mervis (Eds.), The Radiology of Acute Cervical Spine Trauma, third ed., Lippincott Williams & Wilkins, Philadelphia, 1996, pp. 213–244.
[4] J.R. Hoffman, W.R. Mower, A.B. Wolfson, et al., Validity of a set of clinical criteria to rule out injury to the cervical spine in patients with blunt trauma. National Emergency X-Radiography Utilization Study Group, N. Engl. J. Med. 343 (2000) 94–99.
[5] R.W. Hurst, Vascular disorders of the spine and spinal cord, in: S.W. Atlas (Ed.), Magnetic Resonance Imaging of the Brain and Spine, third ed., Lippincott Williams & Wilkins, Philadelphia, 2002, pp. 1825–1854.
[6] T.P. Naidich, S.I. Blaser, B.N. Delman, et al., Congenital anomalies of the spine and spinal cord: embryology and malformations, in: S.W. Atlas (Ed.), Magnetic Resonance Imaging of the Brain and Spine, third ed., Lippincott Williams & Wilkins, Philadelphia, 2002, pp. 1527–1632.
[7] A.G. Osborn, Nonneoplastic disorders of the spine and spinal cord, in: A.G. Osborn (Ed.), Diagnostic Neuroradiology, Mosby, St. Louis, 1994, pp. 820–875.
[8] A.G. Osborn, Normal anatomy and congenital anomalies of the spine and spinal cord, in: A.G. Osborn (Ed.), Diagnostic Neuroradiology, Mosby, St. Louis, 1994, pp. 785–819.
[9] G. Sze, Neoplastic disease of the spine and spinal cord, in: S.W. Atlas (Ed.), Magnetic Resonance Imaging of the Brain and Spine, third ed., Lippincott Williams & Wilkins, Philadelphia, 2002, pp. 1715–1768.
[10] I.G. Stiell, G.A. Wells, K. Vandemheen, et al., The Canadian C-Spine Rule for radiography in alert and stable trauma patients, JAMA 286 (2001) 1841–1848.

CHAPTER 51

HEAD AND NECK: PART I

Mary Scanlon, MD, and
Laurie A. Loevner, MD

1. The hyoid bone divides the neck into two distinct regions. Name them.

The hyoid bone divides the neck into the *suprahyoid neck* (extending from the skull base to the hyoid bone) and the *infrahyoid neck* (extending from the hyoid to the cervicothoracic junction) (Fig. 51-1). The hyoid bone is a logical dividing point because its fascial attachments functionally cleave the neck into these two distinct anatomic regions.

2. What imaging modalities are used to evaluate lesions in the two regions of the neck?

Magnetic resonance imaging (MRI) is the study of choice for the evaluation of lesions in the suprahyoid neck. The superior soft tissue contrast and multiplanar capabilities of MRI enable excellent evaluation of the skull base and evaluation for intracranial extent of disease from direct growth and from perineural and meningeal spread. In the infrahyoid neck, where there is abundance of fat and less complex anatomy, computed tomography (CT) is the imaging study of choice.

3. What are the three subdivisions of the pharynx?

The three subdivisions of the pharynx are nasopharynx, oropharynx, and hypopharynx (see Fig. 51-1). The *nasopharynx* extends from the base of the skull to the superior surface of the soft palate. The *oropharynx* extends from the soft palate to the hyoid bone. The *hypopharynx* extends from the hyoid bone to the inferior aspect of the cricoid cartilage. The oral cavity is a separate anatomic compartment distinct from the pharynx. It is located anterior to the oropharynx, from which it is anatomically demarcated by a ring of structures that include the circumvallate papillae of the tongue, anterior tonsillar pillars, and soft palate (Fig. 51-2).

4. What are the boundaries of the nasopharynx?

The nasopharynx is divided into three subsites: the posterior-superior wall, lateral wall (also known as Rosenmüller fossa), and anterior-inferior wall (which is the superior surface of the soft palate). Laterally, the torus tubarius serves as the cartilaginous opening of the eustachian tube (Fig. 51-3).

5. What structures are part of the oropharynx?

The oropharynx includes the posterior third of the tongue (base of tongue), vallecula, palatine tonsils and tonsillar fossa, soft palate, and uvula.

6. What structures are part of the hypopharynx?

The hypopharynx includes the piriform sinuses laterally, postcricoid region inferiorly (essentially the anterior wall of the hypopharynx), and posterior pharyngeal wall.

7. What structures are part of the oral cavity?

The oral cavity includes the lips, anterior two thirds of the tongue, buccal mucosa, gingiva, hard palate, retromolar trigone, and floor of the mouth.

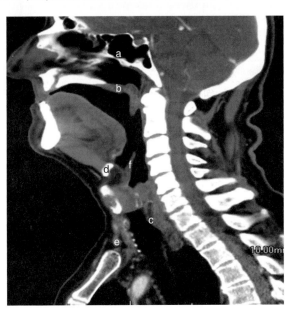

Figure 51-1. Contrast-enhanced midline sagittal CT scan of the neck. Hyoid bone (*d*) divides the neck into the suprahyoid neck extending from the skull base (*a*) to the hyoid bone, and the infrahyoid neck extending from the hyoid to the cervicothoracic junction (*e*). The nasopharynx extends from the skull base to the superior soft palate (*b*). The oropharynx extends from the soft palate to the hyoid bone. The hypopharynx extends from the hyoid to the inferior cricoid (*c*). The larynx (comprising the supraglottis, glottis, and subglottis) extends from the hyoid bone to the inferior cricoid cartilage. Epiglottis (*f*) is part of the supraglottic larynx.

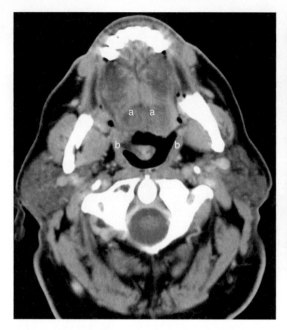

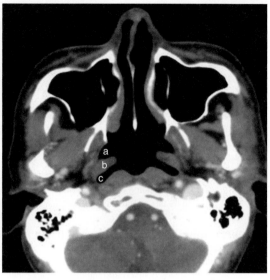

Figure 51-2. Axial unenhanced CT scan showing the anterior tonsillar pillars (*b*) and the circumvallate papillae (*a*), which along with the soft palate separate the oral cavity anteriorly from the oropharynx posteriorly.

Figure 51-3. Contrast-enhanced axial CT scan through the nasopharynx showing the opening of the eustachian tube (*a*), the torus tubarius (*b*), and the lateral wall of the nasopharynx, also known as Rosenmüller fossa (*c*). This is the most common site of origin of nasopharyngeal cancers.

8. Name the three anatomic subsites of the larynx.

The supraglottis, glottis, and subglottis are the three anatomic subsites of the larynx. The soft tissues of the larynx are supported by a cartilaginous framework that includes the cricoid, thyroid, and arytenoid cartilages.

9. What are the boundaries of the supraglottis?

The superior extent of the supraglottis is the tip of the epiglottis, and the supraglottis extends inferiorly to the laryngeal ventricle (which separates the false from the true vocal cords) (Fig. 51-4). The supraglottis includes the epiglottis, false vocal cords, aryepiglottic folds, and arytenoid cartilage. The laryngeal ventricle separates the false vocal cords of the supraglottis from the true vocal cords of the glottis. The aryepiglottic folds separate the supraglottic airway from the laterally situated piriform sinus of the hypopharynx.

10. What structures compose the glottis?

The glottis is composed of the true vocal cords and the anterior and posterior commissures.

11. Where is the subglottis located?

The subglottis is the region of the larynx that extends from the undersurface of the true vocal cords through the inferior surface of the cricoid cartilage.

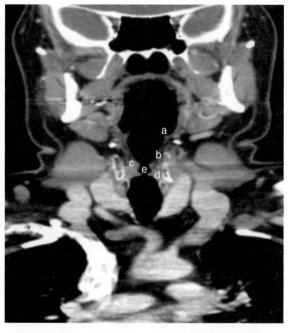

Figure 51-4. Contrast-enhanced coronal CT scan through the larynx. The supraglottis extends from the tip of the epiglottis inferiorly to the laryngeal ventricle (*e*). The laryngeal ventricle separates the false cords (*c*) of the supraglottis from the true cords (*d*) of the glottis. The aryepiglottic folds (*a*) separate the supraglottic airway from the lateral piriform sinus of the hypopharynx. Tumor can spread in the fat of the submucosal paraglottic space transglottically (*b*). The mucosal surface or the paraglottic space may serve as conduits of spread of laryngeal cancer from one part of the larynx to another (i.e., supraglottic cancer may spread to the glottis and subglottis).

12. Name and identify the extramucosal spaces of the head and neck in Fig. 51-5.

Lateral to the pharyngeal airway are the parapharyngeal space (PPS), masticator space (MS), parotid space (PS), and carotid space (CS). Posterior to the pharyngeal airway are the retropharyngeal space (RPS) and the perivertebral space (PVS). The PPS is the central, primarily fat-containing space around which the other extramucosal spaces are located. The PPS contains fat, lymphatics, nerves, and minor salivary gland tissue. The MS contains the muscles of mastication (lateral and medial pterygoid and masseter and temporalis muscles), the ascending ramus of the mandible, and the V3 branch of the trigeminal nerve. The PS includes the parotid gland, facial nerve, retromandibular vein, external carotid branches, and intraparotid lymph nodes. The CS includes the internal carotid artery, internal jugular vein, cranial nerves IX through XII, sympathetic plexus, and lymph nodes of the deep cervical chain. The RPS includes predominately fat and lymph nodes. The PVS includes the longus colli/capitis muscle complex, paraspinal musculature, vertebral body, posterior triangle of the neck, neurovascular structures within the spinal canal, and brachial plexus. The transverse process of the vertebral bodies divides this space further into the prevertebral portion anteriorly and the paraspinal portion posteriorly.

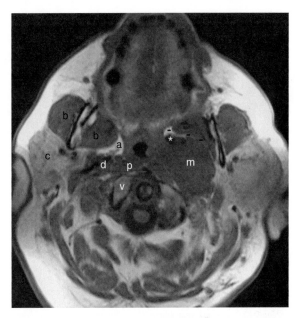

Figure 51-5. Unenhanced axial T1-weighted MR image of the suprahyoid neck, showing the normal extramucosal spaces on the right side of the neck. On the left, note the large carotid space mass (*m*) with characteristic anterior displacement of the fat in the parapharyngeal space (*a*). The retropharynx is a "potential space" that sits anterior to the prevertebral space (*p*), and behind the pharyngeal constrictor muscles. Anterior displacement of the carotid (*asterisk*) places this mass in the carotid space (*d*). (*b*, masticator space; *c*, parotid space; *v*, vertebral space.)

13. Describe how displacement of the fat in the PPS helps to localize lesions or masses to their correct anatomic subsite in the extramucosal compartment.

The PPS is the central, primarily fat-containing space that is surrounded by the MS anteriorly, CS posteriorly, PS laterally, and pharyngeal mucosal space medially. Deviation of the fat in the PPS can help localize large masses to one of these four spaces. Large MS lesions deviate the PPS fat posteromedially, a mass in the PS deviates it medially, a CS mass deviates the PPS fat anteriorly, and submucosal extension of a pharyngeal mucosal mass deviates the fat medially (see Fig. 51-5).

14. Displacement of the longus colli/longus capitis prevertebral muscle complex helps differentiate masses in what two extramucosal spaces?

Displacement of the longus colli/longus capitis prevertebral muscle complex helps differentiate masses in the RPS and PVS. If these muscles are depressed posteriorly, the mass is arising either from the pharyngeal mucosal space or from the RPS. If the muscle is elevated anteriorly off of the spine, the lesion is arising from the PVS (usually the bone). If one can localize a mass to the correct extramucosal space, and if the anatomic components of that space are known, a differential diagnosis can be readily formulated.

15. Displacement of the cervical internal carotid artery helps differentiate masses in what two extramucosal spaces?

Displacement of the cervical internal carotid artery helps differentiate masses in the PPS (prestyloid) and CS (poststyloid). Masses in the PPS, when large enough, displace the adjacent internal carotid artery posteriorly, whereas masses in the CS elevate the adjacent internal carotid artery anteriorly (see Fig. 51-5).

16. What are the imaging criteria for diagnosis of a pathologic lymph node?

Imaging criteria for pathologic nodes are based on nodal size and architecture. Any lymph node, regardless of size, that exhibits central low density (necrosis or cystic degeneration) is pathologic until proven otherwise (Fig. 51-6). The size criteria used depend on nodal location. The cervical nodes are anatomically classified by a grading system (I to VII), as follows:

- Level I nodes are the submental and submandibular nodes.
- Levels II, III, and IV are the nodes in the internal jugular chain; level II nodes are located from the base of the skull to the hyoid bone, level III nodes are located between the hyoid bone and cricoid cartilage, and level IV nodes are located below the cricoid cartilage.

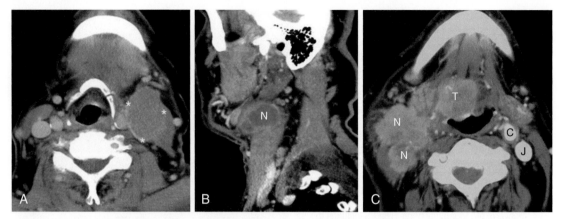

Figure 51-6. Pathologic lymph nodes resulting from metastatic thyroid cancer and metastatic head and neck cancer. **A,** Low-density cystic node with barely perceptible contrast-enhancing wall (*asterisk*). In a child, a cystic mass behind the angle of the mandible is most likely a branchial cleft cyst. In an adult, a cystic neck mass is a pathologic node until proven otherwise. In the differential diagnosis of cystic nodal masses in adults, one must consider metastatic nodes from papillary thyroid cancer and metastatic disease from oropharyngeal squamous cell carcinomas arising from the base of tongue or tonsil. **B,** Necrotic lymph node from metastatic head and neck squamous cell carcinoma. Low-attenuation center with thick irregular contrast-enhancing wall (*N*) is the characteristic appearance on imaging of a necrotic lymph node. **C,** Solid conglomerate lymph node mass (*N*) with encasement and occlusion of carotid artery and jugular vein. Note the primary tumor in base of tongue (*T*) and the normal carotid (*C*) and jugular vein (*J*) in the contralateral neck.

- Level V nodes are posterior to the sternocleidomastoid muscle.
- Level VI nodes are in the deep visceral chain.
- Level VII nodes are in the superior mediastinum.

Level II to VII nodes are considered pathologic in size if they are greater than 1 cm. Level I and the jugulodigastric nodes (the only named level II node) are considered pathologic if they are greater than 1.5 cm.

17. What is the best cross-sectional imaging study to identify pathologic nodes?

If the only clinical question is whether there is pathologic lymphadenopathy in the neck, CT is the study of choice. It is more accurate than MRI in detecting nodal necrosis, especially in nodes of normal size.

Key Points: Neck Lesions

1. Neck lesions above the hyoid bone should be studied first with MRI. Pathologic conditions of the neck below the hyoid bone should be imaged first with CT scanning.
2. The most common cause of a cystic neck mass in an adult is metastatic adenopathy.

---

18. What is the most common cause of a calcified cervical lymph node?

In an adult, the most common cause is metastatic papillary thyroid carcinoma. In a child, metastatic neuroblastoma is the most common cause of calcified lymph nodes. Other, less common causes of calcified lymph nodes include tuberculosis, other nontubercular granulomatous infections, sarcoid, and treated lymphoma.

19. What is the most common cause of a cystic mass in the lateral neck of an adult?

Metastatic nodal disease is the most common cause of a cystic mass in the lateral neck of an adult. Causes of such metastases include papillary thyroid cancer and squamous cell carcinoma (see Fig. 51-6). Carcinoma of the base of the tongue and tonsillar carcinoma are the most common primary head and neck carcinomas that result in cystic metastases. Metastatic cancer should always be the primary consideration of a cystic neck mass in adults. Branchial cleft cysts are usually diagnosed in young patients. They most often are found at the angle of the jaw anterior to the sternocleidomastoid muscle and just touching the posterior aspect of the submandibular gland.

20. What are the most common causes of cervical lymph node metastases in an adult?

In 85% of patients older than 40 years, lymph node metastases from squamous cell carcinoma of the head and neck are most common. In patients 20 to 40 years old, the major differential diagnosis includes lymphoma, metastatic squamous cell carcinoma, metastatic thyroid cancer, and inflammatory adenitis.

21. In patients with head and neck cancer, how does the presence of metastatic adenopathy affect prognosis?

The presence of nodes dramatically reduces the 5-year survival of patients with squamous cell carcinoma. It follows the rule of 50%. The presence of a single lymph node reduces the 5-year survival by 50%. If the nodes are bilateral, 5-year survival is reduced by another 50%. If there is nodal fixation or extracapsular extension of tumor, expected survival goes down yet another 50%. Fixation of nodes (nonmobility) is probably best determined clinically. Extranodal spread can be suggested on CT by the demonstration of shaggy, irregular margins to the nodes; the presence of soft tissue stranding in the neck fat around the nodes; and enlarging nodal size. Extracapsular extension occurs in 75% of nodes 3 cm or greater in dimension.

22. What is the role of the radiologist in the evaluation and staging of head and neck cancer?

The clinician and radiologist must work together as a team. The clinician/endoscopist can accurately assess the mucosa of the aerodigestive tract. The radiologist, with cross-sectional imaging, sees the submucosa. When clinical and radiologic data are combined, there is 85% accuracy in staging patients. The radiologist is best at assessing submucosal spread of tumor, identifying necrosis in normal-sized nodes, and identifying retropharyngeal nodes (generally clinically occult).

23. Describe the most common neck masses in a child.

Inflammatory adenitis and congenital mass lesions are the two most common causes of neck masses in children. Malignancy is third. Lateral neck masses include cystic hygroma, branchial cleft cysts, inflammatory adenitis, and lymphoma. Midline masses include thyroglossal duct cysts, hemangiomas, and dermoids/epidermoids.

The most common congenital neck mass is a thyroglossal duct cyst. It can occur anywhere from the foramen cecum at the base of the tongue to the natural location of the thyroid gland. Most are located in the infrahyoid neck (65%), but they can occur at the hyoid (15%) or above (20%); 75% are located in the midline. The more inferior the cyst, the more likely it is to be off-midline (Fig. 51-7).

Thyroid carcinoma, usually papillary, arises in less than 1% of thyroglossal duct cysts. The presence of a nodule or calcification associated with the cyst should raise suspicion for the presence of carcinoma.

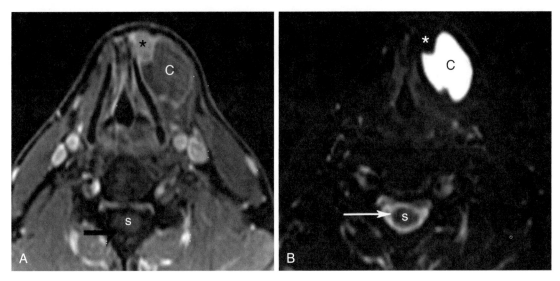

Figure 51-7. Axial MR images through the infrahyoid neck showing the characteristic appearance of a thyroglossal duct cyst (*C*) embedded in the strap muscles. **A,** Axial enhanced T1-weighted MR image shows proteinaceous (fluid hyperintense or "brighter" than the cerebrospinal fluid [*arrow*] around the spinal cord [*S*]) cystic left paramedian neck mass (*C*). Also note the solid nodule (*asterisk*) along the anteromedial aspect of the cyst. This nodule reflects papillary cancer in the thyroglossal duct cyst, which is seen in approximately 1% of these lesions. The presence of solid tissue or calcification within a thyroglossal duct cyst is usually indicative of coexistent papillary cancer within the cyst. **B,** Axial T2-weighted MR image shows hyperintense "bright" fluid of the cyst (*C*), similar to cerebrospinal fluid (*arrow*).

BIBLIOGRAPHY

[1] B.F. Branstetter IV, J.L. Weissman, Infection of the facial area, oral cavity, oropharynx, and retropharynx, Neuroimaging Clin. North Am. 13 (2003) 393–410.

[2] D.M. Gor, J.E. Langer, L.A. Loevner, Imaging of cervical lymph nodes in head and neck cancer: the basics, Radiol. Clin. North Am. 44 (2006) 101–110.

[3] P. Henrot, A. Blum, B. Toussaint, et al., Dynamic maneuvers in local staging of head and neck malignancies with current imaging techniques: principles and clinical applications, RadioGraphics 23 (2003) 1201–1213.

[4] L.A. Loevner, S. Kaplan, M. Cunnane, G. Moonis, Cross-sectional imaging of the thyroid gland, Neuroimaging Clin. N. Am. 18 (2008) 445–461.

[5] M.G. Mack, J.O. Balzer, C. Herzog, T.J. Vogl, Multi-detector CT: head and neck imaging, Eur. Radiol. 13 (Suppl. 5) (2003) M121–M126.

HEAD AND NECK: PART II

Mary Scanlon, MD, and
Laurie A. Loevner, MD

CHAPTER 52

PARANASAL SINUSES

1. Through what structure do the maxillary, frontal, and anterior ethmoid air cells drain?

The ostiomeatal complex is the common drainage pathway for the paranasal sinuses. It refers to the uncinate process, a small bone around which mucus and secretions drain through the maxillary sinus ostium, infundibulum, hiatus semilunaris, and middle meatus (Fig. 52-1). The posterior ethmoid and sphenoid sinuses drain via the sphenoethmoidal recess into the superior meatus. Only the lacrimal duct drains into the inferior meatus. Acute bouts of sinusitis are typically treated medically, and diagnosis is made on clinical grounds. Imaging is reserved for patients who have chronic symptoms despite maximal medical therapy. Computed tomography (CT) is never performed during acute infection, but rather after 4 to 6 weeks of maximal medical therapy. Delineation of ostiomeatal complex anatomy and the identification of any anatomic variants that narrow this common drainage pathway are key for the ear, nose, and throat surgeon (otorhinolaryngologist) to plan possible surgical correction.

2. In which paranasal sinus does malignancy most commonly arise?

The most common site involved is the maxillary sinus, followed by the nasal cavity and the ethmoid air cells. It is rare to have a malignancy arise within the frontal or sphenoid sinus. The role of the radiologist is not, however, to be the histologist, but rather to map the extent of disease so that the surgeon can plan his or her surgical approach. Of sinonasal malignancies, 80% are squamous cell carcinomas. Another 10% are adenocarcinomas and adenoid cystic carcinomas arising from minor salivary gland rests. Other cell types include melanoma and olfactory neuroblastomas (esthesioneuroblastoma). The hallmark of squamous cell carcinoma is bony destruction.

3. On an unenhanced CT scan, what are common causes of hyperdense tissue within the paranasal sinuses?

The big three are inspissated secretions, mycetoma (fungus ball), and blood. Inspissated secretions resulting from chronic sinusitis are the most common of these entities. These dense secretions may also be seen within chronic polyps of the sinonasal cavity. With polyposis, there is expansion and bony remodeling. The dense appearance on CT is due to high protein content and viscosity. Blood within a paranasal sinus usually shows an air-fluid-hemorrhage level.

4. What classic radiologic finding supports the diagnosis of acute sinusitis in the appropriate clinical setting?

An air-fluid level in a paranasal sinus, in the absence of trauma or sinus irrigation, is the characteristic finding in acute sinusitis.

5. Name the three major salivary glands and the ducts that drain them.

The three major salivary glands are the parotid, submandibular, and sublingual.

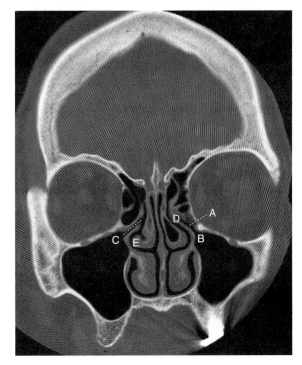

Figure 52-1. Coronal unenhanced CT scan of paranasal sinuses at the level of the ostiomeatal unit performed using bone algorithm. *A,* uncinate process (*dotted line*); *B,* maxillary sinus ostia; *C,* infundibulum (*dotted line*); *D,* hiatus semilunaris; *E,* middle meatus.

- The parotid gland is drained by Stensen duct, which courses from the parotid gland and passes over the masseter muscle to insert into the cheek at the level of the second maxillary molar.
- The submandibular gland is drained by Wharton duct, which drains on either side of the frenulum in the floor of the mouth (Fig. 52-2).
- The sublingual glands consist of 12 to 18 small, paired glands located in the sublingual space in the floor of the mouth. The sublingual glands have many draining ducts, known as the ducts of Rivinus, which drain into the floor of the mouth. If there is a dominant sublingual duct opening into Wharton duct, it is called the duct of Bartholin.

6. What salivary gland has the highest incidence of calculi/stones, and why?

By 4:1, it is most common to have calculi/stones in the submandibular gland (see Fig. 52-2). The submandibular gland is more prone to stone formation because of its more alkaline and viscous secretions. In addition, its draining duct is wider, has a narrower orifice, and takes an upward course. On thin-cut unenhanced CT, more than 90% of these stones are radiopaque.

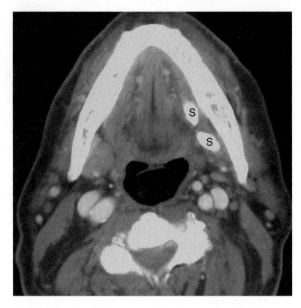

Figure 52-2. Contrast-enhanced axial CT scan through the floor of mouth showing multiple calculi (*S*) in the submandibular (Wharton) duct.

7. Which salivary gland contains lymphoid tissue? What is the significance of this tissue?

The parotid gland is the first salivary gland to form and the last to encapsulate. As such, it is the only salivary gland to contain lymphoid tissue. For this reason, it is the only salivary gland that has the potential for lymphadenopathy from systemic diseases (e.g., rheumatoid arthritis, Sjögren syndrome, human immunodeficiency virus [HIV] infection), metastases to intraglandular nodes (usually from skin cancer of the scalp), lymphoma, and Warthin tumors. A major lymphatic drainage pathway of the scalp is to the lymph nodes in the parotid gland.

8. What is the most common benign tumor of the salivary glands?

The most common benign tumor of the salivary glands is pleomorphic adenoma (mixed benign tumor), which is seen most often in the parotid gland, where it represents approximately 80% of all parotid masses. Parotid gland masses follow the 80% rule: 80% are benign, 80% are pleomorphic adenomas, 80% occur in the superficial lobe, and approximately 80% of untreated pleomorphic adenomas remain benign (20% may undergo malignant degeneration to squamous cell carcinoma).

9. What are the most common malignancies of the salivary glands?

The most common malignant lesion of the parotid gland is mucoepidermoid carcinoma. In the submandibular, sublingual, and minor salivary glands, the most common malignancy is adenoid cystic carcinoma.

10. How is the size of the salivary gland related to the likelihood of a mass in the gland being malignant?

In an adult, the rule is that the larger the salivary gland, the lower the likelihood that a mass within it would be malignant. The reverse is true in pediatric patients. In an adult, a parotid mass has a rate of malignancy of about 15% to 20%; the submandibular gland, 40% to 50%; and the sublingual glands, greater than 50%.

11. What imaging features distinguish a benign thyroid mass from a malignant thyroid mass?

There is nothing specific about the appearance of an intrathyroidal mass (e.g., calcification, low attenuation, or hemorrhage) that distinguishes a benign nodule from a malignant nodule (Fig. 52-3). Any thyroid mass that measures 1.2 to 1.5 cm in two planes should be studied further with histologic analysis. Tissue for cytology is usually obtained by fine-needle aspiration in the physician's office for palpable lesions and under ultrasound guidance in the radiology department for lesions that are nonpalpable. Missed cancers that are 1.2 cm or larger in two planes tend to have a higher incidence of unfavorable biologic behavior (i.e., lymphatic spread and angioinvasion).

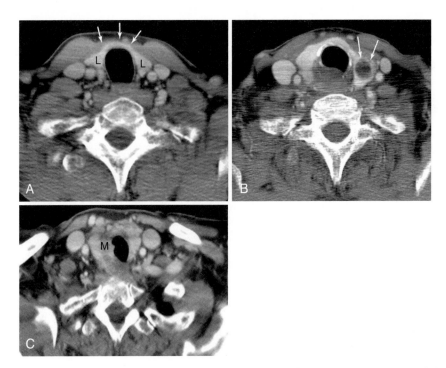

Figure 52-3. Normal thyroid gland and thyroid mass. **A,** Contrast-enhanced axial neck CT image at the level of the thyroid gland. Note normal right and left lobes of the thyroid gland (*L*) and the isthmus (*arrows*). **B,** Contrast-enhanced axial neck CT image in a different patient shows 1.3-cm, low-density mass in the left thyroid lobe (*arrows*). This is nonspecific regarding benign (i.e., goiter or adenoma) versus malignant disease (cancer). **C,** Contrast-enhanced axial neck CT image in a different patient shows low-density mass in the right lobe of the thyroid (*M*) with direct extension into the airway. Only secondary findings of extension of a thyroid mass outside the thyroid capsule and into adjacent soft tissues, the trachea or larynx, and the vessels in the carotid sheath or pathologic cervical lymphadenopathy are usually indicative of a malignant mass. CT and MRI features of an isolated mass in the thyroid gland are themselves not indicative of benign versus malignant thyroid pathology.

Other findings on cross-sectional imaging that suggest a thyroid mass is malignant include the presence of pathologic lymphadenopathy in the neck, extension of the thyroid mass outside of the thyroid capsule, and vascular invasion (spread into the adjacent internal jugular vein) (see Fig. 52-3C). Of thyroid carcinomas, 80% to 90% are papillary carcinoma. Other malignant tumors of the thyroid gland include anaplastic carcinoma, follicular cancer, medullary carcinoma, and primary lymphoma. Rarely, metastatic disease to the thyroid gland occurs (from primary lung, breast, and renal cell carcinomas).

12. What is the most common cause of proptosis in an adult?

Graves disease is the most common cause of unilateral or bilateral proptosis secondary to increased orbital fat and extraocular muscle enlargement. The extraocular muscle bellies are typically involved with characteristic sparing of the tendon insertions (Fig. 52-4). In contrast, the pattern of involvement with orbital pseudotumor (the second most common cause of proptosis), includes the tendons. Patients do not have to be hyperthyroid to have Graves ophthalmopathy. It may occur before, during, or after treatment. The key clinical feature of orbital pseudotumor is eye pain associated with the proptosis. Ocular lymphoma and metastatic disease are other common causes of proptosis

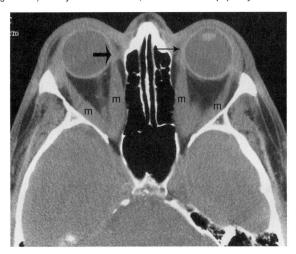

Figure 52-4. Unenhanced axial CT scan through the orbit showing bilateral enlargement of medial and lateral rectus muscles (*m*). Note the characteristic pattern of involvement—enlargement of the muscle bellies with sparing of the tendinous insertions (*arrows*). This feature helps distinguish Graves disease from orbital pseudotumor. Clinical presentation is also important. Pseudotumor typically manifests with eye pain.

13. Which metastatic lesion to the orbit is classically associated with enophthalmos?
Intraorbital, retrobulbar (behind the globe) metastatic breast carcinoma is commonly associated with enophthalmos. This association is due to the frequent scirrhous reaction of breast carcinoma that results in retraction of adjacent tissues, similar to what is commonly seen in the breast (retraction and dimpling of skin).

14. What is the most common primary ocular malignancy in a child and in an adult?
- In a child, retinoblastoma is the most common malignant tumor, and 95% of these masses are calcified. CT is best for detection of calcification (which can be difficult to see with magnetic resonance imaging [MRI]), whereas MRI is best for detecting intracranial extension.
- In an adult, the most common primary ocular malignancy is melanoma, although overall, the most common intraocular malignancy in an adult is a metastasis. The uveal tract is involved with both. Melanomas may grow along the optic nerve and into the subarachnoid space, with resultant dissemination throughout the neural axis.

In children and adults, malignant masses are commonly associated with a retinal detachment. Whenever a nontraumatic retinal detachment is identified, there must be careful evaluation for the presence of an associated intraocular mass.

15. What key clinical and imaging features distinguish an optic nerve glioma from an optic nerve meningioma?
The age of the patient and appearance of the optic nerve distinguish an optic nerve glioma from an optic nerve meningioma. Meningiomas occur in middle-aged adults, whereas optic nerve gliomas occur in children (mean age 8 to 9 years). Meningiomas straighten the optic nerve because they arise from the surrounding dura of the optic nerve sheath complex, whereas gliomas kink the nerve as the tumor arises from the nerve itself. With meningiomas, the mass can be separated from the optic nerve. Both can occur in children with neurofibromatosis, but optic nerve gliomas are the most common.

16. Hearing loss is classified into what two major subtypes?
The two major subtypes of hearing loss are sensorineural and conductive. MRI is the best imaging study to evaluate unilateral or asymmetric sensorineural hearing loss in an adult. The most common neoplasm associated with this hearing loss is an acoustic (vestibular) schwannoma, and thin-section MRI with contrast enhancement should be obtained through the internal auditory canal and cerebellopontine angle. The remainder of the acoustic pathway, including the cochlear nuclear complex, medulla, and thalami, and the temporal lobes should also be evaluated. High-resolution, thin-section unenhanced CT of the temporal bones is the best imaging study for sensorineural hearing loss in patients younger than 15 years because congenital anomalies or atresias involving the otic capsule, semicircular canals, and vestibular aqueduct are commonly the cause. CT is the study of choice in patients with conductive hearing loss at any age because it is best for showing the sequela of chronic otitis media or cholesteatoma.

> **Key Points: Sinusitis and Hearing Loss**
> 1. The best predictor of acute sinusitis in the appropriate clinical setting (facial pain, nasal drainage, fever) is the presence of an air-fluid level on a CT scan.
> 2. CT is the imaging modality of choice for conductive hearing loss.
> 3. MRI is the imaging modality of choice in adult-onset sensorineural hearing loss.

17. How is tinnitus clinically subcategorized?
Tinnitus is classified as pulsatile or nonpulsatile. Pulsatile tinnitus is divided further into *subjective* (patient hears beating) and *objective* (patient hears beating and so does the physician with a stethoscope). Pulsatile tinnitus is most often secondary to a vascular problem, including masses, malformations, or an anomaly. Causes include glomus tumor, dural arteriovenous fistula, aberrant internal carotid artery, or a high-riding jugular bulb. In subjective pulsatile tinnitus, CT is the first imaging study to perform. In objective pulsatile tinnitus, one may perform MRI, although patients are often assessed with conventional catheter angiography because the most concerning potential diagnosis is dural fistula. The most common cause of pulsatile tinnitus reported in the neurologic literature is benign intracranial hypertension (pseudotumor cerebri). Tinnitus without a pulsatile quality may be an early symptom of an acoustic tumor or otosclerosis. Other causes include cholesteatomas, noise damage, and old age. Relatively rare causes include multiple sclerosis and Arnold-Chiari I malformation.

18. Cholesteatoma is commonly noted to be a "pearly white" mass seen in the middle ear on otoscopic examination. What is a cholesteatoma?
Cholesteatomas can be acquired or congenital. Acquired cholesteatomas are basically an ingrowth of skin through a perforation in the tympanic membrane (TM). Patients have a history of chronic otitis media with TM rupture, and often have a history of myringotomy tube placements. The ingrowth of skin results in accumulation of squamous and keratin

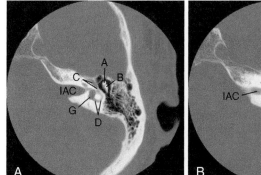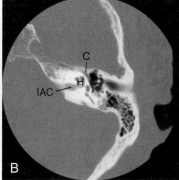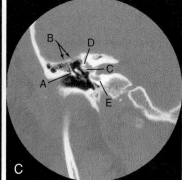

Figure 52-5. Normal temporal bone anatomy. **A,** and **B,** Unenhanced axial CT images (*A,* head of malleus; *B,* body of incus; *C,* tympanic portion of facial nerve; *D,* semicircular canals; *G,* vestibule; *H,* cochlea; *IAC,* internal auditory canal). **C** Unenhanced coronal CT image (*A,* scutum; *B,* tegmen tympani; *C,* tympanic portion of facial nerve; *D,* lateral semicircular canal; *E,* basal turn of the cochlea).

debris in the middle ear. The presence of associated osseous erosions on CT imaging is key to the diagnosis. One must be familiar with the normal anatomy of this region (Fig. 52-5). In the absence of such erosions, a cholesteatoma can look exactly like chronic granulation tissue or chronic otitis media. Most commonly, cholesteatomas occur through a defect superiorly in the pars flaccida portion of the TM. Tissue first fills Prussak space in the epitympanicum and erodes the scutum, then the ossicles, and may eventually progress to erode through the roof of the epitympanicum/tegmen tympani or undergo fistulization to the lateral semicircular canal or facial canal. Less commonly, cholesteatomas occur through a defect inferiorly in the pars tensa portion of the TM.

19. What neoplasms occur in the jugular foramen?

Glomus tumors, neural neoplasms (schwannoma), meningioma, and metastatic disease occur in the jugular foramen. Glomus jugulare tumors are the most common. They arise from Arnold nerve, a branch of cranial nerve X, which resides in the pars vascularis compartment of the jugular foramen. The jugular foramen is composed of two parts separated by a bony spur, the jugular spine. Anteriorly is the pars nervosa, which contains cranial nerve IX; posteriorly is the pars vascularis, which contains the internal jugular vein and cranial nerves X and XI. Glomus tumors, when large, erode the jugular spur and cause permeative bony changes (in contrast to the smooth osseous scalloping seen with schwannomas). In addition, in contrast to the other masses in this location that may compress the internal jugular vein, glomus tumors commonly grow directly into the jugular vein (Fig. 52-6).

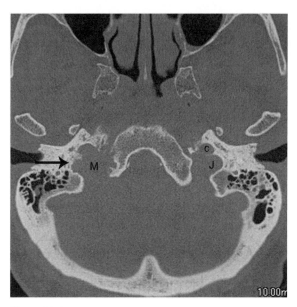

Figure 52-6. Unenhanced axial CT scan through the skull base showing normal jugular foramen on the left. The internal carotid artery canal (*c*) and the pars vascularis (*j*) are separated by a thin bony spur (caroticojugular spine). On the right, the jugular foramen is expanded by a mass (*M*) with permeative bony changes (*arrow*), and the jugular spine is eroded. These findings are most suggestive of a glomus tumor. Metastatic disease can also have this appearance.

20. Unilateral middle air fluid in an adult should trigger the search for what lesion?

Unilateral middle air fluid in an adult should raise suspicion for nasopharyngeal carcinoma, which most often arises from the lateral wall of the nasopharynx (fossa of Rosenmüller). Infiltration of the levator veli palatini muscle leads to eustachian tube dysfunction and serous otitis media. Nasopharyngeal carcinomas can infiltrate widely in all directions. Superiorly, they can extend into the clivus, sphenoid sinus, and neural foramina and osseous structures of the skull base.

BIBLIOGRAPHY

[1] G. Moonis, Imaging of sinonasal anatomy and inflammatory disorders, Crit. Rev. Comput. Tomogr. 44 (2003) 187–228.

[2] M. Okahara, H. Kiyosue, Y. Hori, et al., Parotid tumors: MR imaging with pathological correlation, Eur. Radiol. 13 (Suppl. 4) (2003) L25–L33.

[3] G.V. Shah, N.J. Fischbein, R. Patel, S.K. Mukherji, Newer MR imaging techniques for head and neck, Magn. Reson. Imaging Clin. N. Am. 11 (2003) 449–469.

POSITRON EMISSION TOMOGRAPHY

CHAPTER 53

Andrew Newberg, MD

1. **What instructions do patients need to prepare for positron emission tomography (PET) scan with fluorodeoxyglucose (FDG)?**
   The most important issue regarding a PET scan is that FDG competes with nonradioactive glucose. If a patient has recently eaten or has diabetes with a blood glucose level greater than 150 mg/dL, the sensitivity of the PET scan would be diminished. Typically, blood glucose levels greater than 200 mg/dL should exclude a patient from having a PET scan. Nondiabetic patients should have nothing by mouth (NPO) overnight or at least for 4 to 6 hours if their scan is later in the day. Diabetic patients should be managed carefully because some have difficulty forgoing eating. Also, insulin drives glucose, including FDG, into the muscles, so care should be taken regarding the administration of insulin too close to the scan time. It is preferred that the patient not inject insulin or eat before the PET scan, but if this is impossible, the referring physician must balance glucose levels, eating, and insulin in the diabetic patient. The scan itself takes place approximately 30 minutes after the intravenous injection of FDG, and performance of a whole-body scan takes an additional 30 to 60 minutes, depending on the type of scanner.

2. **Is bowel activity normal on the FDG PET scan in Fig. 53-1?**
   Generally, bowel activity can be a normal finding on a PET scan, which sometimes makes the evaluation of cancer in the bowel more difficult. Some centers recommend a bowel preparation to minimize constipation, which might result in substantial smooth muscle uptake in the bowel. Bowel uptake that is very focal and intense should raise suspicion, but it is very important to correlate such findings with either anatomic imaging or endoscopy.

3. **What structures in the head and neck normally take up FDG? Is the neck uptake normal in Fig. 53-2?**
   Normal uptake in the head and neck can be observed in the facial muscles, tongue (especially when patients are talking at the time of injection), neck muscles, brown fat, thyroid tissue, and vocal cords. The uptake of FDG can be very intense and can mimic or obscure cancer in these regions. Minimizing talking and patient movement and keeping the environment quiet and dimly lit during injection and for approximately 15 to 20 minutes after injection may help to diminish uptake in these areas.

4. **Is the lung nodule in the right upper lobe benign or malignant in Fig. 53-3?**
   A lung nodule that has a moderate amount of uptake needs to be evaluated further for malignancy. Typically, a standardized uptake value (SUV), a quantity that incorporates the patient's size and the injected dose, that is more than 2.0 is considered to be suggestive of malignancy, whereas lesions with SUVs less than this value are considered to be benign. The SUV of this nodule in the right upper lobe is 4.0. Benign lesions include inflammatory or infectious etiologies. There are examples, however, in which active infectious or inflammatory processes may result in SUVs comparable to SUVs observed in malignant disease, so clinical history and anatomic correlation are required for adequately assessing any finding on FDG PET.

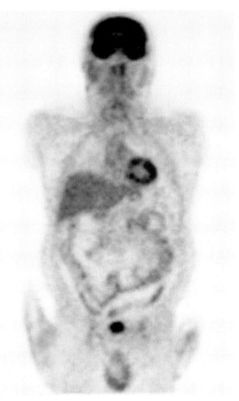

Figure 53-1. Normal FDG PET scan shows mild diffuse uptake throughout the bowel (normal variant), mild uptake in the liver, significant uptake in the brain and heart, and marked uptake in the bladder.

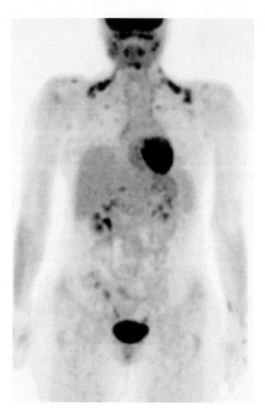

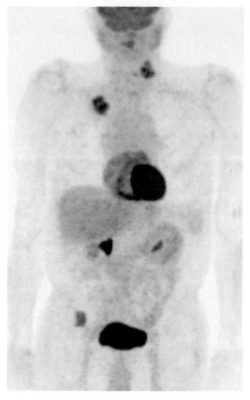

Figure 53-2. The neck uptake in this patient is related to muscle uptake or brown fat. Other structures normally seen in the neck include salivary glands, oropharynx, tongue, vocal cords, and sometimes the thyroid. Uptake in the heart, brain, kidneys, and bladder is normal. There are several small foci of mildly increased uptake in the lungs, which suggests an active metabolic process, such as neoplasm.

Figure 53-3. FDG PET scan of a patient with lung cancer shows intense uptake in the right upper lobe with a SUV of 4.0. Additional areas of increased uptake in the left supraclavicular region and the right inguinal region are also concerning for malignancy, and would require additional follow-up. Uptake in the heart, kidneys, and bladder is normal.

5. **Is the patient in Fig. 53-3 a good surgical candidate?**

One of the important uses of FDG PET is presurgical evaluation of patients with known lung cancer. If FDG PET scan shows malignant lesions on the contralateral hilar regions or distant metastases, the patient no longer is a surgical candidate and would proceed to systemic therapy. In this particular patient, there are additional areas of uptake that are concerning for malignancy in the left supraclavicular region and the right inguinal region, which would require additional follow-up. If these areas are confirmed to be malignant, the patient would no longer be a surgical candidate.

6. **How can FDG PET change the management of patients with lung cancer?**

Studies have revealed that FDG PET changes the surgical management of patients in 40% of cases. In some cases, distant metastases or restaging indicates that the cancer is inoperable, preventing surgery that would not have been useful. In 20% of patients, PET shows that enlarged nodes that may have prevented surgery from being considered are benign, so that surgery can be performed. This ability to change management has also contributed to the discovery that FDG PET is cost-effective in the management of patients with lung cancer because it can greatly alter the management and guide appropriate treatment.

Key Points: Indications for PET

1. *Oncologic staging*: St aging or restaging of non–small cell lung cancer, breast cancer, colorectal cancer, melanoma, lymphoma, head and neck cancer, and esophageal cancer (this indication is approved by Medicare)
2. *Brain tumors*: Differentiation of residual or recurrent brain tumor from radiation necrosis
3. *Seizures*: Presurgical, interictal identification of refractory brain seizure foci
4. *Cardiac imaging*: Metabolic assessment of myocardial viability

7. What are potential confounding diseases that can mimic lung cancer?

Several nonmalignant diseases can mimic lung cancer by appearing as focally intense areas of increased uptake on FDG PET scan. Most infectious processes, such as pneumonia, active tuberculosis, or other abscesses, can appear as focal areas of increased activity. Sarcoidosis and other granulomatous diseases can also manifest as focally increased uptake (Fig. 53-4). Iatrogenic causes, such as postsurgical or postradiation therapy, can have increased activity, although radiation changes are usually more diffuse, involving most of the radiation field.

8. How is dual time point imaging used?

The physiology of glucose uptake is such that malignant cells continue to take up more and more glucose over time, whereas normal tissues establish an equilibrium. By taking FDG PET images at several time points, the later time point images should reveal malignant regions as increasing in intensity, especially compared with the background levels. Dual time point imaging can contribute to making more accurate diagnoses, especially when FDG uptake is borderline high on earlier images and increases on later images.

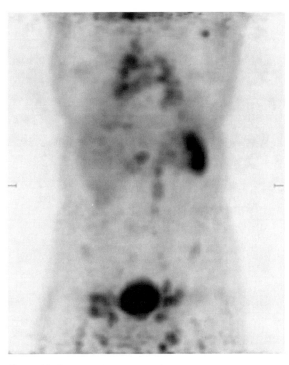

Figure 53-4. FDG PET scan of a patient with sarcoidosis shows multiple areas of intensely increased activity in the hilar regions; these findings appear similar to findings in lung cancer. This scan also shows increased activity in other regions, such as the left axilla, abdominal, and pelvic lymph nodes.

9. How important prognostically is FDG PET scan with negative results after treatment for lymphoma?

Studies evaluating the prognostic value of PET imaging for lymphoma after therapy have been quite dramatic. Patients with a PET scan with negative results have generally been shown to have greater than a 90% cure rate with excellent long-term survival. Patients with PET scans with positive results after therapy have less than a 10% chance of cure, and most have a survival of less than 2 to 3 years. FDG PET after chemotherapy for patients with lymphoma has very important prognostic implications and may suggest additional therapy for patients with scans with positive results (Fig. 53-5).

10. What are the current indications for FDG PET in patients with lymphoma?

Currently, FDG PET scans are recommended for initial staging, especially to evaluate whether there is disease above and below the diaphragm. PET imaging can also be valuable in the early stages of therapy to assess whether the particular intervention is working. PET can be used to obtain prognostic information after therapy. PET can be used to evaluate the possibility of recurrence of disease and can be a primary means of long-term follow-up of patients. PET can also be used for restaging if tumor recurrence is already observed.

11. How useful is PET in the evaluation of colon cancer?

A meta-analysis of studies evaluating almost 600 patients with colorectal cancer showed a sensitivity and specificity of whole-body FDG PET of 97% and 75%. The specificity was found to be greater for local recurrence and hepatic metastases (>95%). FDG PET imaging was responsible for a change in patient management in almost 30% of cases.

12. How does correlation with anatomic imaging help in detecting cancer accurately?

Fusing computed tomography (CT) and PET images has significant advantages over PET or CT alone. Studies have suggested that combining CT with PET may increase the diagnostic accuracy in 40% of patients compared with PET or CT alone. Specific advantages of fusing CT and PET images include discriminating metastases from physiologic foci of activity, improving lesion detection on PET and CT, precisely localizing metastatic foci, differentiating bone from soft tissue, differentiating liver from adjacent bowel, and identifying specific structures of the neck. These advantages have led to a change in management in 10% to 20% of patients over PET alone.

13. How does PET help with patient planning for radiation therapy?

FDG PET can play several roles with respect to planning for radiation therapy. Because PET can detect distant metastatic disease, it may change the need for performing radiation therapy in the first place. PET can also be beneficial in helping to evaluate the area that requires radiation. Numerous studies have shown that PET may show that the area of

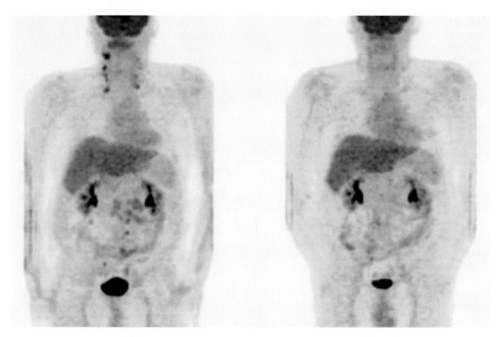

Figure 53-5. FDG PET scans in a patient with lymphoma before (*left*) and after (*right*) chemotherapy. The scan before chemotherapy shows multiple foci of increased activity in the neck and abdominal lymph node chains. The scan after chemotherapy reveals complete resolution of these findings, suggesting a good response to therapy and good overall prognosis.

increased metabolism extends beyond the abnormal region on anatomic imaging, which would result in expanding the target volume for radiation treatment. Alternatively, PET may show that some areas believed to be involved with cancer on anatomic imaging are hypometabolic and are not actively neoplastic. In this setting, the radiation volume can be reduced. Such changes in the plan for radiation therapy can occur in 25% of patients.

14. Is FDG PET useful for evaluating peritoneal seeding?

FDG PET can detect peritoneal seeding, but the sensitivity and specificity of PET for making such a diagnosis are much less than for other, more focal lesions. Peritoneal seeding can be difficult to detect on other imaging modalities as well; PET can still be useful when CT or magnetic resonance imaging (MRI) findings are equivocal because diffusely increased FDG uptake in various abdominal areas can suggest peritoneal seeding. PET can often show negative results, however, in patients with peritoneal seeding.

15. How useful is FDG PET in the evaluation of osteomyelitis?

FDG PET has been shown to be useful for evaluating infections in bones and soft tissues. Studies have suggested that FDG PET has a high sensitivity (90% to 100%) and specificity (81% to 89%) for detecting osteomyelitis in lower limb prostheses. Similar sensitivities and specificities have been reported in the detection of chronic osteomyelitis. Areas of osteomyelitis typically have intense uptake that is localized in the bone itself. More recently, PET has been used to evaluate soft tissue infectious or inflammatory disease, such as vascular graft infection, inflammatory bowel disease, and fever of unknown origin (Fig. 53-6).

16. How is PET used in the interictal evaluation of patients with seizure disorders?

FDG PET scans are commonly used to evaluate seizure patients who are refractory to medications before surgery is performed to remove specific seizure foci. FDG PET scan findings are also correlated with other clinical findings, such as electroencephalography, Wada test, MRI findings, and neuropsychologic tests. FDG PET has a sensitivity of more than 70% in the detection of seizure foci. The most common approach is to perform an interictal scan in which a seizure focus is expected to have reduced glucose metabolism. A clearly observed seizure focus on FDG PET can confirm the location of the seizure focus so that surgery can be performed. In Fig. 53-7, there is hypometabolism in the left temporal lobe, which is consistent with a seizure focus.

17. What are the most common areas for seizure foci, and what are the implications for finding multiple abnormal areas?

The temporal lobe is the most common focus of partial epilepsy and is the region that can be most accurately evaluated with FDG PET. The frontal lobes are the next most common area where seizure foci arise. This area is also relatively easy

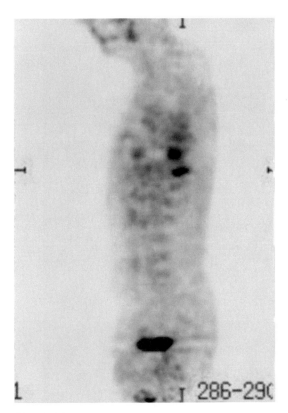

Figure 53-6. FDG PET scan of a patient with suspected osteomyelitis of the spine reveals intense activity in two adjacent mid-thoracic vertebral bodies. This finding is consistent with osteomyelitis.

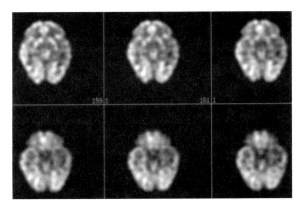

Figure 53-7. Interictal FDG PET brain scan in a patient with seizures reveals decreased metabolism in the left temporal lobe, consistent with a seizure focus.

to observe on FDG PET, and the sensitivity and specificity for the detection of seizure foci in both regions are similar. On scans in which more than one area appears to be involved, or when the regions of hypometabolism extend to other structures, the likelihood of resolution of seizures after surgery is typically diminished, sometimes substantially.

18. How useful is FDG PET for the evaluation of primary brain tumors or new metastatic disease?

FDG PET has generally not been useful for detecting primary brain or new metastatic tumors because the normal brain has such a high metabolism, and it is often difficult to find a tumor embedded in areas that already have high metabolism. Some studies have suggested, however, that the degree of hypermetabolism in tumors that have been detected may have prognostic implications because highly metabolic tumors tend to be the most aggressive and portend the worse prognosis. Low-grade tumors have lower metabolism and have an overall better prognosis.

19. What are the sensitivity and specificity for differentiating tumor recurrence from radiation necrosis in patients with brain cancer?

Although FDG PET seems to be useful in grading brain tumors and determining their prognosis, the major use of PET imaging is its ability to distinguish radiation necrosis from tumor recurrence. The ability to differentiate these two entities has critical clinical implications and is often difficult with MRI or CT. Generally, radiation necrosis should have virtually no metabolism, whereas recurrent tumor has increased metabolism. The ability to detect tumor recurrence is enhanced by the contrast of the tumor over the background hypometabolism induced by the radiation therapy (or surgery). Reports have generally scored the sensitivity and specificity of PET for detecting tumor recurrence as approximately 85% and 60% (Fig. 53-8).

20. What are the characteristic features of Alzheimer disease on FDG PET in Fig. 53-9?

The classic pattern of Alzheimer disease on FDG PET is hypometabolism in the temporoparietal regions; this may also involve the posterior cingulate gyrus. The subcortical areas, sensorimotor area, visual cortex, and cerebellum are generally less affected. More recent studies have shown, however, that other areas may be hypometabolic, particularly when the patient has specific neurocognitive deficits. Temporoparietal hypometabolism can also be observed in other conditions, including Parkinson disease, bilateral parietal subdural hematomas, bilateral parietal stroke, and bilateral parietal radiation therapy ports.

21. What is the typical metabolic pattern in the PET study of a patient with depression (Fig. 53-10)?

FDG PET studies of depressed patients usually show decreased metabolism, which can be global or affect more specific regions, such as the frontal lobes. More recent studies have suggested that certain areas may have increased activity, such as the limbic regions. This more global pattern can usually be distinguished from specific neurodegenerative diseases, such as Alzheimer or Pick disease, which typically affect the temporoparietal (Alzheimer disease) and frontal (Pick disease) lobes.

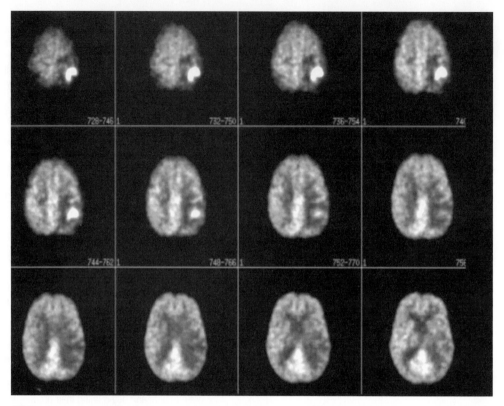

Figure 53-8. FDG PET brain scan in a patient after radiation therapy of a tumor in the left parietal region reveals decreased metabolism in the left parietal lobe with an intense region of activity centrally. These findings are consistent with recurrent brain tumor in the setting of radiation necrosis.

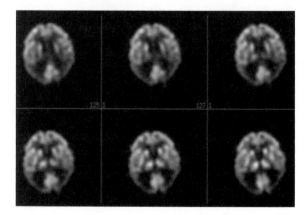

Figure 53-9. FDG PET brain scan in a patient with Alzheimer disease shows bilateral temporoparietal hypometabolism. This is the most typical feature in Alzheimer disease, although other structures, including the frontal lobes and visual cortex, can also be involved.

22. How is cardiac PET used clinically?

Cardiac PET usually uses two different tracers during a stress test. One tracer (ammonia N 13 or rubidium-82) typically evaluates perfusion, and FDG evaluates metabolism. In ischemia, perfusion is decreased in the affected area. In the heart, ischemic areas switch from use of fatty acids to glucose for energy, however, so the FDG scan shows preserved or increased uptake. PET scans also can help show viability because preserved FDG uptake suggests ischemic but viable tissue, whereas decreased perfusion and metabolism suggests infarcted tissue.

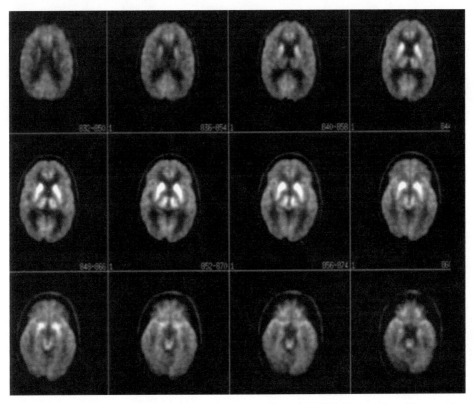

Figure 53-10. FDG PET brain scan in a patient with moderate depression reveals globally decreased cerebral glucose metabolism compared with the subcortical structures of the basal ganglia and thalami.

BIBLIOGRAPHY

[1] R. Hustinx, F. Benard, A. Alavi, Whole-body FDG-PET imaging in the management of patients with cancer, Semin. Nucl. Med. 32 (2002) 35–46.

[2] L. Kostakoglu, S.J. Goldsmith, 18F-FDG PET evaluation of the response to therapy for lymphoma and for breast, lung, and colorectal carcinoma, J. Nucl. Med. 44 (2003) 224–239.

[3] A.B. Newberg, A. Alavi, Role of positron emission tomography in the investigation of neuropsychiatric disorders, in: M.P. Sandler, R.E. Coleman, J.A. Patton, et al. (Eds.), Diagnostic Nuclear Medicine, fourth ed., Lippincott Williams & Wilkins, Philadelphia, 2003, pp. 783–819.

[4] P.E. Valk, D.L. Bailey, D.W. Townsend, M.N. Maisey (Eds.), Positron Emission Tomography: Basic Science and Clinical Practice, London, Springer, 2003.

[5] H. Zhuang, A. Alavi, 18-Fluorodeoxyglucose positron emission tomographic imaging in the detection and monitoring of infection and inflammation, Semin. Nucl. Med. 32 (2002) 47–59.

BONE SCANS

Andrew Newberg, MD

1. What should a patient know about a bone scan?

A bone scan requires the intravenous injection of a small amount of a radioactive tracer (e.g., technetium [Tc]-99m) that is absorbed into the bones. The tracer carries a relatively low dose of radioactivity and is extremely unlikely to result in any allergic or adverse reactions. The patient can eat and take medicines regularly and is able to continue all daily activities before and after the scan. The scan itself occurs approximately 2 hours after injection of the tracer, and the scan time is approximately 45 minutes for a whole-body scan. Three-phase bone scans require scanning for approximately 20 minutes at the time of the injection.

2. What are the normal structures observed on a bone scan? Describe the typical nonmalignant findings in asymptomatic patients.

Normally, all of the bones should be visible on a bone scan, including individual vertebrae and ribs. The kidneys and bladder are also seen in most patients. Normal soft tissue uptake can occur in the breasts and sometimes in vascular structures such as the uterus. Calcified cartilage is also commonly seen in the costochondral and thyroid cartilage. Common nonmalignant findings in asymptomatic patients include degenerative disease in the spine or joints, dental or sinus disease, calcification of atherosclerotic disease, and prior fractures (Fig. 54-1).

3. Why is a "superscan" associated with a negative prognosis in the patient with prostate cancer shown in Fig. 54-2?

A "superscan" implies that so much of the methylene diphosphate (MDP) is taken up by the bones that there is no significant excretion in the kidneys and bladder or uptake in the soft tissues. The scan appears almost too good with high contrast between the bones and other tissues. The most common causes of a "superscan" are

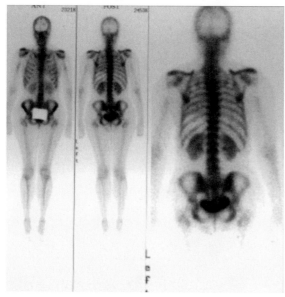

Figure 54-1. Anterior and posterior projections of a normal bone scan using Tc-99m–labeled MDP show uniform activity throughout the bones, kidney, and bladder, and mild degenerative changes.

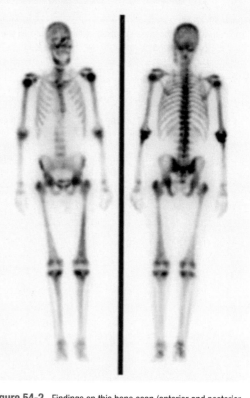

Figure 54-2. Findings on this bone scan (anterior and posterior projections) are consistent with a "superscan," in which there is intense activity throughout virtually all of the bones with no significant excretion in the kidneys or bladder. Some areas, such as the proximal humeri and left femur, are particularly intense. This patient had widespread metastatic prostate cancer.

renal failure, hyperparathyroidism, metabolic bone disease, Paget disease, or widespread metastatic disease. In a patient with cancer, a "superscan" implies widespread osseous metastases that cannot be individually distinguished, but rather occupy almost the entire skeleton.

4. **Is there a way to treat successfully a patient with bone pain associated with multiple osteoblastic metastases?**
Patients with bone pain from osteoblastic metastases can be treated primarily with four modalities: cancer-specific chemotherapy, radiation therapy, narcotic pain management, or beta-emitting radiopharmaceutical agents that target bone. The last option is often the best when multiple sites are involved that cannot be easily targeted by radiation therapy or would result in excessive radiation to uninvolved tissues or the whole body. Radiopharmaceutical agents, such as strontium-89 (Metastron) or samarium-153 (Quadramet), can be injected intravenously in patients with osteoblastic metastases for relief of pain. Studies suggest that 80% of patients experience some pain relief, and almost 50% have complete relief. Pain relief lasts a mean of 6 to 8 months, and patients can be retreated with similar pain relief. Although these treatments are not considered a cure, they can substantially improve a patient's quality of life and decrease reliance on narcotic medications.

5. **Fig. 54-3 shows a scan of a patient complaining of swelling and pain in the distal arm after a recent traumatic event. What is the diagnosis?**
Patients with such symptoms after a traumatic event typically have either osseous or soft tissue uptake characteristic of focal injury. In these patients, a three-phase bone scan helps make that determination. The first two phases—the blood flow, or vascular, phase and the blood pool, or tissue, phase—help to show whether there is soft tissue edema. If there is also focal uptake on the delayed bone images, an osseous injury is suspected, which may be superimposed on soft tissue injury. The scan in Fig. 54-3 shows diffusely increased uptake on all three phases, however, which is suggestive of reflex sympathetic dystrophy. Reflex sympathetic dystrophy is a response to a traumatic event and results from autonomic dysfunction in the extremity, causing altered regulation of blood flow. On a bone scan, the typical result is increased flow and uptake on all three phases. Other patterns have also been described. Regardless, the findings are almost always diffuse because they affect the entire extremity, including all of the fingers and distal arm.

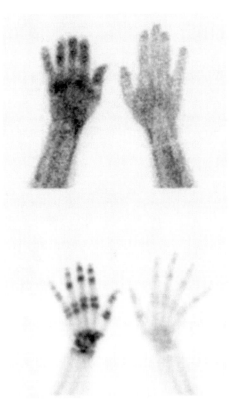

Figure 54-3. Bone scan shows diffusely increased activity throughout the entire right (*left side of image*) arm and hand on the blood pool images (*top*) and delayed images (*bottom*). These findings are consistent with reflex sympathetic dystrophy.

6. **What causes a bone scan that does not show the bones clearly?**
Usually a suboptimal bone scan is related to technical factors, such as not waiting at least 2 hours between the injection and the scan, poor preparation of the MDP, a significantly infiltrated injection dose, patient motion, or the camera being set to the incorrect energy window (e.g., for iodine-123 rather than Tc-99m). Physiologic reasons for suboptimal scans include large patient size, resulting in significant photon attenuation, or poor circulation states, such as congestive heart failure in which the tracer is not adequately delivered to the bones. Finally, patients with osteoporosis simply do not have enough bone for good visualization of osseous structures, and patients with iron overload have inhibited uptake of the tracer.

7. **Is a bone scan an appropriate study for a 65-year-old patient with multiple myeloma?**
Bone scans generally are not sensitive for lytic bone lesions, and patients who show multiple myeloma or lytic abnormalities on computed tomography (CT) or x-ray should not be referred for a bone scan. These patients should undergo a bone survey with multiple plain film x-rays. Patients with certain cancers that can have mixed lytic and blastic bone metastases may still benefit from a bone scan. Also, a patient with multiple myeloma with lytic disease in weight-bearing bones that might be susceptible to pathologic fracture may benefit because the fracture would show up as a focus of increased uptake. If a nuclear medicine scan is needed to differentiate bone metastases better, fluorodeoxyglucose positron emission tomography (FDG PET) scan may be the most appropriate choice.

8. **Does a bone scan that shows a worsened condition after chemotherapy portend a bad prognosis?**

Although a bone scan that shows apparent worsening abnormalities, characterized by increased activity in known lesions or the observation of new lesions, can be suggestive of progression of disease, the apparent worsening abnormalities may also be associated with the "flare" phenomenon. The flare phenomenon results from increased osteoblastic activity in lesions that is associated with the bone's healing response after chemotherapy. The flare response is associated with a good prognosis, suggesting effective therapy. The flare response can occur 2 to 6 months after chemotherapy. A patient with a bone scan that shows apparent worsening abnormalities in this time period should be followed up with another bone scan 4 to 6 months later to determine whether the lesions subsequently regress. If there is improvement on the latter scan, the previous scan can be considered to be related to a flare response associated with effective treatment.

9. **What are the most common findings on a bone scan that suggest metastatic disease?**

Bone scan findings of metastatic disease most commonly have intensely increased activity and may be either a solitary focus or multiple foci (Fig. 54-4). Widespread disease may appear as a "superscan," in which all of the bones have diffusely intense uptake (see question 3). Cold, or photopenic, defects can be observed in patients with lytic bone metastases. Because the sensitivity of bone scans is not 100%, scans can have negative results in the face of metastatic disease. Finally, metastatic disease can be observed in the soft tissues, including organs such as the lungs or liver.

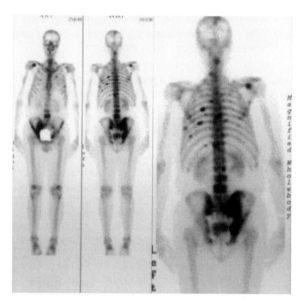

Figure 54-4. Anterior and posterior views of a bone scan show a patient with multiple foci of intense activity throughout the axial skeleton, consistent with prostate cancer. In particular, there are foci of intense uptake in multiple ribs, throughout the spine, in the skull, in the right scapula, and in the pelvis.

10. **What are the causes of "cold," or photopenic, defects on bone scans?**

There are numerous benign and malignant reasons for photopenic regions on a bone scan. Bones with avascular necrosis or infarct in the early stage have photopenia. Lytic bone tumors or metastases can be cold because there is an absence of osteoblastic activity. Any metal objects—either external, such as jewelry, or internal, such as a pacemaker or joint prosthesis—can attenuate or block photons. Bone can also be affected by disuse or radiation therapy, in which there is an overall decrease in uptake in a focal area. Finally, there have been several reports of cold defects in acute osteomyelitis.

Key Points: Common Findings of Metastatic Disease on Bone Scans

1. Solitary focal lesions
2. Multiple focal lesions
3. "Superscan"
4. Photon-deficient ("cold" defect) lesions
5. Normal findings (false-negative scan)
6. Soft tissue uptake

---

11. **Are three-phase bone scans alone useful for the diagnosis of osteomyelitis?**

Three-phase bone scans can be positive for osteomyelitis if there is a focal area of intense uptake. This is particularly true when a patient has a superficial area of infection, such as an ulcer or cellulitis. In such a case, the question to be answered is whether the underlying bone is affected, which can be readily detected on a three-phase bone scan. Increased uptake on all three phases of a bone scan can also occur in acute fractures, surgical manipulation, metastatic disease, avascular necrosis, and Paget disease. If any of these other conditions are potentially expected, a three-phase bone scan by itself is not likely to be useful because of poor specificity.

12. What other scans can be used to improve diagnostic accuracy?

Studies to consider in addition to three-phase bone scan are an indium-labeled white blood cell scan for the extremities; a gallium scan for the spine; or a PET scan, which can be used for any site of suspected osteomyelitis. Because these three studies evaluate infectious or inflammatory processes rather than response of the bone, they have higher specificity than a bone scan.

Key Points: Causes of Cold Defects on a Bone Scan
1. Avascular necrosis
2. Malignant bone tumors
3. Metastases
4. Prosthesis, pacemaker, jewelry, lead shield
5. Barium in colon
6. Disuse atrophy
7. External radiation therapy
8. Early osteomyelitis

13. Is lung uptake normal on a bone scan?

Lung uptake is almost never normal on a bone scan and is usually associated with malignant pleural effusions, large tumors, inflammatory processes, or metastatic disease. Metastatic osteosarcoma has particularly intense uptake when involving the lungs. Lung uptake itself is usually detected by comparing the left hemithorax and right hemithorax, observing for increased uptake in the intercostal spaces.

14. Can Paget disease be distinguished from cancer in the bones?

Paget disease typically is associated with focal areas of intensely increased uptake in the flat bones and the ends of the long bones. The uptake is usually diffuse, although there can be focal areas of increased uptake. There is no definitive way to exclude metastatic disease or primary bone tumors from Paget disease on the basis of uptake in the bones. The pattern of Paget disease in terms of its distribution and appearance may help in the diagnosis, however. It is less likely that an individual would have an entire hemipelvis as the only site of metastatic disease, but this can commonly be a presentation of Paget disease.

15. What is the "Mickey Mouse" sign?

In the spine, the "Mickey Mouse" sign refers to foci in which there is uptake in the entire vertebral body and the spinous process, which is almost always Paget disease, rather than metastatic disease (Fig. 54-5).

16. Intense activity on a bone scan in multiple joints can be the result of which disorders?

Polyarticular uptake on a bone scan is typically associated with arthritic conditions, such as osteoarthritis, rheumatoid arthritis, psoriatic arthritis, gout, or ankylosing spondylitis. The diagnosis of these different disorders can be suggested by the specific joints involved, such as the knees, acromioclavicular joints, and interphalangeal joints in osteoarthritis; the metacarpophalangeal joints in rheumatoid arthritis; and involvement of the great toe in gout.

17. Can shin splints be differentiated from stress fractures on a bone scan?

Shin splints generally show linear increased activity primarily on the delayed bone images in the posterior tibia (Fig. 54-6). Stress fractures should be more focally increased with intense uptake on delayed bone scans and are often more anterior in their location. Stress fractures commonly show

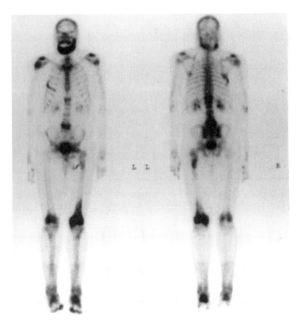

Figure 54-5. Anterior and posterior views of a bone scan show a patient with Paget disease associated with multiple areas of intense MDP uptake in the mandible, proximal humeri, femurs, right rib, and spine. The increased activity in the distal femurs can be distinguished from degenerative changes because Paget disease involves much of the femur, rather than only the joint area, which would be typical of osteoarthritis.

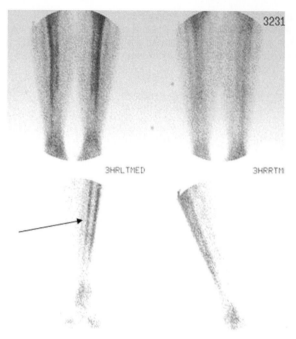

Figure 54-6. Bone scan showing linear uptake along the posterior tibia (*arrow*) consistent with shin splints. There is no evidence of focal uptake that would suggest a stress fracture.

increased activity on the first two phases of the bone scan, so any patient being referred for stress fractures should have a three-phase bone scan.

18. Is a prostate-specific antigen (PSA) level relevant to bone scan findings in patients with prostate cancer?
Several studies have shown that a low PSA level (<10 ng/dL) is associated with a very low chance of having bone metastases. Some authorities have suggested that for low-risk patients with a PSA of less than 10 ng/dL, bone scintigraphy may be unnecessary. PSA levels greater than 20 ng/dL are associated with a significantly greater chance of bone metastases. Most large trials have still revealed relatively low occurrence of abnormalities on bone scans in the early work-up of patients with prostate cancer, however. Knowledge of the PSA level is beneficial because equivocal findings may be considered less likely to be metastases in a patient with a very low PSA level.

19. What is the significance of a single rib lesion in a patient being evaluated for metastatic disease from a known primary cancer?
The traditional view is that a single rib lesion has approximately an 8% to 10% chance of being a metastasis; this can be modified by the characteristics of the finding. Typically, linear areas of increased activity that appear to extend along the rib are more suggestive of metastatic disease, whereas small, macular lesions are more likely the result of trauma. In addition, the patient's history might reveal a recent fall, which would also more likely suggest that the finding is the result of trauma.

20. Which benign bone tumors have increased uptake on a bone scan?
Osteoid osteomas have increased uptake on delayed bone scan images and may have an observable photopenic center. They commonly arise in the femur or spine. Uptake is also very intense for osteochondromas and chondroblastomas. Enchondromas do not typically have significantly increased uptake on a bone scan.

21. Do bone scans have a role in the evaluation of child abuse?
A bone scan may be an important study in the evaluation of potential child abuse because it enables a ready evaluation of all of the bones in one scan and can often show old or occult fractures. Even if a child does not complain of pain in a particular bone, the bone scan can reveal prior trauma. If there are multiple fracture sites that would not occur from a typical fall or disease process, child abuse might be suspected as the cause.

22. Are planar bone scans sufficient for the evaluation of spondylolysis?
Patients with back pain and suspected spondylolysis can undergo bone scans for the evaluation of abnormalities in the spine. Planar imaging may be sufficient to show a focus of increased uptake in the region of the posterior elements of the vertebra. A tomographic image is often necessary for diagnosis, however, if the planar scan has negative or equivocal results. Studies suggest that single photon emission computed tomography (SPECT) imaging enhances the sensitivity of planar bone scans. The usual findings are focal increased uptake in the posterior elements of the vertebra, which can be unilateral or bilateral. Uptake can be seen on the affected side because of the remodeling or on the contralateral side owing to altered biomechanics.

23. Is increased uptake in the kidneys a clinically relevant finding on a bone scan?
If one or both kidneys have increased uptake on a bone scan, this finding can be clinically relevant because such a finding can occur in the setting of hydronephrosis and obstruction. Increased uptake on a bone scan may also be the result of the effects of chemotherapy or from the involvement of tumor, nephrocalcinosis, radiation nephritis, or acute tubular necrosis. A patient with abnormally increased uptake in one or both kidneys should be followed up with additional imaging, including anatomic and scintigraphic if clinically indicated.

24. What are the causes of liver uptake on a bone scan?

The most problematic cause of liver uptake on a bone scan is the presence of hepatic metastases, which most likely are associated with melanoma or cancers of the colon, breast, or lung. Sometimes there can be increased activity in the liver associated with overlying soft tissue activity, in which case the liver is not the actual source of the increased activity. Diffuse hepatic necrosis, although rare, can result in increased liver uptake on a bone scan. Finally, a colloid formation of the tracer because of poor preparation techniques can result in the equivalent of a sulfur colloid (liver/spleen) scan.

25. What can cause uptake in the muscles on the scan in Fig. 54-7?

Increased uptake in the muscles on a bone scan usually implies some type of inflammatory process, such as myositis, which was the case in this patient. Other considerations include rhabdomyolysis, hypercalcemia, hematomas, and tumors. The latter two conditions are usually more focal. There are technical factors, such as poor preparation of the radiopharmaceutical agent, or possibly not waiting long enough after injection before imaging. The intensity and diffuseness of the uptake on this scan is indicative of myositis.

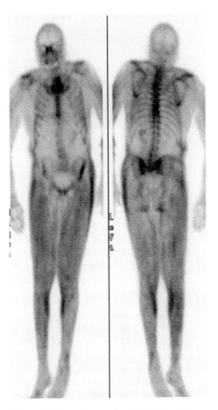

Figure 54-7. Anterior and posterior views of a bone scan show diffuse, intense uptake throughout most of the skeletal muscle groups. This finding is consistent with widespread myositis.

BIBLIOGRAPHY

[1] H.M. Abdel-Dayem, The role of nuclear medicine in primary bone and soft tissue tumors, Semin. Nucl. Med. 27 (1997) 355–363.
[2] R.M. Atkins, W. Tindale, D. Bickerstaff, J.A. Kanis, Quantitative bone scintigraphy in reflex sympathetic dystrophy, Br. J. Rheumatol. 32 (1993) 41–45.
[3] B.D. Collier, I. Fogelman, I. Rosenthal (Eds.), Skeletal Nuclear Medicine, Mosby, St. Louis, 1996.
[4] S. Haukaas, J. Roervik, O.J. Halvorsen, M. Foelling, When is bone scintigraphy necessary in the assessment of newly diagnosed, untreated prostate cancer? Br. J. Urol. 79 (1997) 770–776.
[5] I. Sarikaya, A. Sarikaya, L.E. Holder, The role of single photon emission computed tomography in bone imaging, Semin. Nucl. Med. 31 (2001) 3–16.

VENTILATION-PERFUSION (V̇/Q̇) SCANS

Andrew Newberg, MD

1. How would you prepare a patient for a ventilation-perfusion V̇/Q̇ scan?

Patients should be informed that the test takes approximately 20 to 30 minutes and consists of two parts. During the ventilation part, the patient has a facemask placed over the mouth and nose and is asked to inhale an odorless radioactive gas. The mask is left on for approximately 5 to 10 minutes, and images of the lungs are acquired. The patient is then asked to lie down to receive an intravenous injection of a radioactive material (macroaggregated albumin [MAA]) to measure the blood flow to the lungs. Images are acquired in multiple projections around the body over approximately 20 minutes. There is no specific preparation for the patient. The patient does not need to be without food. Although patients can receive oxygen, subjects who require oxygen by facemask are unlikely to be able to perform the ventilation component of the study successfully.

2. In what order should radiographic studies be obtained in the work-up of a patient with acute shortness of breath?

The first radiologic study in any patient with shortness of breath should be a chest x-ray. The chest x-ray excludes many causes and is necessary for adequate evaluation of V̇/Q̇ scans. The next study depends on numerous variables, which include the current protocols for an individual hospital, but, more importantly, on whether the patient has normal or abnormal x-ray findings. Many hospitals now use helical contrast-enhanced, multidetector-row computed tomography (CT) scanning to evaluate patients for pulmonary embolism (PE), whereas others use V̇/Q̇ scan. In patients with significant abnormalities on x-ray, it is more likely that V̇/Q̇ scan would result in an intermediate scan result that would not provide additional clinical information. Only patients with relatively unremarkable chest x-rays should proceed to V̇/Q̇ scans in the current medical setting. If CT or V̇/Q̇ scan or both are equivocal, pulmonary angiogram is the gold standard for the detection of PE.

3. How do aerosols compare with xenon (Xe)-133 for ventilation scans?

Xe-133 is a radioactive isotope of a noble gas. It can be inhaled into the lungs and washes out quickly in a normal lung, although there is persistent activity (gas trapping) in parts of the lung affected by airway disease, such as asthma or chronic obstructive pulmonary disease (COPD). Xe-133 is the ventilatory agent used for the large Prospective Investigation of Pulmonary Embolism Diagnosis (PIOPED) study of V̇/Q̇ scanning, so there are more data supporting the use of Xe-133 in the evaluation of ventilation. Radioaerosols are typically technetium (Tc)-99m–labeled particles, such as diethylenetriaminepentaacetic acid (DTPA), suspended in air. Such aerosols are deposited on the lining of the alveolar spaces and do not wash out. Although gas trapping cannot be assessed because the particles remain in the lungs, particles have the advantage of allowing for imaging in multiple projections, which can be more easily compared with the perfusion images.

4. What are normal findings on V̇/Q̇ scan?

Normal findings consist of uniform ventilation throughout both lung fields (Fig. 55-1). On Xe-133 ventilation scan, there is usually good inflow of the gas; uniform activity during the equilibrium phase, which lasts approximately 3 minutes while the patient breathes into the closed system of the machine; and rapid and uniform washout within about 1 to 2 minutes. Perfusion should also be uniform throughout, with the exception of the cardiac silhouette. No activity should be observed in the brain because this would suggest a right-to-left shunt.

5. What findings are necessary to classify V̇/Q̇ scan as "high probability" for PE?

The PIOPED study, which prospectively evaluated patients with suspected PE, helped establish the criteria by which V̇/Q̇ scans are currently read. A high probability for PE requires that V̇/Q̇ scan have the equivalent of two or more large segmental perfusion defects (75% to 100% involvement of the segment) that are not matched by ventilatory abnormalities. Four or more moderately sized perfusion defects (25% to 75% involvement of the segment) would also represent a high probability for PE. The implication of a high-probability scan is that the patient has a greater than 80% chance of having PE (Fig. 55-2).

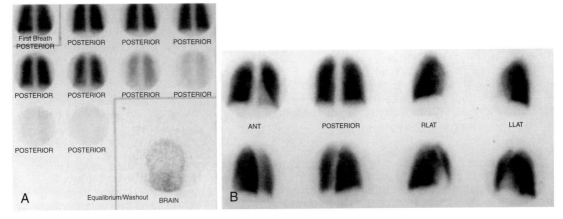

Figure 55-1. **A,** Normal V̇/Q̇ scan with ventilation that shows uniform activity on the initial first breath (*upper left*), followed by an equilibrium phase, and then a washout phase (each view represents 45 seconds). Just below the ventilation scan is the image of the brain that is used to observe whether there is any right-to-left shunt. **B,** Perfusion images are shown in multiple projections (*top row,* anterior, posterior, right lateral, and left lateral projections; *bottom row,* left posterior oblique, right posterior oblique, right anterior oblique, and left anterior oblique projections), and also show uniform activity throughout both lungs.

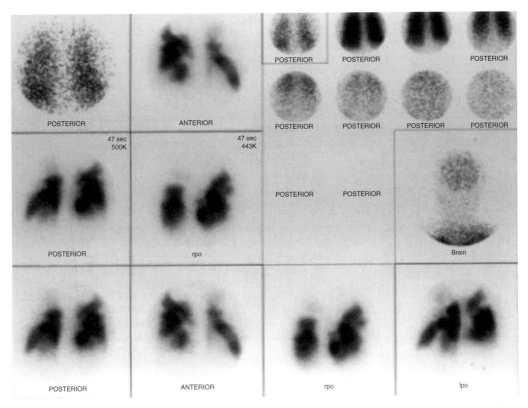

Figure 55-2. V̇/Q̇ scan shows high probability for PE. There is relatively uniform ventilation (*upper right corner of scan*) with only mild gas trapping in the upper lobes. There are multiple wedge-shaped perfusion defects throughout both lungs that are mismatched (i.e., no corresponding ventilation defect). Also there is mild uptake in the brain, consistent with a right-to-left shunt (see question 18).

6. What are the causes of gas trapping on V̇/Q̇ scan?

Gas trapping refers to radioactive gas that persists in certain areas of the lungs during the washout phase of the ventilation scan. Potential causes for gas trapping are asthma, COPD, chronic bronchitis, mucous plug, cystic fibrosis, smoke inhalation, tumors (e.g., carcinoma, adenoma), and foreign body. The implication of gas trapping is that there is an airway process that is contributing to the patient's symptoms. If the airway abnormality can be treated by medication or surgical interventions, the gas trapping should also be resolved.

> ### Key Points: Potential Causes of Gas Trapping on V̇/Q̇ Scan
>
> 1. Asthma
> 2. COPD
> 3. Chronic bronchitis
> 4. Mucous plug
> 5. Cystic fibrosis
> 6. Smoke inhalation
> 7. Tumors (e.g., carcinoma, adenoma)
> 8. Foreign body

7. How does a quantitative V̇/Q̇ scan assist in preparing patients for lung surgery?

Quantitative V̇/Q̇ scans help in the preoperative assessment of patients by showing the areas of the lung that have the poorest overall function. This information may help direct surgeons to resect preferentially areas that have the worst function. Perhaps more importantly, the quantitative analysis provides a percentage of function for the various lobes and for the overall lung. When this percentage is multiplied by the forced expiratory volume in 1 second (FEV_1), the surgeon can predict how much overall lung function would be left if certain parts of the lung are removed. If a patient requires an upper and middle right lobectomy for lung cancer, and the remaining lower lobe of the right lung and the whole left lung account for 70% of the lung function, the surgeon can determine whether the patient would have adequate pulmonary function after surgery. Generally, the remaining FEV_1 should be at least 700 mL/min. In the case described, the patient needs to have a preoperative FEV_1 of at least 1000 mL/min so that the remaining 70% would provide the necessary function for postoperative survival.

8. What is the significance of a "triple match" on V̇/Q̇ scan and chest x-ray?

A triple match refers to a ventilation defect and perfusion defect on a V̇/Q̇ scan that match each other and are matched to an opacification on the corresponding chest x-ray. The implication of such a finding is that it might represent a pulmonary infarct resulting from PE. The revised PIOPED data indicate that a triple match defect in the upper or middle lung zones is still associated with a low probability for PE, but in the lower lung zone, it is associated with an intermediate probability.

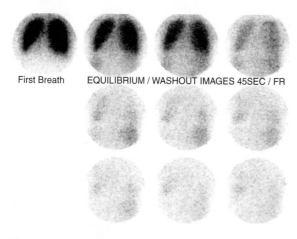

First Breath   EQUILIBRIUM / WASHOUT IMAGES 45SEC / FR

Figure 55-3. First breath, equilibrium, and washout phases of Xe-133 ventilation scan showing increased uptake below the diaphragm in liver and spleen.

9. What can cause liver and splenic uptake on Xe-133 ventilation scan?

The primary cause of uptake in the liver and spleen on a ventilation scan is fatty infiltration of these organs because Xe-133 is lipid-soluble, and a small percentage crosses the alveolar lining and enters into the bloodstream. Uptake in the liver or spleen does not usually result in a poor prognosis and has no bearing on the diagnosis of PE. It is a common finding on V̇/Q̇ scans, however (Fig. 55-3).

10. If the clinical suspicion for PE is high, and V̇/Q̇ scan result is low probability, what is the patient's actual probability for having PE?

A high clinical suspicion for PE may occur in the setting of factors including predisposing conditions such as cancer or immobility, a sudden onset of shortness of breath, sudden requirement for oxygen, or abnormalities on electrocardiogram (ECG) or chest x-ray suggesting PE. In such a case, a low probability result on V̇/Q̇ scan still indicates a 40% chance of PE. A corroborative test, such as pulmonary angiogram, would be necessary. A high-probability V̇/Q̇ scan result would indicate more than a 95% chance of PE and would be enough to support the initiation of anticoagulant therapy.

11. Name the causes of mismatched perfusion defects on V̇/Q̇ scan.

Although mismatched perfusion defects (a region with normal ventilation but no perfusion) are most likely to be associated with PE, other potential causes should be excluded, including the following:

- Acute PE
- Chronic PE
- Other emboli (drug abuse, iatrogenic, fat)
- Vascular-obstructive tumor or obstructive adenopathy
- Idiopathic pulmonary fibrosis
- Hypoplasia of the pulmonary artery

- Swyer-James syndrome
- Vasculitis (post–external radiation therapy, collagen vascular)

12. How can V̇/Q̇ scans be used in the evaluation of chronic PE?

Patients who have pulmonary hypertension or some other pulmonary process that might list chronic PE as a potential etiologic factor can undergo V̇/Q̇ scans to assess for mismatched perfusion defects. V̇/Q̇ scan cannot be easily used to determine the age of perfusion defects, and there is no way to state definitively whether a perfusion defect is attributable to chronic or acute PE. In the setting of a chronic disease process, such a finding would be consistent with chronic PE. If there is evidence for PE, anticoagulant treatment can be started.

13. Why is α_1-antitrypsin deficiency the most likely cause of the perfusion scan findings in Fig. 55-4?

Generally, the upper lung zones in patients with airway disease related to COPD or asthma typically are more affected than the lower lobes. Most of the lung becomes affected over time, however. On V̇/Q̇ scan, the result is a markedly heterogeneous perfusion pattern that shows the greatest decreases in the upper lung zones. In contrast, α_1-antitrypsin deficiency typically affects the lower lung zones first. V̇/Q̇ scan findings usually show markedly decreased and heterogeneous perfusion in the lower lung zones, such as is the case in this patient with α_1-antitrypsin deficiency.

14. Can idiopathic pulmonary fibrosis (IPF) be easily distinguished from PE?

As shown in Fig. 55-5, IPF can commonly result in perfusion defects that are often mismatched to the ventilation pattern. IPF usually results in multiple nonsegmental defects and can be distinguished from PE. When such defects appear in a segmental pattern, PE cannot be excluded. Because one of the criteria for an intermediate-probability V̇/Q̇ scan is a scan that cannot be classified as high or low probability, many scans of patients with IPF would be considered to be of intermediate probability.

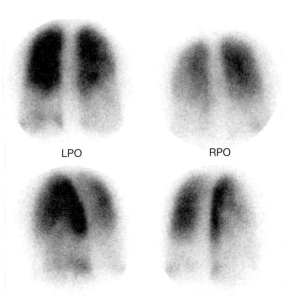

LPO   RPO

Figure 55-4. Perfusion scan (*clockwise from top left:* posterior, anterior, left posterior oblique, and right posterior oblique views) of a patient with α_1-antitrypsin deficiency shows characteristic abnormal flow in lower lung zones compared with upper lungs. The upper lungs have relatively uniform and preserved perfusion.

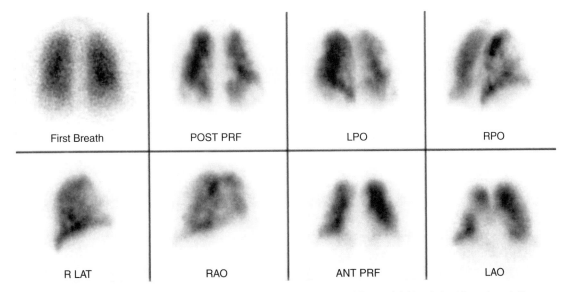

First Breath   POST PRF   LPO   RPO

R LAT   RAO   ANT PRF   LAO

Figure 55-5. Perfusion scan (*top row,* first breath ventilation, posterior, left posterior oblique, and right posterior oblique views; *bottom row,* right lateral, right anterior oblique, anterior, and left anterior oblique views) of a patient with pulmonary fibrosis shows multiple areas of decreased perfusion. Most of these abnormal areas appear nonsegmental, and all of them are mismatched compared with the ventilation.

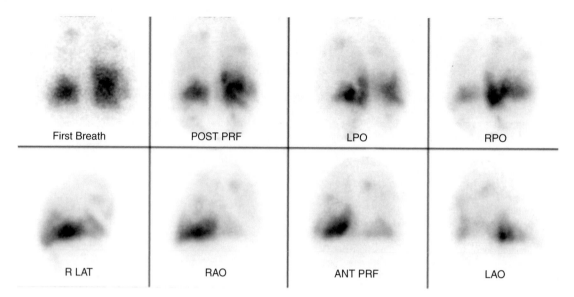

| First Breath | POST PRF | LPO | RPO |
| R LAT | RAO | ANT PRF | LAO |

Figure 55-6. Perfusion scan (*top row,* first breath ventilation, posterior, left posterior oblique, and right posterior oblique views; *bottom row,* right lateral, right anterior oblique, anterior, and left anterior oblique views) of a patient with severe COPD primarily affecting the upper lung and mid-lung zones. Abnormal areas on perfusion images appear to match the ventilation abnormalities on the first breath image.

15. Does the severe airway disease depicted in Fig. 55-6 prevent adequate interpretation of V̇/Q̇ scans?

This is a common problem because many patients with relatively severe COPD are referred for V̇/Q̇ scan because of worsening shortness of breath, and the question is whether the clinical symptoms are associated with a COPD flare or PE. Initial analysis of the PIOPED data suggested that severe airway disease usually associated with nonuniform matched perfusion and ventilation patterns made adequate assessment of PE too difficult. Such scans were read as intermediate or indeterminate. Subsequent analysis has shown, however, that if all of the perfusion abnormalities can be matched to the ventilatory findings, the scan can be interpreted as a low-probability scan. Although airway disease makes interpretation difficult, it is still possible to provide clinically relevant information using V̇/Q̇ scan.

16. Could the V̇/Q̇ scan in Fig. 55-7 result from a lung tumor?

Lung tumors, if small, can elude detection, with no significant abnormality on V̇/Q̇ scan observed. Larger tumors can appear as cold or photopenic defects on V̇/Q̇ scan because the tumor is a region that is not receiving blood in the same manner as the rest of the lung or is closed off from the other ventilatory areas. Large central or hilar tumors can preferentially obstruct the pulmonary vasculature, rather than the bronchi, resulting in an entire lung having decreased or absent perfusion with relatively preserved ventilation. Endobronchial lesions typically result in matched ventilation and perfusion defects because the airways are obstructed to that part of the lung.

17. Can V̇/Q̇ scans be performed in pregnant women?

V̇/Q̇ scans generally can be performed in pregnant women, especially because most of the radioactivity is confined to the lungs rather than the abdomen or pelvis. It is important to establish the need for V̇/Q̇ scan in this setting so that the patient can be informed that the risks of PE outweigh the minor risks of low levels of radiation to the fetus from the scan. It is sometimes protocol to decrease the dose of MAA by half to diminish further the radiation exposure to the fetus.

18. What does activity in the brain or kidneys imply on V̇/Q̇ scan?

Most nuclear medicine departments image the brain or kidneys to evaluate for a mechanical right-to-left shunt. Because MAA is too large to pass through the capillary beds of the lungs, all of the injected material should remain in the lungs, unless there is a shunt that bypasses the lungs. Such a shunt is most commonly found in the heart (i.e., an atrial septal defect) or possibly as arteriovenous malformations in the lungs. Although the shunt can be detected on V̇/Q̇ scan, it is difficult to assess adequately the severity of the shunt, which typically requires additional studies using other radiographic or ultrasound techniques.

19. How quickly do perfusion defects associated with PE resolve?

Studies have reported varying rates of resolution of perfusion defects associated with PE. Some perfusion defects can resolve within 24 hours, whereas others may persist indefinitely. For this reason, some clinicians recommend obtaining V̇/Q̇ scan approximately 3 months after treatment of PE to determine the new "baseline" perfusion pattern of the patient. This scan can be compared with future scans if a determination of new PE is needed because of acute pulmonary symptoms.

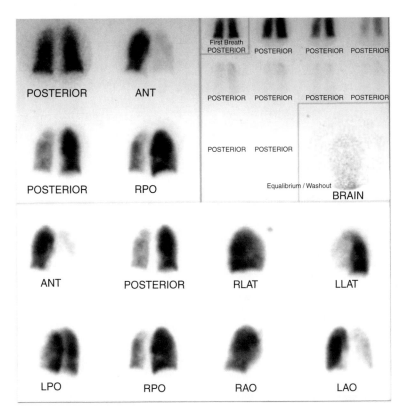

Figure 55-7. V̇/Q̇ scan shows relatively uniform ventilation (*upper right corner*) with a mild decrease in the left lung. Perfusion images in the lower two rows (*uppermost row*, anterior, posterior, right lateral, and left lateral projections; *lower row*, left posterior oblique, right posterior oblique, right anterior oblique, and left anterior oblique projections) show markedly reduced perfusion in the entire left lung, which is much worse than the corresponding ventilation abnormality.

20. How are V̇/Q̇ scans used in patients who have had lung transplants?

In the immediate postoperative period, V̇/Q̇ scan can be used to assess the transplanted lung for overall function and to confirm that it is working adequately. V̇/Q̇ scans can also be used to assess patients for PE in the transplanted lung, in the same way they are used in nontransplant patients. V̇/Q̇ scans can also be helpful to assess patients for worsening function that may be attributable to rejection or infection. Although the exact V̇/Q̇ findings are nonspecific, rejection can result in small perfusion defects that are associated with small vessel abnormalities. Worsening ventilation and perfusion can also be observed in transplant patients who are developing bronchiolitis obliterans, although the chest x-ray may be unremarkable.

21. What is a "stripe" sign, and what does it signify on V̇/Q̇ scan?

A "stripe" sign is a rim of activity that surrounds the edge of a perfusion defect, as shown in Fig. 55-8. The implication of this sign is that a perfusion defect that is bordered by the "stripe" sign is not the result of PE. The physiologic basis of this interpretation is that perfusion defects related to PE should extend all the way to the periphery of the lung. If there is a stripe of perfused tissue distal to the perfusion defect, it most likely does not represent PE.

22. What are the causes of matched ventilation and perfusion defects?

Most conditions associated with matched ventilation and perfusion defects arise from diseases affecting the airways with subsequent physiologic shunting away from the underventilated regions. The most common causes of matched defects include COPD, bronchitis and bronchiectasis, and asthma. Other causes include pleural effusions, mucous plugging, tumors, blebs and bullae, and pneumonia.

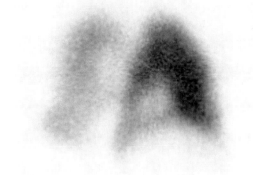

Figure 55-8. Perfusion image in right posterior projection shows a "stripe" sign, in which there is decreased activity centrally with a rim around the activity posteriorly and inferiorly. The implication is that this does not represent a PE because PE should result in a perfusion defect that extends to the periphery of the lung.

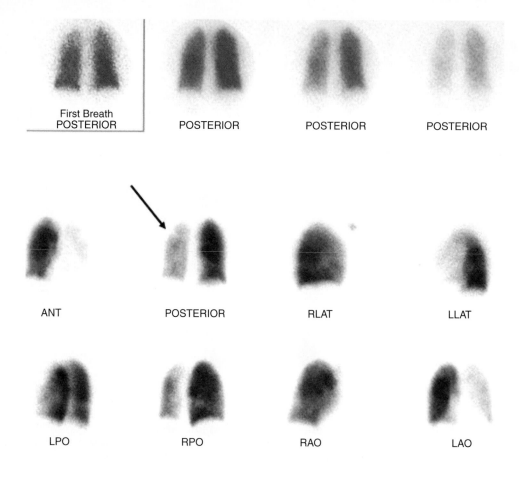

First Breath
POSTERIOR

POSTERIOR

POSTERIOR

POSTERIOR

ANT

POSTERIOR

RLAT

LLAT

LPO

RPO

RAO

LAO

Figure 55-9. Ventilation (*top row*) is relatively normal with perhaps mildly decreased ventilation in the left lung. There is substantially decreased perfusion to the entire left lung (*arrow*).

23. What are possible causes of unilateral decreases in lung perfusion with relatively preserved ventilation as shown in Fig. 55-9?

The most common cause of unilaterally decreased lung perfusion is a proximal mass lesion, such as lung cancer, which affects perfusion more than ventilation owing to the more compressible nature of blood vessels compared with that of the rigid bronchi. Patients with congenital heart disease, such as Blalock-Taussig shunt or an absent pulmonary artery, can have a similar pattern. PE in the central pulmonary artery is another cause of unilateral perfusion decrease. A similar pattern can also be observed in patients who have undergone unilateral lung transplant. The perfusion pressure in the pulmonary arteries of patients with COPD may be normal, and the perfusion in the transplanted lung in the immediate postoperative period may be only 50% to 60%, but increases with time. Patients with pulmonary hypertension have significant improvement with the lung transplant, which can receive 90% of the perfusion in the early postoperative period.

BIBLIOGRAPHY

[1] A.F. Jacobson, N. Patel, D.H. Lewis, Clinical outcome of patients with intermediate probability lung scans during six-month follow up, J. Nucl. Med. 38 (1997) 1593–1596.

[2] PIOPED Investigators, Value of the ventilation/perfusion in acute pulmonary embolism: results of the Prospective Investigation of Pulmonary Embolism Diagnosis (PIOPED), JAMA 263 (1990) 2753–2759.

[3] M. Remy-Jardin, J. Remy, F. Deschildre, et al., Diagnosis of pulmonary embolism with spiral CT: comparison with pulmonary angiography and scintigraphy, Radiology 200 (1996) 699–706.

[4] N.P. Trujillo, J.P. Pratt, S. Tahisani, et al., DTPA aerosol in ventilation/perfusion scintigraphy for diagnosing pulmonary embolism, J. Nucl. Med. 38 (1997) 1781–1783.

[5] D.F. Worsley, A. Alavi, Radionuclide imaging of acute pulmonary embolism, Semin. Nucl. Med. 33 (2003) 259–278.

What patient preparation is required before thyroid scanning?
Patients should fast after midnight or, at a minimum, for 4 hours before receiving the radioactive iodine (I)-123 pill to maximize absorption through the gut. Patients should also avoid ingesting foods containing high amounts of iodine because they would saturate the iodine stores in the body and thyroid and diminish the uptake of the radioactive iodine. Foods such as shellfish and seaweed and supplements containing large amounts of iodine should be avoided. Patients should also discontinue taking any medication that would affect thyroid function, particularly thyroid replacement medication (for at least 2 weeks); thyroid-blocking medication (propylthiouracil or methimazole for at least 5 days); and other medications, such as amiodarone, that contain substantial amounts of iodine. Finally, patients should not undergo scanning if they have received iodinated contrast agents as recently as 1 month before the scan (although sometimes the effects of such contrast agents on the thyroid can be seen 3 months later).

2. Which isotopes can be used for imaging the thyroid, and how do they compare physiologically?
The most common radioactive materials used in thyroid imaging are the various isotopes of iodine. I-123 is the most commonly used isotope because of its excellent image quality and relatively low radiation exposure. Isotopes I-125 and I-127 are not typically used because of their high radiation exposure and poorer image quality. I-131 is still used for thyroid imaging in patients with thyroid cancer. Its higher photon energy theoretically makes it easier to detect cancer foci in the deep soft tissues in the body. I-131 releases a higher radiation exposure to patients, however, and the image quality is not *typically* as good as I-123. All of the iodine tracers are trapped by the thyroid and undergo organification into the thyroid hormones. The other primary tracer for thyroid imaging is technetium (Tc)-99m pertechnetate. This material is trapped (not organified) by the thyroid and can provide high-quality images. The amount of uptake of the Tc-99m tracer cannot be used to plan I-131 therapy, however, as is the case with the iodine tracers.

3. What are normal thyroid scan and iodine uptake results?
Thyroid images are obtained 24 hours after the administration of I-123 or approximately 30 minutes after Tc-99m. The gland should appear uniform throughout with smooth contours. The isthmus and pyramidal lobes can be observed, although they are more commonly seen in patients with Graves disease. Iodine uptake values are usually obtained at 2 and 24 hours after administration of the I-123 pill. The 2-hour uptake should be 2% to 10%, and the 24-hour uptake is usually 10% to 30%. These values may differ slightly, depending on the uptake probe that is used, so it is always important to know what a particular institution considers to be the normal range (Fig. 56-1).

4. Can a patient with normal I-123 uptake still have Graves disease?
The iodine uptake refers to the activity of the gland and not to whether the patient is hyperthyroid. Although a patient may have normal scan results and uptake values, if the thyroid function tests indicate that the patient is hyperthyroid, a normal iodine uptake is still too high. A hyperthyroid patient should have a gland that is almost completely shut down. An uptake of 20% to 30% is too high if a patient is hyperthyroid with an undetectable thyroid-stimulating hormone (TSH) level. In such a setting, a patient with normal scan results can still have Graves disease.

5. What are possible outcomes after I-131 therapy for Graves disease?
There are three possible outcomes:

- A patient may be hypothyroid if the dose is sufficient to destroy most of the thyroid tissue and function.
- A patient may be euthyroid if the dose diminishes the function of the thyroid, but there is sufficient activity to maintain normal circulating levels of thyroid hormone.
- A patient may be undertreated (i.e., remain hyperthyroid), with the gland continuing to produce high levels of thyroid hormone.

In the hypothyroid case, patients typically begin undergoing thyroid replacement therapy. In the hyperthyroid case, patients usually require retreatment with a higher dose of I-131. The likelihood of each outcome depends on the range of doses given. Lower doses result in fewer hypothyroid patients, with more patients requiring retreatment for

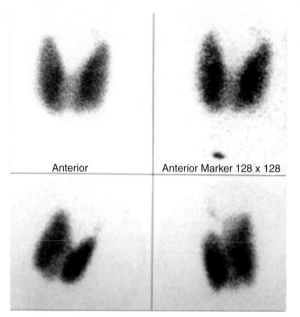

Figure 56-1. Normal thyroid scan (*clockwise from top left*: anterior view, anterior view with marker in sternal notch, right anterior oblique view, and left anterior oblique view).

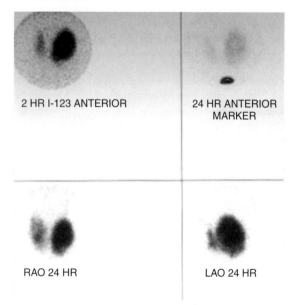

Figure 56-2. Thyroid scan shows large "hot" nodule in left lobe with suppression of right lobe (*clockwise from top left*: anterior view, anterior view with marker in sternal notch, right anterior oblique view, and left anterior oblique view).

persistent hyperthyroidism. Higher doses result in more patients being hypothyroid, and fewer needing to be retreated.

6. How is a patient with a hot nodule treated for hyperthyroidism?
Hot nodules are typically treated with I-131 therapy, but are more resistant. It is usually recommended that the dose be higher than that used for treating a patient with Graves disease. The overall approach to therapy is similar, however, including the preparation and radiation precautions that are followed after the dose is given.

7. Why is a patient with a hot nodule more likely to end up euthyroid?
Patients with hot nodules have a higher likelihood of ending up euthyroid because the hot nodule typically causes a suppression of the remainder of the gland. This suppression protects the gland from I-131 therapy. When the nodule is eliminated by I-131, the patient's thyroid function decreases, and eventually the TSH level begins to increase. This increased TSH stimulates the remaining thyroid tissue to begin producing thyroid hormone again. Because most of the suppressed tissue was protected, the patient may be able to make normal amounts of thyroid hormone (Fig. 56-2).

8. What are the typical radiation safety precautions that patients must follow after I-131 therapy?
For approximately 5 days, patients treated with I-131 must do the following: sleep alone, if possible; avoid kissing and sexual intercourse; minimize time with pregnant women and young children; minimize close contact with others; use good hygiene habits; wash hands thoroughly after each toilet use; use a separate bathroom, if possible; flush the toilet two times after each use; drink plenty of liquids; use disposable eating utensils; use separate bath linens; launder linens and underclothing separately initially; maintain a toothbrush in a separate holder; if possible, not prepare food for others; not apply cosmetics or lip balm; and wipe the telephone mouthpiece with a tissue after each use. In addition, nursing women should completely discontinue breastfeeding until their next child, and all women should not attempt to become pregnant for at least 90 days.

9. When should a patient with multinodular goiter be treated with I-131?
Typical indications are either symptomatic hyperthyroidism or symptomatic mass effect related to the enlarged thyroid. Hyperthyroid patients can usually be treated with I-131, although with usually two to three times the dose as that for a patient with Graves disease because the multinodular gland can be more refractory to the effects of I-131. Patients with compression of the airway or other vital structures in the neck or chest from an enlarged thyroid can be treated either surgically or with I-131. I-131 therapy is much less invasive and usually results in substantial shrinkage of the gland, which may obviate the need for surgery. Some clinicians are concerned, however, that potential inflammatory response from high levels of I-131 may result in clinical worsening (Fig. 56-3).

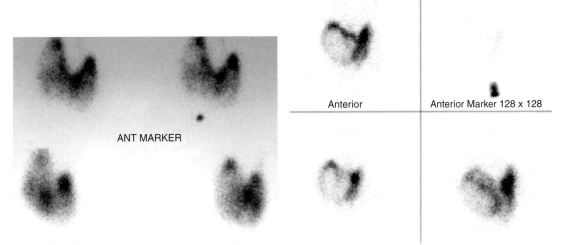

Figure 56-3. Thyroid scan shows multinodular goiter with numerous hot and cold regions (*clockwise from top left*: anterior view, anterior view with marker in sternal notch, right anterior oblique view, and left anterior oblique view).

Figure 56-4. Thyroid scan shows large cold nodule in the right pole (*clockwise from top left*: anterior view, anterior view with marker in sternal notch, right anterior oblique view, and left anterior oblique view).

10. What factors affect the likelihood that a cold nodule represents thyroid cancer?

Several factors relating to patient demographics, patient history, and features of the nodule affect the probability that a cold nodule may harbor cancer. Younger male patients with cold nodules are more likely to have cancer than older female patients with similar findings. Exposure to radiation in the neck is an important risk factor for cancer. Cold nodules in the setting of a multinodular goiter are substantially less likely to be cancer than other cold nodules. Finally, ultrasound findings of mixed cystic and solid components within a cold nodule are also more suggestive of thyroid cancer (Fig. 56-4).

11. Why can I-131 be used to treat thyroid cancer if the original nodule is cold?

Although a cold nodule does not appear to take up any of the radioactive iodine on scintigraphy, its inactive appearance is in comparison to the background activity of the normal gland. Thyroid cancer cells generally take up the iodine, but not as well as normal tissues. For this reason, thyroid cancer appears cold on the scan, but it can still take up enough iodine for therapy to be effective. To enhance the therapeutic effects of I-131 therapy, the normal thyroid is surgically removed. By eliminating much of the normal thyroid tissue, there is a better chance for any remaining thyroid cancer cells to take up I-131. The hope is that by removing the thyroid and keeping the patient off thyroid replacement hormones, the TSH level would be greater than 30 IU/L, which should maximally stimulate any thyroid cancer cells to take up I-131. Patients are also usually prescribed a low-iodine diet to "starve" any thyroid cells, maximizing uptake of I-131 further.

12. What foods should be avoided as part of a low-iodine diet?

A low-iodine diet is highly restrictive because many foods contain iodine. Foods to be avoided include most dairy products (milk, yogurt, ice cream, cheese), luncheon meats, bacon, hot dogs, fish, shellfish, noodles, pasta, cereals, pastry, breads, packaged rice, canned juices, canned fruits, canned or frozen vegetables, cocoa mixes, diet bars, jams/jellies, nuts, mustard, olives, candy, pretzels, and any snack foods. Patients can eat small portions fresh chicken, fresh potatoes, fresh fruit, all fresh vegetables except spinach, sweet butter, vegetable oils, onion or garlic powder, fresh herbs, and popcorn with no salt.

13. What is the general management plan for patients diagnosed with thyroid cancer?

Usually, patients who are diagnosed with thyroid cancer initially undergo surgery to remove the gland. Occasionally, one lobe is removed first, and then, if cancer is detected, the other lobe is removed. Most of the time, when cancer has already been definitively diagnosed with biopsy, as much of the gland is removed as possible. The patient goes to the nuclear medicine department for a scan and therapy. The pretherapy scan usually shows some uptake in the thyroid bed because it is difficult to remove all of the gland surgically, especially when it is adjacent to critical structures in the neck. Therapy is performed using I-131, given as an oral dose. The purpose of this therapeutic dose is to ablate any remaining normal thyroid tissue (some of which is usually left by the surgeon because of its proximity to critical structures in the neck) and to eliminate any remaining thyroid cancer cells. Patients are followed up at regular intervals with neck and whole-body iodine scans and serum measures of thyroglobulins. Patients can be retreated with I-131 if there is a recurrence (Fig. 56-5).

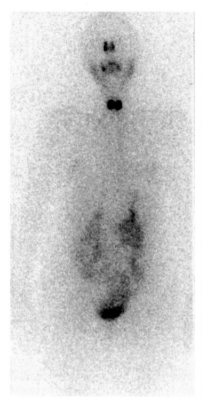

Figure 56-5. Anterior view of I-123 whole-body scan of a patient with thyroid cancer after surgical resection. The scan of this patient who is now presenting for I-131 therapy shows two foci in the neck of residual thyroid tissue. The activity in the nasopharyngeal area, gut, and bladder represents areas of normal excretion of I-123.

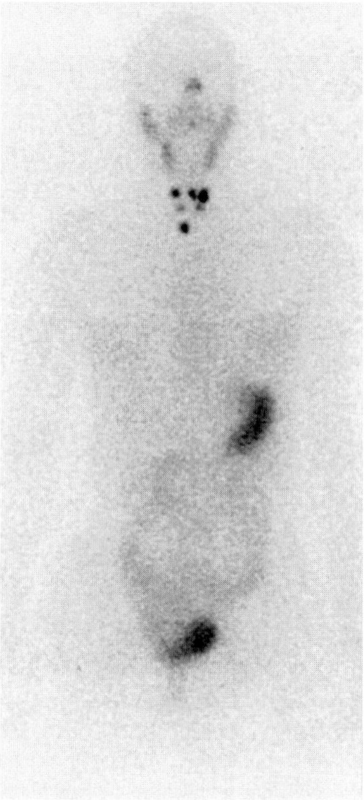

Figure 56-6. Anterior view of I-123 whole-body scan of a patient with thyroid cancer after surgical resection. The scan of this patient who is now presenting for I-131 therapy shows multiple foci in the neck, which are consistent with lymph node involvement.

14. What does "stunning" mean with regard to I-131 scanning?

Several studies have suggested that a typical I-131 imaging dose of 4 mCi actually has a small therapeutic effect on the thyroid and "stuns" the thyroid cells, making them slightly resistant to the larger therapeutic dose. For this reason, some clinicians have recommended using I-123 for whole-body imaging before I-131 therapy to avoid this effect.

15. What range of doses of I-131 is typically recommended for therapy for thyroid cancer in patients with the scans in Figs. 56-6 and 56-7?

The range of doses given to patients being treated for thyroid cancer depends on the extent of the cancer and the institution. Either way, there is usually a graded scale of doses that increases for worsening extent of disease.

Key Points: Typical Dose Ranges for I-131 Therapy for Thyroid Cancer
1. 60 to 100 mCi for low-risk disease
2. 125 mCi for lymph node involvement
3. 150 mCi for lung involvement
4. 175 mCi for bone involvement

16. How does a recombinant human thyrotropin alfa (Thyrogen) scan work?

A Thyrogen scan is usually performed in the second year of follow-up for patients treated with I-131 for thyroid cancer. A Thyrogen scan is performed by subcutaneously administering a synthetic version of TSH on 2 consecutive days and then performing the iodine scan to detect thyroid tissue. Usually, patients stop taking thyroid medications to ensure that the TSH is maximally stimulating any residual thyroid tissue so that it can be detected on the scan. By giving the patient TSH, a similar physiologic state is obtained.

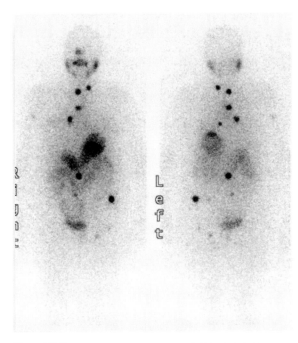

Figure 56-7. Anterior and posterior views of I-123 whole-body scan of a patient with thyroid cancer after surgical resection who is now presenting for I-131 therapy. The scan shows multiple foci of intense activity in the neck, mediastinum, thorax, abdomen, and right humerus. These findings suggest widespread disease with bone involvement.

17. What are possible causes of a thyroid scan in which there is no uptake or minimal uptake by the thyroid?

When there is no uptake observed on a scan, there are several potential causes. Patients may have thyroiditis, in which the inflammatory process has destroyed most functioning tissue. Such patients can be hyperthyroid or hypothyroid. Other causes of minimal uptake in the thyroid gland include exogenous sources of thyroid hormone (some patients take thyroid hormone as a form of diet pill) or iodine (e.g., recent iodinated contrast agent administration, ingestion of drugs containing iodine such as amiodarone, consumption of high-salt or seafood diets, and ingestion of alternative medicine supplements). Exogenous sources of thyroid tissue, such as struma ovarii (thyroid tissue in a monodermal ovarian teratoma), should also be considered in such patients.

18. How is fluorodeoxyglucose positron emission tomography (FDG PET) useful in the management of thyroid cancer?

In general, PET has no application in the initial diagnosis of thyroid carcinoma because there is overlap of FDG uptake between benign and malignant thyroid tumors. PET can be very useful, however, in patients previously treated for thyroid cancer who now have increasing tumor markers and an I-131 scan with negative results. FDG PET can be a useful adjunct imaging modality to help detect sites of tumor recurrence. The sensitivity for detection of recurrence with FDG PET is improved with hormonal withdrawal or administration of recombinant TSH. FDG PET also has a role in the management of patients with anaplastic, Hürthle cell, or medullary carcinoma because these tumors are not iodine avid.

BIBLIOGRAPHY

[1] N.S. Alnafisi, A.A. Driedger, G. Coates, et al., FDG PET of recurrent or metastatic ^{131}I-negative papillary thyroid carcinoma, J. Nucl. Med. 41 (2000) 1010–1015.

[2] H.J. Dworkin, D.A. Meier, M. Kaplan, Advances in the management of patients with thyroid disease, Semin. Nucl. Med. 25 (1995) 205–220.

[3] W.D. Leslie, A.C. Peterdy, J.O. Dupont, Radioiodine treatment outcomes in thyroid glands previously irradiated for Graves' hyperthyroidism, J. Nucl. Med. 39 (1998) 712–716.

[4] L.K. Shankar, A.J. Yamamoto, A. Alavi, et al., Comparison of I 131 scintigraphy at 5 and 24 hours in patients with differentiated thyroid cancer, J. Nucl. Med. 43 (2002) 72–76.

[5] P.A. Singer, D.S. Cooper, G.H. Daniels, et al., Treatment guidelines for patients with thyroid nodules and well differentiated thyroid cancer, Arch. Intern. Med. 156 (1996) 2165–2172.

GASTROINTESTINAL AND GENITOURINARY SCINTIGRAPHY

Andrew Newberg, MD

1. What should patients know about a renal scan, and what preparation should they be given?

In general, there is little in the way of patient preparation for a renal scan, although patients should be well hydrated. Patients should refrain from taking furosemide, which is sometimes given during the scan to help evaluate for obstruction. Angiotensin-converting enzyme (ACE) inhibitors should also be avoided because they can alter the kidney's ability to regulate perfusion; however, captopril may be given during the study to help assess for renovascular disease. The scan itself usually takes approximately 30 minutes and begins with an injection of a radiopharmaceutical agent followed by imaging in the posterior view for native kidneys and the anterior view for transplants.

2. What are the normal findings in a renal scan?

The perfusion component, measured during the first minute after injection of the tracer, should reveal renal perfusion occurring within several seconds of the aortic activity. Renal blood flow should be symmetric and greater than that in the spleen and liver (each kidney receives approximately 10% of cardiac output compared with <5% for the liver and spleen). Cortical images are obtained usually every minute for approximately 25 minutes. Cortical uptake should be symmetric with no focal defects. Activity should be observed entering the collecting system by 5 minutes (*cortical transit time* [how long it takes for urine to appear in the collecting system]). Urine should flow freely into the bladder without significant retention or obstruction (Fig. 57-1).

3. What are causes of focal areas of decreased flow within a kidney?

Most causes involve a mass effect, such as a cyst, abscess, or tumor (benign or malignant), that has altered renal morphologic features. Scarring in the kidney can result from chronic pyelonephritis or chronic ureteral reflux. Other causes of focal decreases in blood flow include infarction of part of the kidney or a hematoma associated with trauma or surgery. Such abnormalities can be either unifocal or multifocal, and all should be evaluated with anatomic imaging such as ultrasound (US) or computed tomography (CT).

4. An increase in size of one or both kidneys may be associated with what processes?

A common cause of a unilateral large kidney is compensatory hypertrophy for an absent or poorly functioning contralateral kidney. Hydronephrosis can also result in an enlarged kidney and may affect one or both kidneys. Patients with polycystic disease can also have kidneys that appear enlarged

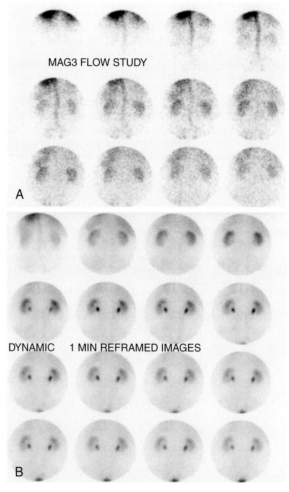

MAG3 FLOW STUDY

A

DYNAMIC   1 MIN REFRAMED IMAGES

B

Figure 57-1. A, Normal renal scan (posterior view) with symmetric and prompt flow into both kidneys on the blood flow phase. **B,** Delayed images show activity entering into the collecting systems by 4 minutes with adequate and symmetric excretion into the bladder. There is only mild retention of activity in the collecting systems on the last image.

and often have multiple cold defects associated with cysts. Renal vein thrombosis can also result in enlargement of a kidney related to the engorgement of blood associated with the obstruction on the venous side.

5. List the causes of a unilateral small kidney on the renal scan.

- Dysplastic kidney
- Postinflammatory atrophy
- Postobstructive atrophy
- Renal artery stenosis
- Radiation nephritis

Correlation with clinical history and anatomic imaging such as US or CT can help to differentiate the etiologic factor. Bilateral small kidneys are usually a manifestation of end-stage renal disease, which can be caused by many processes.

6. Describe potential causes of nonvisualization of a kidney.

Nonvisualization of a kidney on renal scan can be expected when a patient has had a nephrectomy, renal agenesis, post-traumatic or postsurgical damage to the kidney's vascular supply, or other vascular or obstructive processes. Vascular disorders that result in nonvisualization of a kidney include renal artery occlusion, which can be in the artery itself or from an abdominal aortic aneurysm, and renal vein occlusion. Neoplastic disease can also impair renal function or perfusion, resulting in nonvisualization. Finally, chronic obstruction, such as ureteropelvic junction obstruction, can eventually result in absent flow and function in a kidney (Fig. 57-2).

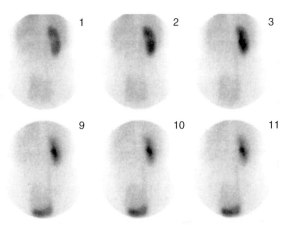

Figure 57-2. There is no visualization of the left kidney in this renal scan of a patient after nephrectomy for renal cell carcinoma. The right kidney appears slightly enlarged and has a normal cortical transit time.

7. How do processes that decrease the activity in both kidneys differ from processes that affect a single kidney?

Processes affecting both kidneys are often more systemic. Glomerulonephritis can cause decreased flow in both kidneys. Acute or chronic renal failure also results in decreased flow and function in both kidneys. Acute tubular necrosis (ATN) similarly results in decreased flow and function in the kidneys, although the function is typically more severely impaired. There can always be bilateral vascular or obstructive processes, and these should also be considered. Finally, technical factors, such as injecting the wrong tracer or acquiring images on the wrong photopeak, can be considered if the kidneys are not visualized (Fig. 57-3).

8. How is a captopril renal scan used to evaluate for renal artery stenosis?

A renal scan in a patient with renal artery stenosis often appears normal because the renin-angiotensin system causes a vasoconstriction of the efferent arterioles, which helps maintain the pressure across the glomeruli, preserving renal function. A renal scan performed after the administration of captopril or another ACE inhibitor reveals abnormal flow and function because the regulatory mechanism of angiotensin is blocked by the ACE inhibitor. A scan using diethylenetriaminepentaacetic acid (DTPA) after captopril should show evidence of diminished

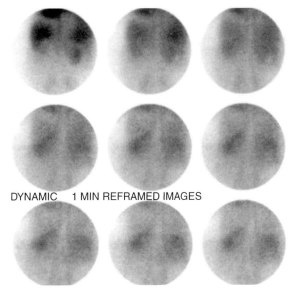

DYNAMIC   1 MIN REFRAMED IMAGES

Figure 57-3. Delayed images from a renal scan in a patient with chronic renal failure show bilaterally decreased uptake in the kidneys and no clear evidence of function. The kidneys have less activity than the liver and spleen, confirming the overall poor renal flow and function. Typically, each kidney receives approximately 10% of cardiac output, whereas the liver and spleen each receive less than 5%. Normal kidneys should have more activity than that in the liver and spleen.

flow and function in a kidney with renal artery stenosis compared with the renal scan without captopril. Generally, the overall sensitivity and specificity of this test have been approximately 90% and 95%. With the advent of magnetic resonance angiography (MRA), there has been considerably less use of the captopril renal scan, but it is still sometimes helpful in evaluating the functional relevance of partially stenotic renal arteries.

9. Why are renal scans obtained 1 day after transplant?

A renal scan within 1 day of surgical transplant can be very useful for detecting overall flow in the transplanted kidney to ensure that the artery is patent. The renal scan can also be used to help evaluate the extent of ATN, which occurs in virtually every transplant, although it is much more common and severe in cadaveric transplants compared with living related transplants. ATN on a renal scan typically is diagnosed when there is normal flow but diminished cortical transit of the tracer. The normal cortical transit time is usually less than 5 minutes; ATN can be evaluated based on the delay in cortical transit, with severe ATN showing no significant cortical function. A renal scan can also help with the evaluation of hyperacute rejection, which would appear as near-absent perfusion of the kidney. Renal scans can also provide information regarding possible obstruction or leak of urine (leaks most often occur several days after transplant) (Fig. 57-4).

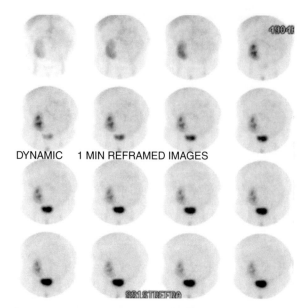

DYNAMIC   1 MIN REFRAMED IMAGES

Figure 57-4. Renal scan (anterior projection) in a patient 1 day after transplant from a living related donor. The uptake is good, and the cortical transit is within 5 minutes with good excretion into the bladder.

10. How is ATN differentiated from rejection in transplant patients?

Clinically, ATN occurs almost immediately, whereas chronic rejection occurs over several days to weeks or longer. ATN can occur later, although it is usually associated with some specific event that might damage the kidney. ATN usually takes several weeks or months to resolve after transplantation. Renal scan findings are often different for ATN and rejection, with ATN having normal or only slightly diminished perfusion of the kidney with a delayed cortical transit time. Rejection usually is associated with diminished flow with mildly impaired cortical function. In severe rejection, flow and function are markedly reduced. In both cases, when minimal or no urine is produced, it is impossible to exclude a leak or urinary tract obstruction because both of these entities require some radioactive urine to be produced. It is also possible to have ATN and rejection superimposed, and this is particularly the case when a bone scan reveals diminished flow and function. A clinician may have to treat such patients for both conditions (Fig. 57-5).

11. What type of renal scan is used to evaluate for cortical scarring related to pyelonephritis or vesicoureteral reflux? How does it work?

Pyelonephritis can result in scarring, hypertension, proteinuria, and renal failure. Renal scarring from vesicoureteral reflux accounts for 10% to 20% of patients with end-stage renal disease. A renal scan with dimercaptosuccinic acid (DMSA) is more sensitive than US or intravenous urography for the detection of parenchymal involvement. DMSA binds to the renal cortex and is essentially not excreted into the urine. This allows for imaging of the cortex to evaluate for areas of abnormally decreased activity. Imaging typically is performed approximately 20 minutes after injection, and single photon emission computed tomography (SPECT) imaging is performed to provide tomographic images for evaluation.

12. What are the current uses of a liver/spleen scan?

In current nuclear medicine practice, liver/spleen scans are primarily used to evaluate liver function associated with cirrhosis, in which there is decreased uptake in the liver and a "colloid shift" to the spleen and bone marrow. Liver/spleen scans can help to assess patients for focal nodular hyperplasia, which results in focal areas of increased uptake in the liver. Liver/spleen scans can also be used to assess splenic function. This last indication may be in the setting of trauma or surgery that may have damaged the spleen, or it may be used to seek out additional splenic tissue in patients with heterotaxia (Fig. 57-6).

13. What conditions result in a hot quadrate lobe and a hot caudate lobe on a liver/spleen scan?

Superior vena cava obstruction results in increased activity in the quadrate lobe; this occurs because collateral thoracic and abdominal vessels communicate with a recanalized umbilical vein, resulting in a hot quadrate lobe relative to the other areas of the liver. Budd-Chiari syndrome (hepatic vein thrombosis) appears as increased uptake in the caudate

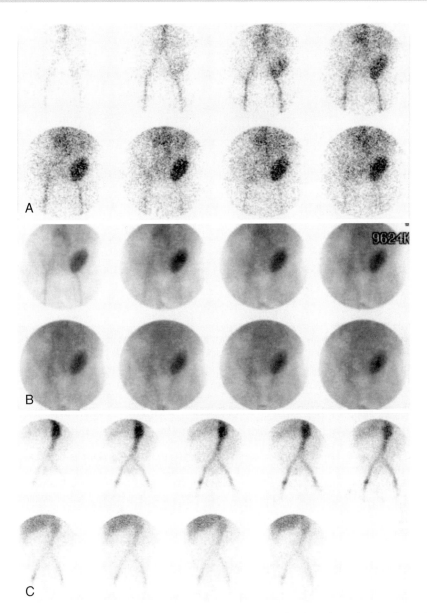

Figure 57-5. **A** and **B,** DTPA renal scan (anterior projection) in a patient 1 day after cadaveric renal transplant showing good flow (**A**), but no clear evidence of function (**B**). This constellation of findings is consistent with ATN. An obstruction or a leak cannot be adequately assessed on this scan because of the overall poor renal function. **C,** Chronic rejection (in a different patient) typically reduces flow and function to the point that severe rejection exhibits no significant flow in the transplanted kidney.

lobe, which has preserved function owing to direct venous drainage into the inferior vena cava. The remainder of the liver has decreased activity because of impaired function.

14. What is the diagnostic pattern of activity on a red blood cell (RBC) scan in a patient with a hemangioma in the liver?

The diagnosis of hemangiomas in the liver using tagged RBC imaging is based on identifying an early photopenic area with delayed filling because of the altered vasculature in the hemangioma. As blood slowly accumulates in the hemangioma, however, it has difficulty exiting the lesion because of the altered vasculature of the hemangioma. The same area eventually has increased activity on delayed images. The reported sensitivity for planar imaging is approximately 55% and for tomographic imaging is 88%.

15. What is the best test for the detection of splenic tissue?

The heat denatured RBC scan is the most sensitive and specific for evaluation of splenic tissue. Autologous RBCs are incubated at 50° C for 30 minutes and then reinjected. The main indications for performing such a study are to evaluate

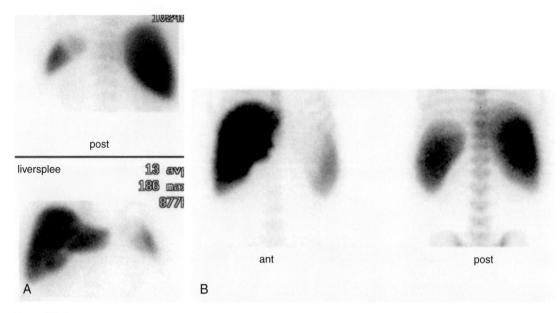

post

liversplee

13 avg
186 max
8771

ant

post

A   B

Figure 57-6. **A,** Normal colloid distribution on anterior and posterior projections of a liver/spleen scan with the most activity in the liver, followed by the spleen. Only approximately 5% of the activity is in the bone marrow. **B,** This can be compared with a patient with mild colloid shift with a larger spleen with similar uptake to the liver and overall more prominent bone marrow activity.

patients with heterotaxia, patients who may have ectopic splenic tissue, and patients with sickle cell disease to assess for splenic function.

16. What functions of the hepatobiliary system can be evaluated using iminodiacetic acid tracers?

Hepatocellular function can be evaluated because the tracer uptake by the liver depends on overall function. If the activity in the cardiac blood pool disappears within 5 minutes, hepatocellular function is considered to be normal. A longer time to clearance suggests hepatocellular dysfunction. The patency of the common bile duct and cystic duct can also be evaluated. This helps to diagnose acute and chronic cholecystitis. Finally, a leak or extrabiliary collection can be assessed (Fig. 57-7).

17. When should cholecystokinin (CCK) or morphine sulfate be used in relation to a hepatobiliary scan?

CCK should be used before the administration of a radiopharmaceutical agent when a patient has not eaten in more than 24 hours. The reason for the use of CCK is that the gallbladder can become filled with sludge with prolonged fasting, and this can result in false-positive scans. The intravenous infusion of CCK over about 15 to 30 minutes

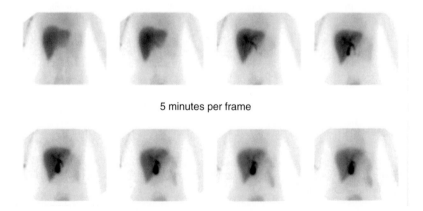

5 minutes per frame

Figure 57-7. Normal hepatobiliary scan (5 minutes per image) using Tc-99m mebrofenin (Choletec) shows good hepatocellular function associated with elimination of the cardiac blood pool by 5 minutes. The gallbladder is observed by 20 minutes, and activity is observed in the bowel by 25 minutes.

(faster infusions can result in nausea and vomiting) before beginning the hepatobiliary scan causes contraction of the gallbladder, which then fills with the radioactive tracer as it expands. Morphine augmentation is used if, after the 1-hour scan, there is nonvisualization of the gallbladder, and there is activity entering into the small bowel. If only the liver is seen without any activity entering the small bowel, morphine should not be given because the common bile duct may not be patent. Morphine causes contraction of the sphincter of Oddi, which results in a back pressure that can open a functionally closed cystic duct. If there is still nonvisualization of the gallbladder at the end of an additional 30 minutes of imaging after morphine is given, the result is consistent with acute cholecystitis.

18. What can a gallbladder ejection fraction study show?
A gallbladder ejection fraction study can be performed in patients with a normally filling gallbladder who continue to have right upper quadrant symptoms. At the end of the standard hepatobiliary scan, CCK (or sometimes a fatty meal) is administered, and images are obtained for another 30 minutes. The counts in the pre-CCK and post-CCK scans can be compared to provide a gallbladder ejection fraction. A normal value is considered to be greater than 30% to 35%; however, the distribution of values makes a normal range difficult to determine. If the ejection fraction is less than this value, gallbladder dysfunction is suspected. Cystic duct syndrome is considered if the gallbladder does not contract in a uniform manner or even expands after administration of CCK.

19. What are the causes of nonvisualization of the gallbladder on a hepatobiliary scan?
The most common cause is *acute cholecystitis* (Fig. 57-8). Many other potential causes, including various diseases and congenital problems, must be considered, however, in the evaluation:

- Acalculous cholecystitis
- Chronic cholecystitis
- Complete common duct obstruction
- Prolonged fasting
- Severe hepatocellular disease
- Acute pancreatitis
- Cholecystectomy
- Agenesis of gallbladder

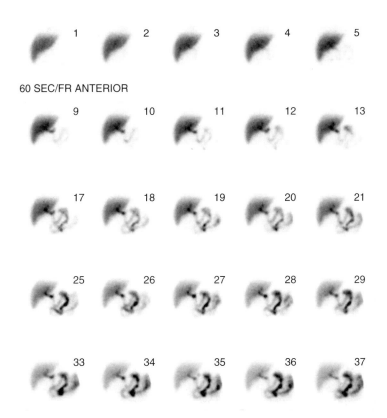

Figure 57-8. Hepatobiliary scan shows good liver uptake, but no evidence of gallbladder activity. If the gallbladder is still not visualized on morphine augmentation or delayed images, the scan findings are highly suggestive of acute cholecystitis.

20. Discuss the causes of a false-negative scan (i.e., visualization of the gallbladder in the presence of acute cholecystitis).

There are several reasons why the gallbladder, or a structure appearing to be the gallbladder, can be observed on a hepatobiliary scan. False-negative results occur most commonly when the patient has acalculous cholecystitis. Several other structures, such as the bowel, a duplicate gallbladder, or another abnormality of the biliary tree, can show activity in the region of the gallbladder even though the patient actually has acute cholecystitis. Another cause of false-negative results is perforation of the gallbladder, which subsequently reduces the pressure and relieves the obstruction, allowing the radioactive tracer to enter into the gallbladder region.

Key Points: Causes of False-Negative Hepatobiliary Scans

1. Acalculous cholecystitis
2. Loop of bowel
3. Dual gallbladder
4. Biliary duplication cyst
5. Right hydronephrosis
6. Gangrenous cholecystitis after perforation
7. Partial cystic duct obstruction
8. Intermittent obstruction from stone

---

21. What is the "rim" sign, and what does it imply?

The "rim" sign refers to an area of increased activity in the region of the liver surrounding the gallbladder. The implication is that there is hyperemia or inflammation associated with acute cholecystitis. This hyperemia appears as a rim of increased activity immediately adjacent to the gallbladder. The diagnosis of acute cholecystitis still depends, however, on nonvisualization of the gallbladder.

22. When a biliary leak occurs, where are the possible sites to observe the leak?

A biliary leak can occur anywhere along the biliary tree. However, Leaks usually occur, however, in areas of surgical interventions or anastomoses. When performing a hepatobiliary scan to look for a leak, it is important to perform the test in the standard manner. Additional images of surgical drains and anterior views with the patient in lateral decubitus positions help to assess for subtle leaks. Surgical drains should be evaluated for activity, and it is important to know where these drains are actually located. Drains in the surgical bed that have activity suggest a leak in that area. Drains in the biliary tree should naturally have activity. Decubitus views are obtained to assess for activity in free abdominal fluid, which would help to confirm a leak (Fig. 57-9).

23. How is biliary atresia differentiated from neonatal hepatitis on a hepatobiliary scan?

In both disorders, the bilirubin level is extremely high, making adequate visualization of activity entering into the small bowel difficult to assess. During the initial hour of imaging, activity is usually seen in the liver with persistent cardiac blood pool activity. Delayed imaging at 4 hours and sometimes 24 hours is required to determine whether any activity is observed entering into the bowel. If any activity does enter the bowel, biliary atresia can be excluded, and the diagnosis of neonatal hepatitis can be made. Absence of activity in the small bowel can still be related to either disorder, however, because if insufficient activity is sent into the biliary system by the liver, it is impossible to evaluate for potential complete obstruction.

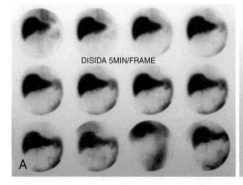

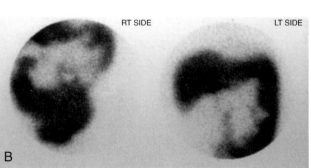

Figure 57-9. **A,** Hepatobiliary scan in a patient after liver transplant. The liver has preserved function. The gallbladder is not visualized secondary to the surgery. There is an accumulation of activity lateral to the left lobe of the liver that appears to be filling the left colic gutter. **B,** Anterior images taken with the patient in lateral decubitus position reveal radioactivity in the free fluid in the abdomen, which is consistent with a large leak.

24. What are the typical findings of a positive gastrointestinal (GI) bleed?

A positive GI bleeding scan generally requires that there be a focus of growing intensity that moves through the bowel. A focus that only increases in activity can sometimes be a false-positive finding and attributable to kidney activity or hyperemia in the bowel or some other vascular structure. It is also important to observe the initial site in which the focus occurs because the primary importance of this study is to determine localization of the bleed.

25. Contrast the differences between the sulfur colloid scan and the tagged RBC scan for detecting GI bleeding.

Both radiopharmaceutical agents are labeled with technetium (Tc)-99m. *Sulfur colloid scans* can be started immediately when the patient arrives in the nuclear medicine department because the agent can be prepared ahead of time. The sulfur colloid remains in the intravascular space for approximately 25 minutes. An active bleed can be detected quickly. An intermittent bleed might be missed if the patient bleeds after more than 25 minutes following injection of the sulfur colloid. Because sulfur colloid does not remain in the intravascular space, if there is a negative scan the first time, a repeat scan can be performed any time when the patient begins to bleed again.

A tagged RBC scan requires drawing some of the patient's blood, which must be labeled, a process that takes 15 to 20 minutes. After injection of Tc-99m–labeled RBCs, the activity persists in the intravascular space, and imaging can be performed continuously for several hours after injection; this can help to detect intermittent bleeds. If the initial scan results are negative, however, a repeat scan cannot be performed for approximately 24 hours so that the Tc-99m decays sufficiently. Otherwise, the bowel would have too much activity.

26. How does a gastric emptying study work?

A gastric emptying study involves the ingestion of a standardized meal consisting of some food source that is tagged with a radioactive label. The most common meal today consists of egg whites tagged with Tc-99m–labeled sulfur colloid. Meals must be standardized for content and calories so that an adequate comparison is made. Imaging usually is performed over 90 to 180 minutes. Images may be obtained throughout that time period or at regular intervals. Images are usually obtained in either the anterior and posterior views or a single left anterior oblique view. The importance of these views is that food enters the stomach posteriorly and moves anteriorly. Images must take into account movement within the stomach and differentiate it from actual emptying.

27. What are the normal rates for gastric emptying?

The rate of gastric emptying depends on the particular methods and meal used, but the normal half emptying time of the stomach is usually 50 to 100 minutes (Fig. 57-10).

28. What physiologic factors normally affect gastric emptying?

Numerous factors can affect gastric emptying. Factors that increase the gastric emptying rate include the patient positioned upright, younger male patients, higher liquid content of food, smaller size of food particles, larger volume of food, and lower fat content. Factors that can slow the rate include the patient positioned supine, older female patients, higher solid content of food, larger size of food particles, smaller volume of food, and higher fat content. Other factors that can cause variable responses include the hormonal and metabolic state of the patient, stress, and drugs. For these reasons, it is imperative that a standardized meal and acquisition protocol be used and compared with normal values established for that specific technique.

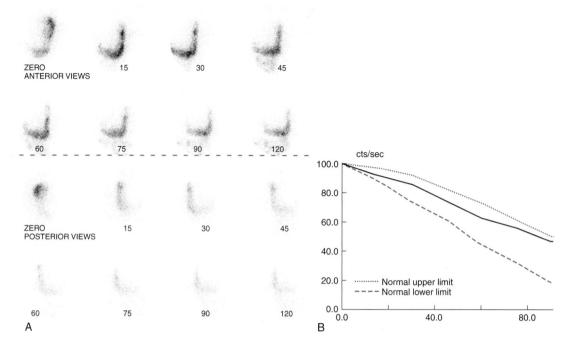

Figure 57-10. A, Normal gastric emptying study showing adequate transit of the tracer in anterior and posterior images. Anterior and posterior imaging is required because food moves from the posterior aspect of the stomach anteriorly over time, and without both projections, gastric emptying calculations may be inaccurate. **B,** Graph shows the rate of gastric emptying over 1.5 hours in the same patient with the upper and lower limits of normal shown for comparison.

BIBLIOGRAPHY

[1] F.L. Datz, Considerations for accurately measuring gastric emptying, J. Nucl. Med. 32 (1991) 881–884.

[2] E.V. Dubovsky, C.D. Russell, A. Bischof-Delaloye, et al., Report of the Radionuclides in Nephrourology Committee for evaluation of transplanted kidney (review of techniques), Semin. Nucl. Med. 29 (1999) 175–188.

[3] J.T. Emslie, K. Zarnegar, M.E. Siegel, et al., Technetium-99m-labeled red blood cell scans in the investigation of gastrointestinal bleeding, Dis. Colon Rectum. 39 (1996) 750–754.

[4] S. Krishnamurthy, G.T. Krishnamurthy, Biliary dyskinesia: role of the sphincter of Oddi, gallbladder and cholecystokinin, J. Nucl. Med. 38 (1997) 1824–1830.

[5] P. O'Reilly, M. Aurell, K. Britton, et al., Consensus report on diuresis renography for investigating the dilated upper urinary tract, J. Nucl. Med. 37 (1996) 1872–1876.

[6] F. Ponzo, H. Zhuang, F.M. Liu, et al., Tc-99m sulfur colloid and Tc-99m tagged red blood cell methods are comparable for detecting lower gastrointestinal bleeding in clinical practice, Clin. Nucl. Med. 27 (2002) 405–409.

[7] A. Taylor, J. Nally, M. Aurell, et al., Consensus report on ACE inhibitor renography for detecting renovascular hypertension, J. Nucl. Med. 37 (1996) 1876–1882.

NUCLEAR CARDIOLOGY

Andrew Newberg, MD

CHAPTER 58

1. How do you prepare a patient for a nuclear medicine stress test?

Patients should be informed that the test takes approximately a half day and consists of two parts. There is typically a resting part and a stress part. The placement of an intravenous catheter (usually inserted at the beginning of the day) is required to administer the radiopharmaceutical agent. The order of the study can be either rest-stress or stress-rest, although the higher dose is given for the second scan, and the stress test is often performed second to have the best image quality. Scans are obtained approximately 30 to 60 minutes after injection of the radiopharmaceutical agent, and each scan takes approximately 15 to 30 minutes. The patient should not eat or drink the night before the examination. Patients are commonly asked to stop taking their medications unless there is some reason (e.g., very high blood pressure or serious arrhythmias) that requires the stress test to be performed while the patient continues to take medications.

2. What are the different types of radiopharmaceutical agents available for stress testing?

There are three basic categories: thallium, technetium (Tc)-99m–labeled compounds, and positron emission tomography (PET) compounds. Table 58-1 compares thallium and Tc-99m compounds. The most commonly used Tc-99m compounds are tetrofosmin and sestamibi, which have similar imaging and chemical characteristics. Tc-99m compounds generally provide more flexibility in terms of imaging times. Because of the photon energy and the number of photons emitted, Tc-99m compounds are generally easier to use for image acquisition and analysis. PET radiopharmaceutical agents, such as ammonia N 13 and fluorodeoxyglucose (FDG), can be used to evaluate myocardial perfusion and glucose metabolism. Ammonia N 13 has a short (20-minute) half-life, so there are some logistical limitations in using PET for cardiac imaging.

3. What are the three types of stress tests?

The three basic types of stress tests are exercise, dipyridamole (Persantine) or adenosine, and dobutamine.

- *Exercise stress tests* are typically performed using a treadmill with several possible protocols that sequentially increase the speed and grade of the treadmill. An alternative exercise test uses a stationary bicycle. The goal is to increase heart rate to 85% of the patient's age-predicted maximum, although others have used a combination of heart rate and blood pressure as a target.
- *Dipyridamole (Persantine)* is an inhibitor of adenosine deaminase that results in increased adenosine within the epicardial coronary arteries. The result is a relative decrease in perfusion to areas in which there is a significant obstruction in the coronary arteries.
- *Dobutamine,* an adrenergic agonist, causes increased heart rate and increased inotropic contraction of the heart, simulating exercise.

4. What are contraindications for an exercise stress test?

Any patient with significant musculoskeletal problems that would prevent him or her from achieving maximal heart rate should undergo pharmacologic stress testing. Patients with certain ongoing arrhythmias, such as ventricular

Table 58-1. Comparison of Technetium (Tc)-99m Compounds and Thallium for Cardiac Imaging

	TC-99M COMPOUNDS	THALLIUM
Energy	140 keV (ideal for gamma camera)	69-83 keV (suboptimal for gamma camera)
First-pass studies of ventricular function	Possible with these agents	Not feasible
Gated imaging	Readily accomplished	Count rate marginal for gated imaging
Stress-rest imaging	Two injections required	Can be accomplished with one injection

tachycardia, supraventricular tachycardia, new-onset atrial fibrillation, or heart block, should receive treatment for those arrhythmias before the stress test is rescheduled. Known atrial fibrillation that is adequately treated is not a contraindication. Patients with severe pulmonary disease, severe hypertension (i.e., systolic blood pressure >210 mm Hg and diastolic blood pressure >110 mm Hg), abdominal aortic aneurysms, symptomatic aortic stenosis, unstable angina, or active ischemia on electrocardiogram (ECG) should also be excluded.

5. What are the contraindications for pharmacologic stress tests?

Persantine stress tests should not be performed in patients with severe reactive airway disease, particularly when a patient has active wheezing on physical examination. Patients who use inhalers but who otherwise have stable airway disease can often safely undergo Persantine stress tests. Any patient taking Persantine or methylxanthines should not have a Persantine stress test, unless the medication can be stopped for at least 24 to 48 hours. All patients who are to undergo Persantine studies should abstain from caffeine for 24 hours because caffeine blocks the effect of Persantine and adenosine. Dobutamine stress tests have similar contraindications to those of exercise testing except that musculoskeletal problems are not an issue.

6. Should patients taking medications that can affect the heart be given stress tests?

Generally, any patient can undergo a cardiac stress test. In patients taking medications for blood pressure, such as β-blockers or calcium channel blockers, the medication may prevent the patient from achieving the necessary heart rate. In such patients, it is recommended that the medications be stopped for approximately 24 hours before the study. If a patient has severe hypertension, the patient may need to be tested while taking the medication for this condition because without the medication, the blood pressure would be too high to proceed safely with the study.

7. List the conditions under which an exercise stress test should be stopped.

- The patient cannot continue because of dyspnea, chest pain, fatigue, or musculoskeletal problems.
- The patient has a hypertensive response.
- The patient develops ST segment depressions greater than 3 mm.
- The patient develops ST segment elevation, heralding a possible myocardial infarction.
- The patient develops the onset of a potentially dangerous arrhythmia, such as ventricular tachycardia, ventricular fibrillation, very rapid supraventricular tachycardia, or heart block.

8. Which territories are supplied by which coronary arteries?

The three main branches of the coronary arteries are the left anterior descending artery, the left circumflex artery, and the right coronary artery. The left anterior descending artery supplies the anterior wall, including the anterolateral region; septum; and, in most cases, the apex. The right coronary artery supplies the inferior wall and, in a "right dominant" system, can wrap around the apex to include part of the inferoapical wall. The left circumflex artery supplies the lateral wall. Smaller branches of these major arteries can supply smaller segments of individual walls (Fig. 58-1).

9. What is the implication of a "fixed" defect?

A fixed defect implies that there is a lack of perfusion during the rest and stress components of the scan (i.e., there is no difference between the two scans). Fixed defects can often be caused by artifact, such as when part of the heart is attenuated, or blocked, by a structure between the heart and the scanner. The most common structures that cause fixed defects via attenuation include the diaphragm (inferior wall) and breast tissue (anterior wall and apex). When fixed defects are associated with an actual cardiac pathologic condition, they are related to scarring or infarction. An infarct should have decreased perfusion during stress and rest images because it is dead tissue (Figs. 58-2 and 58-3).

10. What methods are available to correct for attenuation artifact?

Two common methods are used to correct for attenuation artifact. One method directly corrects this problem by using an external radioactive source that is transmitted through the patient. This source is used to map the patient's body structures to assess their ability to attenuate radioactive photons. By creating an attenuation map, the computer can combine the attenuation map with the emission images to correct for missing counts. The resulting image appears to "fill in" the areas that have attenuation artifact and eliminate the defects altogether.

A second method involves performing an ECG-gated study, obtaining images throughout the cardiac cycle. The ECG is monitored, and the R–R interval is divided into 8 or 16 equal segments during which the scan is acquired. The result is a sequence of images that can be played back to back to observe the wall motion throughout the R–R cycle. By obtaining the end-diastolic and end-systolic volumes, ejection fraction and regional wall motion can be determined. If a fixed defect is observed to move and thicken normally, it is most likely normal myocardium that has an apparent defect related to attenuation. If a fixed defect does not appear to move, it is most likely related to a scar. Gating helps to assess whether a defect is related to attenuation artifact or whether it is a real perfusion defect.

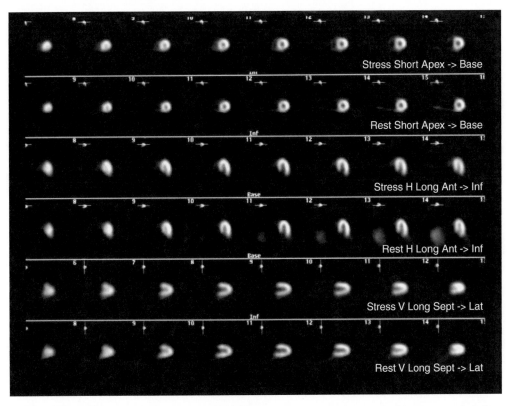

Figure 58-1. Normal cardiac perfusion scan with Tc-99m sestamibi. Stress images are on the top and rest images are on the bottom of each pair of projections. The short-axis view (from apex to base) shows the classic "doughnut" appearance, with the anterior wall at the top of the cardiac image, the lateral wall to the right, the inferior wall at the bottom, and the septum to the left. The horizontal long-axis view shows the septum on the left of the cardiac image, the apex at the top of the image, and the lateral wall to the right. The vertical long-axis view shows the anterior wall on the top of the image, the apex at the right of the image, and the inferior wall at the bottom. On this normal scan, the level of activity is uniform throughout all walls.

11. How do stress imaging studies compare with routine stress ECG studies in the evaluation of coronary artery disease (CAD)?

Generally, a routine stress ECG is sensitive, with positive ECG stress test results indicating a high likelihood for CAD. The accuracy is significantly reduced, however, in patients with abnormal baseline ECGs or a previous history of CAD, or if a patient does not achieve 85% of the maximal heart rate for patient age. In these patients, a stress imaging study has a sensitivity of approximately 92% and a specificity of approximately 72% for detecting CAD. The relative prevalence of CAD in the specific patient population is also a factor. Women have a much higher rate of false-positive stress test results because their prestudy risk is much lower than that for men.

12. What is the implication of a reversible defect?

A reversible defect implies a lack of perfusion during the stress component, but normal perfusion during rest. Reversible defects can be caused by attenuation artifact, but must always be assumed to be related to CAD, in which the stenotic artery cannot accommodate the extra perfusion demand during stress. The importance of a reversible defect is that the myocardium is intact, but is at risk for coronary events. It typically requires a stenosis of at least 50% to 70% for perfusion to be affected during the stress test. Reversible defects also usually mandate further study with coronary angiography to assess for the extent of blockage of the artery (Fig. 58-4).

Key Points: Reversible Defect on Cardiac Nuclear Scanning

1. Reversible defect equals lack of perfusion during stress and normal perfusion during rest.
2. Reversible defect implies vessel stenosis of at least 50% to 70%.
3. Coronary angiography is indicated for further evaluation.

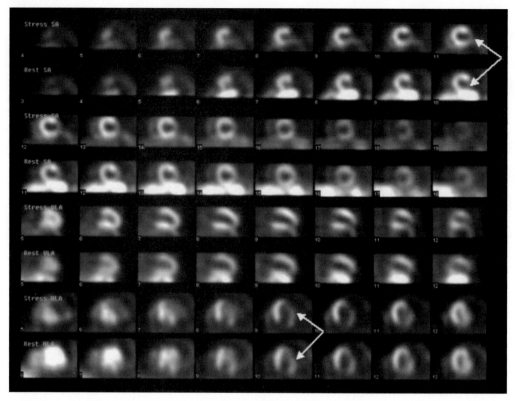

Figure 58-2. Cardiac perfusion scan with Tc-99m sestamibi reveals a lateral wall perfusion defect on the stress and rest images in the short-axis view and the horizontal long-axis view (*arrows*). Because this perfusion defect is observed on stress and rest images, it is a fixed defect and implies a prior infarct with near-absent perfusion in the scar.

13. Why is transient left ventricular cavity dilation a poor prognostic sign?

Transient left ventricular cavity dilation refers to the cavity appearing larger on stress images than on resting images. This is in contrast to *fixed cavity dilation,* which may be associated with a cardiomyopathy. Transient left ventricular cavity dilation indicates that during stress, the perfusion abnormalities result in worsening myocardial function such that the heart cannot maintain its usual contractile state and then dilation occurs. Transient left ventricular cavity dilation is a poor prognostic sign because significant cardiac function and structure is at risk for an ischemic event.

14. How might a left bundle-branch block (LBBB) on ECG affect imaging findings?

LBBB on ECG can cause perfusion defects in the septum during exercise. A reversible defect can be observed in patients with LBBB. The cause of this defect has not been completely elucidated, although it may be associated with altered depolarization of the septum owing to the conduction abnormality or related to left ventricular dilation and dysfunction associated with LBBB. To minimize the problem of perfusion defects associated with LBBB, a Persantine or adenosine stress test can be performed.

15. How is a thallium resting-redistribution scan performed, and how are the results of a resting-redistribution scan used clinically?

In a resting-redistribution scan, the patient receives an injection of thallium at rest and undergoes scanning approximately 15 minutes later. The patient is scanned again approximately 4 hours later and sometimes 24 hours after injection. Images are reconstructed in the typical tomographic projections. The images are evaluated for perfusion and for reversibility of defects observed on the initial scan. The general idea is that a patient with known CAD has several segments of the myocardium that have undergone ischemic injury. The question is whether these segments are viable, which can be determined because they either have some perfusion on initial images or show some degree of reversibility. Areas of the myocardium that show this type of viability typically respond well after revascularization by regaining some degree of function. Areas that are not viable typically do not respond to revascularization. Resting-redistribution studies can help to determine what parts of the heart, and what vessels, might be the best targets for revascularization.

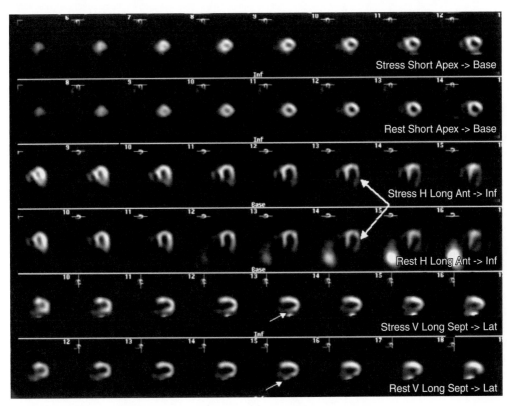

Figure 58-3. Cardiac perfusion scan with Tc-99m sestamibi reveals a fixed inferolateral wall perfusion defect. There is decreased perfusion in the lateral wall on the horizontal long-axis view (*large arrows*) and decreased perfusion in the inferior wall on the vertical long-axis view (*small arrows*). The defect can also be observed on the short-axis views. It is typically important to confirm any finding on other projections to ensure that it is a real defect rather than from artifact. This fixed defect represents a prior infarction.

16. What is the difference between hibernating and stunned myocardium?

- *Stunned myocardium* refers to relatively preserved myocardial perfusion as measured by single photon emission computed tomography (SPECT) or PET imaging, normal or decreased glucose metabolism on FDG PET scans, and decreased wall motion on echocardiography. The implication is that there was an ischemic event that caused a reduction in myocardial wall function, although perfusion and metabolism are now re-established. The stunning should resolve as long as perfusion is maintained.
- *Hibernating myocardium* refers to decreased perfusion with relatively preserved glucose metabolism and decreased wall motion. The implication is that chronic ischemia is resulting in decreased flow and function, although the myocardium is still viable. Hibernating myocardium should respond well to attempts to revascularize the region, which would return flow and eventually reverse the functional deficits.

17. How is a multiple-gated acquisition (MUGA) scan performed?

MUGA scan involves the radioactive tagging of the patient's red blood cells (RBCs) so that the blood pool remains radioactive throughout the study (Fig. 58-5). Labeling can be performed either in vitro or in vivo. In vitro labeling requires blood to be drawn from the patient first; the labeling is performed in the laboratory, and blood is reinjected into the patient. Alternatively, the RBCs can be labeled in the patient by first injecting stannous pyrophosphate, which allows the RBCs to take up Tc-99m. When the patient's RBCs are labeled, images are usually acquired in the left anterior oblique projection and the anterior projection for approximately 15 minutes while the ECG is monitored. The R–R interval is divided into 8 or 16 segments, during which image acquisition occurs. The result is that the activity in the ventricle can be measured throughout the cardiac cycle, and the end-diastolic (ED) and end-systolic (ES) activity levels and regional wall motion can be assessed. The ejection fraction is calculated based on the following equation:

$$(ED - ES) / (ED - BG)$$

The background (BG) counts are also important because placement of the background region over an area with significant activity (e.g., the aorta) would result in a falsely elevated calculated ejection fraction.

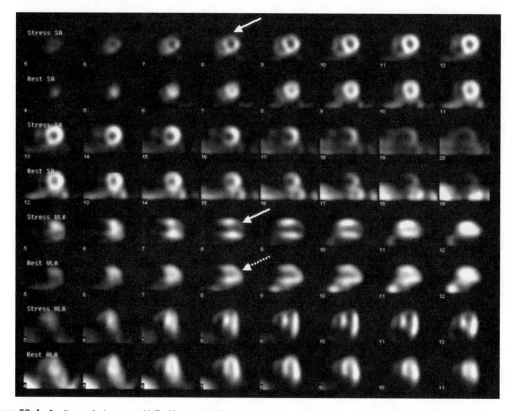

Figure 58-4. Cardiac perfusion scan with Tc-99m sestamibi shows a perfusion defect in the anterior and apical regions on the stress images in the short-axis view and vertical long-axis view (*solid arrows*). The site of the stress perfusion defect appears to be normal on the resting images (*dotted arrow*), suggesting that the defect is reversible. The implication is that there is significant atherosclerosis in the artery supplying this territory, which in this case is the left anterior descending artery. The overall left ventricular cavity size appears dilated on the stress images compared with the resting images (see in particular the short-axis and vertical long-axis images), a finding that implies left ventricular dysfunction during stress.

18. How is MUGA scan used clinically?

MUGA scan is primarily used in the evaluation of myocardial wall motion and determination of left ventricular ejection fraction. Both of these can now be assessed with echocardiography, which can also be used to evaluate the structure and function of the heart's valves. For this reason, MUGA scans are used infrequently. The principal use is for the determination of ejection fraction in cancer patients before and after they undergo chemotherapy. Patients taking chemotherapeutic agents that can affect cardiac function, such as doxorubicin (Adriamycin), need to have serial measures of cardiac function with the initial scan before therapy. MUGA scans provide true quantitative information regarding ejection fraction because the actual counts of activity within the left ventricular cavity can be assessed (echocardiography determines ejection fraction by estimation). General guidelines suggest that if the ejection fraction declines to less than 40% or has a decrease of more than 15%, the patient should not continue chemotherapy with the same agent.

19. How does FDG PET scan of the heart as shown in Fig. 58-6 help evaluate myocardial viability?

The primary energy substrate of the myocardium is free fatty acids rather than glucose. During ischemia, there is a switch in the myocardium to glucose use. If there is decreased perfusion but preserved FDG uptake, that area of the myocardium is considered viable. If there is decreased perfusion and metabolism, that area of the myocardium is considered to be a scar. In Fig. 58-6, FDG PET shows that the heart is enlarged, with preserved metabolism throughout the myocardium with the exception of the apex. The apex would be considered to be scar, but the rest of the myocardium is viable tissue.

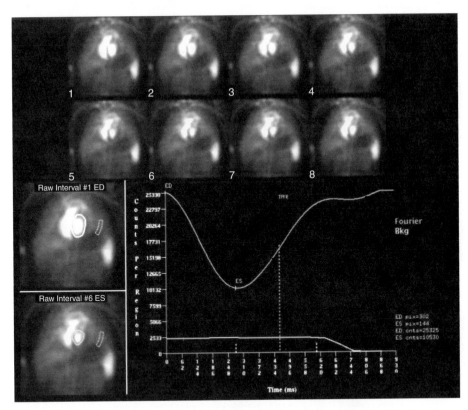

Figure 58-5. Normal MUGA scan showing eight images (*top*) ranging from end diastole (ED) to end systole (ES) with a subsequent decrease in the overall cavity size and counts. To the left are two images that include regions drawn around the left ventricle on ED and ES, and a background region. These regions help to establish the curve that represents the normal number of counts throughout the cardiac cycle. The background counts are the curve at the bottom. The ejection fraction is calculated on the basis of the ED and ES counts in the left ventricle, which in this case was 61%.

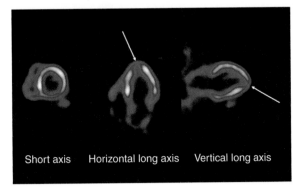

Figure 58-6. FDG PET scan of the heart showing an enlarged left ventricle with preserved metabolism in all segments except for the apex. The areas of preserved metabolism represent viable myocardium, whereas the apex (*arrows*) is considered to be scar.

BIBLIOGRAPHY

[1] R. Bolli, Myocardial 'stunning' in man, Circulation 86 (1992) 1671–1691.
[2] K.A. Brown, E. Altland, M. Rowen, Prognostic value of normal technetium-99m-sestamibi cardiac imaging, J. Nucl. Med. 14 (1994) 554–557.
[3] L.M. Freeman, M.D. Blaufox, Cardiovascular nuclear medicine, parts 1 and 2, Semin. Nucl. Med. 19 (1999).
[4] S.H. Rahimtoola, The hibernating myocardium, Am. Heart. J. 117 (1989) 211–221.
[5] C. Santano-Boado, J. Candell-Riera, J. Castell-Conesa, et al., Diagnostic accuracy of technetium-99m-MIBI myocardial SPECT in women and men, J. Nucl. Med. 39 (1998) 751–755.
[6] M. Schwaiger, Myocardial perfusion imaging with PET, J. Nucl. Med. 35 (1994) 693–698.

PEDIATRIC THORACIC RADIOLOGY

CHAPTER 59

D. Andrew Mong, MD

1. What is the embryologic relationship between the lungs and the gastrointestinal tract?
The lung bud is an outpouching of the primitive foregut, appearing during the fourth week of development. This intricate relationship is the basis for tracheoesophageal fistulas (see Chapter 60).

2. Describe the histologic stages of lung development.
The lung bud progressively ramifies during embryologic development, undergoing a pseudoglandular stage (weeks 5 to 17); a canalicular stage (weeks 16 to 25); a terminal sac stage (weeks 25 to 40); and an alveolar stage, which begins late in fetal life and continues until approximately 8 years.

3. What is surfactant, and why is it important?
Surfactant is produced by type II pneumocytes, which begin to form at approximately 6 months of gestation. It is a complex substance containing phospholipids and apoproteins, which act to reduce surface tension and prevent alveolar collapse.

4. Describe the pertinent findings on a normal neonatal chest radiograph.
- The appearance of the thymus is variable, but it may be visible until 2 years of age. The "sail" sign refers to the thymus creating a triangular shadow of soft tissue along the mediastinal border on chest x-ray.
- Always check for the side of the aortic arch (normally left-sided); this may be difficult to do in newborns, and the side of the aortic arch may need to be inferred by observing that the descending aorta runs to the left of the spine and that the trachea is mildly deviated to the right.
- Look at heart size. In contrast to adults, the cardiac-thoracic ratio may be 60%. The apex of the heart should be on the left (*levocardia*).
- Pulmonary vascularity should be assessed. This assessment may be difficult, but some clues to increased vascularity include seeing vessels behind the liver shadow or noting that the right descending pulmonary artery is larger in diameter than the trachea.
- Look at the bones (especially the vertebrae for any segmental anomalies), and note whether the humeral heads have ossified (this happens at 40 weeks of gestation).
- Look under the diaphragm for organomegaly and the position of the stomach bubble (normally in the left upper quadrant.)
- Because you are not going to forget to look at the lung fields, try to make yourself do that last.

5. What is neonatal respiratory distress syndrome (RDS)?
RDS is a syndrome of premature infants, usually born at less than 36 weeks of gestation, that occurs as a result of surfactant deficiency from underdeveloped type II pneumocytes. This leads to elevated alveolar surface tension and diffuse microatelectasis.

6. How does RDS appear radiographically?
The radiographic appearance of RDS is a diffuse, symmetric ground-glass appearance to the lung parenchyma with low lung volumes (Fig. 59-1).

7. How is RDS treated? What are the potential consequences?
Maternal steroids have been shown to promote surfactant production if preterm delivery is imminent. Exogenous surfactant administration is beneficial. Infants may require intubation. Intubation may lead

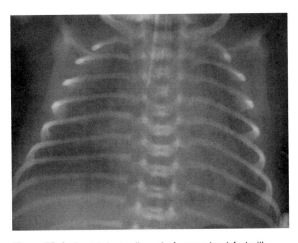

Figure 59-1. Frontal chest radiograph of a premature infant with diffuse ground-glass lung disease and low lung volumes, which is indicative of RDS. (Courtesy of Richard Markowitz, MD, Children's Hospital of Philadelphia.)

413

to air leaks in the form of pneumothoraces; pneumomediastinum; or pulmonary interstitial emphysema, which appears as linear interstitial lucencies. Long-term consequences of barotrauma and increased oxygen exposure include neonatal chronic lung disease, which may manifest as diffuse interstitial thickening and hyperaeration.

8. In addition to RDS, what are other neonatal diffuse lung diseases?
- Transient tachypnea of the newborn (TTN)
- Congestive heart failure (CHF)
- Neonatal pneumonia
- Meconium aspiration

9. How might other neonatal diffuse lung diseases be differentiated clinically?
Neonatal pneumonia may occur in a preterm or term infant. Meconium aspiration and TTN are generally diseases of term infants. CHF and pneumonia may occur in either preterm or term infants.

> **Key Points: Causes of Neonatal Diffuse Lung Disease**
>
> 1. Respiratory distress syndrome (RDS)
> 2. Transient tachypnea of the newborn (TTN)
> 3. Congestive heart failure (CHF)
> 4. Pneumonia
> 5. Meconium aspiration

10. What is the mechanism behind meconium aspiration, and how does it appear radiographically?
Perinatal hypoxia may lead to a deep gasping reflex and premature passage of meconium, which combine to cause aspiration. Meconium aspiration may cause hyperaeration (sometimes the sole radiographic appearance), scattered areas of atelectasis, and ropelike perihilar radiations.

11. What is TTN?
TTN results from inadequate clearance of fetal serum from the lung parenchyma during the transition to aerated lung at birth. A primary stimulus for clearance is passage through the birth canal, so infants delivered by cesarean section are at increased risk. TTN is usually a benign process that resolves within 2 to 3 days, although in rare cases, infants may require intubation.

12. How does TTN appear on a chest radiograph?
Radiographically, TTN appears as mild CHF, with an enlarged heart, increased interstitial markings, and pleural effusions.

13. Name the major causes of CHF in a newborn.
TTN, as described, may look like CHF. Causes of CHF in a newborn include constitutional problems, such as anemia, hypoglycemia, or sepsis; primary pump problems, such as hypoplastic left heart; outflow obstructions, such as aortic stenosis or coarctation of the aorta; inflow problems, such as cor triatriatum or mitral valve stenosis; and extracardiac shunts, such as a vein of Galen malformation or a hepatic hemangioendothelioma.

14. What is the role of the radiologist in assessing suspected congenital heart disease (CHD)?
Although magnetic resonance imaging (MRI) examination of the heart (beyond the scope of this chapter) may be used to assess cardiac chamber size and position, wall thickness, presence of intracardiac shunts, and position of the coronary arteries, the initial role of the radiologist is to evaluate the chest radiograph and to provide an ordered, logical differential diagnosis. It is usually impossible to give a precise diagnosis in these cases.

15. What are the most common acyanotic CHDs?
The first consideration in diagnosing CHD should be whether the infant is clinically cyanotic. Acyanosis implies a left-to-right shunt, and the most common causes include atrial septal defect, ventricular septal defect, patent ductus arteriosus, and endocardial cushion defects. These typically cause enlargement of specific chambers in the heart as a result of decompression of some chambers and overload in others. A ventricular septal defect results in an enlarged right ventricle, main pulmonary artery, and left atrium, but the left ventricle is normal in size as blood is shunted away from it. An atrial septal defect typically results in an enlarged right atrium and right ventricle, but a normal-sized left atrium.

16. **How does assessment of pulmonary blood flow aid in the diagnoses of cyanotic CHD?**

Cyanosis implies either admixture of oxygenated and deoxygenated blood, which would appear as increased blood flow in the heart, or that blood is shunted away from the lungs, which would appear as decreased blood flow. Assessment of blood flow includes looking for shunt vessels at the periphery of the lung fields or behind the liver shadow.

17. **Which CHDs appear with cyanosis and increased pulmonary blood flow?**

These conditions include total anomalous pulmonary venous return, truncus arteriosus, transposition of the great vessels, tricuspid atresia, and single ventricle. Hypoplastic left heart syndrome may also appear with CHF and cyanosis.

18. **What is the importance of a right-sided aortic arch?**

A right-sided arch may show mirror-image branching or an aberrant left subclavian artery (see question 21). A right-sided arch may be associated with tetralogy of Fallot or truncus arteriosus. If you see a right-sided aortic arch, look for other anomalies and consider recommending echocardiography.

19. **What are the major surgical diseases of the neonatal chest?**

Surgical neonatal chest disease is generally a focal process and includes entities such as congenital diaphragmatic hernia (CDH), congenital cystic adenomatoid malformation (CCAM), pulmonary sequestration, and congenital lobar emphysema. Although these entities may appear solid at birth, CDH, CCAM, and congenital lobar emphysema usually aerate over time. Pulmonary sequestrations and certain types of CCAM remain solid unless there is superinfection (Fig. 59-2).

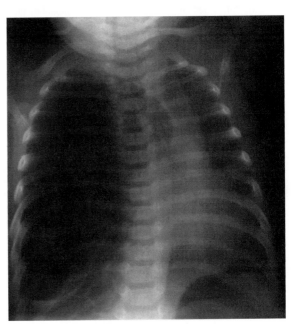

Figure 59-2. CCAM may be seen as several large cysts, multiple small cysts, or microscopic cysts that appear solid. The appearance of this frontal chest radiograph could also be due to congenital lobar emphysema. (Courtesy of Richard Markowitz, MD, Children's Hospital of Philadelphia.)

20. **What is the most common cause of a neonatal pleural effusion?**

A chylothorax is the most common cause of a neonatal pleural effusion. The etiologic factor of these effusions is uncertain, but it may be secondary to birth trauma of the thoracic duct. These are typically treated conservatively, with drainage of the effusion and administration of a medium-chain triglyceride diet.

21. **Describe the two main types of vascular rings.**

Vascular rings may cause constriction of the trachea and esophagus, creating stridor or dysphagia. A ring around the trachea and esophagus may be formed by a double aortic arch or by a right-sided arch with an aberrant left subclavian artery. In the latter case, the ring is completed by the ligamentum arteriosum. A vascular ring may be suspected if lateral compressions on the trachea on a chest radiograph are noted. Traditionally, rings were evaluated with a barium swallow, which would show a posterior external compression on the esophagus (with either type of ring). Today, these are often evaluated with MRI.

Key Points: Causes of Focal Neonatal Lung Disease

1. Congenital diaphragmatic hernia (CDH)
2. Congenital cystic adenomatoid malformation (CCAM)
3. Congenital lobar emphysema
4. Pulmonary sequestration

---

22. **How does a pulmonary sling cause symptoms?**

A pulmonary sling refers to anomalous origin of the left pulmonary artery from the right pulmonary artery, with the left artery coursing abnormally between the trachea and the esophagus. Patients typically present with wheezing or respiratory distress. There is a high association with complete cartilaginous rings of the trachea (as opposed to the incomplete horseshoe cartilaginous components in a normal patient), which are often the cause of the patient's symptoms.

23. How do heterotaxia syndromes manifest in the lungs?

Heterotaxia syndromes refer to *situs ambiguus,* when the organs conform neither to the normal situs solitus confirmation nor to the situs inversus (complete mirror image.) In heterotaxia, the liver is midline, and the stomach bubble may be to the right or left of midline. Heterotaxia syndromes are typically divided into polysplenia and asplenia. In *polysplenia,* the abdomen and chest are "left-sided." Findings include multiple spleens, azygous continuation of the inferior vena cava, and absence of the gallbladder. In the chest, polysplenia syndrome includes two "left-sided lungs," so there are bilateral bilobed lungs with hyparterial bronchi (under the pulmonary arteries). In *asplenia,* the abdomen and chest are right-sided. The spleen is absent. In the chest, asplenia syndrome includes two right-sided lungs that have three lobes and eparterial bronchi (above the pulmonary arteries). Asplenia and polysplenia are associated with gastrointestinal malrotation and CHD, although CHD in polysplenia tends to be milder than in asplenia.

24. Describe how chlamydial pneumonia manifests clinically and radiographically.

Chlamydial pneumonia is a disease of neonates, usually manifesting within the first 2 weeks of life, often with associated conjunctivitis. Chest radiographs usually show hyperinflation and ill-defined linear markings, sometimes creating a shaggy appearance of the cardiac border.

25. What are the pulmonary and extrapulmonary manifestations of cystic fibrosis?

Cystic fibrosis is an autosomal recessive disorder of abnormal chloride ion transport, which results in backup of thick mucous secretions in various organs. In the lungs, cystic fibrosis manifests as repeated infections that result in bronchiectasis, predominantly in the upper lobes. On plain films, bronchiectasis may appear as multiple lucent holes or a tram-track appearance of the bronchi, which may be fluid-filled. On computed tomography (CT) examination, bronchiectasis is defined as bronchi that are larger in diameter than the adjacent pulmonary arteries. Extrapulmonary manifestations include neonatal meconium ileus (small bowel obstruction at the terminal ileum from inspissated meconium), chronic pancreatitis, and cirrhosis. An enlarged spleen may result from portal hypertension. This may be manifest on a chest radiograph as medial deviation of the stomach bubble in the left upper quadrant.

26. What are the findings of primary tuberculosis of the lungs in a pediatric patient?

The findings of primary tuberculosis are nonspecific, as in an adult, but can include mediastinal or hilar adenopathy or both, pulmonary parenchymal disease, and pleural effusion.

27. Whom does acute chest syndrome affect?

Acute chest syndrome affects patients with sickle cell anemia. Acute chest syndrome refers to alveolar edema, which appears radiographically as scattered dense areas of consolidation. This is usually difficult to differentiate from bacteria pneumonia.

28. What is lymphocytic interstitial pneumonia?

Lymphocytic interstitial pneumonia is a lymphoproliferative response in the chest, often to human immunodeficiency virus (HIV). Radiographically, lymphocytic interstitial pneumonia appears as multiple interstitial nodules. This pattern is much more common in children than in adults. The differential diagnosis of multiple pulmonary nodules includes Langerhans cell histiocytosis, miliary infections such as tuberculosis or histoplasmosis, hypersensitivity pneumonitis, viral etiologies such as varicella, and metastatic disease.

29. How should a suspected aspirated foreign body be evaluated?

A nonradiopaque aspirated foreign body in a main stem bronchus may produce a ball-valve effect, trapping air unilaterally and creating a large lucent lung compared with the contralateral normal size. These findings may be subtle, but if suspected, expiratory films may make them more obvious because the unaffected lung would lose volume, whereas the affected lung would not. Decubitus films may also exaggerate this difference, with the unaffected lung losing volume when it is in the dependent position. Air trapping may also be shown by fluoroscopy.

30. What is Swyer-James syndrome?

The hypothesized pathogenesis of Swyer-James syndrome involves a viral infection that arrests growth of an affected lung through an obliterative bronchiolitis. Hyperlucency from air trapping and diminished arterial flow results. Traditionally, this was thought to be a unilateral process, but CT examinations often show scattered areas of bilateral air trapping.

31. What are important structures to identify on a lateral view of the neck?

- Assess the prevertebral soft tissues. Soft tissue swelling in this area could be due to retropharyngeal abscess, edema, hematoma, or soft tissue mass.

- The epiglottis should be triangular or flat, not bulbous or thumblike (which would indicate epiglottitis), and the aryepiglottic folds should not be thickened.
- Look for enlargement of the adenoid tissue and tonsils.
- Assess the caliber of the trachea, which should not change abruptly.
- You may identify sloughed membranes within the lumen from bacterial tracheitis.
- A frontal radiograph is often useful in identifying croup, characterized by symmetric subglottic narrowing that creates the steeple sign from loss of the normal subglottic shoulders (Figs. 59-3 and 59-4).

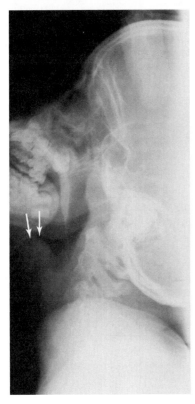

Figure 59-3. Abnormal bulbous thickening of the epiglottis (*arrows*). This finding reflects epiglottitis, an emergency requiring intubation. (Courtesy of Richard Markowitz, MD, Children's Hospital of Philadelphia.)

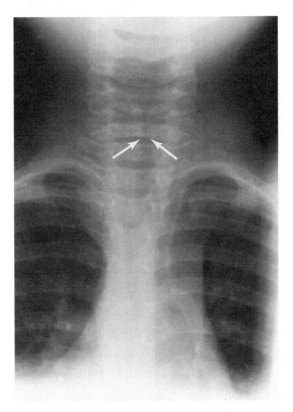

Figure 59-4. Frontal plain film of the soft tissues of the neck shows classic steeple sign (*arrows*) of croup, with loss of the normal subglottic shoulders.

BIBLIOGRAPHY

[1] B.A. Alford, J. McIlhenny, An approach to the asymmetric neonatal chest radiograph, Radiol. Clin. North Am. 37 (1999) 1079–1092.
[2] W.E. Berdon, Rings, slings, and other things: vascular compression of the infant trachea updated from the mid-century to the millennium—the legacy of Robert E. Gross, MD, and Edward B.D. Neuhauser, MD, Radiology 216 (2000) 624–632.
[3] A.T. Gibson, G.M. Steiner, Imaging the neonatal chest, Clin. Radiol. 52 (1997) 172–186.
[4] J.L. Strife, R.W. Sze, Radiographic evaluation of the neonate with congenital heart disease, Radiol. Clin. North Am. 37 (1999) 1093–1107.

PEDIATRIC GASTROINTESTINAL RADIOLOGY

Kerry Bron, MD, and
Avrum N. Pollock, MD

1. What are the most common causes of small bowel obstruction in a child?

AAIIMM is a mnemonic that makes it easy to remember the causes:

- *A* = *A*dhesions, usually postsurgical
- *A* = *A*ppendicitis
- *I* = *I*ntussusception
- *I* = *I*ncarcerated inguinal hernia
- *M* = *M*alrotation with volvulus or bands
- *M* = *M*iscellaneous, such as Meckel diverticulum or intestinal duplication

2. What is intussusception?

Intussusception is a condition in which a proximal portion of the bowel (intussusceptum) telescopes into the adjacent distal bowel (intussuscipiens). When the inner loop and its mesentery become obstructed, a small bowel obstruction occurs.

3. What causes intussusception?

In most cases, intussusception is idiopathic. In less than 5% of cases, the intussusception contains a lead point, such as a polyp, Meckel diverticulum, or hypertrophic lymphatic tissue. Most intussusceptions are ileocolic.

4. Describe the clinical signs of intussusception.

The classic clinical triad of intussusception is intermittent colicky abdominal pain, current jelly stools, and a palpable abdominal mass. Less than 50% of patients present with these symptoms, however. Children often cry and are very irritable during bouts of abdominal pain, and then become drowsy and lethargic. Vomiting and fever may also occur. Intussusception is most common in children 3 months to 4 years old, with a peak incidence at 3 to 9 months. It is more common in boys.

5. How is intussusception diagnosed radiologically?

The most accurate technique for the diagnosis of intussusception is ultrasound (US). The characteristic US appearance is a mass that measures 3 to 5 cm, which is easily detectable. On the transverse scan, the mass has a "target" appearance that contains echogenic fat. The "pseudokidney" sign appears in the longitudinal direction. A barium enema can also be used to diagnose intussusception. Although the plain film has been used in the past to diagnose intussusception by detection of a soft tissue mass in the right upper quadrant and lack of large bowel gas, particularly in the right upper quadrant, studies have shown poor interobserver agreement and predictive value of only approximately 50%.

6. How is an intussusception treated?

An intussusception is treated by air enema with fluoroscopic guidance or hydrostatic enema using barium or water-soluble contrast agent (Fig. 60-1). The advantages of the air enema are that it is quicker, less messy, easier to perform, and delivers less radiation to the patient. The only contraindications to enema reduction of intussusception are pneumoperitoneum or peritonitis. The air enema can generates pressure of 120 mm Hg to reduce the intussusception.

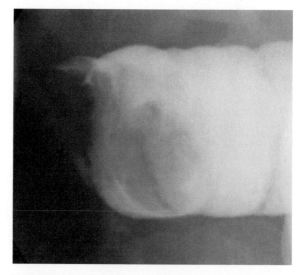

Figure 60-1. Spot radiograph from a contrast enema examination shows intussusception, with the lead point outlined by the barium.

7. How can one tell that an intussusception has been successfully reduced?

If a successful air reduction has been performed, fluid with air bubbles should be seen passing through the ileocecal valve into the terminal ileum. If a successful reduction with contrast agent has been performed, contrast agent must reflux into multiple loops of small bowel. If reflux into the small bowel is not seen, the intussusception may not have been completely reduced, and a distal lead point may have been overlooked.

Key Points: Intussusception

1. Common cause of small bowel obstruction in children
2. Idiopathic in children, in contrast to in adults
3. Usually ileocolic
4. Diagnosed by US
5. Treated with air enema or contrast barium enema

---

8. Describe the "double bubble" sign, and name the conditions in which it is found.

The "double bubble" sign is found on plain radiographs and represents an air-filled or fluid-filled distended stomach and duodenal bulb (Fig. 60-2). It is seen in malrotation, duodenal atresia, and jejunal atresia.

9. What is malrotation of the intestines?

Malrotation of the intestines is a misnomer because it is really *nonrotation* or *incomplete rotation* of the bowel. To understand malrotation, one must first consider normal embryologic rotation of the intestines. During normal embryologic development in the first trimester, the midgut leaves the abdominal cavity, travels into the umbilical cord, and returns to the abdominal cavity. As the intestines return, the proximal and distal parts of the midgut rotate around the superior mesenteric artery axis 270 degrees in a counterclockwise direction. The ligament of Treitz (duodenojejunal junction) lands in the left upper quadrant, and the cecum comes to rest in the right lower quadrant. In malrotation, this intestinal rotation and fixation occur abnormally. If normal rotation does not occur, the cecum is not anchored in the right lower quadrant and may be midline or in the upper abdomen. The small bowel is not anchored in the left upper quadrant and may lie entirely in the right abdomen.

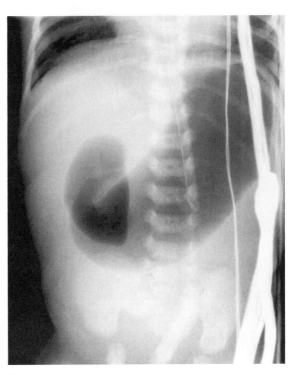

Figure 60-2. Plain film of the abdomen in a child with duodenal atresia, showing a dilated stomach and duodenal bulb—the "double bubble" sign.

10. What are Ladd bands?

Ladd bands are dense peritoneal bands that develop as an attempt to fix the bowel to the abdominal wall in malrotation. They may extend from the malpositioned cecum across the duodenum to the posterolateral abdomen and porta hepatis in either incomplete rotation or nonrotation and can cause extrinsic duodenal obstruction.

11. How does a midgut volvulus occur, and why is this an emergency?

Lack of attachment of the midgut to the posterior abdominal wall allows the midgut to twist on a shortened root mesentery, which results from lack of complete rotation (Fig. 60-3). This twisting is called a *volvulus,* and it causes small bowel obstruction with concomitant obstruction to the lymphatic and venous supply of the bowel and eventually to the arterial supply, which leads to ischemia and necrosis. If it is not repaired within several hours, all of the intestine supplied by the superior mesenteric artery undergoes infarction.

12. Does a patient with malrotation always present with clinical symptoms.

Not all patients with malrotation are symptomatic because not all develop a midgut volvulus or extrinsic duodenal obstruction from Ladd bands.

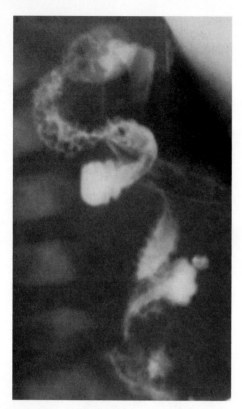

Figure 60-3. Spot radiograph from an upper GI examination showing the "corkscrew" finding of a midgut volvulus.

13. What is the clinical presentation of malrotation?

Patients with incomplete rotation who have intestinal obstruction usually present within the first week or first month of life (75% of patients). They present with an acute onset of bilious vomiting, which is a surgical emergency. Some patients present later in childhood with intermittent mechanical obstruction, which manifests as cyclic vomiting. Malrotation in the remaining patients is often found incidentally when the patients are studied for other complaints.

14. Which study is the gold standard for diagnosing malrotation?

The upper gastrointestinal (GI) examination is the gold standard for diagnosing malrotation. To confirm normal rotation of the bowel, the ligament of Treitz, which attaches the third and fourth parts of the duodenum, must be visualized to the left of midline. If there is malrotation, the ligament of Treitz may be located to the right of midline or in the midline. Often, there is inversion of the superior mesenteric artery and vein, which can be visualized on computed tomography (CT).

15. List other anomalies that are associated with malrotation.

- Duodenal atresia or stenosis
- Meckel diverticulum
- Omphalocele
- Gastroschisis
- Polysplenia/asplenia syndromes
- Situs ambiguus
- Bochdalek hernia
- Renal anomalies

Key Points: Malrotation of the Intestines

1. Malrotation causes small bowel obstruction through a midgut volvulus and Ladd bands.
2. Malrotation causes altered GI anatomy, with the ligament of Treitz not situated in the left upper quadrant and the cecum not in the right lower quadrant.

---

16. Describe the clinical presentation of pyloric stenosis.

Hypertrophic pyloric stenosis, which is the most common GI surgical disease of infancy in the United States, manifests most commonly during the second to sixth weeks of life, with a peak incidence at 3 weeks of age and rare presentation after age 3 months. The major symptom is progressive nonbilious vomiting, which starts as simple regurgitation and progresses to projectile vomiting. This progressive vomiting leads to dehydration and hypochloremic metabolic alkalosis and weight loss. The condition is more common in boys. A palpable "olive" representing the thickened pylorus muscle is present in the right upper quadrant approximately 80% of the time if the infant can be examined in a calm manner with decreased stomach distention.

17. If the "olive" cannot be palpated, how can pyloric stenosis be diagnosed with radiologic studies?

The evaluation can begin with a supine or prone plain film of the abdomen, which can exclude other diagnoses that could be causing similar obstructive symptoms. The plain film would also reveal a markedly dilated stomach, soft tissue mass projecting into the gastric antrum, and paucity of gas in the distal bowel. The suspicion of pyloric stenosis can be confirmed with either US or fluoroscopy. US is the imaging test of choice because it directly visualizes the hypertrophied pylorus muscle without radiation (Fig. 60-4), whereas an upper GI series infers the presence of pyloric stenosis indirectly. With US, the pylorus muscle is seen as a hypoechoic structure greater than 4 mm thick surrounding an echogenic compressed pyloric channel. Although less sensitive, the pyloric channel length is another measurement used to make the diagnosis. A length greater than 17 mm is considered diagnostic for pyloric stenosis.

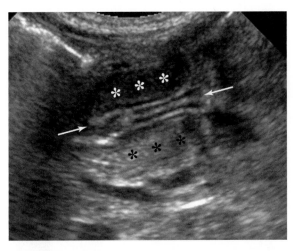

Figure 60-4. US examination of the pylorus shows hypertrophic pyloric stenosis. The thickened walls of the pylorus (*asterisks*) surround the central lumen (*arrows*).

18. **What is Meckel diverticulum?**

    Meckel diverticulum is the most common anomaly of the GI tract. It is a persistence of the omphalomesenteric duct at its junction with the ileum. It can be remembered by the rules of 2: It occurs in 2% of the population, 2% develop complications, complications usually occur before 2 years of age, and it is located within 2 feet of the ileocecal valve. The most common complication of Meckel diverticulum is painless GI bleeding, which occurs secondary to irritation or ulceration from production of hydrochloric acid by the gastric mucosa that lines it.

19. **How is Meckel diverticulum diagnosed?**

    Meckel diverticulum is detected by a nuclear medicine scan with technetium (Tc)-99m pertechnetate. The tracer accumulates within the diverticulum, usually appearing at or approximately at the same time as activity in the stomach, with gradually increasing intensity, which verifies the presence of ectopic gastric mucosa.

20. **What are the most common causes of GI bleeding in children?**

    The differential diagnosis depends on the age of the patient (Table 60-1).

21. **What causes necrotizing enterocolitis (NEC)?**

    NEC is a multifactorial condition that has traditionally been thought to be caused by hypoxia, infection, and enteral feeding. The pathology of NEC resembles that of ischemic necrosis. It may be that the main pathologic trigger in NEC is injury to the intestinal mucosa, which can be caused by different factors in different patients.

22. **Who develops NEC?**

    Approximately 80% of patients who develop NEC are premature infants. Older infants who develop NEC usually have severe underlying medical problems, such as Hirschsprung disease or congenital heart disease. Patients with this condition present with abdominal distention, vomiting, increased gastric residuals, blood in the stool, lethargy, apnea, and temperature instability.

23. **What findings of NEC can be seen on plain x-ray film, and what is the role of the radiologist?**

    The radiographic findings of NEC are nonspecific when the condition is first suspected. Films are obtained serially; the role of the radiologist is to try to diagnose the condition before bowel perforation occurs. In early NEC, the most commonly detected abnormality is diffuse gaseous distention of the intestine. A more useful sign of early NEC is loss of the normal symmetric bowel gas pattern, with a resulting disorganized or asymmetric pattern. In more advanced NEC, the finding

Table 60-1. Common Causes of Gastrointestinal Bleeding in Children

NEWBORN AND NEONATE (<1 MO)	YOUNG INFANT (1-3 MO)	OLDER INFANT (3 MO–1 YR)	CHILD (1-10 YR)
Swallowed maternal blood	Esophagitis	Esophagitis	Esophagitis
Anal fissure	Intussusception	Anal fissure	Esophageal varices
Necrotizing enterocolitis	Anal fissure	Colon polyp	Colon polyp
Hemorrhagic disease of the newborn	Gangrenous bowel	Intussusception	Anal fissure
Allergic or infectious colitis	Meckel diverticulum	Gangrenous bowel	Foreign body
		Foreign body	Crohn disease
			Ulcerative colitis

of pneumatosis intestinalis (intramural gas) is pathognomonic for the condition (Fig. 60-5). Gas in the portal venous system is another pathognomonic finding in NEC, which occurs in 10% to 30% of cases. Infants at risk for imminent perforation often have portal venous gas. They may have the persistent loop sign, which is a dilated loop of intestine that remains unchanged over 24 to 36 hours. Another grave sign is a shift from a pattern of generalized dilation to asymmetric bowel dilation. Ascites is another sign of impending perforation. When pneumoperitoneum develops, this is a definite sign that the bowel has perforated, and the infant must have surgery.

24. What are other causes of pneumoperitoneum in infants and children?

The most common causes are surgery and instrumentation. Pneumoperitoneum can be found after laparotomy, after paracentesis, or after resuscitation. Also, distal bowel obstruction from conditions such as Hirschsprung disease or meconium ileus and dissection of air from pneumomediastinum, a ruptured ulcer, or Meckel diverticulum can cause pneumoperitoneum.

25. What is Hirschsprung disease?

Hirschsprung disease is a condition of distal aganglionic bowel that results from the lack of Auerbach (intermuscular) and Meissner (submucosal) plexuses. Functional obstruction of the distal bowel results. Hirschsprung disease usually manifests in the first 48 hours of life with the failure to pass meconium, or it may manifest with abdominal distention, bilious vomiting, or diarrhea. More than 80% of patients present in the first 6 weeks of life.

26. What are the plain x-ray film findings of Hirschsprung disease?

The most typical plain film finding of Hirschsprung disease is a dilated colon proximal to the distal and smaller aganglionic segment. Radiographs may also show high-grade distal bowel obstruction. Radiologic diagnosis of Hirschsprung disease requires a contrast enema (Fig. 60-6). Spot radiographs are obtained in the lateral and oblique projections, and the examination is stopped after a transition zone has been identified. The barium enema can show the transition zone, which is situated between a narrowed aganglionic segment and the distended proximal bowel. The x-ray transition zone may be visualized more distally than the histologic transition zone secondary to stool dilating the proximal part of the aganglionic segment.

27. Is Hirschsprung disease diagnosed definitively by imaging?

To make a definitive diagnosis of Hirschsprung disease, a rectal biopsy specimen must be obtained that shows lack of ganglion cells.

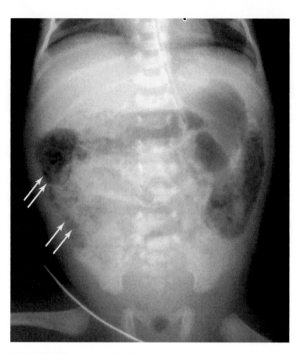

Figure 60-5. Plain film radiograph of the abdomen in a patient with NEC. The mottled pattern of air in the bowel wall (*arrows*) is typical of NEC.

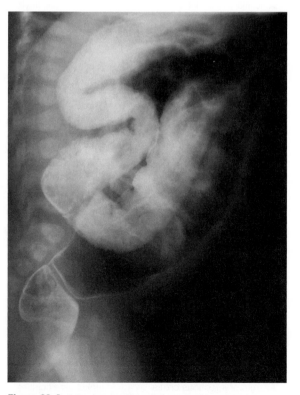

Figure 60-6. Lateral spot radiograph from a barium enema examination in a patient with Hirschsprung disease shows transition zone (from dilated to nondilated bowel) in the distal colon.

28. Name the types of tracheoesophageal fistulas (TEF). How common is each type?

- The most common type of TEF is esophageal atresia with distal esophageal communication with the tracheobronchial tree (Fig. 60-7). This accounts for more than 80% of cases.
- The next most common type is esophageal atresia without a TEF, which accounts for almost 10% of cases.
- H-type fistulas occur between an otherwise intact trachea and esophagus and account for approximately 5% of cases.
- Esophageal atresias occurring with proximal and distal communication with the trachea are found in less than 2% of cases, and esophageal atresia with proximal communication is rare.

TEF is associated with VACTERL syndromes (in which affected patients manifest at least three of the following: vertebral anomalies, anal atresia/imperforate anus, cardiac anomalies, tracheoesophageal fistula, renal anomalies, and limb anomalies).

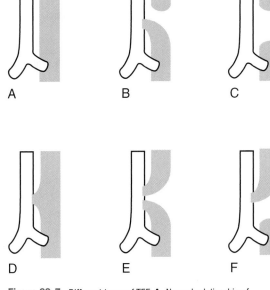

Figure 60-7. Different types of TEF. **A,** Normal relationship of esophagus anterior to trachea—no atresia or fistula. **B,** Esophageal atresia with distal TEF—most common (>80%). **C,** Esophageal atresia with no TEF (approximately 10%). **D,** H-type fistula with no esophageal atresia (approximately 5%). **E,** Esophageal atresia with proximal and distal fistulas (<2%). **F,** Esophageal atresia with a proximal fistula (1%).

29. What are the plain film findings in TEF?

In a patient with esophageal atresia (and no fistula or a proximal fistula), plain film may reveal a gasless abdomen. A nasogastric tube may be seen coiled in the proximal esophagus. Patients with esophageal atresia with a distal TEF or H-type fistula may present with a distended abdomen. Aspiration is a risk for all patients with esophageal atresia.

30. How can a plain film help to differentiate a coin in the esophagus from a coin in the trachea?

On a plain chest film, a coin in the esophagus is visualized as a round object en face (a full circle can be seen) (Fig. 60-8). A coin in the trachea lies sagittally and appears end-on in a posteroanterior film.

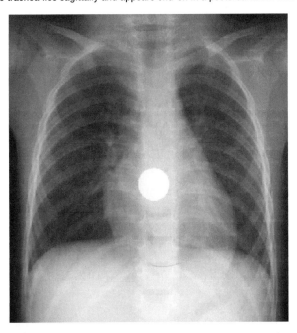

Figure 60-8. Posteroanterior plain film of the chest shows a coin in the esophagus.

BIBLIOGRAPHY

[1] C. Buonomo, The radiology of necrotizing enterocolitis, Radiol. Clin. North Am. 37 (1999) 1187–1197.
[2] A. Daneman, D. Alton, Intussusception: issues and controversies related to diagnosis and reduction, Radiol. Clin. North Am. 34 (1996) 743–755.
[3] K. Hayden, Ultrasonography of the acute pediatric abdomen, Radiol. Clin. North Am. 34 (1996) 791–806.
[4] M. Hernanz-Schulman, Imaging of neonatal gastrointestinal obstruction, Radiol. Clin. North Am. 37 (1999) 1163–1185.
[5] D.R. Kirks, Practical Pediatric Imaging: Diagnostic Imaging of Infants and Children, third ed., Lippincott-Raven, Philadelphia, 1997.
[6] W. McAlister, K. Kronemer, Emergency gastrointestinal radiology of the newborn, Radiol. Clin. North Am. 34 (1996) 819–844.
[7] D. Merten, Practical approaches to pediatric gastrointestinal radiology, Radiol. Clin. North Am. 31 (1993) 1395–1407.

PEDIATRIC URORADIOLOGY

CHAPTER 61

Richard D. Bellah, MD

1. What is the role of the radiologist in pediatric urinary tract infections (UTI)?

UTI that occur and recur in some children are the result of many interrelated factors, most of which the radiologist cannot assess. Generally, UTI results when bacterial virulence outweighs host resistance. One important factor affecting host resistance that the radiologist can assess is whether there is impairment of unidirectional flow of urine out of the urinary tract, resulting in urinary stasis and predisposing infants and children to UTI.

2. What conditions can be detected radiologically that impair normal urinary flow?

Urinary tract obstruction (congenital), vesicoureteral reflux (VUR), and dysfunctional voiding (e.g., neurogenic bladder) (Fig. 61-1) all can be detected radiologically.

3. Which imaging tests should be used to diagnose these conditions?

Renal and bladder ultrasound (US) and voiding cystourethrography (VCUG) should be used to diagnose the above-mentioned conditions.

4. Why is renal and bladder US used?

Renal and bladder US should be used to detect hydronephrosis secondary to obstruction or VUR and to assess for any renal parenchymal damage that may have been caused by prior infections.

5. When should renal and bladder US be performed?

US should be performed within several weeks after an initial UTI is diagnosed, but sooner if the child fails to respond to conventional antibiotic therapy. (Also, as a result of the routine use of prenatal US, hydronephrosis is often detected in utero, and UTI can be prevented by prophylactically administering antibiotics to the infant.)

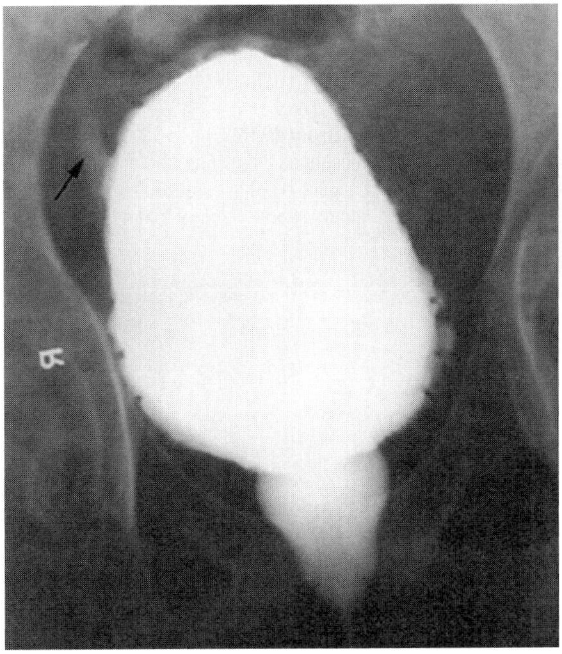

Figure 61-1. Dysfunctional voiding. Fluoroscopic spot view of the bladder and urethra at VCUG shows mild bladder wall trabeculation. A small amount of VUR is seen on the right (*arrow*). The urethra has a "spinning top" configuration.

6. How is VCUG performed?

The bladder is catheterized using sterile technique, and under fluoroscopy, the bladder is filled to capacity with iodinated contrast agent. The catheter is removed, and the child voids on the fluoroscopy table. During the procedure, the anatomy of the lower urinary tract and bladder function are examined, a series of radiographic images is obtained, and the presence or absence of reflux of contrast agent (i.e., VUR) into the ureters is determined.

7. How is VCUG modified in infants?

A cyclic study is typically performed. Infants usually void around the small catheter that is placed through the urethra into the bladder; multiple cycles of voiding and bladder filling are studied. This method also increases the probability that reflux, if present, will be elicited.

8. When should VCUG be performed?

VCUG should be performed after a first UTI in boys and girls and generally after the bladder infection is treated.

- In boys, routine fluoroscopic VCUG is recommended as the initial examination, particularly to study the urethral anatomy (e.g., to look for valves in the posterior urethra, a common cause of lower urinary tract obstruction in young boys).
- In girls, either routine VCUG can be done or a voiding urethrogram can be performed by instilling a radionuclide into the bladder. The latter procedure is performed in the nuclear medicine department; images are obtained with a gamma camera, and reflux is detected when the radionuclide (which is diluted in the sterile saline that is placed in the bladder via a catheter) reaches the ureter during the instillation of contrast agent or during voiding.

9. What are the pros and cons of a radionuclide cystogram compared with fluoroscopic VCUG?

Fluoroscopic VCUG provides anatomic detail, but at a much higher radiation dose. Radionuclide cystogram is highly sensitive for detecting reflux because the child is continuously monitored by the gamma camera, but at the expense of good anatomic detail. Radionuclide cystogram is particularly useful for follow-up studies that assess for resolution of previously detected VUR and is useful for screening siblings of patients with known reflux.

10. What is primary VUR?

VUR occurs either primarily or secondarily. Primary reflux is due to "immaturity" or abnormality of the ureterovesical junction (UVJ), which allows urine to ascend into the ureters during bladder filling or voiding. Generally, reflux is related to ureteral orifice size and the length of the ureter as it tunnels into the bladder.

11. What is secondary VUR?

Secondary reflux occurs as the result of an abnormality of the UVJ, such as a distal ureteral diverticulum or a ureterocele (an outpouching of the ureter that extends into the bladder). Secondary reflux may also occur as a result of bladder outlet obstruction or secondary to a neurogenic bladder.

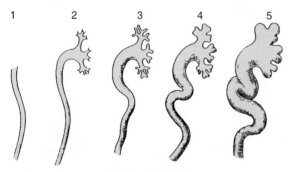

Grades of reflux

Figure 61-2. Grading of primary VUR. Reflux is graded according to the degree of ureteral and pyelocalyceal filling. The higher the grade, the less likelihood of spontaneous resolution.

12. How is primary reflux graded?

Primary reflux is graded on a scale of 1 to 5, based on the degree of ureteral and pyelocalyceal (renal collecting system) filling and dilation (Fig. 61-2). In addition to providing the referring physician with a visual description of the degree of reflux, assigning a grade also gives the clinician an idea of the likelihood of spontaneous resolution (e.g., 80% of cases of grade 2 reflux resolve within 3 years).

13. What is dysfunctional voiding?

Dysfunctional voiding may be due to a neurogenic bladder or the so-called pediatric unstable bladder. The bladder may show variable degrees of thickening, trabeculation, and alteration in contour and storage capacity (see Fig. 61-1). Bladder-sphincter dyssynergia may be indicated by the presence of a dilated posterior urethra caused by the external sphincter failing to relax as the bladder neck opens. This condition often leads to high-pressure voiding, incomplete emptying, and urine retention.

14. What diagnostic tests are useful for the detection of acute and chronic pyelonephritis in children?

Renal cortical scintigraphy (nuclear scan), contrast-enhanced computed tomography (CT), and renal US are used to detect acute and chronic pyelonephritis in children. Pyelonephritis may be difficult to diagnose accurately, especially in infants and young children who cannot give a history. It may be difficult to distinguish between uncomplicated UTI and pyelonephritis (with or without subsequent complications such as renal abscess) on the basis of physical examination, history, and laboratory studies. Imaging plays an important role in the work-up of children with known or suspected UTI.

15. What are the findings on a renal nuclear scan in acute and chronic infection?

A renal cortical nuclear scan reveals parenchymal defects in children with acute infection secondary to focal areas of edema and inflammation. These defects revert to normal if the process completely resolves. In chronic infection or chronic pyelonephritis secondary to reflux nephropathy, residual areas of scar appear as persistent cortical defects on follow-up examinations.

16. What are the CT findings associated with pyelonephritis?

Contrast-enhanced CT scan is less sensitive than a renal cortical nuclear scan for the detection of acute infection. Acute infection is seen as wedge-shaped areas of decreased density in the kidney. Areas of scar related to prior infection can also be identified. CT is particularly helpful when abscess formation is suspected.

17. How useful is renal US in the work-up of suspected pyelonephritis?

Gray-scale US is limited in its ability to depict acute pyelonephritis. The sensitivity of US is increased, however, when power Doppler US is used (Fig. 61-3). The latter technique is an advance in Doppler US that depicts normal and abnormal blood flow in a manner that is independent of the direction of the flow; power Doppler is more sensitive than routine color Doppler. Renal US may also be used to assess for significant renal scarring secondary to chronic pyelonephritis. Small focal scars may be difficult to detect with US.

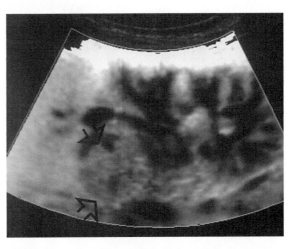

Figure 61-3. Acute pyelonephritis. Power Doppler US shows focal area of decreased perfusion within the upper pole of the kidney (*arrows*). This finding corresponds to an area of pyelonephritis.

18. List the most common forms of congenital hydronephrosis.

- Ureteropelvic junction (UPJ) obstruction
- UVJ obstruction, commonly referred to as *primary obstructive megaureter*
- VUR
- Renal and ureteral duplication anomalies
- Posterior urethral valves
- Prune-belly syndrome

19. When should a postnatal renal and bladder US examination be obtained in a patient with congenital hydronephrosis?

A postnatal renal and bladder US examination should be performed on any infant with dilation of the renal pelvis that is detected prenatally on US, if the renal pelvis measures 4 mm or greater before 33 weeks of gestation and 7 mm or greater after 33 weeks of gestation. A renal pelvic diameter less than 4 mm seen on US at birth has been shown to normalize spontaneously within 1 year. In boys with bilateral hydroureteronephrosis, US should be obtained soon after birth to assess for posterior urethral valves. Otherwise, the initial US examination should be done at 5 to 7 days after birth (when the glomerular filtration rate is greater than it is immediately after birth).

20. What are the roles of nuclear medicine, VCUG, intravenous urography, and magnetic resonance imaging (MRI) in congenital hydronephrosis?

VCUG should be performed to assess for reflux and to determine whether posterior urethral valves are present (in boys). Use of nuclear renal scintigraphy and intravenous urography varies from patient to patient and from institution to institution. Renal scintigraphy provides quantitative information regarding the effect of obstruction on renal function; the function of the obstructed kidney can be compared with the opposite kidney before and after surgical treatment. IV urography provides less quantitative information, but provides better anatomic detail. It serves best as a road map for the surgeon and gives information about anatomy and function after surgery. More recent studies have shown that functional MRI with gadolinium is a promising technique, not only because it provides the advantage of exquisite anatomic detail, but also, similar to renal scintigraphy, it can provide information of differential perfusion and function.

21. What are posterior urethral valves?

At the distal end of the verumontanum, several folds, or plicae, arise and pass caudally to encircle a portion of the membranous urethra. These plicae occur normally and vary in the extent to which they encircle the urethra. When they fuse anteriorly, they form the most common type of posterior urethral valves (type 1) (Fig. 61-4). Type 2 posterior urethral valves are mucosal folds that extend from the proximal end of the verumontanum toward the bladder neck; their very existence is controversial. Type 3 valves refer to a urethral diaphragm that occurs below the caudal end of the verumontanum.

22. How are posterior urethral valves detected?

Posterior urethral valves, which are the most common cause of bladder outlet obstruction in infant boys, cause changes in the bladder that are detected by US and cystography. These changes include enlargement, thickening, sacculation, and trabeculation of the bladder. Dilation of the posterior (prostatic) urethra above the valve can be seen on prenatal and postnatal US scans and with VCUG. Hydroureteronephrosis is often present, owing to either reflux or high pressures

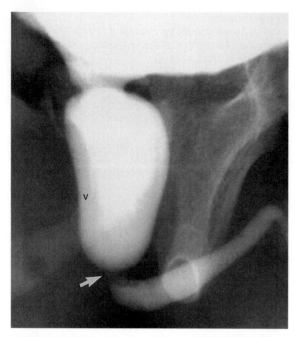

Figure 61-4. Posterior urethral valves. Fluoroscopic spot view shows dilated posterior urethra. Valves (*arrow*) are identified at the distal end of the verumontanum (*v*).

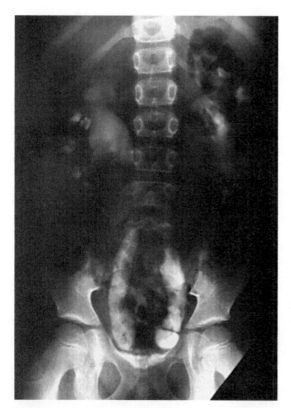

Figure 61-5. Primary obstructive megaureter. Intravenous urogram shows mild bilateral pyelocaliectasis. Moderate ureterectasis is most significant in the distal one half of the ureters.

in the bladder. If rupture of a calyceal fornix occurs, urinary ascites or a urinoma or both can develop. Posterior urethral valves are confirmed cystoscopically and are treated with fulguration or incision.

23. What is primary megaureter?

Primary megaureter results from an abnormal proportion of muscle fibers and fibrous tissue in the distal-most 3 to 4 cm of the ureter. When primary megaureter is obstructive, the degree of obstruction is variable and seems to improve in many cases over time. Most often, this condition is detected incidentally on prenatal US. Postnatal US and urography reveal a variable degree of dilation of the ureter and collecting system on the affected side (Fig. 61-5). Occasionally, a short, narrow segment of ureter may be seen through US at the UVJ. VCUG typically shows absence of reflux, although reflux may be present in 10% of cases.

24. What are common forms of a duplex kidney?

A *duplex kidney* (duplication of the kidney, collecting system, and ureters) arises from abnormal development of the ureteric bud. Although various degrees of duplication may be present, in the full-blown condition, the kidney is large, and there are separate collecting systems and ureters that drain the upper and lower poles of the kidney.

25. What is the Weigert-Meyer rule?

According to the Weigert-Meyer rule, when there is a complete duplication of the kidney, the lower pole ureter inserts normally into the bladder. The upper pole ureter inserts ectopically into the bladder, in a location that is medial and caudal to the insertion of the lower pole ureter.

26. Are the collecting systems and ureters dilated in a duplicated system?

The appearance depends on whether there is reflux into the lower pole ureter and the exact site of the ectopically inserting upper pole ureter. In the typical situation, which is often bilateral, the distal ureters are contained within a common sheath and either come together or insert separately, but are close together in the trigone of the bladder. If the upper pole ureter is associated with a ureterocele (a localized dilation of the distal ureter), the ureterocele can protrude through the bladder to the urethra and manifest as a perineal mass. If a ureterocele is present, the upper pole of the kidney may be obstructed (the "drooping lily" effect on the lower pole collecting system) or may be small and dysplastic, causing little or no effect on the lower pole. If a ureterocele is not present, the upper pole moiety may insert in an ectopic location and have a stenotic insertion, causing obstruction (boys and girls), or may manifest with urinary dribbling (girls only) owing to an ectopic insertion into the urethra, vagina, or perineum.

27. What is the most common cause of a scrotal mass?
The most common cause of a scrotal mass is probably a hydrocele, which is a collection of fluid outside the testicle, between layers of the tunica vaginalis. It may be congenital or may be associated with trauma, torsion, or hemorrhage.

28. What are the main differential considerations of a painful scrotum?
The main differential considerations of a painful scrotum are testicular torsion and epididymitis or orchitis. Testicular torsion is a surgical emergency and can be confirmed or excluded with color Doppler US or nuclear scan (using technetium [Tc]-99m pertechnetate as the radiopharmaceutical agent). Epididymitis is much more common in postpubescent boys than in younger boys and is identified on US by swelling of and increased flow in the epididymis. The cause of epididymitis is often bacterial, and there may be associated infection in the testicle.

Key Points: Pediatric Uroradiology

1. Congenital urinary tract obstruction, VUR, and dysfunctional voiding can be diagnosed with renal and bladder US and VCUG.
2. Primary VUR is graded on a scale of 1 to 5, depending on the degree of ureteral and pyelocalyceal filling and dilation.
3. Renal cortical scintigraphy, contrast-enhanced CT, and renal US may be used to diagnose pyelonephritis in children.
4. US and cystography can detect bladder outlet obstruction owing to posterior urethral valves, which are the most common cause of bladder outlet obstruction in boys.
5. The main differential considerations of a painful scrotum are testicular torsion and epididymitis or orchitis.
6. Testicular torsion is a surgical emergency and can be confirmed or excluded with color Doppler US or a nuclear scan with Tc-99m pertechnetate.

---

29. If epididymitis is present in an infant, what should be suspected as the etiologic factor?
Epididymitis is rare in infants and is usually associated with an anatomic abnormality of the genitourinary system, such as a dysplastic kidney with an ectopic ureter. Renal and bladder US and VCUG are indicated.

30. What is the most common testicular tumor in children?
Yolk sac tumor is the most common testicular tumor in children. Yolk sac tumors occur more commonly than teratomas and are seen primarily during the first 2 years of life. Most children with yolk sac tumors have elevated α-fetoprotein levels, whereas children with teratomas do not have elevated levels.

31. What are the most common testicular tumors in adolescents?
Germ cell tumors (Fig. 61-6) are the most common testicular tumors in adolescents, but the most common histologic types are seminomas, choriocarcinomas, teratocarcinomas, and tumors with mixed histologies.

32. What urinary problems occur in children with spina bifida?
There is an increased incidence of renal anomalies in children with myelomeningocele, including fusion anomalies (e.g., horseshoe kidney), renal dysplasia, and agenesis. The most significant problems relate to the abnormal innervation of the bladder.

33. Name the specific problems in spina bifida that are related to neurogenic bladder.
The neurogenic bladder fails to store urine correctly, which may cause leaking; does not empty properly because of bladder-sphincter dyssynergia; and experiences uninhibited contractions, which may also cause leaking (Fig. 61-7). High storage pressures can result in reflux and hydronephrosis.

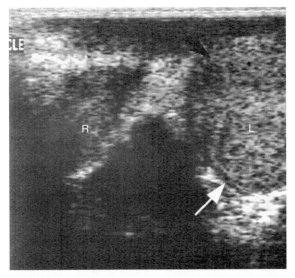

Figure 61-6. Testicular germ cell tumor. Transverse US of the scrotum in an infant shows normal right (*R*) testis and massive enlargement of the left (*L*) testis (*arrows*).

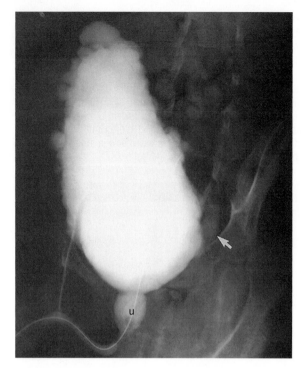

Figure 61-7. Neurogenic bladder. VCUG in a patient with meningomyelocele shows a "pine-cone" bladder with marked trabeculation and sacculation. When the patient attempts to void, there is dilation of the posterior urethra (*u*) with contraction of the external sphincter. A small amount of reflux is seen in the distal left ureter (*arrow*).

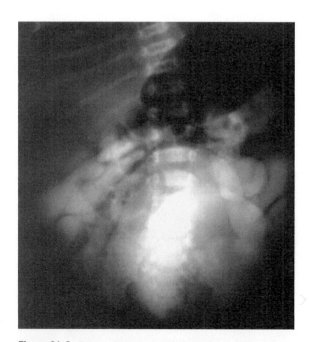

Figure 61-8. Prune-belly syndrome. VCUG shows megacystis and bilateral pyelocaliectasis and ureterectasis with significant ureteral tortuosity.

34. Discuss the goals of therapy for urinary tract dysfunction in a patient with spina bifida.

The goals are to decrease storage pressure, with frequent intermittent catheterization, vesicostomy, or bladder augmentation, and to keep the patient "dry" through continent diversion. Cystography is performed to assess bladder size, storage capacity, and the volume at which leakage occurs, and to detect any reflux. Renal and bladder US is routinely performed every 6 months to assess for hydronephrosis, stones, and the ability of the patient to empty the bladder with self-catheterization.

35. What is the triad of prune-belly syndrome?

The triad of prune-belly syndrome is absent or deficient abdominal musculature, cryptorchidism, and urinary tract abnormalities (Fig. 61-8).

36. What urinary tract abnormalities are associated with prune-belly syndrome?

They are diverse and include marked hydroureteronephrosis and marked bladder and urethral dilation, reflux, renal dysplasia, prostatic hypoplasia, urachal abnormalities, and microphallus. The clinical features often parallel the degree of urinary tract involvement. Newborns with severe renal dysplasia may have Potter syndrome (oligohydramnios, pulmonary hypoplasia). Children with urinary tract dilation or reflux or both need to be closely monitored for infection.

37. What is a basic classification for cystic kidney diseases affecting infants, children, and adolescents?

Cystic renal diseases can be classified as genetic or nongenetic. The most common cause of nongenetic cystic disease is multicystic dysplastic kidney (MCDK).

38. What is the most common US appearance of MCDK?

Most commonly, MCDK is the result of atresia of the renal pelvis, and the kidney appears on US as multiple cysts of varying sizes that do not communicate with each other; there is no definable renal pelvis. The less common form is the hydronephrotic form, which has a central renal cyst. MCDK is associated with other abnormalities of the urinary tract, especially a contralateral UPJ obstruction and contralateral VUR.

39. List the other forms of nongenetic cystic renal disease.

- Simple renal cyst (rare in children)
- Medullary cystic disease
- Calyceal diverticulum
- Cystic renal dysplasia (associated with urinary tract obstruction)

40. Name the genetic forms of cystic renal disease.
- Autosomal dominant polycystic kidney disease (ADPCKD)
- Autosomal recessive polycystic kidney disease (ARPCKD)
- Glomerulocystic kidney disease
- Congenital nephrosis
- Cystic kidney disease associated with syndromes (e.g., tuberous sclerosis)

41. Does "adult-type" ADPCKD occur in infants and young children?
ADPCKD has been recognized on US prenatally and postnatally. The appearance can closely mimic ARPCKD, in which both kidneys can appear large and echogenic. Small, sonographically resolvable cysts can be seen in either syndrome in the newborn period. More commonly, ADPCKD is suspected if US reveals progressive development of multiple cortical and medullary renal cysts; this may be found incidentally or in a child referred for hypertension and hematuria. Careful examination of the family history and US screening of the family are recommended to detect any evidence of cystic kidney disease in parents who may be unaware of their own subclinical disease.

42. What imaging findings may help distinguish ADPCKD from ARPCKD in an infant or young child (Fig. 61-9)?
The renal US appearance of ADPCKD and ARPCKD can be quite similar. The kidneys are often large and echogenic with each syndrome. Careful inspection with US can occasionally detect tubular ectasia in echogenic renal pyramids, which is typical of ARPCKD. Sonographically resolvable cysts are more suggestive of autosomal dominant disease. Additionally, the liver should be examined for abnormal echotexture caused by hepatic fibrosis and biliary ectasia, which is often associated with autosomal recessive disease. In adolescents with ARPCKD, the renal involvement is less marked than the liver disease, which causes portal hypertension and splenomegaly. Excretory urography (or CT) can occasionally be helpful to distinguish the recessive from the dominant disease. In ARPCKD, there is delay and prolongation of the nephrogram; the contrast agent is taken up by dilated tubules and has a spoked-wheel appearance. These findings are typically absent in ADPCKD, in which excretion is prompt.

43. Name five hereditary syndromes associated with renal cysts.
- Tuberous sclerosis
- von Hippel-Lindau disease
- Zellweger (cerebrohepatorenal) syndrome
- Jeune syndrome (thoracic asphyxiating dystrophy)
- Meckel-Gruber syndrome

44. What conditions cause echogenic renal pyramids in infants?
- Nephrocalcinosis (owing to renal tubular acidosis, hypercalcemia, or furosemide therapy)
- Renal tubular ectasia (ARPCKD)
- Tamm-Horsfall protein deposition (transient phenomenon)

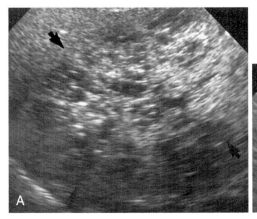
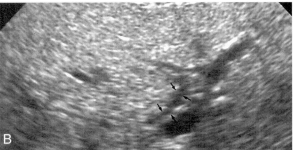

Figure 61-9. Autosomal recessive polycystic kidney disease. **A,** Sagittal US of right kidney (*arrows*) shows marked enlargement with heterogeneous echogenicity. Small (1 mm) cystic elements are seen within renal parenchyma. **B,** Transverse US of liver. Parenchyma shows increased liver echotexture owing to hepatic fibrosis. Minimal ectasia of intrahepatic biliary tree (*arrows*) can be seen adjacent to left portal vein.

45. What is the most common solid renal mass in infants?

The most common solid renal mass in infants is fetal renal hamartoma, also known as *mesoblastic nephroma*. Infants usually present with a palpable renal mass. Hematuria, hypertension, and hypercalcemia may also be present. The tumor is composed of monotonous sheets of spindle-shaped cells and usually occupies most of the kidney. The tumor appears large and solid on US. The mass is usually resected, and the prognosis is excellent. Less common causes of solitary renal masses in infants include nephroblastomatosis and malignant rhabdoid tumor.

46. What is the role of imaging in infants with ambiguous genitalia?

Evaluation is indicated when the testes cannot be palpated and when there is severe hypospadias, incomplete scrotal fusion, fused labia, a micropenis, or clitoral enlargement. These conditions can be classified as true hermaphroditism, female pseudohermaphroditism, male pseudohermaphroditism, and gonadal dysgenesis, depending on further clinical, laboratory, and surgical investigations. US is the simplest method of identifying the internal anatomy by detecting the presence or absence of a uterus and gonads. US is usually combined with a retrograde genitogram performed under fluoroscopy that defines further the relationship of the urogenital sinus to the urethra and vagina (Fig. 61-10).

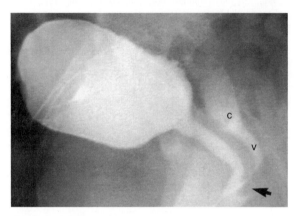

Figure 61-10. Urogenital sinus in ambiguous genitalia. Retrograde genitogram shows low confluence (*arrow*) of the urethra and the vagina (*v*) and cervical impression (*c*).

47. What is nephroblastomatosis?

Nephroblastomatosis refers to multiple or diffuse rests of nephrogenic tissue. They are persistent embryonal remnants in the kidney that are apparent precursors to Wilms tumor. The involved kidneys are typically enlarged and have a lobulated configuration. US, CT, and MRI can be used to identify and monitor nephroblastomatosis (Fig. 61-11). The following are several conditions in which children may have nephroblastomatosis and can develop Wilms tumor: hemihypertrophy, Drash syndrome (pseudohermaphroditism), aniridia, and a positive family history of Wilms tumor or nephroblastomatosis.

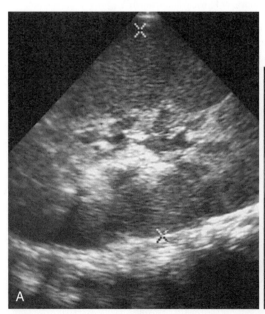 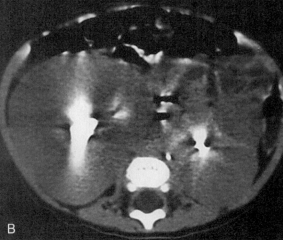

Figure 61-11. Nephroblastomatosis. **A,** US of right kidney shows significant renal enlargement with loss of normal corticomedullary differentiation (left kidney has a smaller appearance). **B,** CT (enhanced) shows loss of normal intrarenal architecture with diffuse infiltration of both kidneys by intralobar nephroblastomatosis.

48. What are the two major types of nephroblastomatosis?

Perilobar and intralobar are the two major types of nephroblastomatosis. The perilobar form is limited to the periphery of the kidney, whereas the intralobar form can be found anywhere within a renal lobe and within the renal pelvis and collecting system. Nephroblastomatosis may remain dormant, mature, involute, develop hyperplastic overgrowth, or become neoplastic (Wilms tumor).

49. How can nephroblastomatosis be distinguished from Wilms tumor?

Generally, Wilms tumor is suspected when a lesion noted by either US or CT is greater than 3 cm and has a spherical configuration. Many lesions previously thought to be small or medium-sized Wilms tumors, especially in cases of bilateral or multicentric tumor, may represent hyperplastic nephroblastomatosis. Biopsy is of limited value in distinguishing the hyperplastic form from Wilms tumor, and serial imaging is crucial in determining whether surgery should be performed.

50. What is Mayer-Rokitansky-Küster-Hauser syndrome?

Mayer-Rokitansky-Küster-Hauser syndrome refers to vaginal atresia with other variable müllerian duct abnormalities such as a bicornuate or septated uterus. The fallopian tubes, ovaries, and broad ligaments are normal. Unilateral renal and skeletal anomalies are associated in 50% and 12% of cases.

51. How is pelvic US used in the evaluation of a child with precocious puberty?

Uterine and ovarian volumes are larger than normal in true isosexual precocious puberty, whereas enlargement of only the ovary has been reported with pseudosexual precocity. True isosexual precocity is due to the premature activation of the hypothalamic pituitary gonadal axis, whereas pseudosexual precocity refers to pubertal changes occurring independent of these actions, as in the case of a functional ovarian cyst or tumor. Multiple, small (<1 cm) cysts can be seen in the ovaries of normal children and in children who have precocious puberty. The best predictor of true precocious puberty is bilateral ovarian enlargement, but unilateral ovarian enlargement associated with larger cysts is more related to pseudosexual precocity.

BIBLIOGRAPHY

[1] J.B. Beckwith, Precursor lesions of Wilms' tumor: clinical and biological implications, Med. Pediatr. Oncol. 21 (1993) 158–168.

[2] E. Bjorgvinsson, M. Majd, K.D. Eggli, Diagnosis of acute pyelonephritis in children: comparison of sonography and Tc99m-DMSA scintigraphy, AJR. Am. J. Roentgenol. 157 (1991) 539–543.

[3] J.G. Blickman, R.L. Lebowitz, The coexistence of primary megaureter and reflux, AJR. Am. J. Roentgenol. 143 (1984) 1053–1057.

[4] J.E. Corteville, D.L. Gray, J.P. Crane, Congenital hydronephrosis: correlations of fetal ultrasonographic findings with infant outcome, Am. J. Obstet. Gynecol. 165 (1991) 384.

[5] B.J. Cremin, A review of ultrasonic appearances of posterior urethral valves and ureteroceles, Pediatr. Radiol. 16 (1986) 357–364.

[6] R. Fotter, W. Kopp, E. Skein, et al., Unstable bladder in children: functional evaluation by modified voiding cystography, Radiology 161 (1986) 811–813.

[7] F.J. Greskovich III, L.M. Nyberg Jr., The prune belly syndrome: a review of its etiology, defects, treatment and prognosis, J. Urol. 140 (1988) 707–712.

[8] M. Jain, G.W. LeQuesne, A.J. Bourne, P. Henning, High-resolution ultrasonography in the differential diagnosis of cystic diseases of the kidney in infancy and childhood: preliminary experience, J. Ultrasound Med. 16 (1997) 235–240.

[9] B.S. Kaplan, P. Kaplan, H.K. Rosenberg, et al., Polycystic kidney diseases in childhood, J. Pediatr. 115 (1989) 867–879.

[10] L.R. King, M.J. Siegel, A.L. Solomon, Usefulness of ovarian volume and cysts in female isosexual precocious puberty, J. Ultrasound Med. 12 (1993) 577–581.

[11] R.L. Lebowitz, J. Mandell, Urinary tract infection in children: putting radiology in its place, Radiology 165 (1987) 1–9.

[12] I.N. Nunn, F.D. Stephens, The triad syndrome: a composite anomaly of the abdominal wall, urinary system, and testes, J. Urol. 86 (1961) 782–794.

[13] H.K. Rosenberg, N.H. Sherman, W.F. Tarry, et al., Mayer-Rokitansky-Kuster-Hauser syndrome: US aid and diagnosis, Radiology 161 (1986) 815–819.

[14] H.M. Saxton, M. Borzyskowski, A.R. Mundy, G.C. Vivian, Spinning top urethra: not a normal variant, Radiology 168 (1988) 147–150.

[15] R.S. Sutherland, R.A. Mevorach, L.S. Baskin, B.A. Kogan, Spinal dysraphism in children: an overview and an approach to prevent complications, Urology 46 (1995) 294–304.

CHAPTER 62

PEDIATRIC NEURORADIOLOGY

D. Andrew Mong, MD, and
Avrum N. Pollock, MD

1. **How does myelinated brain differ from nonmyelinated brain on an infant magnetic resonance imaging (MRI) examination? Where do you expect to see myelinization occur first?**

   Myelinated brain white matter, as in adults, appears hyperintense relative to gray matter on T1-weighted MR images and hypointense on T2-weighted images. In nonmyelinated brain, this pattern is reversed. Myelinization of the infant brain occurs in a predictable pattern, beginning in the brainstem and cerebellum and progressing to the posterior limb of the internal capsule, optic pathways, and parietal lobes. This pattern of change occurs from caudal to cephalad, dorsal to ventral, and central to peripheral. Myelinization should appear complete on MRI by 24 months, but may be incomplete in the terminal zones up to approximately 4 to 5 years of age and in rare cases not until the first decade.

2. **What are migrational anomalies of the central nervous system (CNS)?**

   Normal neuronal migration occurs during fetal brain development as neurons migrate from the germinal matrix to the cortex along radial glial fibers. Partial or total arrest of this process leads to a migrational anomaly. These anomalies include the following:

   - Subependymal heterotopias (abnormal gray matter lining the ventricles)
   - Band heterotopias (an extra band of gray matter exists partially or completely underneath a normal-appearing cortex and a strip of white matter)
   - Schizencephaly (a cleft lined by gray matter extending from the outer cortex to the ventricles)
   - Polymicrogyria (too many gyri)
   - Pachygyria (abnormally thickened gyri)
   - Lissencephaly (complete absence of gyri).

   Children typically present with developmental delay or seizures (Fig. 62-1).

3. **Name the three kinds of holoprosencephaly.**

   Holoprosencephaly refers to incomplete differentiation of the fetal prosencephalon (forebrain) into separate ventricles. Holoprosencephaly may manifest as *alobar,* resulting in one ventricle and fusion of the thalami; *semilobar,* two hemispheres posteriorly but not anteriorly; or *lobar,* the mildest form, which may manifest with only mild midline abnormalities, such as absence of the septum pellucidum and subtle incomplete visualization of the interhemispheric fissure associated with an azygous anterior cerebral artery. The mildest form along the continuum is thought to include septo-optic dysplasia.

4. **What is the differential diagnosis for what appears to be massively dilated ventricles on a prenatal ultrasound (US) examination?**

   The appearance of massively dilated ventricles may be secondary to holoprosencephaly, hydranencephaly, or hydrocephalus. Hydranencephaly results from massive necrosis of the cerebral hemispheres and may be

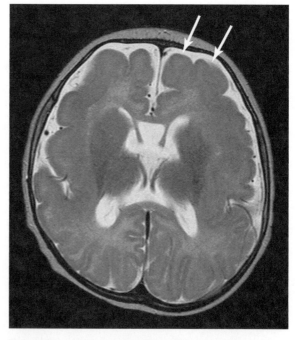

Figure 62-1. Axial T2-weighted MR image through the level of the basal ganglia shows abnormally thickened and enlarged large gyri (*arrows*) of the frontal cortex, which is consistent with pachygyria.

secondary to vascular disease with bilateral internal carotid occlusion, infection, or trauma with severe hydrocephalus. There is usually a thin residual remnant of cerebral cortex applied to the inner table of the calvaria. The most common causes of prenatal hydrocephalus include Arnold-Chiari malformation II, intracranial hemorrhage, aqueductal stenosis, and Dandy-Walker malformation.

5. Describe the classification of germinal matrix hemorrhage.

The germinal matrix lies in the caudothalamic groove. This is a highly vascular region of the prenatal and premature brain and is prone to hemorrhage, with rupture of the thin venules subsequent to decreased perfusion or oxygenation. Morbidity and mortality can be predicted based on the grade of the hemorrhage:

- Grade I hemorrhage is confined to the germinal matrix.
- Grade II hemorrhage extends into the lateral ventricle.
- Grade III hemorrhage expands into and dilates the lateral ventricle.
- Grade IV hemorrhage extends into the adjacent parenchyma.

US of the premature infant's head through the anterior fontanelle is the modality of choice for diagnosis and follow-up of germinal matrix hemorrhage.

> **Key Points: Grading of Germinal Matrix Hemorrhage in Neonates**
> 1. *Grade I:* Confined to the caudothalamic groove
> 2. *Grade II:* Extension into the lateral ventricle
> 3. *Grade III:* Extension into and dilation of the lateral ventricle
> 4. *Grade IV:* Extension into the adjacent parenchyma

6. How does the premature brain respond to ischemic injury?

Periventricular leukomalacia is characterized by ischemia in an endarterial distribution—in the watershed regions of white matter that surround the ventricles. US examination may show increase in periventricular echogenicity soon after the initial insult. Cystic change in these regions can be seen later in the subacute stage, as the white matter begins to be resorbed. MRI shows abnormal periventricular signal intensity and volume loss. Before 28 weeks of gestation, the developing brain does not display a leukomalacic response, and only volume loss results. This volume loss may take the form of dilated ventricles and expanded extra-axial spaces or even porencephalic cysts (expanded cystlike dilations from the ventricles, which may reach the cortex). A porencephalic cyst can be differentiated from schizencephaly by noting that, in the former entity, there is no gray matter lining the cyst.

7. Describe the three main types of Chiari malformation.

- *Chiari I malformation* involves herniation of the cerebellar tonsils into the foramen magnum (>5 mm in patients <15 years old) (Fig. 62-2).
- *Chiari II malformation* is more severe, involving herniation of the medulla and vermis and elongation and downward displacement of the brainstem. Chiari II is virtually always associated with a meningomyelocele. Prenatal US may show crowding of the posterior fossa ("banana" sign appearance of the cerebellar hemispheres as they wrap around the brainstem). Lacunar skull (lückenschädel) may also be shown in Chiari II, but is thought to be due to a bony dysplasia, rather than the copper-beaten appearance associated with increase in intracranial pressure. Lacunar skull appears on plain film as multiple focal areas of thinning in the skull, which resolves with age.
- *Chiari III malformation* involves herniation of contents of the posterior fossa through the occiput or upper cervical canal via a bony defect (i.e., akin to an encephalocele).

8. How does the corpus callosum develop, and why is this important?

The corpus callosum develops front to back except for the rostrum (anterior genu, body, splenium, and rostrum last). This is important because an in utero insult may result in destruction of part of the corpus callosum. If posterior portions of the corpus callosum are present and anterior portions are not, this means that they were present at one point and were destroyed. If posterior portions are absent instead, this may mean that they did not develop.

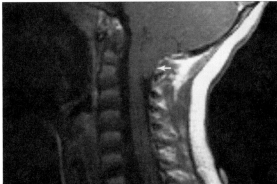

Figure 62-2. Sagittal T1-weighted MR image through the craniocervical junction shows inferior displacement of the cerebellar tonsils (*arrow*) below the level of the foramen magnum.

9. What entity does not follow the normal rule of corpus callosum development?

Holoprosencephaly, previously described, may follow an atypical pattern of corpus callosum development, in which the posterior portions develop and the anterior portions do not. This is termed *atypical callosal dysgenesis.*

10. What are TORCH infections?

The *TORCH* acronym stands for infections caused by *t*oxoplasmosis, *o*ther (varicella), *r*ubella, *c*ytomegalovirus (CMV), and *h*erpes/human immunodeficiency virus (HIV).

11. How do TORCH infections appear radiographically?

It is often impossible to distinguish TORCH infections radiographically. Intracranial calcification patterns may aid in differentiating them. CMV calcifications are classically present only in the periventricular (circumventricular) regions, whereas toxoplasmosis and rubella also have basal ganglia and cortical calcifications. CMV may also be associated with migrational abnormalities previously discussed. HIV infection may manifest as atrophy with bilateral basal ganglia calcifications. Cerebral atrophy may be present in any infection.

12. Discuss the CNS manifestations of neurofibromatosis type 1 (NF1).

Patients with NF1 may have plexiform neurofibromas, which are present along a nerve distribution and insinuate within the fascial planes of the head and neck. Sphenoid wing dysplasia, with its resultant harlequin eye appearance, is also a common finding. Nonspecific areas of high T2 signal may be present (NF spots) in the basal ganglia, brainstem, and cerebellum, and are referred to as *spongiform dysplasia.* Gliomas may develop anywhere along the optic pathway.

In the spine, patients with NF1 may develop lateral meningoceles, which herniate from the thecal sac into the thorax. Plain films of the spine may also show posterior vertebral body scalloping (from dural ectasia) or enlargement of the neural foramina (from neurofibromas) and inferior rib notching/remodeling secondary to the growth of the neurofibromas along the course of the intercostal nerves.

> **Key Points: Central Nervous System Manifestations of Neurofibromatosis Type 1**
>
> 1. Plexiform neurofibromas
> 2. Optic pathway gliomas
> 3. NF spots in the basal ganglia
> 4. Sphenoid wing dysplasia
> 5. Lateral meningoceles
> 6. Dural ectasia and posterior vertebral scalloping
> 7. Enlargement of the neural foramina from neurofibromas

13. How is neurofibromatosis type 2 (NF2) different from NF1?

The gene for NF2 is on chromosome 22, as opposed to chromosome 17 for NF1. NF2 tumors can be remembered with the mnemonic *MISME,* which stands for *m*ultiple *i*nherited *s*chwannomas, *m*eningiomas, and *e*pendymomas. Classically, these appear as bilateral cerebellopontine angle tumors, representing bilateral acoustic schwannomas (but may involve any of the cranial nerves), which is diagnostic of NF2.

14. What is tuberous sclerosis?

Tuberous sclerosis is an autosomal dominant disorder with variable expressivity, which manifests as hamartomatous lesions in multiple organ systems. Tuberous sclerosis consists of the clinical triad of seizures, adenoma sebaceum, and mental retardation. In the CNS, subependymal nodules and subcortical tubers occur. The tubers have a typical appearance of wispy high signal on T2-weighted images in the subcortical white matter. Giant cell astrocytomas may occur at the foramen of Monro and cause an obstructive hydrocephalus. Involvement outside of the CNS includes angiomyolipomas (fat-containing masses) in the kidneys, rhabdomyomas of the heart, cystic lung disease, and bony involvement (Fig. 62-3).

15. Describe the manifestations of Sturge-Weber syndrome.

Sturge-Weber syndrome, also known as *encephalotrigeminal angiomatosis,* includes venous angiomatous malformations within the leptomeninges and choroid plexus with an associated port-wine stain in the distribution of a branch of the trigeminal nerve on the side of the hemispheric involvement. On cross-sectional imaging, there is a focal region of leptomeningeal enhancement, often overlying a region of cortical atrophy. There is usually also abnormal enhancement in the enlarged ipsilateral choroid plexus. Computed tomography (CT) examination also detects "tram-track" subcortical calcifications and ipsilateral hemispheric volume loss, which is not seen in early infancy because they take some time to occur.

16. What are the most common brain tumors in infants?

Although pediatric tumors generally are more likely to occur in the posterior fossa, in infants 2 years old or younger, the most common individual tumors are supratentorial. These include teratoma, astrocytomas (e.g., glioblastoma multiforme), choroid plexus papilloma and carcinomas (in the lateral ventricles), and primitive neuroectodermal tumors.

17. Name the major posterior fossa tumors in children.

Most pediatric brain tumors are infratentorial. These include pilocytic astrocytoma, fibrillary astrocytoma, medulloblastoma, and ependymomas.

18. Describe the typical tumors that occur in the suprasellar region of a child.

Craniopharyngiomas are cystic lesions that often contain calcium (Fig. 62-4). These may be confused with Rathke cleft cysts, which are remnants of Rathke pouch, the structure that forms the anterior portion of the pituitary gland. Other tumors include tumors of hypothalamic origin (gliomas or hamartomas), optic nerve tumors (e.g., tumors seen in NF1), germinomas arising from the pituitary stalk, and pituitary adenomas. Langerhans cell histiocytosis (eosinophilic granuloma) can manifest as thickening of the infundibulum and loss of visualization of the normal posterior pituitary bright spot and is associated with a clinical history of growth delay.

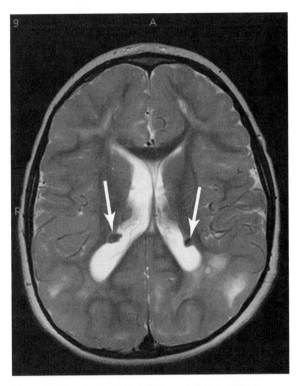

Figure 62-3. Axial T2-weighted MR image through the brain shows dark subependymal nodules (*arrows*) lining the lateral ventricles and wispy high signal in scattered subcortical areas, representing hamartomas.

19. Why is thickening of the pituitary stalk an important finding?

The pituitary stalk is considered thickened if it is greater than 2 mm at the insertion of the gland. Close interval follow-up is warranted because this thickening may be a manifestation of a germinoma or Langerhans cell histiocytosis. Alternatively, the thickening may be idiopathic.

20. What is the differential diagnosis for a pediatric cystic neck mass?

This is a broad differential that may be narrowed by location. Type II branchial cleft cysts (the most common) are suprahyoid lesions that classically push the sternocleidomastoid muscle posteriorly and have a tongue of tissue arising between the external and internal carotid arteries. Thyroglossal duct cysts are remnants of the thyroglossal duct and are found in the midline, usually at or below the hyoid bone beneath the strap muscles. Teratomas or dermoids may occur anywhere, but can be identified by the presence of fat or calcium or both. Lymphangiomas have a typical appearance of a cystic mass, often with septations, that insinuates through fascial planes (sometimes inferiorly into the mediastinum).

21. What is the differential diagnosis for leukocoria?

Leukocoria is defined as an abnormal white papillary reflex. Retinoblastoma is the most concerning cause. Other causes include congenital

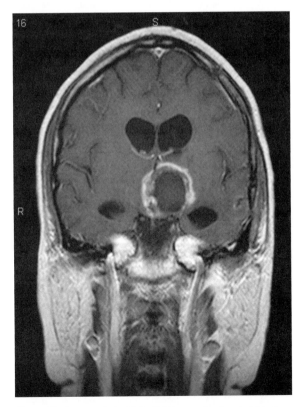

Figure 62-4. Coronal T1-weighted MR image after the administration of intravenous contrast agent shows ring-enhancing craniopharyngioma in the suprasellar region.

cataract, infection (e.g., toxocariasis), persistent hyperplastic primary vitreous, retinopathy of prematurity, and Coats disease (fusiform dilation of retinal vessels, often with associated retinal detachment and subretinal exudate). Historical clues are helpful in differentiating these entities. The average age of patients with retinoblastoma is 13 months, whereas Coats disease generally occurs in boys older than 4 years old, and toxocariasis occurs generally after 6 years of age. The presence of calcification may aid in the diagnosis on CT because 95% of retinoblastomas contain calcium.

22. What is meant by *trilateral retinoblastoma*?

Bilateral retinoblastomas often occur in the familial form of the disease, which is characterized genetically as a mutation in the *Rb1* tumor suppressor gene. These patients are also at risk for developing a third primitive intracranial neoplasm, usually in the pineal gland, the so-called third-eye. *Trilateral retinoblastoma* involves tumor in both eyes and in the pineal gland. As in the retina, even a fleck of calcium in the pineal gland of a child younger than 6 years old should be considered suggestive of neoplasm.

23. What is fibromatosis colli? Describe its imaging characteristics.

Fibromatosis colli is benign focal or fusiform enlargement of the sternocleidomastoid muscle in infants that usually regresses by 6 to 8 months of age and is thought to be due to trauma to the sternocleidomastoid muscle or to an in utero positioning abnormality. US of the muscle shows either diffuse enlargement or a focal hyperechoic mass. If there is question about the diagnosis, MRI may be useful. MRI should show low signal on T2-weighted images, which represents fibrosis in the sternocleidomastoid muscle.

24. Where do cholesteatomas typically arise, and what is the role of the radiologist in their evaluation?

A cholesteatoma is squamous epithelium that is trapped in the skull base, often creating expansion and erosion of adjacent bony structures. Cholesteatomas may be congenital, in which case they are well defined and rounded, and typically occur in the anterior mesotympanum or in the region of the eustachian tube, near the cochlear promontory. Cholesteatomas may also occur as a result of tympanic membrane perforation (i.e., acquired), in which case they typically occur in the epitympanum, adjacent to the scutum and involving Prussak space, or into the posterior middle ear. CT examination of the temporal bones often cannot be used to distinguish between cholesteatoma and fluid or inflammatory tissue, but it is often helpful in defining whether there are effects on adjacent bony structures. Radiologists may comment on the integrity of the ossicles, erosion of the scutum, the presence or absence of labyrinthine fistulas, or defects in the roof of the middle ear (tegmen tympani). MRI is not as helpful for evaluating bony structures, but may be an important problem-solving tool if there are questions concerning intracranial extension.

25. What is the role of the radiologist in the evaluation of sacrococcygeal teratoma?

The presence of a sacrococcygeal teratoma may be detected in utero with US or fetal MRI. Because the mass may be cystic, the differential diagnosis may include a meningocele (outpouching of meninges through a defect in the posterior elements in the lumbosacral spine). High-output cardiac failure caused by a teratoma may result from flow to the mass, leading to hydrops fetalis; placentomegaly; and polyhydramnios, which may necessitate cesarean section or fetal surgery. MRI may be useful in the evaluation of these masses because the prognosis and surgical approach may depend on which components of the mass are within the abdomen and pelvis. Lesions confined to the true pelvis tend to be benign histologically, whereas lesions that extend beyond the confines of the sacrum tend to be malignant.

BIBLIOGRAPHY

[1] C. Parazzini, C. Baldoli, G. Scotti, F. Triulzi, Terminal zones of myelination: MR evaluation of children aged 20–40 months, AJNR Am. J. Neuroradiol. 23 (2002) 1669–1673.
[2] E.S. Roach, Neurocutaneous syndromes, Pediatr. Clin. North Am. 39 (1992) 591–620.
[3] E.H. Roland, A. Hill, Germinal matrix-intraventricular hemorrhage in the premature newborn: management and outcome, Neurol. Clin. 21: 833–851, vi-vii, (2003).
[4] A.P. Truhan, P.A. Filipek, Magnetic resonance imaging: its role in the neuroradiologic evaluation of neurofibromatosis, tuberous sclerosis, and Sturge-Weber syndrome, Arch. Dermatol. 129 (1993) 219–226.
[5] L.G. Vezina, Diagnostic imaging in neuro-oncology, Pediatr. Clin. North Am. 44 (1997) 701–719.

CHAPTER 63

PEDIATRIC MUSCULOSKELETAL RADIOLOGY

D. Andrew Mong, MD

1. How does growing bone respond to trauma, and how is this different from mature bone?

The cartilaginous physis separates the epiphysis from the metaphysis. Pediatric ligaments and tendons are relatively stronger than growing bone (in contrast to adults). Given an equivalent force applied to growing and mature bone, the growing bone has a higher likelihood of fracture. In addition, immature bone has a propensity to bow instead of break, which may cause buckles in one side of the cortex (torus fractures) or greenstick fractures (fracture of one cortex and bowing of the other). These patterns are not seen in mature bone.

2. What is the significance of fractures of the physis?

The cartilaginous physis is vulnerable to injury, especially at its attachment to the metaphysis. Disruption of the physis may result in slower growth and premature fusion, leading to limb length discrepancy.

3. How are fractures of the physis classified?

Physeal injuries are classified in the Salter-Harris scheme, increasing in severity from I to V. Type I is a fracture through the physis. The fracture line in type II includes the metaphysis and physis. Type III fracture includes the epiphysis and the physis. Type IV fracture involves the metaphysis, physis, and epiphysis. Type V fracture is a crush injury of the physis. Follow-up for Salter-Harris fractures may include magnetic resonance imaging (MRI), which can delineate an abnormally fused physis in the healing phase that may need to be disrupted to allow future osseous growth (Fig. 63-1).

4. What are secondary ossification centers?

Secondary ossification centers appear and then fuse later with the primary ossification center on plain radiographs at predictable times during skeletal maturation. Multiple secondary ossification centers are around the elbow and appear at different ages. Their usual sequence can be remembered by the mnemonic *C-R-I-T-O-E*: *c*apitellum (1 year), *r*adial head (3 years), *i*nternal (medial) epicondyle (5 years), *t*rochlea (7 years), *o*lecranon (9 years), and *e*xternal (lateral) epicondyle (11 years) (Fig. 63-2).

5. Why are secondary ossification centers particularly important to understand in the setting of elbow trauma?

One important reason to understand this sequence is that a type I Salter-Harris fracture through the physis of the medial epicondyle may cause displacement of this ossification center into the region of the trochlea. This displacement might create the false impression that the trochlear ossification center is present, whereas the medial epicondylar ossification center has not yet appeared. Knowledge of this sequence allows one to identify this appearance appropriately as a displaced fracture.

6. How may subtle supracondylar fractures of the elbow be diagnosed?

Pediatric elbow fractures often occur in the supracondylar region, where the humerus is relatively flat. The anterior humeral line, drawn on the lateral view of the elbow along the anterior humerus, normally intersects the middle third of the capitellum. This intersection is likely to be disrupted in supracondylar fractures. The presence of a joint effusion (hemarthrosis) is also extremely helpful and can be assessed by the presence of an elevated posterior fat pad, which is displaced and visible on the lateral view if there is blood in the joint. Displacement of the anterior fat pad ("sail" sign) may also be seen with hemarthrosis, but this finding is less specific.

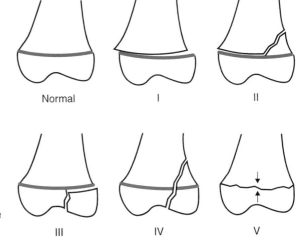

Figure 63-1. Salter-Harris fractures of the distal femur.

7. Describe nursemaid's elbow.

Nursemaid's elbow is caused by radial head subluxation through the annular ligament of the elbow, resulting in abnormal positioning of the ligament between the radial head and capitellum. It is often caused by sudden traction on the forearm in a child 1 to 3 years old. Radiographs may have normal results, but are obtained to exclude fractures.

8. List risk factors for developmental dysplasia of the hip (DDH).

- White race
- Female gender
- Torticollis
- Clubfoot
- Breech birth

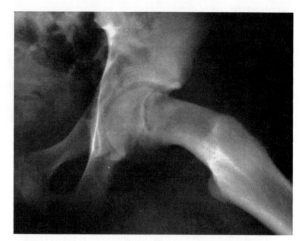

Figure 63-2. Frog-leg view of the left hip shows open physis with inferior displacement of the femoral capital epiphysis compared with the metaphysis. (Courtesy of Richard Markowitz, MD, Children's Hospital of Philadelphia.)

9. When is DDH suspected clinically?

It is difficult to diagnose DDH in newborns 4 weeks old or younger because of normal joint laxity, but this condition is suspected in infants with leg length discrepancy and asymmetric thigh creases. The Barlow maneuver on physical examination dislocates the femoral head rearward, and the Ortolani maneuver reduces the recently dislocated hip, often with a resultant "clunk."

10. Name the potential complications of untreated DDH.

- Leg length discrepancy
- Osteoarthritis
- Pain
- Gait disturbance
- Decrease in agility

11. How is DDH diagnosed radiographically?

Traditionally, plain films have been used to diagnose DDH. Although the femoral head begins to ossify during the first year (usually between 3 and 6 months), its location must be inferred in infants. The acetabulum is divided into quadrants by the horizontal Hilgenreiner line, drawn through both triradiate cartilages, and the vertical Perkin line, drawn through the lateral rim of the acetabulum. A normal femoral head should fall within the inner lower quadrant of these intersecting lines, whereas a femoral head in DDH would be displaced superolaterally. The acetabular angle should also be evaluated, drawn between Hilgenreiner line and a line connecting the superolateral ridge of the acetabulum with the triradiate cartilage. This angle should be less than 30 degrees in neonates.

12. How is DDH diagnosed on ultrasound (US)?

US is now the preferred method of diagnosing DDH in children younger than 1 year old. The hip is studied in the coronal plane. The alpha angle is measured between the straight lateral margin of the ilium and a line from the inferior point of the ilium tangential to the acetabulum. This is a measure of acetabular depth and should be greater than 60 degrees. At least half of the femoral head should be seated within the acetabulum.

13. What is Legg-Calvé-Perthes disease?

Legg-Calvé-Perthes disease refers to idiopathic osteonecrosis of the femoral head, usually affecting children 3 to 12 years old with a mean age of 7 years. Plain radiographic findings include a small femoral head epiphysis, which may become fragmented, and widening of the articular space, which may be due to an associated joint effusion.

14. Describe slipped capital femoral epiphysis (SCFE).

SCFE is a hip disease of early adolescence (10 to 15 years old), characterized by idiopathic posterior and inferior slippage of the capital femoral epiphysis on the femoral neck metaphysis. Complications include avascular necrosis of the femoral head or chondrolysis. Anteroposterior and frog-leg views of both hips should be obtained because the condition can be bilateral in 40% of cases. On the frog-leg view, a normal epiphysis projects superior to Klein line, which is drawn along the superior surface of the femoral neck. In early SCFE, the epiphysis is flush with this line (see Fig. 63-2).

> **Key Points: Characteristic Ages of Pediatric Hip Disorders**
> 1. Developmental dysplasia is a disorder of infants.
> 2. Legg-Calvé-Perthes disease occurs in children 3 to 12 years old.
> 3. SCFE occurs in children 10 to 15 years old. This disorder cannot occur after the physes have fused.

15. How is SCFE treated?

Treatment goals include the prevention of further slippage and physeal plate closure. SCFE may be treated with internal fixation, bone graft, osteotomy, and cast immobilization. There is no attempt to reduce the slip because this may cause avascular necrosis.

16. What are coxa vara and coxa valga?

Coxa vara and coxa valga are abnormalities of the femoral shaft-to-neck ratio. The normal ratio is 150 degrees at birth, decreasing to 120 to 135 degrees in adults. Coxa vara is an angle less than 120 degrees and may be secondary to trauma, tumor, SCFE, or a congenital abnormality. Coxa valga (>150 degrees) is usually neuromuscular in origin but may also be seen in blood dyscrasias such as thalassemia.

17. Describe Blount disease.

Blount disease is a varus deformity of the knee (i.e., the tibia is abnormally directed medially compared with the femur), resulting from growth disturbance of the medial aspect of the proximal tibial metaphysis. This deformity may occur in infants, in which case it is often bilateral, or in adolescents. Tibial osteotomy may be required for treatment because growth disturbance may result from abnormal tibial bowing.

18. What is Osgood-Schlatter disease?

Osgood-Schlatter disease is a common cause of knee pain in adolescence (11 to 14 years old) that is thought to result from repetitive traction through the patellar tendon onto the developing tibial tubercle. This traction can lead to partial avulsion through the ossification center and heterotopic bone formation. Although the diagnosis may be made clinically, radiographs may aid in the exclusion of other etiologies of knee pain. Lateral radiographs may reveal irregular ossification of the proximal tibial tubercle, calcification and thickening of the patellar tendon, and soft tissue swelling.

19. What is the difference between a triplane fracture and a juvenile Tillaux fracture of the ankle?

Both fractures occur after partial closure of the distal tibial physis. On frontal radiographs, a triplane fracture appears as a Salter III fracture through the epiphysis, and on the lateral radiograph, it appears as a Salter II fracture through the metaphysis. A juvenile Tillaux fracture is simply a Salter III fracture that occurs at the anterolateral aspect of the distal tibia. The physis fuses from medial to lateral, leaving the lateral aspect more vulnerable to injury.

20. What is Freiberg infraction?

Freiberg infraction is an idiopathic osteochondrosis of the head of a metatarsal bone (usually the second), which results in flattening and osteosclerosis of the metatarsal head. It is usually seen in adolescents (13 to 18 years old).

21. What are craniosynostoses?

A craniosynostosis represents premature closure of a suture of the skull. This premature closure results in cessation of growth of the skull perpendicular to the suture line and abnormal compensatory growth along the axis of the closed suture. For this reason, sagittal craniosynostosis results in an elongated skull in the anteroposterior dimension (scaphocephaly) (Fig. 63-3). Plagiocephaly results from premature closure of one coronal suture, resulting in abnormal bulging on the opposite forehead. Premature closure of the metopic suture results in trigonocephaly, which appears as a triangular keel-shaped forehead. Cloverleaf skull (kleeblattschädel) results from premature closure of the coronal, lambdoid, and posterior sagittal sutures, with bulging of the vertex of the brain through the squamosal, anterior sagittal, and metopic sutures.

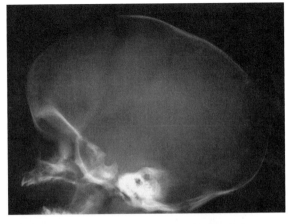

Figure 63-3. Markedly increased anteroposterior diameter from premature closure of sagittal suture, creating a boat-shaped skull, or scaphocephaly.

22. Give the differential diagnosis for vertebra plana.

Flattening of a vertebral body (vertebra plana) in a child should first bring to mind the diagnosis of Langerhans cell histiocytosis. Other diagnostic possibilities in pediatric patients include leukemia, lymphoma, metastatic disease, infection, and storage diseases.

23. When and where do pediatric primary tumors of bone occur?

Ewing sarcoma and osteosarcoma are the most common primary pediatric bone tumors and typically occur between ages 10 and 25 years. The most common sites are the pelvis, thigh, lower leg, upper arm, and ribs, but soft tissue may also be the primary site of involvement. Ewing sarcoma typically does not have a matrix and appears as a permeative aggressive lesion, often with associated periosteal reaction. Most osteosarcomas occur in the metaphysis, typically around the knee. Although the appearance of osteosarcomas is variable, they often produce a characteristic fluffy osteoid matrix.

24. How should a suspected osteoid osteoma be evaluated?

Osteoid osteoma is a benign neoplasm with a nidus of osteoid-rich tissue that typically causes an intense sclerotic reaction in surrounding bone. An osteoid osteoma may occur in the cortical, cancellous, or periosteal regions of any bone (or rarely in adjacent soft tissues). Most patients are between ages 10 and 30 years and often give a typical history of night pain relieved by aspirin. Radionuclide bone scan may point to the abnormality before any changes are apparent on plain film and should be performed on any patient with a painful scoliosis in whom osteoid osteoma in the spine is the working diagnosis. If plain films do not reveal the lucent nidus surrounded by sclerotic bone, a computed tomography (CT) scan is the preferred next step because intracortical tumors may be missed on MRI.

25. What is rickets?

Rickets is a relative or absolute deficiency in vitamin D, which causes a decrease in ossification. It is almost exclusively seen in children younger than 2 years.

26. How does rickets appear radiographically?

Bone density is overall decreased. More specific signs include loss of the zone of provisional calcification within the metaphysis of long bones; this leads to metaphyseal irregularity, cupping, and fraying with an associated widened physis. These changes are seen best in the distal radius, which is why films of the wrists are ordered to evaluate rickets (Fig. 63-4). Another classic appearance is the "rachitic rosary," which is enlargement of the costochondral joints in the chest.

27. Describe the bony changes of sickle cell anemia.

Sickle cell anemia is secondary to a disorder of "sickling" of red blood cells resulting from abnormal hemoglobin molecules. Clumped, sickled cells form venous (and sometimes arterial) thromboses, affecting multiple organs. Osseous manifestations include patchy sclerotic changes in bone from infarctions. A more specific sign includes a "Lincoln log" appearance of the vertebral bodies, with squarelike depressions seen in the superior and inferior end plates on a lateral spine film. Avascular necrosis of the hips may also be seen. Affected patients

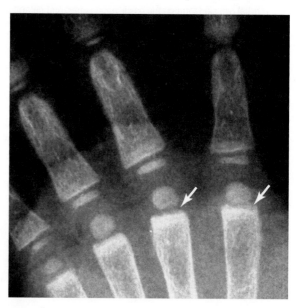

Figure 63-4. Frontal plain film of the hand shows cupping and fraying of metaphyses (*arrows*) from rickets. (Courtesy of Richard Markowitz, MD, Children's Hospital of Philadelphia.)

are prone to osteomyelitis from *Staphylococcus aureus* and *Salmonella*. On MRI, it can be difficult to distinguish infarction from osteomyelitis because both may produce signal abnormalities in marrow (bright T2 signal) along with adjacent soft tissue changes. *Dactylitis* is a nonspecific term referring to inflammation of a digit, which may also be seen in sickle cell anemia and be secondary to infarction or infection. Finally, because of the chronic anemia, patients with sickle cell anemia have an increased red-to-yellow marrow ratio, which may be inferred on a lateral skull radiograph by the widening of the diploic space (Fig. 63-5).

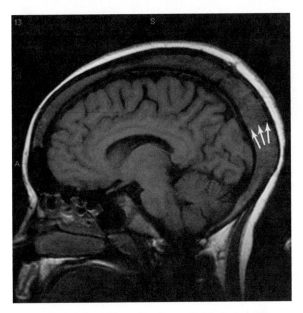

Figure 63-5. Sagittal T1-weighted MR image of the brain shows widening of the diploic space (*arrows*) of the skull from marrow expansion in a patient with sickle cell anemia. This finding is not specific for sickle cell anemia and may be found in other severe anemias, such as thalassemia or iron deficiency anemia.

28. What is the most common type of dwarfism, and what are its manifestations?

The most common type of dwarfism is achondroplasia. This is a rhizomelic (shortening of the proximal bones) autosomal dominant disorder. Typical characteristics include a large head with frontal bossing, a trident configuration of the hands, genu varum (bowed legs), and an exaggerated lumbar lordosis (with posterior scalloping of the vertebral bodies). On a frontal radiograph of the lumbosacral spine in a normal patient, the distance between the pedicles gradually widens from L1 to L5, whereas an achondroplastic dwarf shows a decrease in the interpedicular distance of the caudal spine. Other radiographic findings include a notchlike sacroiliac groove and metaphyseal flaring of the long bones.

29. What is the differential diagnosis for dense metaphyseal bands? How does one know when they are abnormally dense?

Dense metaphyseal bands may be a normal variant, so it is important to look at areas that do not have a lot of bone turnover to see whether they are affected as well. Specifically, the metaphyses of the fibula are good areas to check. A major concern is heavy metal poisoning (specifically lead intoxication). Lead poisoning can be diagnosed by noting not only the metaphyseal bands, but also the radiopaque lead chips seen on a frontal plain view of the abdomen floating in the child's intestines. Other etiologic factors include stress lines, treated rickets, scurvy, hypervitaminosis D, or treated leukemia.

BIBLIOGRAPHY

[1] S.P. England, S. Sundberg, Management of common pediatric fractures, Pediatr. Clin. North Am. 43 (1996) 991–1012.
[2] S.C. Kao, W.L. Smith, Skeletal injuries in the pediatric patient, Radiol. Clin. North Am. 35 (1997) 727–746.
[3] E. Lemyre, E.M. Azouz, A.S. Teebi, et al., Bone dysplasia series: achondroplasia, hypochondroplasia and thanatophoric dysplasia: review and update, Can. Assoc. Radiol. J. 50 (1999) 185–197.
[4] R.E. Lins, R.W. Simovitch, P.M. Waters, Pediatric elbow trauma, Orthop. Clin. North Am. 30 (1999) 119–132.

64 CHAPTER

IMAGING OF CHILD ABUSE

D. Andrew Mong, MD, and
Avrum N. Pollock, MD

1. What are key history and physical examination findings that may raise suspicion of the possibility of nonaccidental trauma (NAT)?

Red flags from the history that should lead the clinician and radiologist to consider child abuse include injuries that are not commensurate with the development of the child, a delay in seeking care, or vague or changing stories given by caretakers. Superficial physical examination findings that the clinician may convey to the radiologist include bruises in various stages of healing; "pattern injuries," such as from cigarette burns; and signs of neglect.

2. What diagnostic algorithm might the clinician and radiologist apply if skeletal injury from child abuse is suspected?

In addition to radiographs of specific injuries, a skeletal survey should be performed on all children younger than 2 years. This survey includes plain frontal radiographs of the chest, arms, hands, pelvis, legs, ankles, and feet, and frontal and lateral radiographs of the skull and entire spine. A "babygram" (frontal radiograph of the chest and abdomen) is inadequate. A nuclear medicine bone scan may be performed if these findings are equivocal for abuse, or if there is a high index of clinical suspicion, and the skeletal survey does not reveal an abnormality (Fig. 64-1).

3. Describe shaken infant syndrome.

Shaken infant syndrome occurs when an infant or young child is shaken forcefully. This creates shearing forces that may cause classic patterns of injury seen in the chest and brain. Long bone injuries with resultant metaphyseal corner fractures are due to twisting/torsion–type injuries, which can occur with or without shaken baby or shaken impact syndrome, but are a separate injury, mechanism, and type of NAT.

4. What are metaphyseal corner fractures?

Metaphyseal fractures result from shearing forces of NAT and appear as metaphyseal corner fractures or bucket-handle fractures, the same fractures seen in different projections or obliquities. These fractures may heal quickly. They typically appear as lucent areas extending across the metaphysis, nearly perpendicular to the long axis of the bone. They are highly specific for child abuse (Fig. 64-2).

5. Name other pediatric fractures with high specificity for child abuse.

Posterior rib fractures are another aspect of shaken infant syndrome that occur when adult hands forcefully grab the infant's chest while shaking the infant, resulting in a levering or fulcruming effect of the posterior ribs against the costal processes of the adjacent vertebral bodies. These fractures are specific for abuse and may be detected incidentally on a routine chest radiograph obtained for an unrelated reason, or when the patient presents with dyspnea or respiratory distress secondary to the underlying central nervous system injury sustained secondary to violent shaking. Other suspicious fractures include fractures of the scapula, spinous processes, or sternum or compression fractures of the vertebral bodies (Fig. 64-3).

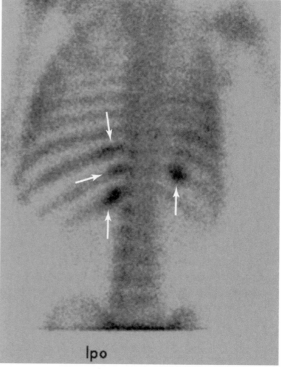

Figure 64-1. Posterior view of technetium-(Tc)-99m–labeled methylene diphosphonate bone scan shows multiple posterior rib fractures (*arrows*).

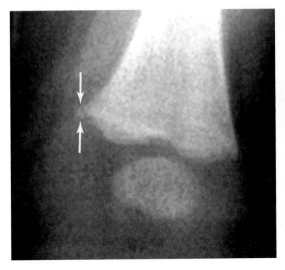

Figure 64-2. Typical metaphyseal corner fracture (*arrows*) of distal tibia.

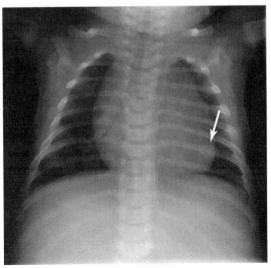

Figure 64-3. Posterior rib fractures (*arrow*).

6. What fractures have low specificity for child abuse?

Fractures of the long bones, clavicular fractures, and linear skull fractures have low specificity for child abuse.

7. What features of skull fractures increase the likelihood of NAT?

Branching, multiple, depressed, or distracted fractures and fractures that cross suture lines are more likely to be caused by abuse than are linear skull fractures.

8. What features of a fracture are useful in estimating its age?

Features that may be useful to the radiologist include sclerosis at the fracture margin, the presence or absence of periosteal reaction, callus formation, bony bridging, and bony remodeling. Multiple fractures of different ages are *highly* suggestive of NAT.

9. Summarize common findings of head trauma in shaken infant syndrome.

Shearing forces may create subdural hematomas. Interhemispheric subdural hematoma and posterior fossa/tentorial subdural hematoma are very suspicious areas of involvement. Severe cerebral edema, which may result from asphyxiation, has a typical appearance on unenhanced head computed tomography (CT), with loss of gray-white matter differentiation and edema of the cerebral cortex and central gray structures (basal ganglia and thalami). The cerebrum appears diffusely low in attenuation (Fig. 64-4).

10. What is the most common cause of death in a patient who has sustained NAT?

Injury to the central nervous system is the most common cause of death.

11. How should imaging of the brain be applied in the setting of suspected abuse?

Any child younger than 2 years in whom there is a clinical suspicion of abuse, even if asymptomatic, should receive a head CT scan

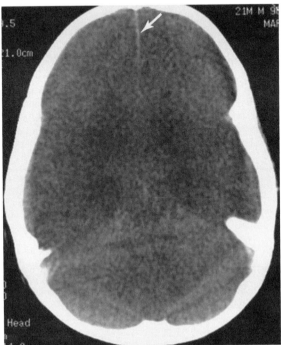

Figure 64-4. Midline subdural hematoma (*arrow*), which is in a typical location seen in cases of NAT. There is diffuse cerebral edema with loss of gray-white differentiation.

because of the high incidence of occult brain trauma. Brain imaging should also be considered in older children. Irritability, vomiting, altered state of consciousness, and irregular respirations are strong indications for imaging the brain. Magnetic resonance imaging (MRI) of the brain can be performed to detect more subtle shear-type injuries of the white matter not visible or evident on head CT, and can be used to date areas of hemorrhage with greater accuracy.

12. How is the age of intracranial blood determined on MRI examinations?

Evolving blood products in cerebral or subdural hematomas go through various stages of signal intensity on T1-weighted and T2-weighted MR images. Hyperacute hemorrhage (oxyhemoglobin) is dark on T1 and bright on T2. Acute hemorrhage (deoxyhemoglobin) is dark on T1 and T2. Early subacute hematoma (intracellular methemoglobin) is bright on T1 and dark on T2. Late subacute hematoma (extracellular methemoglobin) is bright on T1 and T2. Chronic hematoma (hemosiderin) is dark on both sequences.

13. Describe possible bowel findings in cases of abuse.

Bowel injuries typically occur in children older than 2 years who may have been punched or kicked, with resultant compression of the bowel loops against the spinal column. The duodenum and proximal small bowel are the most commonly affected areas of the small bowel and may show lacerations or intramural hematomas, which can cause obstruction if bleeding is severe. These injuries can be studied with an upper gastrointestinal or CT scan.

14. What is the most common cause of pediatric pancreatitis?

The most common cause of pediatric pancreatitis is accidental or nonaccidental trauma. Pancreatic injury may be suspected with abdominal pain, fever, and vomiting. Pancreatitis may be detected with an elevation of amylase and lipase levels without any radiographic findings.

15. Describe radiologic manifestations of pediatric pancreatitis.

On CT examination, pancreatitis may manifest as fullness of the pancreatic tissues, stranding in the adjacent mesenteric fat, or frank peripancreatic fluid collections. On CT examination, pancreatic lacerations appear as areas of linear discontinuation of pancreatic tissue, usually with surrounding fluid.

Key Points: Lesions That Should Prompt a Work-up for Child Abuse

1. Metaphyseal corner fractures (highly specific and sensitive for abuse)
2. Posterior rib fractures
3. Fractures of spinous processes, scapula, or sternum or compression fractures of vertebral bodies
4. Subdural hematomas, especially midline
5. Duodenal hematoma and pancreatitis

---

16. Are multiple bruises and skeletal injuries always diagnostic of child abuse?

No. Systemic disorders can also be responsible for multiple bruises and skeletal injuries. Abnormalities of coagulation including entities such as leukemia, hemophilia, idiopathic thrombocytopenic purpura, and Henoch-Schönlein purpura may mimic abuse. Metabolic/congenital abnormalities are also important mimickers to consider, including osteogenesis imperfecta, Menkes kinky hair syndrome, Ehlers-Danlos syndrome, congenital syphilis, and rickets.

17. How does congenital syphilis mimic child abuse?

Both may produce metaphyseal fractures. In congenital syphilis, these are pathologic fractures secondary to fragmentation of the metaphysis from osteomyelitis. These findings are usually symmetric in a child with syphilis and asymmetric in an abused child. Syphilis may also be differentiated from child abuse through noting concomitant diaphyseal diffuse periosteal reaction along long bones, splenomegaly, and positive serologic test results.

18. What is the differential diagnosis of periosteal reaction in a newborn?

In addition to fractures from NAT, the differential diagnosis includes congenital infection (e.g., syphilis), neuroblastoma metastases, physiologic periosteal new bone formation, prostaglandin treatment, and Caffey disease. Caffey disease is a benign, self-limited periosteal reaction of uncertain etiology, usually involving the mandible, clavicles, and long bones.

19. When does physiologic periosteal new bone formation occur?

Periosteal new bone formation can occur symmetrically along shafts of long bones in newborns and resolves by 3 months of age. It is thought to be due to handling of the infant. There are no associated fractures.

20. Can a metaphyseal corner fracture look like a metaphyseal lucent band?

Yes. If a lucent metaphyseal band is identified, additional projections may identify it as a corner fracture. The differential diagnosis of a lucent metaphyseal band includes leukemia, lymphoma, metastatic disease (neuroblastoma), congenital infection, and scurvy.

21. What is the legal responsibility of any U.S. physician who suspects child abuse?

Child protection ordinances exist in all 50 states and require medical professionals to report suspected abuse to the local child protective service agency. Radiologists must ensure that high-quality films are obtained for the skeletal survey, which may be used in court.

BIBLIOGRAPHY

[1] G.J. Lonergan, A.M. Baker, M.K. Morey, S.C. Boos, From the archives of the AFIP. Child abuse: radiologic-pathologic correlation, RadioGraphics 23 (2003) 811–845.

[2] K.I. Mogbo, T.L. Slovis, A.I. Canady, et al., Appropriate imaging in children with skull fractures and suspicion of abuse, Radiology 208 (1998) 521–524.

[3] K. Nimkin, P.K. Kleinman, Imaging of child abuse, Radiol. Clin. North Am. 39 (2001) 843–864.

SOLITARY AND MULTIPLE PULMONARY NODULES

Drew A. Torigian, MD, MA, and
Charles T. Lau, MD

1. What is a solitary pulmonary nodule (SPN)?

SPN is a solitary focal lesion in the lung that measures 3 cm or less. A solitary focal lesion that is greater than 3 cm is considered to be a mass, and most masses are malignant. Approximately 150,000 SPNs are detected annually in the United States, often incidentally on imaging. About 60% are benign, but 40% can be malignant. The goal of radiologic evaluation of SPN is to differentiate noninvasively whether it is benign or malignant as accurately as possible. SPN is the initial radiographic finding in 30% of patients with lung cancer, and the prognosis depends partly on the stage at presentation.

2. List some causes of pulmonary nodules.

Primary lung carcinoma is the most common cause of SPN; pulmonary granuloma is the second most common overall cause; and pulmonary hamartoma the third most common cause. Table 65-1 provides a more complete list. Many other entities can cause SPNs or multiple pulmonary nodules, including tumors (e.g., metastatic disease), infections, vasculitis, and inflammatory diseases (e.g., sarcoidosis, rheumatoid arthritis, or inhalational lung disease). Be careful about a "confluence of shadows" or overlap of normal vascular and osseous structures that appears to represent a nodule. Nipple shadows can also appear as nodules, but are usually seen at a similar level bilaterally.

3. What is the general approach to the evaluation of SPN?

The initial step is to determine whether a visualized "nodule" on chest radiography is truly a pulmonary nodule or a pseudolesion that mimics a nodule (some of the causes of a pseudolesion are listed in Table 65-1). If a "nodule" is actually a pseudolesion associated with bone, such as a rib fracture, it would have the same anatomic relationship to its bone of origin on radiographs with multiple views, whereas a true pulmonary nodule that overlaps with osseous structures on one view would appear to move apart from these osseous structures on other views. Radiopaque nipple markers can be used to distinguish pseudolesions that are actually nipples from true pulmonary nodules. When a true SPN has been confirmed, a more detailed investigation begins.

4. What further diagnostic steps may be implemented in the work-up of indeterminate pulmonary nodules?

Thin-section unenhanced computed tomography (CT), CT nodule densitometry, fluorodeoxyglucose (FDG) positron emission tomography (PET), short-term follow-up chest radiography or CT, and tissue sampling are some of the options available for the work-up of indeterminate pulmonary nodules. The choice is based on several factors, including the pretest probability of malignancy, the morphologic features of the nodules, and the patient's clinical history and current status. Thin-section unenhanced CT is useful for the identification of fat or certain patterns of calcification within a nodule that indicate benignancy.

5. What are some potential blind spots on chest radiography and CT when trying to detect pulmonary nodules?

- On chest radiography, potential blind spots include the lung apices where the clavicles and ribs overlap, the hila and retrocardiac region where superimposed cardiovascular structures are located, and within the lung bases below the level of the anterior portions of the hemidiaphragms where abdominal soft tissue overlaps.
- On CT, potential blind spots include the central portions of the lungs (e.g., the hilar regions and the azygoesophageal recess) and the endoluminal portions of the trachea and bronchi.

6. List some morphologic imaging features of nodules assessed on chest radiography and CT.

- Shape
- Size/volume and change over time
- Margins
- Internal architecture
- Presence of fat
- Presence and pattern of calcification

Table 65-1. Differential Diagnosis of Solitary Pulmonary Nodule (SPN)

Neoplasia

Primary lung carcinoma (No. 1 cause of SPN)

Metastasis

Lymphoma/post-transplant lymphoproliferative disorder

Carcinoid tumor

Primary lung sarcoma

Hamartoma (No. 3 cause of SPN, No. 2 cause of benign SPN)

Infection

Granuloma (No. 2 cause of SPN, No. 1 cause of benign SPN)

Bacterial

Viral

Fungal

Mycobacterial

Parasitic

Septic emboli (often multiple, peripheral, and cavitary)

Vascular

Pulmonary infarction (often peripheral and wedge-shaped, associated with pulmonary embolism)

Vasculitis

Arteriovenous malformation

Pulmonary venous varix (tubular and avidly enhancing on CT)

Pulmonary artery aneurysm

Inflammatory

Sarcoidosis

Inhalational lung disease

Hypersensitivity pneumonitis

Organizing pneumonia

Bronchiolitis

Langerhans cell histiocytosis (associated with upper lobe predominant cystic interstitial lung disease in smokers)

Rheumatoid (necrobiotic) nodule

Inflammatory pseudotumor

Congenital

Intrapulmonary lymph node

Pulmonary sequestration (solid or cystic opacity most often in lower lobes)

Bronchial atresia

Traumatic

Radiation therapy (typically has linear margins and known history of prior radiation therapy)

Pulmonary contusion (associated with traumatic injury to chest)

Pseudonodules

Rounded atelectasis ("folded lung," typically subpleural opacity associated with pleural thickening or effusion and "comet-tail sign" of swirling bronchovascular structures central to opacity)

Pulmonary scarring

Mucoid impaction

Fluid in interlobar fissure (often lenticular in shape on lateral chest radiograph in the location of a fissure)

Healing rib fracture

Bone island

Spinal osteophyte

Skin lesion

Nipple shadow

Pleural lesion

Mediastinal lesion

Overlap of vascular and osseous structures

7. Describe morphologic imaging findings that are suggestive of a benign SPN.

Small size and smooth, well-defined margins suggest a benign SPN, although 15% and 40% of malignant nodules are less than 1 cm and 2 cm in diameter, and 20% of malignant nodules have well-defined margins. Intranodular fat is a reliable indicator of a hamartoma, which is a benign lesion (Fig. 65-1). Central, diffuse solid, laminated, and "popcorn-like" patterns of nodule calcification are indicative of benignancy, with the first three typically seen in calcified granulomas and the last in a pulmonary hamartoma (Fig. 65-2). Other patterns of calcification are nonspecific, and 15% of lung carcinomas may contain amorphous, stippled, or punctate and eccentric calcification. Avidly enhancing serpentine or tubular feeding arteries and an early draining vein associated with an enhancing nidus are pathognomonic of an arteriovenous malformation (Fig. 65-3). Small satellite nodules around the periphery of a smooth dominant nodule strongly suggest a granulomatous infection. Ground-glass opacity surrounding a nodule ("CT halo" sign) is highly suggestive of angioinvasive opportunistic infection, such as by aspergillosis, particularly in the setting of neutropenia (Fig. 65-4). A three-dimensional ratio of the nodule's largest axial diameter to the largest craniocaudal diameter greater than 1.78:1 (i.e., a flattened configuration) is highly suggestive of benignancy. A peripheral rim of enhancement or the "enhancing rim" sign of a nodule also suggests a benign SPN.

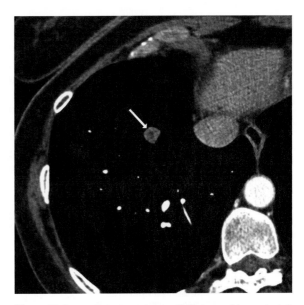

Figure 65-1. Pulmonary hamartoma on CT. Note smoothly marginated round nodule (*arrow*) that contains low-attenuation fat pathognomonic for hamartoma.

8. Describe morphologic imaging findings that are suggestive of a malignant SPN.

Size greater than 2 cm suggests malignancy. Lobulated or spiculated margins with distortion of adjacent vessels are typically associated with malignancy, although a lobulated or spiculated margin is seen in 25% and 10% of benign nodules. The "corona radiata" sign consists of very fine linear strands extending outward from a nodule and is strongly suggestive of malignancy. Partially solid nodules (i.e., nodules composed of ground-glass and solid components) tend to be malignant and are most often due to bronchioloalveolar cell carcinoma (BAC) or adenocarcinoma with BAC features. Internal inhomogeneity, particularly from cystic/bubbly lucencies or pseudocavitation, strongly suggests malignancy, most often from BAC. Cavitary nodules with maximal wall thickness greater than 15 mm and wall irregularity tend to be malignant, whereas nodules with wall thickness 4 mm or less tend to be benign.

9. How does measurement of the doubling time of nodules aid in the determination of a benign SPN?

Doubling time, the time required for a nodule to double in volume (equivalent to an increase of about 26% in diameter), for most malignant nodules is 1 to 15 months. Nodules that double in volume more rapidly or more slowly than this are typically benign. Generally, lack of growth of a nodule over a 2-year period is strongly suggestive of benignancy, although some malignant nodules, such as nodules secondary to BAC, bronchial carcinoid, or some pulmonary metastases, may take longer to grow. Follow-up CT scans for indeterminate pulmonary nodules generally are performed at 3 to 12 months after the initial CT scan to assess for interval growth depending on the size and appearance of the nodule and the presence of risk factors for malignancy, such as a patient history of tobacco use.

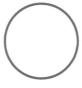

| Central | Diffuse solid | Laminated | Popcorn-like |

Figure 65-2. Four benign patterns of nodule calcification.

10. How does the degree of enhancement of pulmonary nodules on CT aid in the determination of benignancy?

The degree of enhancement of pulmonary nodules is directly related to the likelihood of malignancy and the vascularity of the nodules and may be determined through CT nodule densitometry. Nodule enhancement of less than 15 HU (a measure of density) on CT after intravenous contrast agent administration is strongly predictive of benignancy, whereas enhancement of more than 15 HU may indicate either malignancy or active inflammation. False-negative enhancement studies may occur occasionally when central necrosis, cavitation, or abundant mucin is present within a pulmonary nodule or if a pulmonary nodule is very small.

11. How does FDG PET aid in the differentiation of benign and malignant lung nodules?

Malignant pulmonary nodules generally have increased glucose metabolism with increased uptake, trapping, and accumulation of FDG, a radioisotopic glucose analogue that can be seen on PET. Occasionally, active inflammatory granulomatous pulmonary nodules may show increased uptake of FDG, although not as great in amount as in malignancy. Lack of FDG uptake in a pulmonary nodule measuring 10 mm or more is strongly predictive of benignancy, although malignant nodules that are due to BAC or bronchial carcinoid or that are less than 10 mm may have low or absent FDG uptake. Dual-time point FDG PET with early and delayed imaging can characterize pulmonary nodules further because malignant nodules tend to accumulate radiotracer over time, and benign nodules tend to wash out radiotracer gradually.

12. Describe some clinical features that suggest whether SPN is more likely to be malignant, and whether it is more likely to be due to lung carcinoma or a pulmonary metastasis if there is a history of extrapulmonary primary malignancy.

Older patient age (>35 years old), history of prior malignancy, presence of symptoms and signs of malignancy such as hemoptysis, and history of tobacco use all increase the likelihood that SPN is malignant rather than benign. Most patients with a history of extrapulmonary primary malignancy and SPN have a primary lung carcinoma rather than a pulmonary metastasis or benign lesion, although this varies depending on the type of primary malignancy. A metastasis as the cause of SPN in this setting is more common than primary lung carcinoma when the primary malignancy is due to melanoma, sarcoma, or testicular carcinoma. Multiplicity of pulmonary nodules also tends to make metastases more likely than lung carcinoma. Finally, primary lung carcinoma occurs more commonly in the upper lung fields, whereas pulmonary metastases occur more commonly in the lower lung fields. There are no definitive imaging criteria, however, that can fully separate a pulmonary metastasis from a primary lung carcinoma as the etiologic factor for SPN.

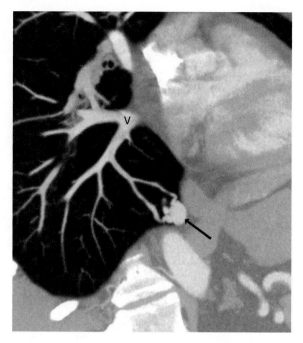

Figure 65-3. Pulmonary arteriovenous malformation on CT. Note tubular nodular nidus in right lung (*arrow*) that has draining veins leading to pulmonary vein (*V*). Other images show enhancing feeding artery to nidus (not shown).

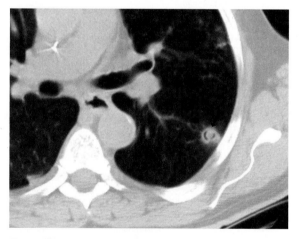

Figure 65-4. Invasive aspergillosis with "CT halo" sign on CT. Note partially cavitary pulmonary nodule (*arrow*) surrounded by faint ground-glass opacity secondary to pulmonary hemorrhage.

13. What minimally invasive procedures may be used to obtain tissue samples from SPN?

Image-guided transthoracic needle biopsy is the procedure of choice for definitive characterization of peripheral pulmonary nodules, whereas bronchoscopic needle biopsy is typically used for the characterization of nodules that involve the central airways and lungs.

14. What are potential complications of transthoracic needle biopsy?

Pneumothorax is the most common complication, occurring in 25% of cases, particularly when severe emphysema is present. Nondiagnostic or false-negative biopsy results, hemoptysis, hemorrhage, pain, infection, air embolus, and tumor seeding are less common complications. Avoiding crossing pulmonary fissures with the biopsy needle or avoiding multiple lung punctures decreases the incidence of pneumothorax.

15. How important is lung carcinoma as a public health issue?

Lung carcinoma is the most common cause of cancer-related death in men and women, and is the second most common cause of cancer in men after prostate cancer and in women after breast cancer. Tobacco use is the number 1 risk factor for lung carcinoma, and 85% of lung carcinoma deaths are due to smoking. The risk of developing lung carcinoma is proportional to the number of pack-years of smoking. Synchronous primary lung carcinomas occur in less than 5% of patients with lung carcinoma, but metachronous primary lung carcinomas may occur in 15%, with a latency of about 4 to 5 years. Overall, survival rates for patients with lung carcinoma are poor (<15% at 5 years), although patients with treated early-stage disease or with a BAC tumor subtype tend to have much better survival rates.

16. What are the major histologic types and subtypes of lung carcinoma?

Histologically, 75% are non–small cell lung carcinomas (NSCLC), for which the prognosis primarily depends on surgical stage at diagnosis, and 25% are small cell lung carcinomas (SCLC), which behave aggressively with early and wide dissemination. NSCLC may be subdivided into adenocarcinoma, squamous cell carcinoma, and large cell carcinoma subtypes, in order of decreasing frequency. BAC is a less aggressive subtype of adenocarcinoma that spreads along preexisting alveolar septa without lung parenchymal invasion.

17. Summarize some of the differing features of the various histologic types and subtypes of lung carcinoma.

- *Adenocarcinoma* is the subtype least closely associated with tobacco use and tends to develop in the lung periphery, whereas *squamous cell carcinoma* is strongly associated with tobacco use, tends to develop centrally within a lobar or segmental bronchus, and is often cavitary.
- *Large cell carcinoma* is a histologic diagnosis of exclusion among the subtypes of lung carcinoma, is strongly associated with tobacco use, and often manifests as a large peripheral lung mass. *Small cell lung carcinoma* usually arises centrally within the chest with extensive metastatic lymphadenopathy involving the hila and mediastinum and only rarely cavitates, but it may manifest in a more limited form in one hemithorax or as SPN.

18. What is a superior sulcus tumor?

Superior sulcus tumor (or *Pancoast tumor*) usually refers to a primary lung carcinoma that is located in the lung apex and involves the adjacent pleura, chest wall, brachial plexus, or subclavian vessels (Fig. 65-5). Typically, this tumor manifests clinically as chest, shoulder, and arm pain with paresthesias, along with Horner syndrome (ipsilateral ptosis, miosis, and anhidrosis) caused by invasion of the stellate ganglion. Squamous cell carcinoma is the most common subtype involved, and adenocarcinoma is the second most common.

19. Describe the major imaging findings related to lung carcinoma.

- A pulmonary or endobronchial nodule or mass is seen that may be associated with obstructive atelectasis or pneumonitis; thoracic lymphadenopathy; pleural, mediastinal, or chest wall involvement; or distant metastatic disease (Fig. 65-6).

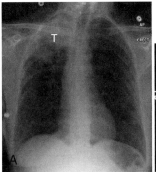
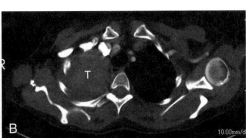
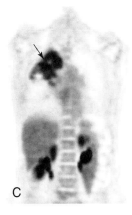

Figure 65-5. A, Pancoast tumor secondary to NSCLC on chest radiograph. Note right apical pulmonary tumor (*T*) with lobulated margins. **B,** Pancoast tumor secondary to NSCLC on CT. Note soft tissue attenuation right apical pulmonary tumor (*T*). **C,** Pancoast tumor secondary to NSCLC on FDG PET. Note avid FDG uptake in right apical pulmonary tumor (*arrow*).

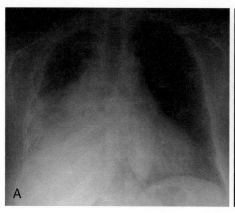
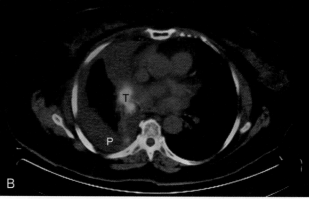

Figure 65-6. **A,** Unresectable NSCLC associated with malignant pleural effusion on chest radiograph. Note soft tissue fullness in right hilum along with obscuration of right hemidiaphragm owing to large right pleural effusion. **B,** Unresectable NSCLC associated with malignant pleural effusion on FDG PET/CT. Note soft tissue tumor (*T*) in right hilum along with large loculated right pleural effusion (*P*) that has areas of FDG uptake.

- Sometimes, obstructive segmental or lobar atelectasis may be the only sign of lung carcinoma on chest radiography, particularly if associated air bronchograms are not present. When obstructive atelectasis is associated with focal convexity centrally owing to the nodule or mass with concavity more distally on chest radiography, an S-shaped smooth fissural margin may be seen that is known as the "S sign of Golden" (Fig. 65-7).
- Unilateral hilar lymphadenopathy; a unilateral pleural effusion (particularly when present on the left); abrupt cutoff of a bronchus (the "bronchial cutoff" sign); and obscuration of a hilar, mediastinal, or diaphragmatic structure (the "silhouette" sign) are other chest radiographic findings of pulmonary malignancy. BAC may appear as a solitary nodule; multiple ground-glass, solid, or mixed-density pulmonary nodules; or solitary, multiple, or diffuse foci of chronic pulmonary consolidation. Cavitation or cystic change may be present (Fig. 65-8).

20. Summarize the tumor node metastasis (TNM) staging system for NSCLC.
See Table 65-2.

21. When is NSCLC generally considered unresectable?
When NSCLC is stage IIIb (i.e., with the presence of invasion of vital mediastinal structures, associated malignant pleural effusion, satellite tumor in the primary tumor lobe, or unresectable lymphadenopathy) or stage IV (i.e., with the presence of distant metastases), it is generally considered unresectable. Symptoms and signs are rarely present until the disease is advanced in stage and more likely to be unresectable.

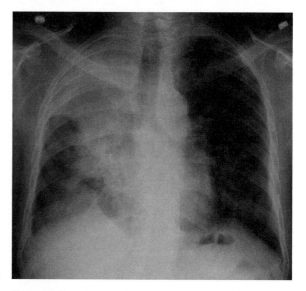

Figure 65-7. NSCLC causing lobar atelectasis with "(reverse) S sign of Golden" on chest radiograph. Note right upper lobe obstructive atelectasis with S-shaped fissural margin with focal convexity centrally owing to central mass and concavity more distally. Note lack of air bronchograms typical of obstructive atelectasis.

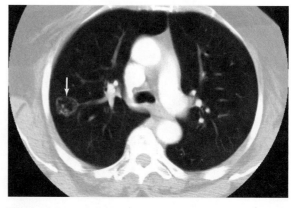

Figure 65-8. BAC subtype of NSCLC on CT. Note SPN (*arrow*) in right lung with cystic or cavitary change.

Table 65-2. TNM Staging System of Non–Small Cell Lung Carcinoma

	T = Primary Tumor
T0	No evidence of primary tumor
T1	≤3 cm, surrounded by lung/visceral pleural, no invasion of main stem bronchus
T2	>3 cm, involvement of main stem bronchus ≥2 cm from carina, invasion of visceral pleura; obstructive atelectasis of part of the lung
T3	Invasion of chest wall, mediastinal pleura, diaphragm, parietal pericardium, main stem bronchus <2 cm from carina; obstructive atelectasis of entire lung
T4	Invasion of mediastinal structures, malignant pleural effusion, or satellite tumor in primary tumor lobe
	N = Regional Lymphadenopathy
N0	No regional lymph node metastases
N1	Ipsilateral hilar, peribronchial, or intrapulmonary lymphadenopathy
N2	Ipsilateral mediastinal or subcarinal lymphadenopathy
N3	Supraclavicular, scalene, contralateral mediastinal, or hilar lymphadenopathy
	M = Distant Metastasis
M0	No distant metastasis
M1	Distant metastasis
	Stage
0	Carcinoma in situ
Ia	T1N0M0
Ib	T2N0M0
IIa	T1N1M0
IIb	T2N1M0, T3N0M0
IIIa	T3N1M0, T1-3N2M0
IIIb	T4N0-3M0, T1-3N3M0
IV	T0-4N0-3M1

Note: Any N2 lesion is at least stage IIIa, any T4 or N3 lesion is at least stage IIIb, and any M1 lesion is stage IV. Patients with stage 0 to IIIa lesions are generally treated with surgery, whereas patients with stage IIIb and IV lesions are generally treated with medical therapy.

22. **Are there any reliable screening tests for lung carcinoma? What is the National Lung Screening Trial (NLST)?**

    At this time, no laboratory or imaging screening test has been shown to decrease lung cancer mortality rates. NLST is an ongoing multicenter prospective trial that is comparing screening with frontal chest radiography with screening with thin-section, low-dose chest CT for a decrease in lung cancer–specific mortality. The trial is expected to be concluded in 2011. Research is also currently ongoing in the search for biomarkers that could potentially be used as screening tools for the presence of lung carcinoma or as indicators of high risk for future development of lung carcinoma.

Key Points: Pulmonary Nodules

1. Be aware of the major blind spots on frontal chest radiography: the lung apices where the clavicles and ribs overlap, the hilar regions where vascular structures abound, the retrocardiac region, and the lung bases where there is superimposition with the upper abdominal soft tissue.
2. If you see lobar or segmental atelectasis on chest radiography, particularly without air bronchograms, be suspicious of an obstructive endobronchial lesion such as a lung carcinoma, and, at the minimum, get a short-term follow-up chest radiograph.
3. If a pulmonary infiltrate does not resolve over time despite treatment with antimicrobial agents, be suspicious of a potential bronchioloalveolar cell subtype of lung carcinoma.
4. The best way to prevent lung cancer is through prevention (i.e., by not smoking).
5. Although mucoid impaction of a bronchus may mimic a pulmonary nodule on chest radiography, one should exclude an endobronchial lesion as the cause for mucus retention in a bronchus if resolution is not seen on follow-up imaging.

23. Name some treatment options for lung carcinoma.

Surgical resection (typically lobectomy with lymph node resection), chemotherapy, and radiation therapy may be used depending on the stage of disease and the histology of the tumor. Cessation of tobacco use is also part of treatment. Newer techniques such as percutaneous ablation of focal lung or bronchial tumors are currently under investigation.

24. Describe the imaging findings of pulmonary metastases.

Solitary or multiple pulmonary and endobronchial nodules or masses are often seen (Fig. 65-9), which may be ill-defined or well circumscribed, ground-glass or solid in density, and often associated with metastases to other thoracic or extrathoracic anatomic locations. Depending on the underlying primary malignancy, the lesions may be

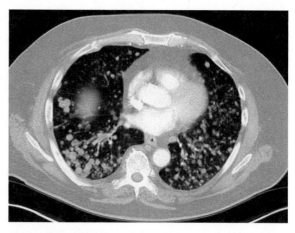

Figure 65-9. Pulmonary metastases are CT. Note multiple, variably sized, smoothly marginated nodules throughout lungs.

homogeneous or heterogeneous with cystic, necrotic, calcific, or hemorrhagic change, and may vary in size from very small (miliary) nodules to very large "cannonball" masses. Pneumothorax is often associated with pulmonary metastatic disease from osteogenic sarcoma. Overall, the lungs are an extremely common site of metastatic disease.

25. What is lymphangitic carcinomatosis?

Lymphangitic carcinomatosis is the hematogenous spread of metastatic disease to lung interstitium with subsequent lymphatic obstruction, interstitial edema, and fibrosis. Primary tumors of the breast, lung, stomach, pancreas, ovary, and cervix are often associated with lymphangitic carcinomatosis. On chest radiography, the lungs may appear clear, or they may show a central linear pattern of interstitial thickening that is commonly bilateral, but asymmetric in distribution between the lungs. On CT, typical smooth or nodular thickening of the interlobular septa is seen often with peribronchovascular thickening and asymmetric involvement of the lungs bilaterally (Fig. 65-10).

26. What are pulmonary carcinoid tumors?

These are rare neuroendocrine neoplasms that range from low-grade typical carcinoids to more aggressive atypical carcinoids. They are not related to tobacco use and occur slightly more commonly in women. Most arise centrally in an endobronchial location and are commonly associated with segmental or lobar obstructive atelectasis or pneumonitis, whereas the remainder appear as well-circumscribed peripheral pulmonary nodules or masses. These lesions typically show avid enhancement, and 40% may be associated with internal calcification. Carcinoid syndrome is rarely associated with pulmonary carcinoid tumors.

27. What is a pulmonary hamartoma?

Pulmonary hamartoma is the most common benign neoplasm of the lung and typically manifests as an asymptomatic well-circumscribed SPN, typically during the fourth through seventh decades of life. Pathologically, these are

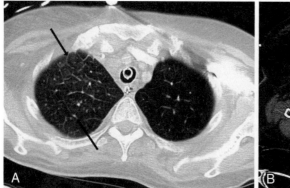
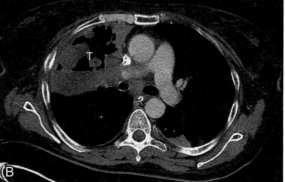

Figure 65-10. A, Lymphangitic carcinomatosis in NSCLC on CT. Note smooth asymmetric thickening of interlobular septa (*arrows*) in right lung. **B,** Lymphangitic carcinomatosis in NSCLC on CT. Note large cavitary tumor (*T*) in right lung secondary to lung carcinoma.

mesenchymal tumors that have foci of mature cartilage separated by islands of fat and bronchial epithelium, often with fibrosis, calcification, or ossification. Typical CT findings include a smoothly marginated SPN that often contains visible fat or dense foci of calcification or ossification or both.

28. What is congenital bronchial atresia?

Congenital bronchial atresia is due to atresia or stenosis of a bronchus at or near its origin, most often seen in the apicoposterior segment of the left upper lobe. Imaging findings include hyperlucency with air trapping and decreased vascularity to the portion of lung supplied by the involved bronchus, along with a nonenhancing hilar mass (bronchocele) or nonenhancing branching soft tissue opacities usually with bronchial dilation owing to mucoid impaction. Congenital bronchial atresia can appear as SPN on chest radiography.

BIBLIOGRAPHY

[1] C.I. Henschke, D.F. Yankelevitz, R. Mirtcheva, et al., CT screening for lung cancer: frequency and significance of part-solid and nonsolid nodules, AJR Am. J. Roentgenol. 178 (2002) 1053–1057.
[2] A. Jemal, R.C. Tiwari, T. Murray, et al., Cancer statistics, 2004, CA Cancer. J. Clin. 54 (2004) 8–29.
[3] J.L. Leef 3rd, J.S. Klein, The solitary pulmonary nodule, Radiol. Clin. North Am. 40 (2002) ix 123–143.
[4] A. Matthies, M. Hickeson, A. Cuchiara, A. Alavi, Dual time point 18F-FDG PET for the evaluation of pulmonary nodules, J. Nucl. Med. 43 (2002) 871–875.
[5] S. Takashima, S. Sone, F. Li, et al., Small solitary pulmonary nodules (l1 cm) detected at population-based CT screening for lung cancer: reliable high-resolution CT features of benign lesions, AJR Am. J. Roentgenol. 180 (2003) 955–964.
[6] B.B. Tan, K.R. Flaherty, E.A. Kazerooni, M.D. lannettoni, The solitary pulmonary nodule, Chest 123 (2003) 89S–96S.
[7] A.W. Tang, H.A. Moss, R.J. Robertson, The solitary pulmonary nodule, Eur. J. Radiol. 45 (2003) 69–77.

66

INTERSTITIAL LUNG DISEASE

*Wallace T. Miller, Jr., MD, and
Drew A. Torigian, MD*

1. **What radiographic features distinguish interstitial diseases from air space diseases?**

   Two primary characteristics radiographically distinguish interstitial from air space diseases. First, interstitial diseases displace little of the air within the lung, whereas air space diseases displace large amounts of air. Interstitial diseases change the overall opacity of the lung very little, whereas air space diseases in most cases dramatically increase the opacity (whiteness) of the lung on chest radiography. Second, interstitial diseases appear as increases in small nodules (generally <5 mm in diameter) or thin lines (<5 mm in width) (or both) within the lung, whereas air space diseases appear as indistinctly marginated patches of opacity. See Fig. 66-1 for the normal appearance of the lungs on frontal chest radiography.

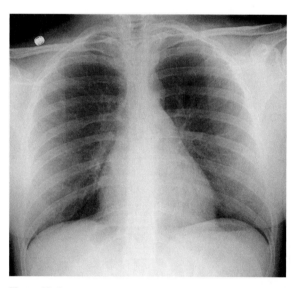

Figure 66-1. Normal frontal chest radiograph of the lungs. Note normal sharp delineation of branching vessels from the bilateral hila outward.

2. **What factors influence the likelihood of one interstitial disease over another interstitial disease?**

   Three primary factors affect the likelihood of a given interstitial disease.

   - The relative incidence of a given disease in the general population. Typical presentations of common diseases are most likely, followed by atypical presentations of common diseases, typical presentations of uncommon diseases, and atypical presentations of uncommon diseases.
   - The clinical history of the patient.
   - The radiographic pattern of the interstitial disease.

3. **What is the most common interstitial abnormality identified on chest radiography?**

   Interstitial pulmonary edema, usually caused by congestive heart failure, is the most common interstitial abnormality encountered in daily practice. A diagnosis of interstitial pulmonary edema should be considered in all cases of interstitial abnormality detected on a chest radiograph. In many cases, it might be advisable to diurese the patient and repeat the chest radiograph as the first diagnostic test.

4. **Name the most common interstitial abnormalities other than interstitial pulmonary edema.**

   Idiopathic pulmonary fibrosis and sarcoidosis are the most common chronic interstitial disorders in the United States and should be among the first diagnoses considered when encountering a chest radiograph with an interstitial abnormality.

5. **What radiographic characteristics help determine the diagnosis of interstitial disorders?**

   Interstitial abnormalities may be roughly subdivided into abnormalities that produce small round opacities (*nodular interstitial diseases*) and abnormalities that produce small networks of holes (*reticular interstitial diseases*). In this chapter, we describe one nodular pattern of interstitial disease and the three following reticular patterns of interstitial disease: the peripheral reticular pattern, the linear pattern, and the cystic pattern.

6. What is the appearance of a nodular interstitial pattern on chest radiography?

A normal chest radiograph typically shows many small nodular opacities that represent normal blood vessels end on. In most cases, these small nodules can be recognized as blood vessels because they overlap with a small line of similar diameter, which represents an adjacent branch of the pulmonary vascular tree. The nodular pattern of interstitial lung disease appears as increased numbers of small nodular opacities (<10 mm in diameter) that are randomly distributed throughout the lung parenchyma. These small nodules do not overlap with the normal vascular lines of the lung (Figs. 66-2 and 66-3).

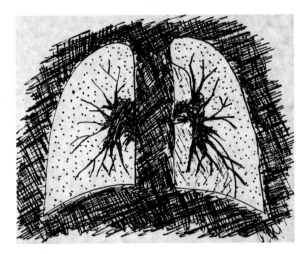

Figure 66-2. Nodular pattern of interstitial lung disease.

7. What disorders cause nodular interstitial diseases?

Three broad groups of disorders cause nodular interstitial diseases:

- Granulomatous lung diseases
- Nodular pneumoconioses
- Small metastases

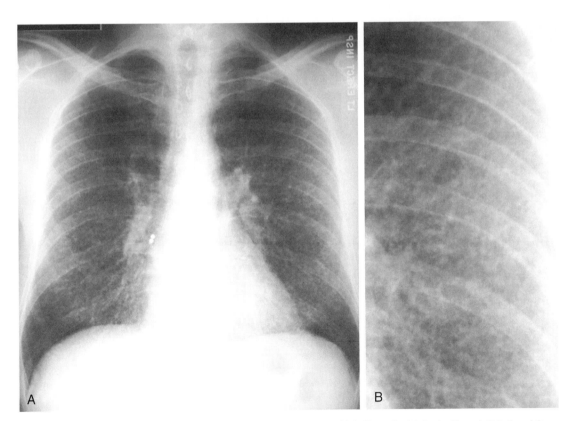

Figure 66-3. A, Nodular pattern of interstitial lung disease caused by cryptococcal infection on frontal chest radiograph. Note the subtle, tiny nodular densities throughout lung fields bilaterally. **B,** Magnified view of chest radiograph. Note the subtle, tiny nodular densities throughout lung.

8. Discuss granulomatous lung diseases that cause nodular interstitial disease.

Sarcoidosis is the most common granulomatous interstitial lung disease to cause a micronodular pattern. This idiopathic disorder typically manifests in middle-aged individuals, especially African Americans. Miliary infections also cause a small nodular pattern and are typified by miliary tuberculosis, but also include miliary spread of histoplasmosis, cryptococcosis, coccidioidomycosis, and blastomycosis. These infections typically affect immunocompromised individuals, such as patients with human immunodeficiency virus (HIV) infection, patients who have undergone organ transplantation, or patients with a history of long-term steroid use. Many physicians are unaware that extrinsic allergic alveolitis or hypersensitivity pneumonitis not only causes a granulomatous interstitial fibrosis, but may also produce an interstitial nodular pattern of lung disease. Langerhans cell histiocytosis, also known as *eosinophilic granuloma of the lung,* may also produce a nodular pattern of interstitial lung disease. In most cases, pulmonary Langerhans cell histiocytosis is associated with a history of smoking, and typically manifests as persistent cough or dyspnea or both in young and middle-aged adults. In the early stages of disease, the patient develops small nodular areas of interstitial fibrosis. As the disorder progresses, cystic lesions may develop in association with an obstructive lung disease.

9. Discuss pneumoconioses and tumors that lead to nodular interstitial lung disease.

Pneumoconioses that may produce a micronodular interstitial pattern are silicosis, coal workers' pneumoconiosis, talcosis, and berylliosis. Pneumoconioses are diffuse interstitial lung diseases caused by inorganic dusts, most often related to occupational exposures. Mining, sandblasting, gravestone engraving, and pottery are some occupations in which workers may be exposed to silica dust with resultant silicosis; as identified in the name, coal workers' pneumoconiosis is seen in coal miners. Berylliosis is an uncommon chronic pneumoconiosis that may be encountered in individuals who mine beryllium, who manufacture beryllium ceramics, or who previously manufactured beryllium lighting (these types of lights are no longer manufactured because of the high risk of acute and chronic berylliosis). Talcosis may occur as a result of the mining of talc or excessive inhalation of talcum powder and in intravenous drug abusers. Thyroid carcinoma is the prototypic tumor that produces thousands of tiny micronodular metastases and may appear as a nodular interstitial lung disease. Breast cancer may also produce this pattern of metastasis; other primary tumors rarely produce a micronodular pattern of lung metastasis.

10. What is the chest radiographic staging system for sarcoidosis, and what is the clinical significance?

Table 66-1 summarizes the staging system for sarcoidosis. The higher the stage of sarcoidosis, the greater the likelihood that the patient will experience chronic respiratory deficits.

Table 66-1. Chest Radiographic Staging System for Sarcoidosis

STAGE	RADIOGRAPHIC APPEARANCE
0	Chest radiograph appears normal
I	Chest radiographic evidence of hilar or mediastinal lymphadenopathy without evidence of interstitial disease
II	Chest radiographic evidence of hilar or mediastinal lymphadenopathy and evidence of interstitial lung disease
III	Chest radiographic evidence of interstitial disease without evidence of hilar or mediastinal lymphadenopathy
IV	Chest radiographic evidence of interstitial fibrosis with distortion of pulmonary structures, such as blood vessels, without evidence of hilar or mediastinal lymphadenopathy

11. Give some examples of hypersensitivity pneumonitis (extrinsic allergic alveolitis).

Farmer's lung is the prototypic example of a hypersensitivity pneumonitis. There are a wide variety of other hypersensitivity pneumonitides; some of the many other causes are listed in Table 66-2. These disorders represent an allergic lung reaction to various organic dusts that can initially manifest as capillary leak pulmonary edema, but chronically result in granulomatous interstitial fibrosis. In most cases, the offending antigens are microorganisms that grow within decaying vegetable matter. Antigens from these organisms are delivered to the lung via inhalation of dust or aerosolized contaminated water. Notable exceptions to this general concept are bird-related hypersensitivity pneumonitides. In bird fancier's lung, hypersensitivity occurs against bird-related antigens, such as those found in bird feathers.

12. Why do intravenous drug abusers get talcosis?

Not all intravenous drug abusers get talcosis. The process that can result in talcosis is the intravenous injection of oral medications. These medications are ground into a fine powder, suspended in fluid, and injected intravenously. Pills contain fillers, including talc and methylcellulose, which are inorganic substances that embolize to the lung

Table 66-2. Causes of Hypersensitivity Pneumonitis

EXPOSURES	CAUSES
Occupational	Organic dust
Farmer's lung	Hay
Baker's lung	Flour
Sugar cane worker's lung	Sugar cane dust
Cotton worker's lung	Cotton dust
Mushroom worker's lung	Mushrooms
Hobbies	
Bird fancier's lung	Bird feathers
Other exposures	
Down pillows and comforters	Bird feathers
Hot tubs	Aerosolized water
Humidifiers	Aerosolized water

microvasculature and result in a foreign body giant cell granulomatous reaction, which may appear as small nodules on chest radiography.

13. **What radiographic feature of nodular pneumoconioses is most strongly associated with respiratory deficits?**

Progressive massive fibrosis (PMF), also know as *conglomerate masses,* is the radiographic feature most strongly associated with respiratory deficits. In PMF, the small nodular areas of fibrosis associated with nodular pneumoconioses progressively coalesce into large (>3 cm) fibrotic masses. These masses are typically found in the upper lung zones and result in fibrotic distortion of the surrounding lung parenchyma. All of the nodular pneumoconioses can cause PMF, but it is most strongly associated with silicosis. Many patients with simple silicosis (nodular interstitial disease without PMF) are clinically asymptomatic. Nearly all patients with complicated silicosis (nodular interstitial disease with PMF) have dyspnea, however. The causes of the nodular interstitial pattern are reviewed in Table 66-3.

Table 66-3. Causes of Nodular Interstitial Lung Disease Pattern

CATEGORY	DISEASES
Granulomatous diseases	Sarcoidosis
	Miliary infections
	Tuberculosis
	Histoplasmosis
	Coccidioidomycosis
	Cryptococcosis
	Blastomycosis
	Hypersensitivity pneumonitis
	LCH (eosinophilic granuloma)
Nodular pneumoconiosis	Silicosis
	Coal workers' pneumoconiosis
	Berylliosis
	Talcosis
Metastasis	Thyroid carcinoma
	Other malignancies

LCH, Langerhans cell histiocytosis.

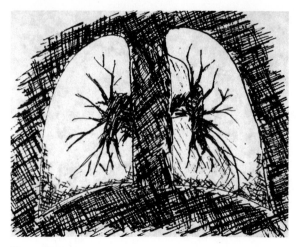

Figure 66-4. Peripheral reticular pattern of interstitial lung disease.

14. What are the radiographic characteristics of the peripheral reticular pattern?

The peripheral reticular pattern has two distinguishing features:

- Small size of the holes (typically <5 mm) seen within a network of fine crisscrossing linear opacities
- Peripheral and basilar distribution of the network

The network typically is seen filling the costophrenic angles on frontal and lateral chest radiographs (Figs. 66-4 and 66-5).

15. Which diseases cause the peripheral reticular pattern?

Although various disorders may occasionally result in the peripheral reticular pattern, most cases are caused by idiopathic pulmonary fibrosis (IPF), a connective tissue disorder, or asbestosis.

16. What demographic features can help distinguish the cause of the peripheral reticular pattern?

Asbestosis and IPF are disorders of elderly patients, usually individuals older than 50, whereas connective tissue disorders tend to affect younger individuals, often in their 30s and 40s. Patients must have had an extensive exposure to asbestos dust to acquire asbestosis. Nearly all patients with asbestosis have an occupational exposure to asbestos, such as from mining, roofing, car brake shoe repair, shipyard work, or boiler making. Asbestosis is almost exclusively seen in men because few women have sufficient asbestos dust exposure to acquire the disease. Connective tissue disorders are more commonly encountered in women, and more patients with connective tissue–related interstitial disease are women.

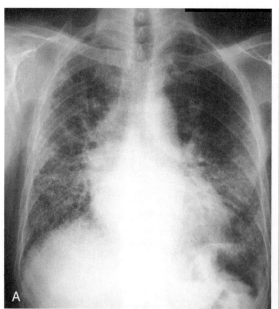
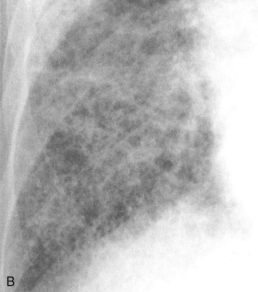

Figure 66-5. A, Peripheral reticular pattern of interstitial lung disease secondary to idiopathic pulmonary fibrosis on frontal chest radiograph. Note peripheral and basilar distribution. **B,** Magnified view of chest radiograph. Note the network of fine crisscrossing linear opacities in peripheral and basilar distribution of the lungs forming small holes between opacities.

17. Which connective tissue disorders can result in interstitial disease?

Scleroderma, or *progressive systemic sclerosis,* has the highest incidence of interstitial fibrosis among all connective tissue disorders. *Rheumatoid arthritis* has the highest prevalence of interstitial disease because it is one of the most common connective tissue disorders and may occasionally cause interstitial fibrosis. *Dermatomyositis/polymyositis* may also result in interstitial fibrosis. By virtue of its potential to overlap with progressive systemic sclerosis, rheumatoid arthritis, or dermatomyositis/polymyositis, *mixed connective tissue disorder* may also cause interstitial fibrosis. *Systemic lupus erythematosus* is one of the most prevalent connective tissue disorders, but only rarely produces clinically significant interstitial fibrosis. Although pathologic and radiologic studies may show mild abnormalities, it is quite rare for patients with systemic lupus erythematosus to have respiratory symptoms related to interstitial fibrosis. When these disorders cause interstitial fibrosis, they produce a peripheral reticular interstitial pattern on chest radiography.

18. Are there any imaging features that can help distinguish the cause of the peripheral reticular pattern?

In most cases, there are no imaging features that help distinguish the different causes of the peripheral reticular pattern. Occasionally, extrapulmonary findings help, however, in the differential diagnosis of the peripheral reticular pattern. Approximately two thirds of patients with asbestosis also have asbestos-related pleural plaques. Patients with progressive systemic sclerosis may have a radiographically identifiable dilated esophagus as a result of CREST syndrome; *CREST* stands for *c*alcinosis cutis, *R*aynaud phenomenon, *e*sophageal dysfunction, *s*clerodactyly, and *t*elangiectasia. Patients with rheumatoid arthritis may have erosions of the distal clavicles as a result of acromioclavicular arthritis. Causes of the peripheral reticular pattern of interstitial lung disease are reviewed in Table 66-4.

Table 66-4. Causes of Peripheral Reticular Interstitial Lung Disease Pattern

Idiopathic pulmonary fibrosis
Connective tissue disorders
Scleroderma, or progressive systemic sclerosis
Rheumatoid arthritis
Polymyositis/dermatomyositis
Mixed connective tissue disorder
Systemic lupus erythematosus
Asbestosis

19. Describe the imaging characteristics of the linear pattern on chest radiography.

The lines visible on a normal chest radiograph represent the branching pulmonary arteries and veins. These begin centrally and radiate from the hilum toward the periphery of the lung. The linear pattern appears as increased numbers of lines radiating from the central hila bilaterally. In addition, the linear pattern may produce Kerley B lines. These are thin horizontal lines 1 to 2 cm long, extending from the lateral chest wall toward the central lung (Figs. 66-6 and 66-7). The most common cause of the linear pattern is congestive heart failure, and to the degree that an interstitial abnormality resembles congestive heart failure, it is more likely to represent the linear pattern of interstitial disease. Novice radiologists should take care not to overdiagnose the linear interstitial pattern. There is a wide variation in the normal appearance of chest radiographs. If one is unsure of whether there is an interstitial abnormality present on a chest radiograph, it is usually best to assume that the examination is normal.

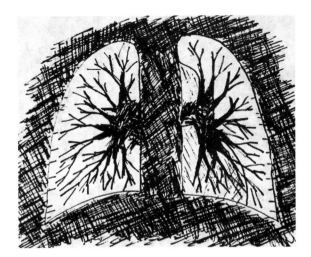

Figure 66-6. Linear pattern of interstitial lung disease.

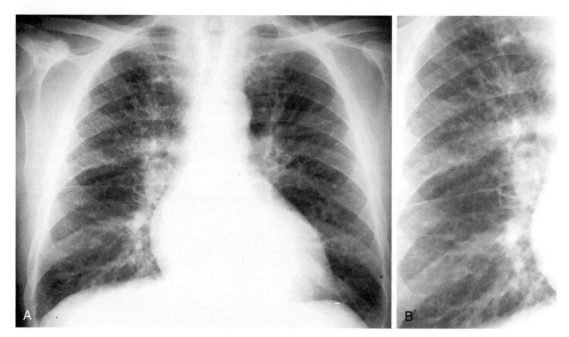

Figure 66-7. A, Linear pattern of interstitial lung disease caused by congestive heart failure on frontal chest radiograph. Note symmetrically increased number of lines radiating from the bilateral hila. **B,** Central linear pattern of interstitial lung disease caused by congestive heart failure on magnified view of chest radiograph. Note the symmetrically increased number of lines radiating from the bilateral hila.

20. What disorders cause the linear pattern of interstitial disease?

Causes of the linear interstitial pattern include:

- Interstitial pulmonary edema
- Lymphangitic carcinomatosis
- Sarcoidosis
- Diffuse pneumonia

Congestive heart failure and other causes of *interstitial pulmonary edema* are the most common causes of the linear pattern. In nearly all cases, the presence of a linear interstitial pattern should be assumed to represent interstitial pulmonary edema. *Lymphangitic carcinomatosis* is the most common chronic cause for the linear pattern. This is a form of hematogenous metastasis that grows along the interstitial framework of the lung, rather than growing concentrically as nodules. Breast and lung cancers are the malignancies most likely to cause a pattern of lymphangitic metastasis. Gastric, pancreatic, and ovarian carcinomas are other causes of lymphangitic carcinomatosis. *Sarcoidosis* typically causes peribronchial granulomas, which may also result in interstitial lung disease with a pattern of lines radiating from the hilum of the lung, producing a linear pattern. Very rarely, some *diffuse pneumonias* such as *Mycoplasma pneumoniae, Pneumocystis carinii (jiroveci)* pneumonia, and viral pneumonia appear as a linear interstitial pattern.

21. Are there any imaging clues that may help to distinguish the cause of the linear interstitial pattern?

In most cases, no imaging clues help to distinguish the cause of the linear pattern of interstitial disease. One notable exception is the recognition of a markedly asymmetric linear pattern, in which one lung is considerably more affected than the other. This imaging finding is virtually always associated with lymphangitic carcinomatosis.

22. What are the imaging characteristics of the cystic pattern of interstitial lung disease?

This pattern is characterized by a group of curved lines that produce a network of fine ring shadows in the more central lung. Although a reticular pattern, the cystic pattern is quite distinct from the peripheral reticular pattern. In the cystic pattern, the holes are, on average, approximately 10 mm in diameter, which are much larger than the holes seen in the peripheral reticular pattern. The rings of the cystic pattern are distributed in the more central lung, whereas the peripheral reticular pattern characteristically affects the subpleural and basilar lung (Figs. 66-8 and 66-9).

23. What disorders produce the cystic interstitial pattern?

The cystic interstitial pattern is the least common of the interstitial patterns on chest radiography, and the most common cause of the cystic pattern is not interstitial lung disease, but emphysema. *Emphysema* usually appears as a decrease in the number and conspicuity of the normal lines seen on chest radiography. It has been recognized for many years, however, that emphysema occasionally appears as an increase in the number and conspicuity of interstitial lines. When emphysema does this, it appears in the cystic interstitial pattern. *Diffuse bronchiectasis* may also appear as many ring shadows distributed throughout the lung parenchyma. Two rare disorders that may also cause this pattern are *Langerhans cell histiocytosis* (which was previously discussed along with the nodular pattern) and lymphangioleiomyomatosis. *Lymphangioleiomyomatosis* is a rare hormonally mediated disorder of young and middle-aged women. Proliferation of interstitial smooth muscle results in air trapping and production of small uniform cystic spaces in the lung. Table 66-5 lists the causes of the cystic interstitial lung disease pattern.

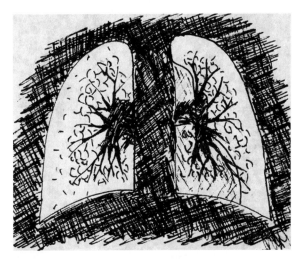

Figure 66-8. Cystic pattern of interstitial lung disease.

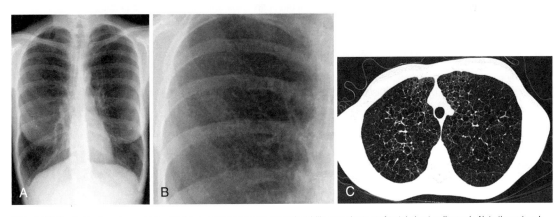

Figure 66-9. A, Cystic pattern of interstitial lung disease caused by eosinophilic granuloma on frontal chest radiograph. Note the network of fine ring shadows in the more central lung and the larger holes between opacities (compared with the smaller holes in peripheral reticular pattern). **B,** Magnified view of chest radiograph. Note the network of fine ring shadows in the more central lung and the larger holes between opacities (compared with the smaller holes in peripheral reticular pattern). **C,** Cystic pattern of interstitial lung disease caused by eosinophilic granuloma on CT. Note the multiple cysts of variable size throughout the lungs.

Table 66-5. Causes of Cystic Interstitial Lung Disease Pattern

Emphysema
Langerhans cell histiocytosis (eosinophilic granuloma)
Lymphangioleiomyomatosis
Diffuse bronchiectasis
Cystic fibrosis
Dysmotile cilia syndrome
Allergic bronchopulmonary aspergillosis
Immunodeficiency states
Common variable immunodeficiency
Hyper-IgE syndrome
Other

Key Points: Interstitial Lung Disease

1. Interstitial pulmonary edema, usually caused by congestive heart failure, is the most common interstitial abnormality encountered in daily practice.
2. The nodular pattern of interstitial lung disease appears as increased numbers of nodular opacities (<10 mm) that are randomly distributed throughout the lung parenchyma. The three broad groups of disorders that cause nodular interstitial disease are granulomatous lung diseases, nodular pneumoconioses, and small metastases.
3. The two distinguishing features of the peripheral reticular pattern of interstitial lung disease are the small size of the holes (typically <5 mm) seen within a network of fine crisscrossing linear opacities and a peripheral and basilar distribution of this network. Most cases are caused by IPF, a connective tissue disorder, or asbestosis.
4. The linear pattern of interstitial lung disease appears as increased numbers of lines radiating from the hila centrally. This pattern also may produce peripheral Kerley B lines. The most common cause of this pattern is congestive heart failure, although lymphangitic carcinomatosis is the most common chronic cause of this pattern.
5. The cystic pattern is characterized by a group of curved lines that produce a network of fine ring shadows in the more central lung with larger holes than are seen in the peripheral reticular pattern. The most common cause of this pattern is emphysema.

24. What disorders cause diffuse bronchiectasis?

Although various disorders may result in bronchiectasis, only a few diseases cause widespread bronchiectasis that involves most of the lung parenchyma. The most common of these is cystic fibrosis. Other diseases include dysmotile cilia syndrome; allergic bronchopulmonary aspergillosis; and various immunodeficiency states, such as common variable immunodeficiency syndrome, natural killer cell deficiency, and hyper-IgE syndrome.

25. Are there any imaging features that help to distinguish the cause of the cystic pattern?

In many cases, the disorders that cause the cystic pattern produce radiographically indistinguishable disease. One notable exception is diffuse bronchiectasis. The cystic spaces caused by bronchiectasis typically produce thick-walled, distinct ring shadows, whereas the other disorders often cause very faint rings (see Table 66-5 for causes of the cystic interstitial pattern).

26. When is computed tomography (CT) scanning indicated for the evaluation of interstitial lung disease?

CT is more sensitive and more specific than chest radiography for interstitial abnormalities. In many advanced cases with obvious chest radiographic findings, no further imaging is necessary. Patients with apparently normal or minimally abnormal chest radiographs in whom there is a clinical suspicion of interstitial lung disease should receive a thin-section chest CT scan to evaluate better for the presence of interstitial lung disease. Patients with chest radiographs that are nonspecific may benefit from a CT study, which in many cases allows the clinician to narrow the differential diagnosis. Lastly, CT provides improved characterization of the extent of disease. In cases in which therapeutic decisions are based on imaging evidence of progression, stability, or regression of disease, CT scanning is indicated.

27. What type of CT scan is indicated for the evaluation of interstitial lung disease?

CT scanning has inherently less spatial resolution than standard chest radiography. Because interstitial diseases are typified by very fine spatial abnormalities, it is necessary to maximize the spatial resolution of CT images. The spatial resolution is done by minimizing the collimation of the CT scanner. Collimation, at most, should be 1.5 mm. Many multislice spiral scanners obtain images at this resolution in nearly all studies, although older single-slice spiral and nonspiral scanners require special imaging protocols to minimize the slice collimation. These imaging protocols are often called high-resolution scans because of the improved spatial resolution that is characteristic of the studies.

BIBLIOGRAPHY

[1] E.A. Kazerooni, High-resolution CT of the lungs, AJR Am. J. Roentgenol. 177 (2001) 501–519.
[2] W.T. Miller Jr., Radiographic evaluation of diffuse interstitial lung disease: review of a dying art, Semin. Ultrasound CT MR 23 (2002) 324–338.
[3] N. Muller, R. Fraser, N. Colman, P.D. Pare, Radiologic Diagnosis of Diseases of the Chest, Saunders, Philadelphia, 2001.
[4] W.R. Webb, N.L. Muller, D. Naidich, High-Resolution CT of the Lung, third ed., Lippincott-Raven, New York, 2001.

MEDIASTINAL DISEASES

Drew A. Torigian, MD, Charles T. Lau, MD, and
Wallace T. Miller, Jr., MD

CHAPTER 67

1. Describe the anatomy of the mediastinum.

The mediastinum is located centrally within the thorax between the pleural cavities laterally, the sternum anteriorly, the spine posteriorly, the thoracic inlet superiorly, and the diaphragm inferiorly. It is usually divided into anterior, middle, and posterior compartments to help categorize tumors and diseases by their site of origin and location. Lesions that arise in these different compartments are generally related to the anatomic structures located within the compartments. Fig. 67-1A shows the normal appearance of the mediastinum on frontal chest radiography.

2. What are the three compartments of the mediastinum?

- The *anterior mediastinal compartment* is the space posterior to the sternum and anterior to the heart and trachea extending from the thoracic inlet to the diaphragm; it contains the thymus gland, thyroid gland, fat, and lymph nodes.
- The *middle mediastinal compartment* is the space that contains the heart and pericardium, and the ascending aorta and aortic arch, brachiocephalic vessels, venae cavae, main pulmonary arteries and veins, trachea and bronchi, fat, and lymph nodes.
- The *posterior mediastinal compartment* is the space posterior to the middle mediastinal compartment that contains the descending thoracic aorta, esophagus, azygos and hemiazygos veins, autonomic ganglia and nerves, thoracic duct, fat, and lymph nodes.

Fig. 67-1B delineates the three compartments of the mediastinum on lateral chest radiography.

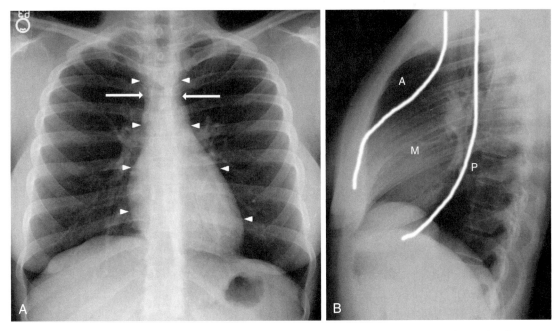

Figure 67-1. A, Normal frontal chest radiograph. Note normal width of mediastinum (*between arrows*) and sharp demarcation of mediastinal contours (*arrowheads*) against adjacent lungs. **B,** Normal lateral chest radiograph. Note lines separating anterior (*A*), middle (*M*), and posterior (*P*) compartments of mediastinum.

3. List the differential diagnosis of major anterior mediastinal lesions.
In the following list, an asterisk (*) indicates the most common causes:

THYMIC MASSES

- Lymphoma*
- Thymoma*
- Thymic carcinoma
- Thymic carcinoid
- Thymolipoma
- Thymic cyst
- Thymic hyperplasia

THYROID MASSES

- Thyroid goiter*
- Thyroid cyst
- Thyroid adenoma
- Thyroid carcinoma

GERM CELL TUMORS

- Teratoma and teratocarcinoma*
- Seminoma
- Mixed germ cell tumors

4. List the differential diagnosis of major middle mediastinal lesions.
In the following list, an asterisk (*) indicates the most common causes:

- Goiter
- Lymphadenopathy
- Metastatic disease* (lung cancer is the most common etiologic factor)
- Lymphoma (non-Hodgkin lymphoma and Hodgkinlymphoma) or leukemia*
- Granulomatous infection (fungus, tuberculosis, nontuberculous mycobacterium)
- Sarcoidosis
- Inhalational lung disease (silicosis, coal workers' pneumoconiosis, or berylliosis)
- Castleman disease
- Aortic abnormalities: aneurysm,* dissection,* traumatic aortic rupture
- Bronchopulmonary foregut cysts
- Tracheal tumor
- Esophageal abnormalities: neoplasms (carcinoma, leiomyoma, leiomyosarcoma), achalasia
- Hiatal hernia* (often contains air-fluid level) (Fig. 67-2)
- Cardiac tumor
- Left ventricular or thoracic aortic aneurysm or pseudoaneurysm
- Pulmonary artery aneurysm
- Neurogenic tumor of the vagus nerve

5. List the differential diagnosis of major posterior mediastinal lesions.
In the following list, an asterisk (*) indicates the most common causes:

- Neurogenic tumors* (peripheral nerve, sympathetic ganglion, or parasympathetic involvement)
- Primary or metastatic bone tumor of the thoracic spine
- Osteomyelitis or paraspinal abscess of the thoracic spine
- Extramedullary hematopoiesis

6. List the differential diagnosis of fat-containing mediastinal lesions.
- Lipoma
- Mature teratoma
- Thymolipoma
- Well-differentiated liposarcoma
- Mediastinal lipomatosis
- Fat-containing hernia (hiatal, Bochdalek, or Morgagni hernia)
- Posterior mediastinal angiomyolipoma

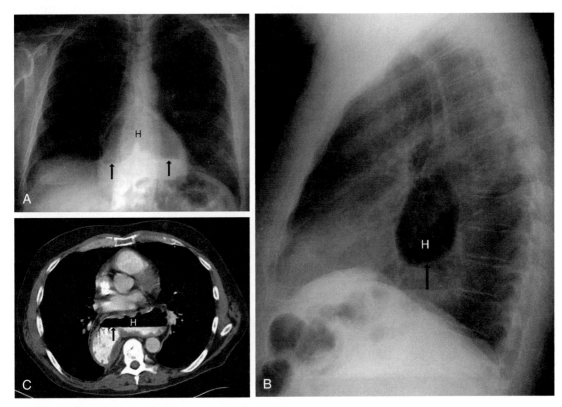

Figure 67-2. A, Hiatal hernia on frontal chest radiograph. Note gas-filled structure (*H*) with air-fluid levels (*arrows*) overlying mediastinum. **B,** Hiatal hernia on lateral chest radiograph. Note gas-filled structure (*H*) with air-fluid levels (*arrow*) posterior to heart in posterior mediastinum. **C,** Hiatal hernia on CT. Note structure filled with gas and oral contrast agent (*H*) lined by rugal folds posterior to the heart in the posterior mediastinum indicating stomach.

7. List the differential diagnosis of cystic mediastinal lesions.

CYSTS WITH THIN, SMOOTH WALL

- Pericardial cyst
- Bronchogenic cyst
- Esophageal duplication cyst
- Thymic cyst
- Neurenteric cyst
- Mediastinal pancreatic pseudocyst
- Intrathoracic meningocele

CYSTS WITH THICK WALL, MURAL NODULARITY, OR INTERNAL SEPTATIONS

- Thymic teratoma
- Any mediastinal tumor with necrosis or cystic change
- Mediastinal abscess

8. Name different collections that may occur within the mediastinum.

- *Fluid*: mediastinal edema or pericardial effusion
- *Blood*: mediastinal hematoma or hemopericardium
- *Pus*: mediastinal abscess, pericardial abscess, or acute mediastinitis
- *Air*: pneumomediastinum and pneumopericardium
- *Fat*: mediastinal lipomatosis
- *Fibrosis*: fibrosing mediastinitis
- *Cells*: mediastinal tumor

9. What clinical symptoms and signs can be associated with mediastinal lesions?

Compression or invasion of the trachea or bronchi, recurrent laryngeal nerve, or esophagus may produce cough, dyspnea, chest pain, respiratory infection, hoarseness, or dysphagia. Compression or invasion of the adjacent cardiovascular structures may produce superior vena cava syndrome; cardiac dysrhythmias; constrictive pathophysiology; cardiac tamponade; or, rarely, sudden death. About 75% of asymptomatic patients with mediastinal tumors have benign lesions, whereas about 66% of symptomatic patients with mediastinal masses have malignant lesions.

10. What is a thymoma?

A thymoma is a rare tumor that is the most common primary tumor of the thymus and the most common primary tumor of the anterior mediastinum. It occurs in men and women equally and most often occurs after age 40. It is an epithelial neoplasm composed of a mixture of epithelial cells and mature lymphocytes. About 33% are invasive, and the remainder are encapsulated. Complete surgical resection is the major treatment for a thymoma. Radiation therapy or chemotherapy may be used for an invasive thymoma, an incompletely resected thymoma, or a disseminated thymoma. Most patients with an encapsulated thymoma are cured with surgical resection, and many with a microscopically invasive thymoma are cured with surgery and adjunctive radiation therapy. Patients with macroscopic invasion often have a prolonged course with slowly growing metastatic disease.

11. Describe the clinical presentation of a thymoma.

Most patients are asymptomatic, although 33% may be symptomatic because of compression or invasion of adjacent structures. Of patients, 50% may have a paraneoplastic syndrome, such as myasthenia gravis, hypogammaglobulinemia, or pure red blood cell aplasia. About 30% to 50% of patients with a thymoma may develop myasthenia gravis, whereas 15% of patients with myasthenia gravis have a thymoma. Ten percent of patients with a thymoma may develop hypogammaglobulinemia, whereas 5% of patients with hypogammaglobulinemia have a thymoma. Five percent of patients with a thymoma may develop red blood cell aplasia, whereas 50% of patients with red blood cell aplasia have a thymoma.

12. Describe the imaging findings of a thymoma.

One typically sees a well-defined, rounded, or lobulated anterosuperior mediastinal soft tissue mass arising from one of the thymic lobes with asymmetric growth toward one side of the midline, often with necrotic, cystic, hemorrhagic, or calcific changes (Fig. 67-3). About 33% of thymomas invade through the capsule with involvement of the mediastinal fat, pleura, pericardium, great vessels, right atrium, or lung, or less commonly with extension through the diaphragm into the peritoneal cavity or retroperitoneum. Metastatic disease is most commonly to the pleura, often mimicking malignant pleural mesothelioma with unilateral pleural thickening, masses, or diffuse nodular circumferential pleural thickening encasing the ipsilateral lung. Uncommonly, pleural effusions, lymphadenopathy, or distant hematogenous metastases are present.

13. What is thymic carcinoma?

Thymic carcinoma is an aggressive epithelial malignancy that often includes early local invasion, lymphadenopathy, and distant metastatic disease. Squamous cell carcinoma and lymphoepithelioma-like carcinoma are the most common cell types and most often occur in middle-aged men. On imaging, thymic carcinomas are commonly large, poorly defined, infiltrative anterior mediastinal masses that may have cystic or necrotic changes, often with pleural and pericardial effusions (Fig. 67-4). Treatment and prognosis depend on the stage and histologic grade of the tumor.

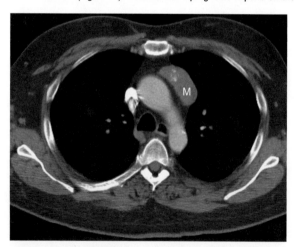

Figure 67-3. Anterior mediastinal mass secondary to thymoma on CT. Note ovoid, partially calcified mass (*M*) anterior to aortic arch within anterior mediastinum.

14. What is thymic carcinoid?

Thymic carcinoid is a rare neuroendocrine tumor that typically affects men in the fourth to fifth decades of life. About 50% of patients have endocrine abnormalities, most commonly Cushing syndrome resulting from ectopic adrenocorticotropic hormone production or multiple endocrine neoplasia syndrome. Classic carcinoid syndrome caused by serotonin secretion is rarely associated with thymic carcinoid. Symptoms and signs secondary to local mass effect and invasion may also occur. A large lobulated and usually invasive anterior mediastinal mass is seen that may be associated with cystic, necrotic, hemorrhagic, or calcific change. Lymphadenopathy and distant metastases may be seen in 75% of cases. Complete surgical excision is the treatment of choice, and radiotherapy and chemotherapy may be used for more advanced disease.

15. What is thymolipoma?

Thymolipoma is a rare, benign, slow-growing thymic neoplasm that may occur in any age group, although young adults are most commonly affected. It is a large, soft, encapsulated mass composed of mature adipose cells and thymic tissue. About 50% of patients are asymptomatic. On imaging, thymolipoma is a large anterior mediastinal mass that commonly droops into the anteroinferior mediastinum, may occupy one or both hemithoraces, and is characterized by its ability to conform to adjacent structures and to change in shape after changes in patient positioning. Predominant fat density and intermixed soft tissue density foci are seen on computed tomography (CT) (Fig. 67-5). Complete surgical resection is curative.

16. What is a mediastinal germ cell tumor?

Mediastinal germ cell tumors are a heterogeneous group of benign and malignant neoplasms that originate from primitive germ cells left in the mediastinum during early embryogenesis. The anterior mediastinum is the most common extragonadal primary site of germ cell tumors. They usually occur in young adults, and although mature teratomas occur equally in men and women, most malignant germ cell tumors occur in men. α-fetoprotein and β-human chorionic gonadotropin serum levels may be positive with malignant mediastinal germ cell tumors. Primary testicular or ovarian germ cell tumor should be excluded when a mediastinal germ cell tumor is discovered because the mediastinum may be a site of metastasis from gonadal germ cell tumors.

17. What is a mediastinal teratoma?

Teratoma is the most common mediastinal germ cell tumor, composed of tissues from more than one of the three primitive germ cell layers (teeth, skin, and hair from ectoderm; cartilage and bone from mesoderm; and bronchial, intestinal, or pancreatic tissue from endoderm). Most teratomas are well differentiated and benign (mature), but rarely contain fetal tissue (when immature, in which case they may recur or metastasize). Mediastinal teratomas occur most commonly in children and young adults. Although usually asymptomatic, large tumors may cause symptoms because of local mass effect. On imaging, mature teratoma appears as a lobulated, well-defined heterogeneous anterior mediastinal mass usually located to one side of the midline with fat density foci, and multilocular cysts, dense teeth, calcification, or bone. The presence of fat, fluid, and soft tissue elements with or without calcification within an anterior mediastinal mass is virtually diagnostic of a mediastinal teratoma. Surgical excision is curative.

18. Name a rare but highly specific clinical presentation of mediastinal teratoma.

Expectoration of hair (trichoptysis) or sebum is a rare but pathognomonic sign of ruptured mediastinal teratoma. This presentation is due to secretion of digestive enzymes by intestinal mucosa or pancreatic tissue in the tumor, precipitating rupture into the bronchi.

19. What is mediastinal thyroid goiter?

Mediastinal thyroid goiter is an encapsulated, lobulated heterogeneous enlargement of part or all of the thyroid gland, most commonly in asymptomatic women with a palpable cervical goiter. Occasionally, local compressive symptoms are present; 20% of lesions extend inferiorly into the thorax, usually into the left anterosuperior mediastinum, and less commonly into the middle or posterior mediastinal compartment. On imaging, a well-defined, lobulated heterogeneous lesion, often in the anterosuperior mediastinum, with areas of cystic, hemorrhagic, or calcific change

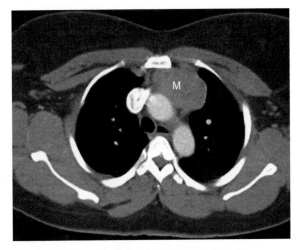

Figure 67-4. Anterior mediastinal mass secondary to thymic carcinoma on CT. Note ovoid soft tissue attenuation mass (*M*) anterior to ascending aorta within anterior mediastinum.

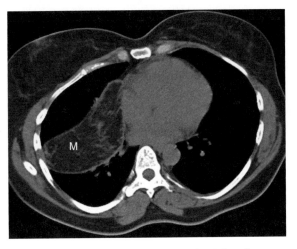

Figure 67-5. Anterior mediastinal mass secondary to thymolipoma on CT. Note predominantly fat attenuation mass (*M*) anterior and to right of heart within anterior mediastinum.

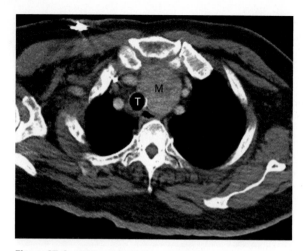

Figure 67-6. Middle mediastinal mass secondary to thyroid goiter on CT. Note soft tissue mass (*M*) within middle mediastinum to left of trachea (*T*). This was seen to be contiguous with inferior aspect of thyroid gland (not shown) confirming thyroid origin.

is seen, often with tracheal displacement in the neck. Tracheal displacement on a chest radiograph indicates a mass of thyroid origin in most cases and represents a goiter. On CT, identification of contiguity of the mass with the thyroid gland establishes origin from the thyroid gland (Fig. 67-6). Surgical resection is the treatment of choice for symptomatic lesions, although most patients with a goiter are asymptomatic and require no therapy other than iodine or hormonal replacement.

20. Define mediastinal lipoma and mediastinal lipomatosis.

- *Mediastinal lipoma* is a benign, well-circumscribed mesenchymal tumor that originates from adipose tissue, predominantly occurring in the anterior mediastinum often without clinical symptoms or signs. On imaging, it is generally a well-circumscribed, oval or round homogeneous fat density lesion.

- *Mediastinal lipomatosis* is due to excessive unencapsulated infiltrative fat deposition within the mediastinum. It is commonly associated with obesity and chronic exogenous corticosteroid administration, and appears as widening of the mediastinum on radiography and as an increase in mediastinal fat on CT.

21. What is Hodgkin lymphoma?

Hodgkin lymphoma accounts for about 25% to 30% of lymphomas. Of patients with mediastinal involvement by lymphoma, 85% may have Hodgkin lymphoma. Hodgkin lymphoma occurs with a bimodal age distribution, with peaks during adolescence and early adulthood and after the fifth decade of life, most often occurring above the diaphragm. The diagnosis is established on pathologic study by identification of Reed-Sternberg cells, generally in a background of inflammation and fibrosis. On imaging, one generally sees enlarged lymph nodes or conglomerate masses, sometimes with hemorrhagic, necrotic, cystic, or calcific change, and almost always involving the anterior mediastinum, often involving contiguous nodal groups. Avid uptake of fluorodeoxyglucose (FDG) on positron emission tomography (PET) imaging is often seen.

22. What is non-Hodgkin lymphoma?

Non-Hodgkin lymphoma may occur in all age groups, although older patients tend to be affected most commonly. Most patients present with advanced disease. On pathologic study, one sees a predominance of malignant lymphocytes that are generally homogeneous and uniformly cellular. On imaging, one may see enlarged lymph nodes anywhere within the thorax, but extranodal disease is common, generally appearing as homogeneous soft tissue masses that may involve nearly any organ in the body. Cystic, necrotic, or calcific changes are uncommon, but may occasionally be seen. Avid uptake of FDG on PET or PET/CT imaging is often present (Fig. 67-7).

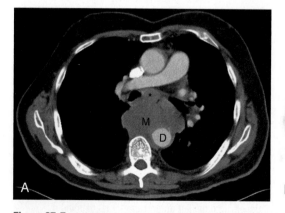
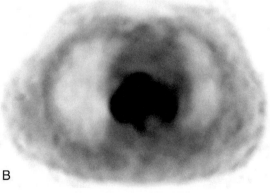

Figure 67-7. A, Middle and posterior mediastinal mass secondary to lymphoma on CT. Note large homogeneous soft tissue attenuation mass (*M*) in subcarinal station of middle mediastinum (*asterisk*) and in posterior mediastinum surrounding descending thoracic aorta (*D*). **B,** Middle and posterior mediastinal mass secondary to lymphoma on FDG PET. Note avid FDG uptake in location of mediastinal mass.

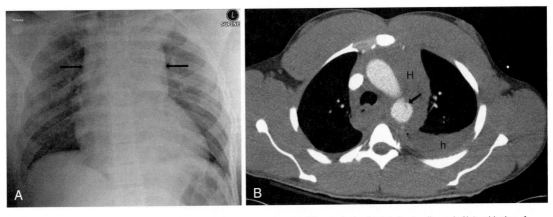

Figure 67-8. A, Mediastinal hematoma secondary to traumatic aortic transection on supine frontal chest radiograph. Note widening of mediastinum (*between arrows*). **B,** Mediastinal hematoma secondary to traumatic aortic transection on CT. Note high-attenuation mediastinal hemorrhage (*H*) and left hemothorax (*h*) along with abnormal contour of transected descending thoracic aorta (*arrow*).

23. What are the most common causes of mediastinal lymphadenopathy?

The four most common causes of radiographically detectable mediastinal lymphadenopathy are sarcoidosis, lymphoma, metastatic tumor, and granulomatous infections. In younger patients with bilateral hilar and mediastinal lymphadenopathy, sarcoidosis should be the diagnosis of exclusion because, by a large margin, it is the most common cause. In older individuals, lymphoma and metastatic tumor are the most common causes of mediastinal lymphadenopathy. It would seem logical that any pulmonary infection could lead to mediastinal lymphadenopathy; however, only granulomatous infections commonly cause mediastinal or hilar lymphadenopathy. These include primary tuberculosis, histoplasmosis, cryptococcosis, and coccidioidomycosis.

24. Which vascular disorders can appear as mediastinal masses?

Aortic aneurysm, aortic dissection, and traumatic aortic rupture can appear as a mediastinal mass, most often projecting from the left side of the mediastinum on chest radiography. Cross-sectional imaging shows enlargement of the aorta in the setting of aortic aneurysm and sometimes in the setting of the latter two conditions. Also, mediastinal hematoma may be seen if aortic rupture has occurred (Fig. 67-8).

25. Describe the congenital foregut cysts.

Bronchogenic cysts represent 50% to 60% of all mediastinal cysts, esophageal duplication cysts represent 5% to 10%, and neurenteric cysts represent 2% to 5%. About 85% of bronchogenic cysts are located close to the trachea, main stem bronchi, or carina, and 15% may occur in the lungs. Esophageal duplication cysts are almost always found within the esophageal wall or adherent to the esophagus. Neurenteric cysts may occur in isolation within the mediastinum or may be connected by a fibrous tract to the spine. On imaging, cysts are generally round, smooth, thin-walled lesions that contain simple fluid or sometimes complex fluid (Fig. 67-9). Symptoms may occur from compression of mediastinal structures or superinfection.

26. What is a mediastinal pancreatic pseudocyst?

A mediastinal pancreatic pseudocyst is an encapsulated collection of pancreatic secretions that does not have an epithelial lining and is almost always located in the inferoposterior mediastinum. A mediastinal pancreatic pseudocyst is due to extension of fluid through the esophageal or aortic hiatus of the diaphragm in the setting of pancreatitis.

27. What is pneumomediastinum?

Pneumomediastinum is air within the mediastinum. On imaging, one sees streaky linear or curvilinear lucent gas in the mediastinum that outlines mediastinal structures (Fig. 67-10).

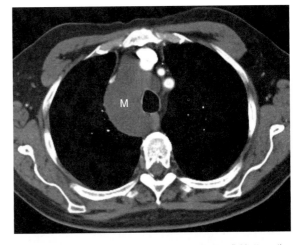

Figure 67-9. Mediastinal bronchogenic cyst on CT. Note fluid attenuation mass (*M*) with lobulated contours in mediastinum.

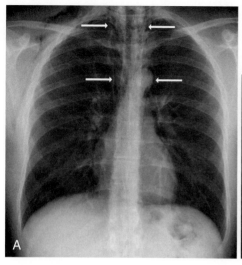
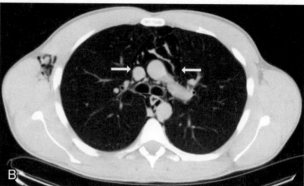

Figure 67-10. A, Pneumomediastinum on frontal chest radiograph. Note streaky linear lucent gas (*arrows*) in mediastinum that outlines mediastinal structures. **B,** Pneumomediastinum on CT. Note very low-attenuation gas (*between arrows*) in mediastinum that outlines mediastinal structures.

Although pneumopericardium (air within the pericardial space) is confined to the distribution of the pericardial reflection, pneumomediastinum may occur anywhere within the mediastinum. The causes of pneumomediastinum include:

- Air trapping from emphysema or asthma
- Straining against a closed glottis from vomiting, parturition, weightlifting, or marijuana use
- Blunt/penetrating trauma or iatrogenic injury to the trachea, bronchi, or esophagus
- Barotrauma from mechanical ventilation, sudden decrease in atmospheric pressure, or coughing
- Erosion of the trachea or esophagus by tumor
- Esophageal rupture from Boerhaave syndrome, alcoholism, or diabetic ketoacidosis
- Extension of air from pneumothorax, pneumoperitoneum, or pneumoretroperitoneum

28. What is a mediastinal abscess?

A mediastinal abscess is a loculated collection of pus. Major causes of mediastinal abscess include surgery, esophageal perforation, tracheobronchial perforation, spread of infection from a contiguous location, or penetrating trauma. On imaging, one may see a loculated fluid collection that tends to have a thick, enhancing wall and that may contain gas. Acute infection of the mediastinum is often fulminant and life-threatening and is treated urgently.

29. What is fibrosing mediastinitis?

Fibrosing mediastinitis is an uncommon benign disorder characterized by proliferation of dense mediastinal fibrous tissue. It typically occurs in young patients who present with symptoms and signs owing to obstruction of vital mediastinal structures. Fibrosing mediastinitis is sometimes related to histoplasmosis infection, but is often idiopathic in etiology. On imaging, one often sees nonspecific mediastinal widening, sometimes with hilar involvement, by focal or diffuse confluent soft tissue that is commonly calcified. Encasement, narrowing, or occlusion of the mediastinal airway or vascular structures is also often seen.

30. What are neurogenic tumors?

Neurogenic tumors are the most common cause of posterior mediastinal masses. Schwannoma and neurofibroma arise from peripheral nerves, more commonly in adults, whereas ganglioneuroma, ganglioneuroblastoma, and neuroblastoma arise from sympathetic ganglia, more commonly in children. Paragangliomas arise from paraganglia and are less common. Schwannomas and neurofibromas are the most common mediastinal neurogenic tumors and are benign. Schwannomas are encapsulated tumors composed of Schwann cells and loose reticular tissue; arise from the nerve sheath; and are often heterogeneous with hemorrhagic, cystic, necrotic, calcific, or fatty change. Neurofibromas are usually homogeneous nonencapsulated tumors composed of Schwann cells, nerve fibers, and fibroblasts.

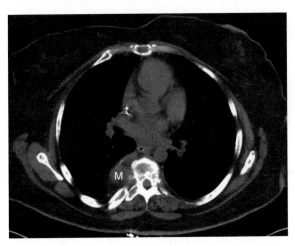

Figure 67-11. Posterior mediastinal mass secondary to ganglioneuroma on CT. Note well-circumscribed mixed soft tissue and fat attenuation mass (*M*) within posterior mediastinum to right of thoracic spine.

31. Describe the imaging appearance of neurogenic tumors.

On imaging, peripheral nerve neurogenic tumors may appear as lobulated spherical or fusiform masses in the paraspinal region of the thorax, sometimes with a dumbbell configuration if there is extension into a neural foramen. A plexiform neurofibroma, pathognomonic for neurofibromatosis type 1 (NF1), usually involves an entire nerve trunk or plexus. Associated smooth pressure erosions of the adjacent inferior rib surfaces and vertebrae or enlargement of the neural foramina may also be seen. Neurogenic tumors that arise from the sympathetic ganglia tend to appear as vertically oriented, elongated paraspinal masses with tapered borders. On CT, fluid attenuation components owing to cystic change or necrosis, soft tissue attenuation components, fat attenuation components secondary to fatty degeneration, and high-attenuation calcification may be visualized (Fig. 67-11).

Key Points: Mediastinal Diseases

1. Lesions that arise in the different compartments of the mediastinum are generally related to the anatomic structures located within the compartments.
2. Most patients with asymptomatic mediastinal tumors have benign tumors, whereas most patients with symptomatic mediastinal tumors have malignant tumors.
3. Thymoma is the most common primary tumor of the anterior mediastinum and of the thymus.
4. Primary testicular or ovarian germ cell tumor should be excluded when a mediastinal germ cell tumor is discovered.
5. Neurogenic tumor is the most common mass of the posterior mediastinum.

32. What is an intrathoracic meningocele?

An intrathoracic meningocele is an anomalous herniation of leptomeninges through an intervertebral foramen or a defect in the vertebral body, commonly associated with NF1. On imaging, one sees a well-circumscribed, smooth, lobulated or round paraspinal cystic lesion with enlargement of the intervertebral foramen or associated vertebral and rib anomalies or scoliosis. Diagnosis is confirmed by filling of the lesion with intraspinal contrast material on CT or fluoroscopy.

33. How do osseous tumors and infection within the posterior mediastinum differ on imaging?

Tumors of the thoracic spine generally are centered on the vertebrae without narrowing of the intervening disc spaces, whereas infections tend to be centered on the intervertebral disc spaces with disc space narrowing and involvement of the adjacent vertebral end plates.

34. What is extramedullary hematopoiesis?

Extramedullary hematopoiesis is due to proliferation of blood-forming elements in patients with thalassemia or other anemias, and occurs most commonly in the liver and spleen and sometimes in the chest. On imaging, multiple lobulated masses along the thoracic spine or along the ribs may be seen with pressure erosions, often with associated osseous abnormalities sometimes with associated splenomegaly. Fat attenuation components that are chronic may be visualized on CT.

BIBLIOGRAPHY

[1] S.C. Gaerte, C.A. Meyer, H.T. Winer-Muram, et al., Fat-containing lesions of the chest, RadioGraphics 22 (Suppl.) (2002) S61–S78.
[2] M.Y. Jeung, B. Gasser, A. Gangi, et al., Imaging of cystic masses of the mediastinum, RadioGraphics 22 (Suppl.) (2002) S79–S93.
[3] N. Muller, R. Fraser, N. Colman, P.D. Pare, Radiologic Diagnosis of Diseases of the Chest, Saunders, Philadelphia, 2001.
[4] S.E. Rossi, H.P. McAdams, M.L. Rosado-de-Christenson, et al., Fibrosing mediastinitis, RadioGraphics 21 (2001) 737–757.
[5] D.C. Strollo, M.L. Rosado-de-Christenson, J.R. Jett, Primary mediastinal tumors, part I: tumors of the anterior mediastinum, Chest 112 (1997) 511–522.
[6] D.C. Strollo, M.L. Rosado-de-Christenson, J.R. Jett, Primary mediastinal tumors, part II: tumors of the middle and posterior mediastinum, Chest 112 (1997) 1344–1357.
[7] C.M. Zylak, J.R. Standen, G.R. Barnes, C.J. Zylak, Pneumomediastinum revisited, RadioGraphics 20 (2000) 1043–1057.

PLEURAL DISEASES

Drew A. Torigian, MD,
Charles T. Lau, MD, and
Wallace T. Miller, Jr., MD

1. Describe the normal pleural anatomy and physiologic features.

The pleural space is a potential space that contains 2 to 10 mL of pleural fluid between visceral and parietal pleural layers that essentially represents interstitial fluid from the parietal pleura (an ultrafiltrate of plasma). The pleural space is contiguous with the interlobar fissures of the lungs. The pleura is a thin, serous layer that covers the lungs (visceral pleura) and is reflected onto the chest wall and pericardium (parietal pleura). The visceral pleura is supplied by the pulmonary arterial system and drains into the pulmonary venous system, whereas the parietal pleura is supplied by the systemic arterial system and drains into the systemic venous system. Fig. 68-1 shows the normal appearance of the pleura on chest radiography.

2. List the major tumors that may affect the pleura.

- Malignant pleural mesothelioma
- Localized solitary fibrous tumor of the pleura
- Pleural metastases
- Pleural lymphoma

3. What are the major substances that may collect within the pleural space?

- *Fluid*: pleural effusion (plasma ultrafiltrate, chyle, bile, urine, gastrointestinal contents, or ascites)
- *Blood*: hemothorax
- *Air*: pneumothorax
- *Pus*: empyema
- *Cells*: pleural tumor
- *Fibrosis*: fibrothorax

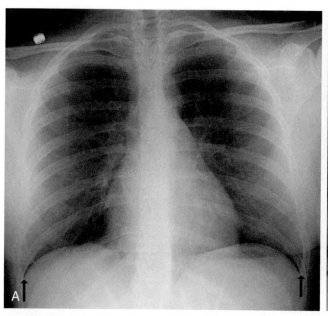
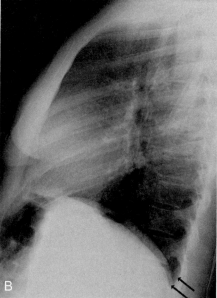

Figure 68-1. A, Normal frontal chest radiograph. Note sharp lateral costophrenic angles (*arrows*) bilaterally and clear demarcation of hemidiaphragms. **B,** Normal lateral chest radiograph. Note sharp posterior costophrenic angles (*arrows*) bilaterally and clear demarcation of hemidiaphragms.

Table 68-1. Differential Diagnosis of Pleural Effusion

Congestive heart failure*
Malignancy
Metastases*
Malignant mesothelioma
Lymphoma
Trauma
Thoracic or abdominal surgery*
Inflammatory disease
Infection (bacterial, mycobacterial, viral, fungal, parasitic)
Parapneumonic effusion*
Empyema
Collagen vascular disease: systemic lupus erythematosus, rheumatoid arthritis, systemic sclerosis
Hypoalbuminemia
Cirrhosis*
Nephrotic syndrome
Acute pulmonary embolism
Abdominal pathologic conditions*
Ascites
Pancreatitis
Peritonitis
Other inflammatory conditions of the abdomen
Other unusual causes
Lymphangioleiomyomatosis (associated with chylous effusions)

*Indicates most common causes.

4. **What is the differential diagnosis of major causes of pleural effusion?**
   See Table 68-1.

5. **List the major mechanisms of pleural effusion formation.**
   - Increased hydrostatic pressure in the microvascular circulation (e.g., congestive heart failure)
   - Decreased oncotic pressure in the microvascular circulation (e.g., hypoalbuminemia)
   - Decreased pressure in the pleural space (e.g., with pulmonary atelectasis or restrictive lung disease)
   - Increased permeability of the microvascular circulation (e.g., from pleural inflammation or neoplasm)
   - Impaired lymphatic drainage from the pleural space caused by blockage in the lymphatic system
   - Transit of fluid from the peritoneal cavity through the diaphragm to the pleural space

6. **What are the two major types of pleural effusion?**
   - *Transudates* are usually caused by increased systemic or pulmonary capillary pressure and decreased osmotic pressure, resulting in increased filtration and decreased absorption of pleural fluid. Major causes are cirrhosis, congestive heart failure, nephrotic syndrome, and protein-losing enteropathy. Protein levels are less than 3 g/dL.
   - *Exudates* occur when the pleural surface is damaged with associated capillary leak and increased permeability to protein, or when there is decreased lymphatic drainage or decreased pleural pressure. Major causes are infection, malignancy, collagen vascular disease, or acute pulmonary embolism. Protein levels are greater than 3 g/dL, the pleural protein-to-serum protein ratio is greater than 0.5, and the pleural lactate dehydrogenase-to-serum lactate dehydrogenase ratio is greater than 0.6.

7. **What are the major imaging findings of simple nonloculated pleural effusions on erect chest radiography?**
   The most common imaging finding of a pleural effusion is blunting of the lateral costophrenic sulcus on erect frontal chest radiography or blunting of the posterior costophrenic sulcus on erect lateral chest radiography. A pleural effusion

usually has a sharply marginated, concave–upward curved border between the lung and pleural space, which is known as the "meniscus" sign. Because the posterior costophrenic angle is more dependent than the lateral costophrenic angle, smaller pleural effusions are more apparent on the lateral view (with >75 mL of fluid) than on the frontal view (with >200 mL of fluid). Moderate to large pleural effusions usually obscure the ipsilateral hemidiaphragm (Fig. 68-2A). Less common manifestations of pleural effusions include apparent elevation and medial flattening of the hemidiaphragm with lateral displacement of the diaphragmatic apex and an increase in distance (>2 cm) between the inferior surface of the lung and the gastric bubble on the left. The lateral decubitus view is the most sensitive radiographic view for detection of a pleural effusion and can detect 5 mL of pleural fluid.

8. **Describe the major imaging findings related to simple nonloculated pleural effusions on portable supine, semierect chest radiography and computed tomography (CT).**

A little understood fact is that blunting of the costophrenic angles is a rare manifestation of pleural effusions on portable supine and semierect chest radiographs. On these views, pleural effusions most often appear as increased opacity of the hemithorax without obscuration of vascular markings or of the ipsilateral hemithorax because fluid layers in the posterior pleural space dependently behind the more anterior nondependent lung. If the patient is supine, this layering appears as a uniform haze of the ipsilateral hemithorax. On semierect radiographs, the density produced by the pleural effusion increases from superior to inferior because free-flowing pleural fluid falls dependently into the more inferior portions of the pleural space. Rarely, if the patient is imaged in the Trendelenburg position, the pleural fluid collects as a crescentic opacity over the lung apex, which is known as an apical cap. On CT, fluid attenuation is seen within the dependent aspect of the pleural space, often with a meniscus along its nondependent aspect (Fig. 68-2B).

9. **What are the major imaging findings associated with complex loculated pleural effusions?**

Complex pleural effusions (often seen with exudative effusions) are often located in nondependent portions of the pleural space and do not shift freely in the pleural space on lateral decubitus chest radiography because of adhesions between the visceral and parietal pleurae. CT scans may also sometimes show associated pleural thickening. Occasionally, loculated pleural fluid in the interlobar fissure may mimic a pseudomass on chest radiography, often appearing as a poorly marginated opacity on frontal chest radiography and as an elliptical opacity in the location of a major or minor interlobar fissure on lateral chest radiography.

10. **List the differential diagnosis of major causes of hemothorax.**
   - Trauma (blunt or penetrating or iatrogenic) (most common cause)
   - Bleeding diathesis (e.g., anticoagulation, protein S or C deficiency)
   - Malignancy
   - Infection
   - Acute pulmonary embolism
   - Thoracic aortic rupture (from [pseudo]aneurysm, dissection, penetrating aortic ulcer, or transection)

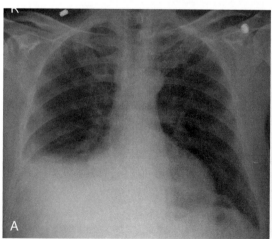
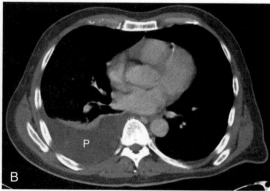

Figure 68-2. A, Simple pleural effusion on frontal erect chest radiograph. Note blunting of right lateral costophrenic angle with meniscus sign and obscuration of right hemidiaphragm. **B,** Simple pleural effusion on CT. Note fluid attenuation pleural effusion (*P*) in dependent right hemithorax. Note higher attenuation mild passive right lower lobe atelectasis of lung anterior to pleural effusion.

11. What is pneumothorax?

Pneumothorax is air within the pleural cavity; this occurs either through a communication between the outside world and the pleural space via a defect in the chest wall or through a communication between the air-containing bronchi or alveoli and the pleural space via a defect in the visceral pleura. Free intrapleural air preferentially moves to the nondependent aspects of the pleural spaces (apicolateral location on erect chest radiography and basilar or anteromedial location on supine chest radiography).

12. What are the radiographic imaging findings of pneumothorax?

The pathognomonic finding is a thin, sharply defined, visceral pleural "white" line between radiolucent lung (with vascular markings) and radiolucent "black" free air in the peripheral pleural space (without vascular markings). On supine chest radiography, one may see sharp visualization of the right cardiac border, superior and inferior vena cavae, left subclavian artery, and anterior junction line; a deep lucent cardiophrenic sulcus ("deep sulcus sign"); hyperlucency at the lung bases; and associated atelectasis of the adjacent lung.

13. How much air in a pneumothorax is required for radiographic visualization?

On erect chest radiographs, small amounts of air (about 50 mL) are generally visible at the lung apex, whereas on supine radiographs, about 500 mL of air is needed to be visible.

14. What radiographic maneuvers can be performed to show a subtle pneumothorax?

Expiratory chest radiography or contralateral decubitus chest radiography (i.e., left side down if looking for a right pneumothorax and vice versa) can often show a small pneumothorax that may not be seen on standard inspiratory frontal chest radiography. Alternatively, cross-table lateral chest radiography with the patient in the supine position can also show a subtle pneumothorax.

15. What is a tension pneumothorax?

Uncommonly, air in the pleural space can develop positive pressure, most often as a result of mechanical ventilation, and can compress the mediastinum with resultant decreased venous return to the heart. This can be a medical emergency because rapid cardiopulmonary compromise and death may ensue if the patient is not immediately treated. The radiographic clues to a tension pneumothorax are the presence of a pneumothorax in association with contralateral mediastinal shift and inferior displacement of the ipsilateral hemidiaphragm (Fig. 68-3). These findings are not diagnostic of a tension pneumothorax, however, which can occur without these findings. The diagnosis is based on radiographic recognition of a pneumothorax and clinical findings of hypotension and tachycardia. Immediate decompression by needle thoracentesis through the second rib interspace in the mid-clavicular line or with chest thoracostomy is typically performed for emergent treatment of a tension pneumothorax.

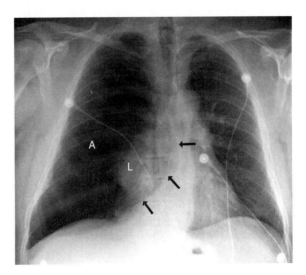

Figure 68-3. Tension pneumothorax on frontal chest radiograph. Note thin, sharply defined visceral pleural "white" line between radiolucent lung (L) and radiolucent "black" free air (A) in right peripheral pleural space, in addition to leftward mediastinal shift (arrows) and inferior right hemidiaphragmatic shift caused by air under tension.

16. What is the differential diagnosis of major causes of pneumothorax?

In the following list, an asterisk (*) indicates the most common causes:

- Idiopathic*: most often because of rupture of an apical bleb
- Trauma*: blunt or penetrating injury, iatrogenic injury (e.g., central venous line placement), barotrauma (mechanical ventilation)
- Obstructive lung disease (e.g., chronic obstructive pulmonary disease, asthma)
- Cystic lung disease (e.g., eosinophilic granuloma, lymphangiomyomatosis, tuberous sclerosis)
- Bronchiectasis or cavitary lung disease (e.g., cystic fibrosis, tuberculosis, *Pneumocystis carinii* (*jiroveci*) pneumonia)
- Advanced interstitial lung disease with honeycombing (e.g., usual interstitial pneumonitis, sarcoidosis, chronic hypersensitivity pneumonitis)
- Adult respiratory distress syndrome

- Endometriosis (e.g., catamenial pneumothorax)
- Bronchopulmonary fistula (e.g., after lung surgery or transplantation)

17. When should treatment of a patient with a pneumothorax be considered?

Many pneumothoraces resolve spontaneously, and only patients at risk for complications of the pneumothorax require intervention. Generally, treatment with chest thoracostomy is necessary if the patient has respiratory compromise as a result of the pneumothorax. Findings such as shortness of breath, dyspnea, hypoxemia, or hypotension indicate the need for drainage of the pneumothorax. If the pneumothorax increases in size on serial chest radiographs, treatment also becomes necessary. If clinical and radiographic findings indicate a tension pneumothorax, decompression and drainage of the pneumothorax are necessary. Finally, most patients receiving positive-pressure ventilation require chest tube drainage because of the increased risk of developing a tension pneumothorax.

18. How is the diagnosis of an empyema obtained?

Diagnosis is made when pleural fluid is grossly purulent, when pleural fluid has a positive Gram stain or culture, or when the white blood cell count is greater than 5×10^9 cells. Anaerobic bacteria, usually streptococci or gram-negative rods, are responsible in about 75% of cases. Chest radiographic findings of empyema are similar to findings of other loculated pleural fluid collections. CT findings may include increased attenuation of the fluid caused by protein, cells, or hemorrhage; septations and loculation; foci of gas; thickened enhancing pleural surfaces (the "split-pleura" sign); or increased attenuation of the extrapleural fat (Fig. 68-4).

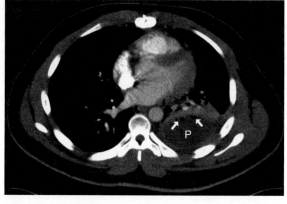

Figure 68-4. Empyema on CT. Note ovoid loculated left pleural effusion (*P*) in left hemithorax surrounded by thickened enhancing visceral and parietal pleural surfaces ("split pleura" sign) and containing nondependent very low-attenuation foci of gas (*arrows*). Note higher attenuation mild passive left lower lobe atelectasis of lung anterior to empyema.

19. When is empyema usually treated?

Empyemas with pH less than 7 or a glucose level less than 40 mg/dL must be treated with chest thoracostomy. If simple drainage fails or if a fibrinous peel forms on the lung, decortication is usually curative.

20. What is empyema necessitatis?

Empyema necessitatis is an uncommon complication of an empyema in which the inflammatory process within the pleural space decompresses and extends into the soft tissues of the chest wall, forming a subcutaneous abscess, which may or may not communicate directly with the skin surface. The most common etiologic factor is tuberculosis, and the most common clinical presentation is a palpable mass in the chest wall, sometimes with a cutaneous fistula. This extension into the chest wall usually is not evident on chest radiographs, but may be detected with CT or magnetic resonance imaging (MRI) of the thorax.

21. List causes of pleural calcification.

- Chronic infection/inflammation (tuberculosis, bacterial empyema)
- Chronic hemothorax
- Asbestos exposure

22. What are pleural plaques?

Pleural plaques are collections of hyalinized collagen in the parietal pleural that are the most common benign finding of prior asbestos exposure. These are virtually pathognomonic for confirming prior asbestos exposure, and typically appear more than 20 years after such exposure. When noncalcified, they appear as small plateau-shaped areas of pleural thickening when seen in profile and may mimic pulmonary nodules when seen en face. They often calcify, however. With a tangential view on chest radiography, a linear or curvilinear calcification along the pleural surface is seen, whereas when seen en face, irregular linear, stippled, or geographic calcification overlying the hemithorax is seen (Fig. 68-5).

23. What is malignant mesothelioma?

Malignant mesothelioma is an uncommon neoplasm that arises from the parietal pleura or, rarely, from the pericardium or peritoneum. Histologic subtypes include epithelioid, sarcomatoid (fibrous), and mixed (biphasic), with epithelioid being the most common. About 2000 to 3000 new cases are diagnosed in the United States each year. This is the most common primary pleural malignancy, and its incidence has been increasing over the past 30 years.

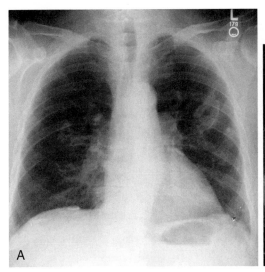
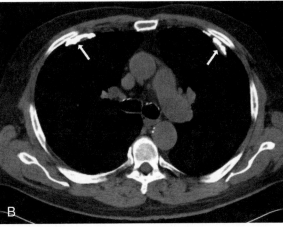

Figure 68-5. **A,** Calcified asbestos-related pleural plaques on frontal chest radiograph. Note linear or curvilinear dense calcifications along inferior aspects of hemithoraces (seen tangentially) and irregular geographic calcifications overlying hemithoraces (seen en face). **B,** Calcified asbestos-related pleural plaques on CT. Note curvilinear dense calcifications (*arrows*) along anterior pleural surfaces.

24. What are risk factors for the development of malignant pleural mesothelioma?

Exposure to asbestos is the most important risk factor (amphibole fibers, including crocidolite and amosite, are the most potent causes). Other minerals and simian virus 40 (SV40) are also risk factors. About 80% of cases occur in patients with a history of asbestos exposure, with a lifetime risk of 10%. The latency period after exposure is an average of 40 years, with a range of approximately 15 to 65 years.

25. Describe symptoms and signs of malignant pleural mesothelioma.

Nonspecific dull chest or shoulder pain, shortness of breath, dyspnea, dry cough, fatigue, weight loss, digital clubbing, hypertrophic osteoarthropathy, superior vena cava syndrome, lymphadenopathy, chest wall masses, dysrhythmias, pleural effusion, pericardial effusion, ascites, or bowel obstruction because of spread to the peritoneal cavity may be seen. Chest wall pain is an important sign of chest wall involvement by tumor. Malignant mesothelioma should be considered in any patient with either pleural effusion or pleural thickening, especially if chest pain is present.

26. What are the imaging findings of malignant pleural mesothelioma?

The most common chest radiographic finding of mesothelioma is a loculated pleural effusion. Unilateral pleural masses and plaquelike or nodular, irregular pleural thickening with encasement of the entire lung are also common findings that are highly suggestive of mesothelioma (Fig. 68-6). Extension into the interlobar fissures, lung,

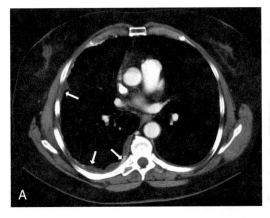
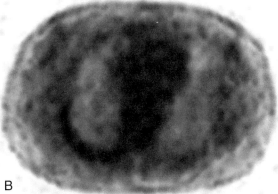

Figure 68-6. **A,** Malignant pleural mesothelioma on CT. Note small right loculated pleural effusion (*arrows*) with several areas of nodular pleural thickening. **B,** Malignant pleural mesothelioma on FDG PET. Note avid FDG uptake in peripheral right hemithorax corresponding to abnormalities on CT.

mediastinum, chest wall, diaphragm, and biopsy tracts may occur. As a result of constriction of the lung by adherent pleural tumor, ipsilateral volume loss of the hemithorax with ipsilateral mediastinal shift, narrowing of the intercostal spaces, and elevation of the ipsilateral hemidiaphragm are commonly present. Pleural calcification resulting from prior asbestos exposure is seen in two thirds of cases, and intrathoracic lymphadenopathy, extension to the peritoneum or retroperitoneum, and hematogenous metastases anywhere in body may be seen on CT or MRI in later stages.

27. What diagnostic tests may be used in the diagnosis or staging of malignant pleural mesothelioma?

Chest radiography, CT, MRI, fluorodeoxyglucose positron emission tomography (FDG PET), ultrasound (US), thoracentesis, and biopsy are used in the diagnosis or staging of malignant pleural mesothelioma. Chest radiography may sometimes have normal results, and negative pleural biopsy and cytology results do not exclude mesothelioma. US, CT, and FDG PET scanning may be used to guide biopsy, however, and increase diagnostic yield. CT and MRI are nearly equivalent in staging accuracy, but MRI is superior to CT for diaphragmatic, endothoracic fascial, or focal chest wall invasion and is often used as a problem-solving tool after CT. FDG PET scanning is also useful in staging and preoperative evaluation and has increased accuracy for detecting malignant lymphadenopathy or occult extrathoracic metastases. Metabolic activity on FDG PET scanning and patient survival are inversely proportional.

28. What is the prognosis for malignant pleural mesothelioma?

Prognosis is generally poor, with a median survival of 8 to 18 months because the tumor is generally progressive. Favorable prognostic factors include limited extent of disease and an epithelioid histologic subtype. Unfavorable prognostic factors include sarcomatoid or mixed histologic subtypes; more advanced stages of disease, such as with intrathoracic lymphadenopathy; extensive pleural involvement; distant metastatic disease; and older age.

29. Describe the general treatment approach to malignant pleural mesothelioma.

Radical surgery (either radical pleurectomy-decortication or extrapleural pneumonectomy with removal of the pleura, mediastinal lymph nodes, ipsilateral pericardium, and diaphragm) is considered when there is epithelioid mesothelioma without lymphadenopathy. Radiotherapy, chemotherapy, and photodynamic therapy may also be used with surgery as adjuvant treatments, but no treatment so far has conclusively improved survival significantly beyond palliative care. Talc pleurodesis or video-assisted thoracoscopic pleurectomy may also be used to control pleural effusions and are safer than open pleurectomy and decortication. Radiotherapy may be used palliatively to relieve pain in about 50% of cases, or can be used prophylactically at biopsy sites to prevent seeding by tumor. Pain medications are used as needed.

30. What is localized fibrous tumor of the pleura?

Localized fibrous tumor of the pleura is a rare mesenchymal neoplasm that most commonly affects the pleura, uncommonly affects the lungs and mediastinum, and rarely involves extrathoracic sites. It is unrelated to asbestos exposure and may be either benign (about 90%) or malignant (about 10%). Most patients present in the fifth through eighth decades of life and have a much better prognosis than patients with malignant pleural mesothelioma. Of these neoplasms, 80% arise from the visceral pleura, and 20% arise from the parietal pleura, although a few are intrapulmonary in location. Of neoplasms, 20% to 50% are pedunculated, and they are composed of spindle-shaped, fibroblast-like cells with a variable amount of collagenous stroma, vascularity, and myxoid or cystic degeneration.

Key Points: Pleural Diseases

1. If a pneumothorax is seen on chest radiography that is associated with contralateral mediastinal shift and inferior displacement of the ipsilateral hemidiaphragm, the physician caring for the patient must be notified immediately because a tension pneumothorax may be present, requiring emergent treatment to prevent rapid death.
2. Malignant mesothelioma is the most common primary malignancy of the pleura and is most often related to prior asbestos exposure.
3. Malignant mesothelioma should be considered in any patient with either pleural effusion or pleural thickening, especially if chest pain is present.
4. Normal chest radiography and negative pleural biopsy and cytology results do not exclude malignant mesothelioma.
5. Paraneoplastic syndromes—such as hypoglycemia, digital clubbing, and hypertrophic osteoarthropathy—may suggest the diagnosis of localized fibrous tumor of the pleura when associated with an intrathoracic mass.

31. Name clinical presentations of localized fibrous tumor of the pleura.

Of localized fibrous tumors of the pleura, 50% may be asymptomatic. Symptoms and signs, when present, may include cough, dyspnea, hemoptysis, chest pain, and sensation of a mass. Paraneoplastic syndromes, such as hypoglycemia, digital clubbing, and hypertrophic osteoarthropathy, are uncommon, but may be associated with an intrathoracic mass.

32. What are the imaging features of localized fibrous tumor of the pleura?

Typically, a well-defined, usually sharply marginated, lobulated, and solitary lesion is identified within the thorax adjacent to the chest wall or diaphragm (Fig. 68-7). It may be very small or massive. When large, it can fill the inferior aspect of the hemithorax and resemble an elevated hemidiaphragm. The tumor typically is connected to the chest wall by a thin pedicle or stalk. Changes in patient positioning, such as with decubitus radiographs, may result in changes in position of the mass within the thorax. On CT or MRI, intense enhancement, myxoid or cystic degeneration, hemorrhage, or calcification may be seen, and no imaging findings other than metastatic disease can help differentiate between benignancy and malignancy of the lesion.

33. What is the treatment for localized fibrous tumor of the pleura?

Treatment involves surgical resection, which is often curative, although some patients have local recurrence, malignant transformation, or distant metastatic disease. Complete surgical excision is overall the best prognostic indicator.

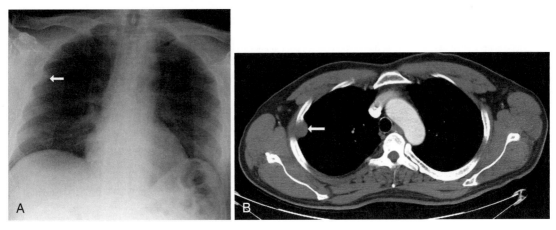

Figure 68-7. A, Localized fibrous tumor of pleura on frontal chest radiograph. Note small, well-defined, sharply marginated solitary lesion (*arrow*) within right hemithorax forming obtuse angle margins with adjacent chest wall. **B,** Localized fibrous tumor of pleura on CT. Note small, well-defined, sharply marginated soft tissue attenuation lesion (*arrow*) within right hemithorax forming obtuse angle margins with adjacent chest wall.

BIBLIOGRAPHY

[1] V.W. Au, M. Thomas, Radiological manifestations of malignant pleural mesothelioma, Australas Radiol 47 (2003) 111–116.
[2] X. Gallardo, E. Castaner, J.M. Mata, Benign pleural diseases, Eur J Radiol 34 (2000) 87–97.
[3] K.H. Lee, K.S. Song, Y. Kwon, et al., Mesenchymal tumours of the thorax: CT findings and pathological features, Clin Radiol 58 (2003) 934–944.
[4] N. Muller, R. Fraser, N. Colman, PD. Pare, Radiologic Diagnosis of Diseases of the Chest, Saunders, Philadelphia, 2001.
[5] C. Parker, E. Neville, Lung cancer, part 8: management of malignant mesothelioma, Thorax 58 (2003) 809–813.
[6] G.J. Peek, S. Morcos, G. Cooper, The pleural cavity, BMJ 320 (2000) 1318–1321.
[7] M.L. Rosado-de-Christenson, G.F. Abbott, H.P. McAdams, et al., From the archives of the AFIP: localized fibrous tumor of the pleura, RadioGraphics 23 (2003) 759–783.
[8] S.A. Sahn, J.E. Heffner, Spontaneous pneumothorax, N. Engl. J. Med. 342 (2000) 868–874.
[9] Statement on malignant mesothelioma in the United Kingdom, Thorax 56 (2001) 250–265.
[10] S. van Ruth, P. Baas, F.A. Zoetmulder, Surgical treatment of malignant pleural mesothelioma: a review, Chest 123 (2003) 551–561.
[11] Z.J. Wang, G.P. Reddy, M.B. Gotway, et al., Malignant pleural mesothelioma: evaluation with CT, MR imaging, and PET, RadioGraphics 24 (2004) 105–119.

TUBES, LINES, AND CATHETERS

Drew A. Torigian, MD, MA, and
Charles T. Lau, MD

1. What is the radiographic appearance of an endotracheal tube (ETT), and where is it optimally placed?

An ETT is usually detected by a thin, radiopaque line along its length, and its position should be determined relative to the carina, which if not seen on chest radiography can be approximated by following the course of the main stem bronchi medially at the T5-T7 level. The tip of the tube should be about 5 to 7 cm above the carina when the patient's head is in neutral position and below the thoracic inlet because flexion and extension of the neck cause the tube to move about 2 cm higher and lower. The optimal width of the tube should be one half to two thirds of the tracheal width (generally <3 cm), and the inflated cuff should not distend the trachea because tracheal injury could occur.

2. Describe how an ETT may be malpositioned; list other potential complications of ETT placement.

If the tube is inserted beyond the carina (i.e., with unilateral bronchial intubation), preferential hyperaeration and potential barotrauma of the intubated lung (more commonly the right) and hypoaeration and atelectasis of the contralateral lung may occur (Fig. 69-1). If the tube is not advanced far enough, inadvertent extubation or possible vocal cord damage because of pressure from the inflated cuff may occur. Esophageal intubation may also be encountered, which is detected clinically by gurgling sounds and distention of the stomach as air is insufflated and radiographically by lateral extension of the tube margins beyond the tracheal margins, visualization of the tracheal air column to the side of the tube, gastric distention, and lung hypoinflation. Other complications include:

- Pharyngeal, laryngeal, or tracheobronchial injury (particularly if placed too high or if the cuff is overinflated)
- Aspiration
- Sinusitis
- Dislodgment of teeth

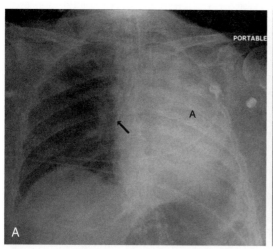
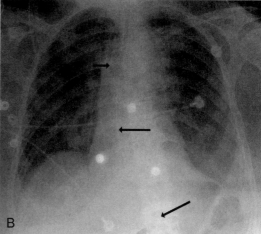

Figure 69-1. A, Malpositioned ETT on frontal chest radiograph. Note tip of ETT within proximal right main stem bronchus (*arrow*) with complete atelectasis (*A*) of the left lung. **B,** Repositioning of ETT on frontal chest radiograph. Note tip of ETT (*arrow*) now appropriately positioned within the distal trachea with resolution of previously noted left lung atelectasis. Also note the normal course of the newly placed NGT (*long arrows*), which follows the expected course of the esophagus before entering the abdomen.

3. What is the optimal positioning of a tracheostomy tube?

A tracheostomy tube tip is optimally located one half to two thirds of the distance from the stoma to the carina. The tube itself should overlie the trachea, and the width of the tube should be about two thirds of the tracheal width.

4. Name potential complications after tracheostomy tube placement.

- Injury of the recurrent laryngeal nerve with resultant vocal cord paralysis
- Injury of the lung apex with pneumothorax or pneumomediastinum formation
- Injury of the trachea with tracheal malacia or stricture formation
- Soft tissue infection, leading to tracheal ulceration and perforation with tracheoinnominate artery fistula, tracheoesophageal fistula, or cervical abscess formation

5. What is the radiographic appearance and ideal positioning of a nasogastric tube (NGT) or orogastric tube?

Radiographically, a thin, radiopaque curvilinear strip is visualized along the entire length of the tube (Fig. 69-2). The tube should extend inferiorly along the midline of the chest, with its tip located at least 10 cm within the stomach because multiple side-holes are usually present from about 10 cm proximal to its distal end.

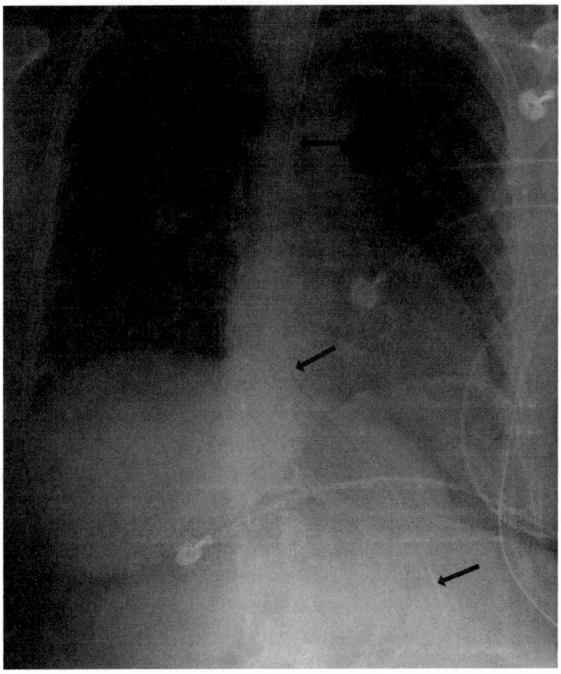

6. Describe the radiographic appearance and optimal location of an enteral feeding tube.

On plain film radiography, a radiopaque marker at the tip of the tube is generally seen and should be located beyond the gastric pylorus within the duodenum, optimally at the duodenojejunal junction (ligament of Treitz). On frontal radiography, the tube generally curves to follow the C-shaped loop of the duodenum, and on lateral radiography, the tube curves posteriorly from the gastric antrum into the duodenum before it enters the retroperitoneal second portion of the duodenum (Fig. 69-3).

Figure 69-2. Appropriately positioned NGT on frontal radiograph. Note the thin radiopaque curvilinear strip along entire length of NGT (*arrows*), which extends inferiorly along the midline of the chest in the expected location of the esophagus with the tip overlying the expected location of the stomach.

7. Discuss ways in which NGT, orogastric tube, or feeding tube may be malpositioned, including other potential complications.

Coiling within the pharynx or esophagus may be seen even if the tip of the tube is in the appropriate position and may lead to vomiting and subsequent aspiration (Fig. 69-4). If a tube is located above the gastroesophageal junction, vomiting and subsequent aspiration may again occur. With tracheobronchial placement, the tube follows the course of the trachea and bronchi, sometimes with lung perforation and location within the pleural space, leading to intrabronchial infusion of feedings, pneumonia, lung abscess, empyema, hydropneumothorax, or pneumothorax (Fig. 69-5). Esophageal perforation is a rare, serious complication, but extraesophageal tube location is not generally appreciated on frontal radiography unless other views or water-soluble contrast agent injection are performed, which typically show a tube that does not follow the expected course of the esophagus, a widened mediastinum, pneumomediastinum, a unilateral pleural effusion, or contrast agent leak from the esophagus into other thoracic compartments.

8. If NGT, orogastric tube, or feeding tube is misplaced within the tracheobronchial tree, what should one do before removing the tube?

One should have a thoracostomy tube set ready at the patient's bedside before removing the tube, just in case a pneumothorax suddenly develops because of lung perforation with a tear in the visceral pleura.

9. When is a thoracostomy tube generally used?

A thoracostomy tube is generally placed for drainage of air (pneumothorax), particularly when persistent (i.e., with a bronchopleural fistula), large, increasing, or symptomatic (i.e., under tension); fluid (pleural effusion); blood (hemothorax); chylous fluid (chylothorax); or pus (empyema) from the pleural space. It may also be placed for drainage of a lung abscess.

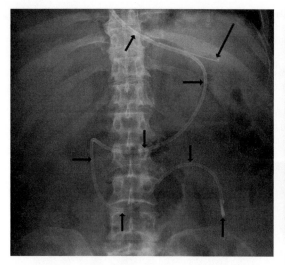

Figure 69-3. Appropriately positioned feeding tube on frontal abdominal radiograph. Note feeding tube (*short arrows*) that curves to follow the C-shaped loop of duodenum with radiopaque marker at the tip overlying the expected located of the duodenojejunal junction (ligament of Treitz). Also note appropriately positioned tip of NGT (*long arrow*) overlying the expected location of the stomach in the left upper quadrant of the abdomen with a thin radiopaque curvilinear strip along its visualized portion.

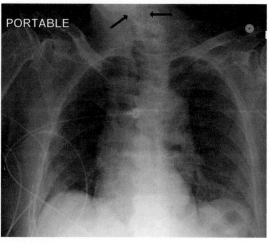

Figure 69-4. Malpositioned feeding tube on frontal chest radiograph. Note portion of feeding tube (*arrows*) curled within the pharynx and upper thoracic esophagus.

10. What is the radiographic appearance of a thoracostomy tube, and where should its tip be located?

A curvilinear radiopaque stripe that has a short-segment interruption in it at the level of its proximal drainage hole is typically seen on radiography; the tube should curve gently within the thorax (Fig. 69-6). For drainage of a pneumothorax, the tube should be positioned near the lung apex at the anterior axillary line and directed anterosuperiorly, whereas for drainage of a pleural effusion, the tube should be positioned at the mid-axillary line and directed posteroinferiorly through the sixth through eighth intercostal spaces. In either case, the proximal side-hole should always be located medial to the ribs within the pleural space. Computed tomography (CT) is indicated when a thoracostomy tube does not drain air or fluid properly, and the chest radiograph is noncontributory.

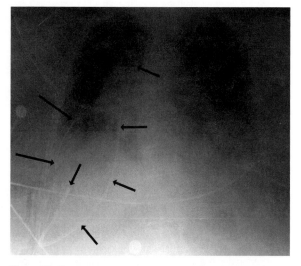

Figure 69-5. Malpositioned feeding tube on frontal chest radiograph. Note feeding tube (*short arrows*) following course of right bronchi and terminating in inferior right hemithorax within pleural space. Also note right thoracostomy tube (*long arrows*) within right pleural space to drain complex pleural fluid.

11. Discuss potential complications of thoracostomy tube placement.

Persistent pneumothorax and extensive subcutaneous emphysema may occur if side-holes are located external to the rib cage and pleural space (Fig. 69-7). Lung laceration with bronchopleural fistula may also occur (Fig. 69-8) with a persistent pneumothorax, pneumomediastinum, and extensive subcutaneous emphysema and is more commonly seen with preexisting lung disease or pleural adhesions. Laceration or injury of an intercostal artery, phrenic nerve, thoracic duct, diaphragm, liver, spleen, stomach, mediastinum, heart, breast, or pectoralis muscle may also occur. Placement within an interlobar fissure is common, may cause poor tube function, and is best seen on CT. Soft tissue or pleural infection may occur adjacent to the tube insertion site. Unilateral re-expansion pulmonary edema may be seen with rapid pleural decompression, and rapid development of an infiltrate at the tip or side-holes may be due to pulmonary infarction from suction of lung tissue. High insertion in the posterior chest wall may lead to Horner syndrome, and recurrence of a pleural collection, pleurocutaneous fistula, or retention of a tube fragment are potential complications after tube removal.

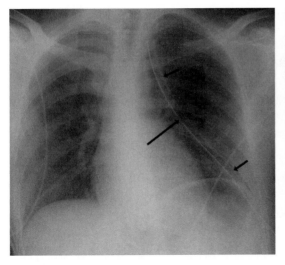

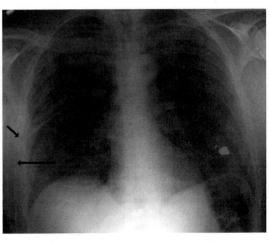

Figure 69-7. Malpositioned thoracostomy tube on frontal chest radiograph. Note thoracostomy tube (*short arrow*) with side-hole (*long arrow*) located external to rib cage.

Figure 69-6. Appropriately positioned thoracostomy tube for pneumothorax on frontal chest radiograph. Note gentle curve of the thoracostomy tube (*short arrows*) with curvilinear radiopaque stripe and short-segment interruption because of side-hole (*long arrow*) with the tip located near the lung apex directed anterosuperiorly.

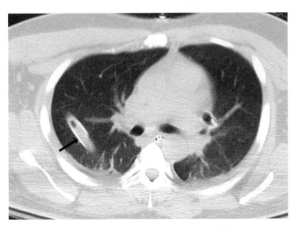

Figure 69-8. Malpositioned thoracostomy tube on CT. Note thoracostomy tube (*arrow*) located within right lung parenchyma instead of pleural space.

12. How can I decrease the chance of injury to an intercostal artery or vein during thoracostomy tube placement?

Place the tube just superior to a rib to avoid the neurovascular bundle that is located at the inferior aspect of each rib.

13. Describe the basic normal venous anatomy of the chest.

The deeply situated brachial veins and the superficially situated basilic and cephalic veins of the upper extremities converge centrally to form the axillary veins. The axillary veins become the subclavian veins beyond the lateral aspects of the first ribs, and the superficially located external jugular veins drain from the neck into the subclavian veins. More centrally, the subclavian veins and internal jugular veins from the neck converge to form the brachiocephalic veins (longer on the left than on the right), which join to form the superior vena cava (SVC), finally leading to the right atrium. The vertical portion of the azygos vein is located to the right of the thoracic spine and drains superiorly to its horizontal portion, which drains into the posterior SVC above the right main stem bronchus. The hemiazygos venous system is located toward the left of the thoracic spine and has variable communication with the azygos system.

14. What is the radiographic appearance and optimal location of a central venous line (CVL) and a peripherally inserted central catheter (PICC)?

A CVL appears as a thin, moderately radiopaque linear or curvilinear tube that extends centrally from a subclavian or internal jugular vein when in the chest (Fig. 69-9), whereas a PICC appears as an even thinner, faintly radiopaque linear or curvilinear tube that extends from the upper extremity (because it is placed peripherally within the lower arm or upper forearm usually via the basilic vein) centrally into the chest. The optimal location of the tip of a CVL and PICC is within the SVC.

15. What are potential complications of CVL or PICC placement?

Early complications include pneumothorax, which is very common and more commonly encountered in the subclavian approach; malpositioning within a vein or artery or in the heart; arterial injury with pseudoaneurysm formation or thromboembolism; venous injury; perforation through a vein with extravascular malpositioning in the pleural space, mediastinum, or soft tissue; cardiac injury with risk of myocardial perforation and cardiac tamponade; hemorrhage or hematoma; air embolism; and catheter knotting, fracture, and embolism. Late complications include catheter occlusion, migration, knotting, fracture, and embolism; venous thrombosis; soft tissue infection; bacteremia/septicemia; and cardiac dysrhythmias, which usually occur with low right atrial placement.

16. List locations where a CVL or PICC may be malpositioned when inserted through a vein.

For a PICC or subclavian vein CVL, malpositioning may occur in the ipsilateral internal jugular vein (Fig. 69-10); contralateral subclavian vein; internal jugular vein; right atrium; right ventricle; pulmonary artery; inferior vena cava; hepatic vein; axillary vein; subclavian vein; brachiocephalic vein; azygos vein; or branch vessels, including the external jugular vein, inferior thyroidal vein, superior intercostal vein, internal thoracic vein, or pericardiacophrenic vein. For an internal jugular vein CVL, malpositioning within the ipsilateral subclavian vein may also occur. Intracardiac malpositioning of a CVL inserted via the subclavian vein approach is more common when inserted on the right (30%) than on the left (12%).

17. Name some clues of inadvertent arterial puncture with CVL, PICC, or Swan-Ganz catheter (SGC).

At the time of catheter placement, bright red and pulsatile backflow of blood may be seen, although in patients with hypoxia or hypotension, the blood may be nonpulsatile and dark, mimicking venous blood. On chest radiography, arterial location of a catheter should be suspected when the course of the catheter follows the expected course of an artery rather than a vein, or when the tip is located in a mid-sternal or left paravertebral location. Confirmation of an arterial puncture may be performed by analysis of blood gas levels of blood samples drawn through the catheter.

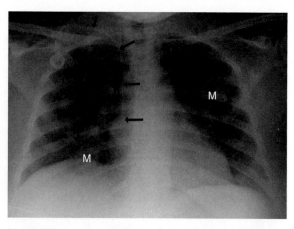

Figure 69-9. Appropriately positioned chemoport CVL for history of uterine sarcoma on frontal chest radiograph. Note thin, moderately radiopaque curvilinear tube (*arrows*) that overlies right internal jugular vein with tip overlying SVC. Also note multiple pulmonary nodules and masses (*M*) in lungs because of metastases.

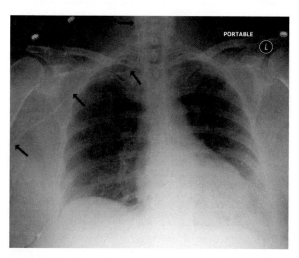

Figure 69-10. Malpositioned PICC on frontal chest radiograph. Note right PICC (*arrows*) seen as thin radiopaque curvilinear tube extending from right upper extremity into the right neck overlying the expected location of the right internal jugular vein.

18. What should one consider in the differential diagnosis for rapid development of an ipsilateral pleural effusion or mediastinal widening after CVL, PICC, or SGC placement?

Rapid development of an ipsilateral pleural effusion or mediastinal widening after venous catheter placement should make one consider (1) perforation of a vein by the catheter, with the tip located in the pleural space or mediastinum after catheter infusion, or (2) vessel injury by the catheter with associated hemithorax or mediastinal hematoma. Pneumothorax is also often associated with vessel injury in this setting.

19. If air embolism is suspected during catheter placement, what should one do to treat the patient?

When air embolism is suspected (usually when a sucking sound during patient inspiration is heard through a catheter at the time of placement or if inadvertent injection of air through a catheter occurs), the patient should immediately be placed in the left lateral decubitus position (i.e., left side down) to keep the air trapped in the right heart chambers, supplemental oxygen should be administered, and vital signs should be monitored.

20. How do I prevent air embolism during catheter placement in the first place?

Air embolism during line placement is easily prevented by keeping a finger over the open end of the catheter until the catheter is flushed with saline and capped.

21. Describe the radiographic appearance of SGC and its optimal location.

SGC (or pulmonary arterial catheter) appears as a thin, moderately radiopaque curvilinear tube that originates centrally from a subclavian or internal jugular vein and passes successively through the brachiocephalic vein, SVC, right atrium, right ventricle, and pulmonary outflow tract, with its tip optimally located in the main, right, or left pulmonary artery or within a proximal lobar pulmonary arterial branch (Fig. 69-11). When a balloon at the tip is inflated for pulmonary capillary wedge pressure measurement, a 1-cm round radiolucency at the catheter tip may be seen radiographically. A thin, short linear tubular radiopacity is also generally seen at the skin entry site, which is the vascular sheath that surrounds the SGC. The SGC can be removed while the sheath still remains in place.

22. What are potential complications of SGC placement?

Potential complications of SGC placement include the complications listed previously for CVL or PICC placement and malpositioning within the right atrium, right ventricle, pulmonary outflow tract, or peripheral pulmonary arterial branch; curling within cardiac chambers (Fig. 69-12) with associated cardiac injury, thrombus formation, or atrial or ventricular cardiac dysrhythmias; tricuspid or pulmonic valve injury; pulmonary arterial injury/rupture, occasionally with formation of either a pseudoaneurysm or a pulmonary artery to bronchial fistula; pulmonary thromboembolism; and pulmonary infarction.

23. Why can pulmonary infarction occur as a complication of SGC placement?

Pulmonary infarction with SGC placement results from obstruction of pulmonary blood flow because of tip placement
too peripherally within a pulmonary arterial branch or persistent inflation of the balloon at the catheter tip. Generally, the extent of pulmonary infarction is directly related to the caliber of the occluded vessel and to the portions of lung supplied by it. Typically, if the tip of the SGC is seen to be more than 2 cm lateral to the pulmonary hilum on frontal chest radiography, it is too peripheral in location and should be pulled back. The balloon should be inflated only during the measurement of wedge pressures.

24. How does an intra-aortic counterpulsation balloon (IACB) work?

An IACB is inserted percutaneously via the common femoral artery and subsequently passes through the external iliac artery, common iliac artery, and abdominal aorta to reach the descending thoracic aorta. A long, inflatable balloon approximately 3 cm long is present around the distal catheter that is repeatedly inflated during early diastole and deflated during early systole at each cardiac cycle. This helps to increase myocardial oxygenation and decrease myocardial oxygenation demand, mainly through improved coronary and peripheral arterial blood flow and decreased cardiac afterload.

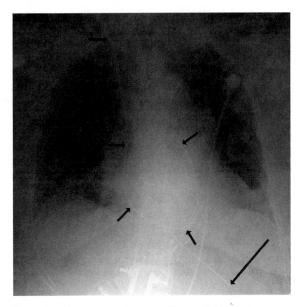

Figure 69-11. Appropriately positioned SGC on frontal chest radiograph. Note thin, moderately radiopaque curvilinear tube (*short arrows*) that overlies right internal jugular vein in the neck and successively follows the course of the right brachiocephalic vein, SVC, right atrium, right ventricle, and pulmonary outflow tract, with the tip located over the main pulmonary artery. Also note the appropriately positioned tip of NGT overlying the stomach in the left upper quadrant of the abdomen (*long arrow*).

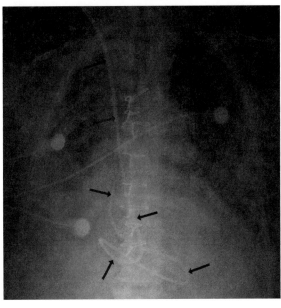

Figure 69-12. Malpositioned SGC on frontal chest radiograph. Note SGC (*arrows*) curled over right heart with tip overlying the superior aspect of the right atrium.

25. What are the major indications and contraindications for placement of IACB?

IACB is often used in critically ill patients with left ventricular failure, unstable angina, acute myocardial ischemia/infarction associated with percutaneous transluminal angioplasty, or severe mitral regurgitation. Major contraindications to IACB placement include severe aortic insufficiency, aortic dissection, severe peripheral vascular disease, or contraindication to systemic anticoagulation.

26. Describe the radiographic appearance of an IACB and its optimal position.

The distal tip of an IACB is seen as a small, radiopaque rectangle and should be located on frontal chest radiography just distal to the left subclavian artery within the proximal descending thoracic aorta below the level of the aortic knob (Fig. 69-13).

27. What are the potential complications of IACB?

Potential complications include arterial injury and hemorrhage; aortic dissection; arterial thromboembolism with secondary limb, visceral, or cerebral ischemia; malpositioning within the aorta proximal to the left subclavian artery or far distal to the aortic arch; venous malpositioning; balloon rupture with potential air embolism if helium gas is used for balloon inflation; thrombocytopenia; soft tissue infection or hematoma formation at the percutaneous site of insertion; or bacteremia/septicemia. When the balloon is located proximal to the left subclavian artery, potential occlusion of the arterial branch vessels of the aortic arch (i.e., innominate, left common carotid, and left subclavian arteries) is possible; when the balloon is located far distal to the aortic arch, counterpulsation is less effective, and potential occlusion of the visceral branch vessels is possible.

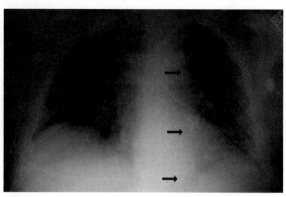

Figure 69-13. Appropriately positioned IACB on frontal chest radiograph. Note linear radiopaque IACB (*arrows*) overlying descending thoracic aorta to the left of midline with small radiopaque rectangle at the tip overlying proximal descending thoracic aorta inferior to the aortic knob.

Key Points: Tubes, Lines, and Catheters

1. If NGT, orogastric tube, or feeding tube is seen to extend into a distal bronchus, lung, or pleural space, the clinical staff should be notified immediately, and the radiologist should suggest that tube removal be performed only after a thoracostomy tube set is at the bedside in case a significant pneumothorax develops.
2. Rapid development of an ipsilateral pleural effusion or mediastinal widening after venous catheter placement should lead one to consider venous perforation, with the tip located in the pleural space or mediastinum after catheter infusion, or vessel injury with associated hemithorax or mediastinal hematoma.
3. When air embolism is suspected during line placement or use, the patient should immediately be placed in the left lateral position to keep the air trapped in the right heart chambers, supplemental oxygen should be administered, and vital signs should be monitored.

---

28. What is the radiographic appearance of a transvenous pacemaker or automatic implantable cardioverter defibrillator (AICD)?

The power/generator pack for a transvenous pacemaker or AICD is located subcutaneously in the pectoral area of the anterior chest wall and appears as a radiopaque, round or ovoid structure that is about 5 cm in diameter on frontal chest radiography. The metallic lead appears as a dense, thin curvilinear radiopacity (associated with thicker short segments of spring defibrillation coils in the case of AICD) that generally extends through the subclavian or internal jugular vein from the generator pack to pass through the brachiocephalic vein and SVC, subsequently terminating in the right atrium, right ventricle, or coronary sinus (Figs. 69-14 and 69-15A).

29. Where should the leads of a transvenous pacemaker or AICD be located?

A right atrial lead (usually in the right atrial appendage) curves around the right side of the heart on frontal chest radiography just below the SVC. On frontal chest radiography, a right ventricular lead should project slightly to the left of midline over the ventricular apex, and on lateral chest radiography it should project anteriorly and inferiorly near the ventricular apex. A lead within the coronary sinus projects superiorly and to the left over the heart on frontal chest radiography, and on lateral chest radiography it is directed posteriorly along the course of the atrioventricular groove.

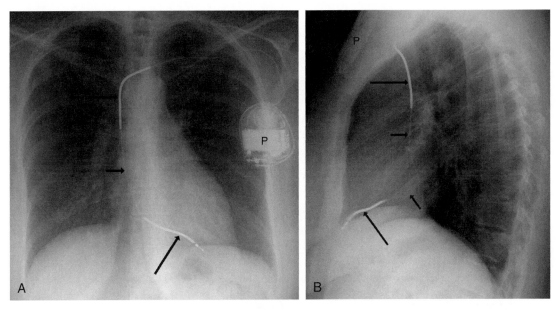

Figure 69-14. A, Appropriately positioned AICD on frontal chest radiograph. Note power/generator pack (*P*) over left pectoral area as radiopaque ovoid structure connected to a thin curvilinear metallic lead (*short arrow*) with the tip overlying the right ventricular apex to the left of midline. Also note the thicker, short segments of spring defibrillation coils (*long arrow*). **B,** Appropriately positioned AICD on lateral chest radiograph. Note power/generator pack (*P*) over anterior chest wall connected to thin curvilinear metallic lead (*short arrows*) with tip overlying the right ventricular apex anteriorly and inferiorly. Also note thicker, short segments of spring defibrillation coils (*long arrows*).

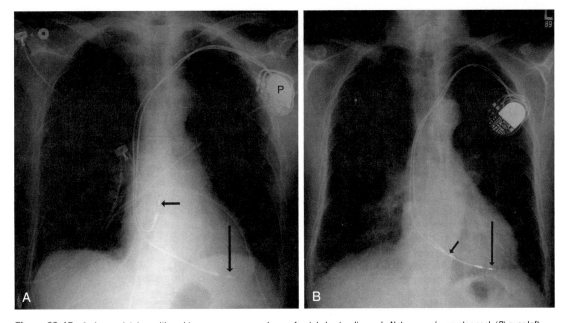

Figure 69-15. A, Appropriately positioned transvenous pacemaker on frontal chest radiograph. Note power/generator pack (*P*) over left pectoral area as a radiopaque ovoid structure connected to leads with tip in the right atrium (*short arrow*) overlying the right side of the heart and tip in the right ventricle (*long arrow*) overlying the ventricular apex. **B,** Subsequent dislodgment of right atrial lead of transvenous pacemaker with migration to the right ventricle on frontal chest radiograph. Note new position of right atrial lead (*short arrow*) compared with **A,** similar to right ventricular lead (*long arrow*).

30. What are potential complications of transvenous pacemaker/AICD placement?

Potential complications of transvenous pacemaker/AICD placement include all the complications of SGC, CVL, and PICC placement previously listed and hematoma or abscess formation around the generator pack; lead malpositioning, redundancy, tautness, dislodgment (Fig. 69-15B), migration, or fracture with or without embolism (Fig. 69-16); twiddler's syndrome; cardiac perforation; loss of pacing or cardioversion/defibrillation function; and induction of cardiac dysrhythmias. Cardiac perforation by a lead should be suspected on chest radiography (particularly on the lateral view) if the lead extends beyond the margin of the cardiac silhouette.

31. What is twiddler's syndrome?

Twiddler's syndrome is a rare disorder in which a patient causes malfunction of a transvenous pacemaker or AICD by manipulating or "twiddling" with the pacing generator pack, which may be facilitated by a large pocket for the generator pack or loose subcutaneous tissue, leading to dislodgment of the pacing leads. Chest radiography is the key to diagnosis and typically shows twisting or coiling of the lead around the axis of the pacemaker and possible lead fracture, displacement, or migration.

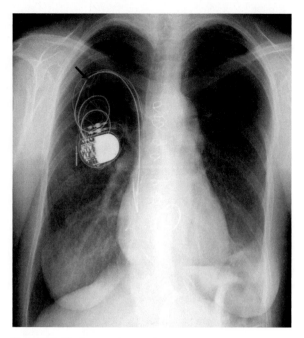

Figure 69-16. Fracture of pacemaker lead on frontal chest radiograph. Note discontinuity (*arrow*) of one pacemaker lead.

BIBLIOGRAPHY

[1] T.Y. Cardall, T.C. Chan, W.J. Brady, et al., Permanent cardiac pacemakers: issues relevant to the emergency physician, part I, J. Emerg. Med. 17 (1999) 479–489.

[2] R.D. Dunbar, Radiologic appearance of compromised thoracic catheters, tubes, and wires, Radiol. Clin. North. Am. 22 (1984) 699–722.

[3] G. Gayer, J. Rozenman, C. Hoffmann, et al., CT diagnosis of malpositioned chest tubes, Br. J. Radiol. 73 (2000) 786–790.

[4] T.B. Gilbert, B.J. McGrath, M. Soberman, Chest tubes: Indications, placement, management, and complications, J. Intensive Care. Med. 8 (1993) 73–86.

[5] C.I. Henschke, D.F. Yankelevitz, A. Wand, et al., Chest radiography in the ICU, Clin. Imaging 21 (1997) 90–103.

[6] H. Levy, Nasogastric and nasoenteric feeding tubes, Gastrointest. Endosc. Clin. North. Am. 8 (1998) 529–549.

[7] J.C. Peterson, D.J. Cook, Intra-aortic balloon counterpulsation pump therapy: a critical appraisal of the evidence for patients with acute myocardial infarction, Crit. Care. 2 (1998) 3–8.

[8] G.W. Stone, E.M. Ohman, M.F. Miller, et al., Contemporary utilization and outcomes of intra-aortic balloon counterpulsation in acute myocardial infarction: the benchmark registry, J. Am. Coll. Cardiol. 41 (2003) 1940–1945.

[9] Z. Zarshenas, R.A. Sparschu, Catheter placement and misplacement, Crit. Care. Clin. 10 (1994) 417–436.

CHAPTER 70

OBSTETRIC ULTRASOUND: FIRST-TRIMESTER IMAGING

Courtney Woodfield, MD, and
Beverly G. Coleman, MD

1. **Should a first-trimester pelvic ultrasound (US) examination be performed transabdominally or transvaginally?**
   Transabdominal pelvic US provides an overall view of the pelvis and is typically performed first, even without a full urinary bladder. If a normal intrauterine pregnancy is identified transabdominally, transvaginal US may be unnecessary. If an intrauterine pregnancy or the adnexa is not well visualized transabdominally, transvaginal US should be performed. The transvaginal approach uses a higher frequency transducer that is placed in closer proximity to the uterus and adnexa, allowing for improved resolution and earlier detection of an intrauterine pregnancy.

2. **What are the indications for first-trimester US?**
   First-trimester US is performed when the pregnancy is high risk (e.g., pregnant by in vitro fertilization or ovulation induction, advanced maternal age, personal or family history of genetic disorders, exposure to teratogens), or when a patient with a positive serum β-human chorionic gonadotropin (β-HCG) level presents with vaginal bleeding, pelvic pain, or an adnexal mass.

3. **List seven causes of vaginal bleeding in the first trimester.**
   - Implantation bleed
   - Subchorionic hemorrhage
   - Embryonic pregnancy/blighted ovum
   - Embryonic demise
   - Spontaneous abortion
   - Ectopic pregnancy
   - Molar pregnancy

4. **Name three possible causes of a positive serum β-HCG level and an empty uterus on US.**
   - Early normal intrauterine pregnancy (<5 weeks)
   - Complete spontaneous abortion
   - Ectopic pregnancy

5. **During a routine first-trimester US examination, what sonographic features should be documented?**
   - Presence and location of a gestational sac
   - Presence or absence of an embryo and yolk sac
   - Sonographic gestational (menstrual) age based on the mean gestational sac diameter and, when possible, the embryonic crown-rump length
   - Embryonic cardiac activity and heart rate
   - Number of gestations
   - Uterine, adnexal, and cul-de-sac findings

6. **When should a gestational sac be seen with transabdominal and transvaginal US?**
   By 5 weeks (serum β-HCG level of 1000 to 2000 mIU/mL), a gestational sac of approximately 5 mm should be seen transabdominally or transvaginally.

Key Points: US Features of Normal Early Intrauterine Pregnancy

1. "Double decidual sac" sign present by 5 to 6 weeks
2. Yolk sac visible by mean gestational sac diameter of 8 mm transvaginally and 20 mm transabdominally
3. Embryo visible by mean gestational sac diameter of 16 mm transvaginally and 25 mm transabdominally
4. Embryonic cardiac activity detected when crown-rump length is 5 mm or greater

---

7. Describe the US features of a normal gestational sac.

Before 5 weeks, a small, hypoechoic saclike structure may be seen within the thickened, echogenic decidual reaction of the endometrium (the "intradecidual sac" sign) (Fig. 70-1). By 5 to 6 weeks, the gestational sac appears as a smooth, round or ovoid, anechoic structure along the upper uterine body surrounded by a 2-mm-thick hyperechoic rim of decidual reaction (the "double decidual sac" sign). The gestational sac grows at a rate of 1.1 mm/day.

8. What constitutes the "double decidual sac" sign?

Visualization of the echogenic decidual reaction of early pregnancy as two or three separate layers is indicative of the "double decidual sac" sign. Decidua vera lines the endometrial cavity, and decidua capsularis surrounds the gestational sac. The decidua basalis arises at the site of implantation and contributes to placental formation. When a small amount of hypoechoic fluid in the endometrial cavity separates the echogenic decidual layers of the endometrium and gestational sac, the "double decidual sac" sign is produced (Fig. 70-2). The "double decidual sac" sign is highly suggestive of an intrauterine pregnancy.

9. When should a yolk sac and an embryo be seen with transabdominal and transvaginal US?

The mean gestational sac sizes at which a yolk sac and an embryo should be seen (also known as the *discriminatory sac sizes*) are outlined in Table 70-1. Fig. 70-3 depicts the normal early gestational US appearance of an embryo and a yolk sac.

10. At what point should embryonic cardiac activity be detected on US?

Embryonic cardiac activity should be detectable transvaginally when the embryonic crown rump length is 5 mm or more. Absence of sonographically detectable embryonic cardiac activity when the crown-rump length is greater than 5 mm is compatible with embryonic demise. Between 5 and 8 weeks, the heart rate is usually 100 beats/min or greater. From 8 weeks to term, the average heart rate is 140 beats/min (range 120 to 180 beats/min). The thresholds for bradycardia based on embryonic size are listed in Table 70-2.

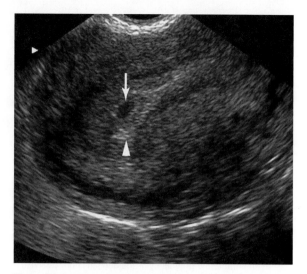

Figure 70-1. Sagittal transvaginal US image of the uterus shows "intradecidual sac" sign of an early intrauterine pregnancy, with a hypoechoic saclike structure (*arrow*) of less than 5 mm located within the thickened, echogenic decidual reaction of the endometrium (*arrowhead*).

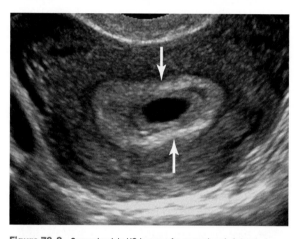

Figure 70-2. Coronal pelvic US image of a normal early intrauterine gestational sac with separation of the hyperechoic decidual endometrial and gestational sac layers, creating "double decidual sac" sign (*arrows*).

Table 70-1. Mean Gestational Sac Sizes at Which a Yolk Sac and an Embryo Should be Seen

	MEAN TRANSVAGINAL GESTATIONAL SAC DIAMETER (mm)	MEAN TRANSABDOMINAL GESTATIONAL SAC DIAMETER (mm)	SERUM β-HCG LEVEL (mIU/mL)*	GESTATIONAL AGE (wk)
Yolk sac visible	8	20	7200	5-6
Embryo visible	16	25	10,000	>6

*Second International Reference Preparation.
β-HCG, β-human chorionic gonadotropin.

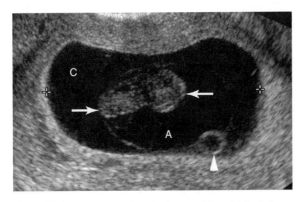

Figure 70-3. Transvaginal US image of a normal 9-week intrauterine pregnancy shows well-defined embryo (*arrows*) and yolk sac (*arrowhead*) with normal separation of the amnion (*A*) and chorionic (*C*) sacs.

11. Describe the US features and significance of an abnormal gestational sac.

On US examination, an irregularly shaped gestational sac that is low-lying and surrounded by a weakly echogenic and thin rim of decidual reaction is 90% to 100% predictive of an abnormal intrauterine pregnancy. A mean gestational sac diameter that is greater than the embryonic crown-rump length by less than 5 mm, which is known as first-trimester oligohydramnios, is also associated with a poor pregnancy outcome. Nonvisualization of an embryo when the mean gestational sac diameter is 25 mm or greater transabdominally and 16 mm or greater transvaginally is reported to be 100% predictive of an abnormal intrauterine pregnancy.

Table 70-2. Thresholds for Bradycardia Based on Embryonic Size	
CROWN-RUMP LENGTH (mm)	**BRADYCARDIA (beats/min)**
<5	<80
5-9	<100
10-15	<110

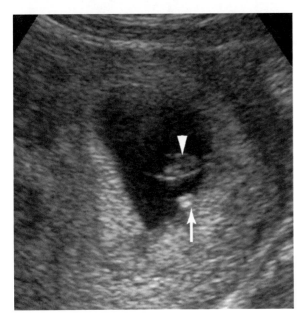

Figure 70-4. Transabdominal pelvic US image of an early failed intrauterine pregnancy with calcified yolk sac (*arrow*) and embryonic remnant (*arrowhead*).

12. What are the US findings of an abnormal yolk sac?

A yolk sac that is large (>6 mm), fragmented, or calcified is suggestive of an abnormal intrauterine pregnancy (Fig. 70-4).

13. Name six types of early pregnancy complications, and describe their US appearances.

See Table 70-3 and Fig. 70-5.

14. What is an ectopic pregnancy?

An ectopic pregnancy refers to a pregnancy located anywhere outside of the endometrial cavity. Ectopic pregnancies occur with a frequency of approximately 14 in 1000 pregnancies. An ectopic pregnancy most commonly occurs in the fallopian tube (95% to 97% of cases), typically in the isthmic or ampullary portion of the tube. Other sites include the interstitial portion of the fallopian tube (2% to 5%), the ovary (1%), the cervix (<0.1%), and the abdominal cavity (<0.1%).

15. Who is at increased risk for an ectopic pregnancy?

Women with a history of prior ectopic pregnancy, pelvic inflammatory disease, fallopian tube surgery, in vitro fertilization, or use of an intrauterine contraceptive device are at increased risk for an ectopic pregnancy.

16. What is the classic clinical presentation of an ectopic pregnancy?

Approximately 45% of patients with ectopic pregnancies present with the clinical triad of vaginal bleeding, pelvic pain, and a palpable adnexal mass.

Table 70-3. Ultrasound Appearance of Six Types of Early Pregnancy Complications

TYPE OF ABORTION	DEFINITION	ULTRASOUND FINDINGS
Threatened abortion	Vaginal bleeding with closed cervical os	Range from live embryo to small, empty gestational sac to normal empty uterus
Abortion in progress	Intrauterine gestation in the process of being expelled	Irregular gestational sac in lower uterus/cervix with or without live embryo
Incomplete abortion	Incomplete passage of gestational tissues	Thickened endometrium with or without fluid and debris; areas of increased endometrial vascularity
Complete abortion	Expulsion of all gestational tissues	Normal empty uterus, which may be mildly vascular
Blighted ovum	Failed or abnormal embryonic development	Empty gestational sac or sac with abnormal yolk sac and no embryo; any abnormal gestational sac development
Embryonic demise	Lack of embryonic growth and absent expected cardiac activity	Embryo without cardiac activity

17. List four possible US findings associated with an ectopic pregnancy.

- Embryo located outside of the uterus (5% to 10% of cases)—100% diagnostic of an ectopic pregnancy
- Complex or solid adnexal mass (Fig. 70-6)
- Moderate to large amount of pelvic free fluid, especially if it is particulate
- Empty uterus in conjunction with serum β-HCG level that is above the level at which a gestational sac should be seen.

18. What is a pseudogestational sac?

In the setting of an ectopic pregnancy, a variable amount of fluid or hypoechoic debris may accumulate within the endometrial cavity, giving rise to a pseudogestational sac of an ectopic pregnancy (Fig. 70-7). This collection of fluid and debris may be surrounded by a single, thin, echogenic rim of decidual reaction because of stimulation of the endometrium by the circulating hormones of an ectopic pregnancy. A pseudogestational sac may be present in 5% of ectopic pregnancies.

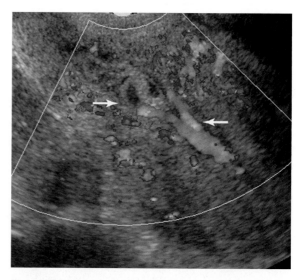

Figure 70-5. Sagittal transvaginal color Doppler US image of an incomplete abortion with increased vascularity, fluid, and echogenic debris (*arrows*) along the endometrium.

19. What is a heterotopic pregnancy?

A heterotopic pregnancy occurs when there are concurrent intrauterine and extrauterine gestations. Patients who are pregnant by in vitro fertilization or the use of ovulation induction have a higher incidence of multiple gestations and are also at increased risk for ectopic and heterotopic pregnancies.

20. How common are heterotopic pregnancies?

The frequency of heterotopic pregnancies in the general population is approximately 1 in 7000 pregnancies. A higher heterotopic pregnancy rate of 1% has been reported in patients pregnant by in vitro fertilization.

Key Points: US Findings Associated with Ectopic Pregnancy

1. Extrauterine embryo (100% diagnostic)
2. Complex or solid adnexal mass
3. Moderate to large amount of particulate pelvic free fluid
4. Empty uterus with extrauterine gestational sac

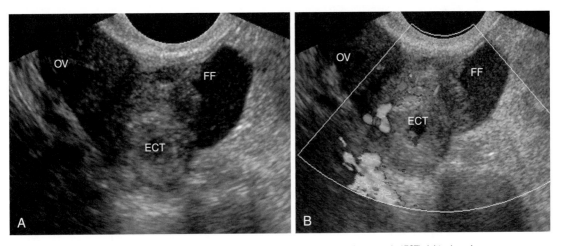

Figure 70-6. A and **B,** Coronal gray-scale (**A**) and Doppler (**B**) transvaginal US images of an ectopic (*ECT*) right adnexal pregnancy seen as a tubal ring separate from the right ovary (*OV*). There is also a small amount of adjacent particulate free fluid (*FF*).

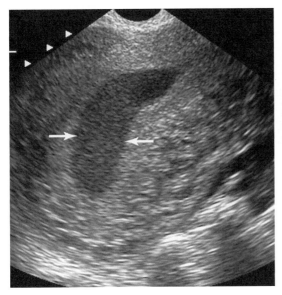

Figure 70-7. Sagittal transvaginal US image of a pseudogestational sac (*arrows*) of an ectopic pregnancy with echogenic material consistent with hemorrhage filling the endometrial cavity.

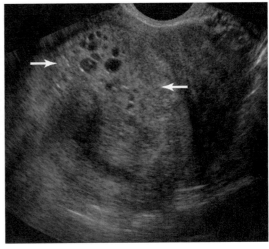

Figure 70-8. Sagittal midline transvaginal pelvic US image of an endometrial cavity filled with heterogeneous cystic and solid placental tissue (*arrows*), which is characteristic of a complete molar pregnancy.

21. What is a molar pregnancy?

A molar pregnancy is the most common and most benign form of gestational trophoblastic disease and is characterized by proliferation of placental tissue after abnormal fertilization of an empty ovum by one (complete mole, no fetus) or two (partial mole, fetus present) sperm. Patients characteristically present with markedly elevated serum β-HCG levels, an enlarged uterus, hyperemesis gravidarum, preeclampsia, or vaginal bleeding, or a combination of these findings.

22. What is the US appearance of a molar pregnancy?

The edematous placental tissue and prominent chorionic villi of a molar pregnancy classically have a "snowstorm" appearance on US. The endometrial canal is filled with hyperechoic placental tissue with good through-transmission and numerous small cystic villi, which may be too small to visualize (Fig. 70-8). A complete mole involves the entire placenta without a fetus. A partial mole involves a portion of the placenta and has an associated fetus, usually with multiple anomalies. Early first-trimester molar pregnancies can mimic blighted ova.

BIBLIOGRAPHY

[1] E. Lazarus, What's new in first trimester ultrasound, Radiol. Clin. North. Am. 41 (2003) 663–679.
[2] E.A. Lyons, C.S. Levi, S.M. Dashefsky, The first trimester, in: C.M. Rumack, S.R. Wilson, J.W. Charboneau (Eds.), Diagnostic Ultrasound, second ed., Mosby, St. Louis, 1998, pp. 975–1011.
[3] W.D. Middleton, A.B. Kurtz, B.S. Hertzberg, The first trimester and ectopic pregnancy, in: Ultrasound: The Requisites, second ed., Mosby, St. Louis, 2003, pp. 342–373.

OBSTETRIC ULTRASOUND: SECOND-TRIMESTER IMAGING

Ross I. Silver, MD, and
Beverly G. Coleman, MD

CHAPTER 71

1. What are the components of the basic (level 1) second-trimester ultrasound (US) examination?

The components of a basic second-trimester US examination include:

- Documentation of the fetal heart rate
- Number and lie of fetuses
- Estimation of the amniotic fluid volume
- Location and appearance of the placenta and its relationship to the internal os
- Gestational age
- Evaluation of the uterus and adnexa
- Assessment of fetal anatomic characteristics, including cerebral ventricles, four-chamber heart, spine, stomach, urinary bladder, umbilical cord, and kidneys

2. How is the normal amniotic fluid volume estimated?

To calculate the amniotic fluid index (AFI), the anteroposterior diameters of the largest empty fluid pocket (no umbilical cord or fetal parts) in each quadrant are added together. The AFI is normally 7 to 25 cm. In addition, each individual pocket of fluid should be 2 to 8 cm. Fluctuations outside of this range define *oligohydramnios* (too little amniotic fluid) or *polyhydramnios* (too much amniotic fluid).

> **Key Points: Components of a Basic Second-Trimester Ultrasound Examination**
>
> 1. Documentation of fetal heart rate and number and lie of fetuses
> 2. Estimation of amniotic fluid volume
> 3. Location and appearance of the placenta and its relationship to the internal os
> 4. Gestational age
> 5. Evaluation of the uterus and adnexa
> 6. Fetal anatomic characteristics

3. What are the major causes of polyhydramnios?

One third of cases of polyhydramnios are idiopathic and not associated with other anomalies. Two thirds of cases are associated with maternal problems, fetal problems, or both. These include gestational diabetes, multiple gestations, structural abnormalities of the fetus that impair swallowing of amniotic fluid (obstruction of the upper gastrointestinal tract, chest narrowing or masses, and severe central nervous system abnormalities), and fetal hydrops.

4. What is the dreaded complication of oligohydramnios?

The lungs need an adequate supply of amniotic fluid for proper development. Oligohydramnios leads to pulmonary hypoplasia, which, depending on the severity, can be a major cause of fetal morbidity and mortality.

5. If the placenta appears to be covering the internal os, what entity may be present?

This is called *placenta previa,* which occurs in 1 in 200 to 400 deliveries, more commonly after a previous cesarean section. If the placenta extends to the edge of the internal os, a marginal previa is present. If the placenta partially covers the os, this is called a *partial previa,* and if it completely covers the internal os, a *complete previa* is present. A fourth type, a *central previa,* occurs when a complete previa is centrally located over the internal os. Placenta previa can lead to maternal hemorrhage secondary to premature detachment of the placenta. It can also be a cause of premature delivery and perinatal mortality (Fig. 71-1).

6. A pregnant woman presents with vaginal bleeding, pelvic pain, and tenderness over the uterus. What entity must be considered?

This is a common presentation of placental abruption, a serious condition that can cause morbidity in the fetus and, less commonly, in the mother. Risk factors include maternal hypertension, collagen vascular disease, and abdominal trauma.

US can detect placental abruption by showing blood behind a placenta that has separated from the uterine wall. Blood has a variable US appearance, depending on the age of the bleed, that ranges from hypoechoic or completely anechoic in the acute and chronic phases to hyperechoic and heterogeneous in the subacute phase.

7. What is an "hourglass" deformity of the cervix?

An "hourglass" deformity is a severe form of incompetent cervix that occurs when the internal cervical os is open, and the endocervical canal is dilated to the external os. Clinically, the amniotic membranes bulge into the vagina. Spontaneous pregnancy loss usually cannot be avoided (Fig. 71-2).

8. Can the presence of a single umbilical artery be normal?

Yes. Normal umbilical cords most commonly have three vessels (two arteries and one vein). A two-vessel cord does not imply fetal abnormality. In single gestations, approximately 50% of two-vessel cords (one artery and one vein) have no associated abnormalities. In multiple gestations, a two-vessel cord is a more common normal variant. Of the abnormalities that may exist with a two-vessel cord, fetal structural abnormalities and growth retardation are the most common. The posterior fossa, face, extremities, and heart should be thoroughly evaluated in pregnancies with a single umbilical artery (Fig. 71-3).

9. What is the most accurate measurement to assess gestational age in the second trimester?

The biparietal diameter (BPD) is accurate from approximately 5 to 7 days up to 24 weeks. It is measured in the transverse plane from the outer edge of the closer temporoparietal bone to the inner edge of the farther temporoparietal bone. The thalamus should be visualized when measuring the BPD. The head circumference is as accurate as the BPD and is measured at the same level. The femur length is as accurate as the BPD after 26 weeks (Fig. 71-4A).

10. How is the abdominal circumference obtained, and why is it used?

The abdominal circumference is measured in the transverse plane at the fetal liver, with the umbilical portion of the left portal vein in the center of the abdomen. The abdominal circumference is not as accurate as the BPD and femur length for estimating gestational age. Instead, it is commonly used to determine proportionality with the head. A head-to-abdominal circumference ratio is used for this purpose. Normally, the head is larger than the body in the second and early third trimesters, with a reversal of this ratio at term (Fig. 71-4B).

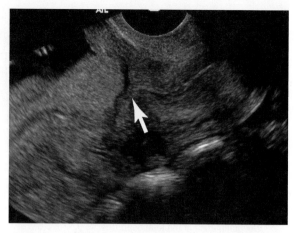

Figure 71-1. Sagittal transvaginal US image shows complete placenta previa. The placenta completely covers the internal os (*arrow*).

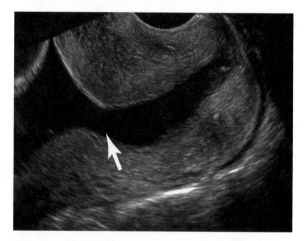

Figure 71-2. Sagittal transvaginal US image shows the "hourglass" deformity of an incompetent cervix (*arrow*).

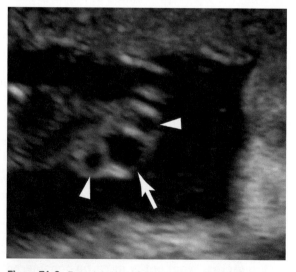

Figure 71-3. Transabdominal US image shows a normal three-vessel cord with single umbilical vein (*arrow*) and two umbilical arteries (*arrowheads*).

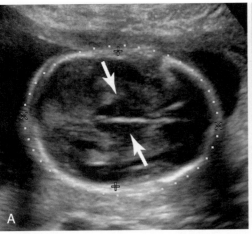 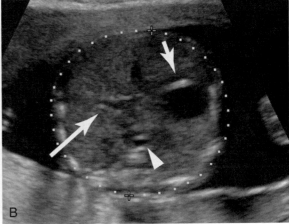

Figure 71-4. Measurements of normal gestational age. **A,** BPD (*plus sign*) and thalami (*arrows*). **B,** Abdominal circumference (*plus sign*), portal vein (*long arrow*), stomach (*short arrow*), and aorta (*arrowhead*).

11. What is the difference between symmetric and asymmetric intrauterine growth retardation (IUGR)?

Asymmetric IUGR constitutes 90% of cases and is due to diminished blood supply and nourishment to the fetus. The abdominal circumference is disproportionately affected compared with the head and femur. It is usually diagnosed in the third trimester. Symmetric IUGR is usually diagnosed in the first or early second trimester and is due to decreased cellular growth, usually secondary to an insult to the mother or fetus early in the pregnancy. The head and body are equally affected in symmetric IUGR.

12. What percentage of cardiac anomalies can be detected by the four-chamber view alone?

Approximately 70% of cardiac anomalies can be detected with the four-chamber view, including abnormalities of cardiac position

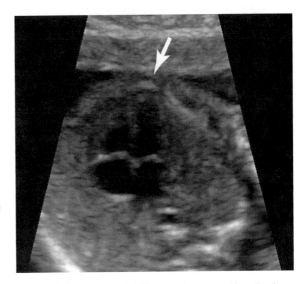

Figure 71-5. Transabdominal US image shows normal four-chamber view of the heart. Apex of the heart (*arrow*).

(situs inversus), septal abnormalities (ventricular septal defect), and masses (rhabdomyomas). The percentage of detected anomalies can be increased to 80% with the addition of a short-axis view of the great vessels at the base of the heart, a view of the right ventricular outflow tract, and a long-axis view of the left ventricular outflow tract (Fig. 71-5).

13. Describe the classic US features of fetal hydrops.

Whether the cause is immune or nonimmune, the appearance of fetal hydrops is the same: fluid in the serous cavities, including ascites; pleural and pericardial effusions; skin thickening; placental enlargement; and polyhydramnios. Not all of these features may be present in any one case, however. In addition, hepatomegaly may be seen, particularly with immune hydrops.

14. What is the most common intrathoracic/extracardiac fetal anomaly?

Congenital diaphragmatic hernia (CDH) occurs in 1 of every 2000 to 3000 live births. Of these, 90% are Bochdalek hernias, which are posterolateral in location. The remaining 10% are Morgagni hernias, which occur in an anteromedial location. With a Bochdalek hernia, US shows the normal stomach bubble located in the chest, and the heart is displaced upward and to the right. The presence of peristaltic, fluid-filled bowel loops in the chest is diagnostic. The spleen and left lobe of the liver may also be present in the thorax. Morgagni hernias are more subtle and difficult to diagnose (Fig. 71-6).

15. Name the four types of anterior abdominal wall defects. Which are most common?

- Omphalocele
- Gastroschisis
- Pentalogy of Cantrell
- Limb–body wall complex

Omphalocele and gastroschisis are the most common, occurring in 1 in 4000 live births (omphalocele) and 1 in 10,000 live births (gastroschisis). The latter two are extremely rare and are associated with a very poor prognosis.

16. Which abdominal wall defect is covered by a membrane?

Omphalocele is defined as the herniation of abdominal contents into the base of the umbilical cord and is covered by a thin amnioperitoneal membrane. Either the liver and small bowel or the small bowel alone can be contained within the defect. Gastroschisis is not covered by a membrane, and the typical appearance is that of free-floating loops of bowel (Fig. 71-7).

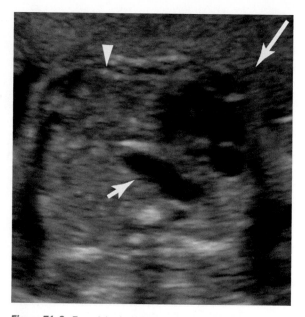

Figure 71-6. Transabdominal US image shows congenital diaphragmatic hernia. The heart (*long arrow*), stomach (*short arrow*), and liver (*arrowhead*) are in the thorax.

17. How can the abdominal cord insertion (ACI) help in the diagnosis of anterior abdominal wall defects?

An omphalocele is centrally located, and the umbilical cord typically inserts into the anterior portion of the defect. A pathognomonic feature of omphalocele is the presence of a "cyst" of Wharton's jelly at the site of cord insertion. A distinguishing feature of gastroschisis is that the defect is paraumbilical, usually to the right of the ACI. Documentation of the ACI is an important part of all second-trimester US examinations. Color flow may be needed to visualize the ACI in some cases (Fig. 71-8).

18. Which has a worse prognosis, omphalocele or gastroschisis?

Omphalocele has a worse prognosis because it is associated with a significantly increased incidence of chromosomal abnormalities (approximately 12%). This is much greater with omphaloceles that contain only bowel. Other structural abnormalities, including cardiac, thoracic, gastrointestinal, genitourinary, and central nervous system, occur in 75% of cases. Gastroschisis is not associated with other abnormalities, although vascular compromise of the extruded bowel (large and small bowel) may occur. Perforation of bowel may lead to an entity called *meconium peritonitis* (Fig. 71-9).

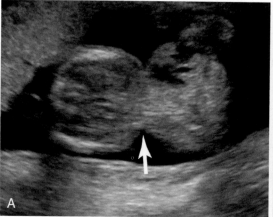 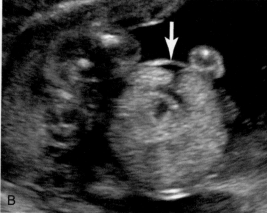

Figure 71-7. A, Transabdominal US image shows abdominal wall defect consistent with omphalocele (*arrow*). **B,** Omphalocele with a covering membrane (*arrow*).

19. Why might the urinary bladder not be visualized?

The bladder should be identified by 16 weeks. Nonvisualization of the urinary bladder is not abnormal, however. Because of the normal cycling of the bladder, rescanning after initial nonvisualization every 15 to 20 minutes for 1 hour is recommended. If the bladder is still not present, an abnormality likely exists, such as impairment of renal function from an intrinsic renal abnormality or upper urinary tract obstruction. Generalized growth retardation can also lead to functional renal impairment. In bladder exstrophy, typically there is an infraumbilical wall defect with nonvisualization of the urinary bladder.

20. A markedly distended bladder and ureters with bilateral hydronephrosis are visualized during a routine second-trimester US of a male fetus. What abnormality may be present?

This is the classic US appearance of a severe, prolonged lower urinary tract obstruction. In a male fetus, this is most commonly caused by posterior urethral valves. In female fetuses, this is likely a result of urethral atresia. Cases of severe lower urinary tract obstruction are usually fatal because of marked oligohydramnios and the pulmonary hypoplasia that results (Fig. 71-10).

21. Name the four patterns of limb shortening seen with skeletal dysplasias.

Skeletal dysplasias can be differentiated by determining which portion of the limb is affected. A *micromelic pattern* of shortening affects the proximal and the distal limbs. If only the proximal segment is shortened, a *rhizomelic type* of dysplasia is present. Less common patterns of dysplasia include the *mesomelic pattern,* in which only the forearm and foreleg are shortened, and

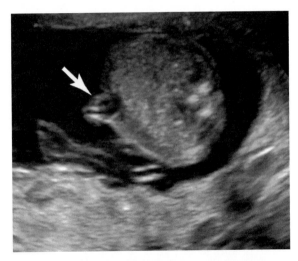

Figure 71-8. Transabdominal US image shows normal ACI (*arrow*).

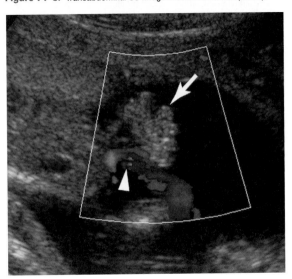

Figure 71-9. Transabdominal US image shows gastroschisis. Free floating bowel loops are seen (*arrow*). Doppler flow shows umbilical cord inserting to the side of the defect (*arrowhead*).

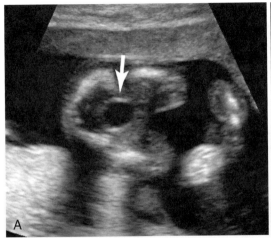
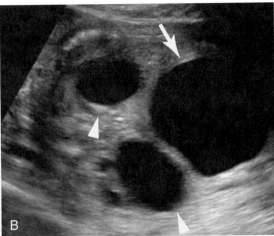

Figure 71-10. A, Transabdominal US image shows normal bladder (*arrow*). **B,** Lower urinary tract obstruction with distended bladder (*arrow*) and ureters (*arrowheads*).

the *acromelic pattern,* in which only the distal segment is shortened. The most common type of skeletal dysplasia, *heterozygous achondroplastic dysplasia,* is characterized by a rhizomelic pattern of shortening.

22. What would produce an enlarged cisterna magna on US?

A Dandy-Walker malformation causes an enlarged cisterna magna. From the inside of the occiput to the back of the cerebellar vermis, the cisterna magna normally measures 2 to 10 mm. Dandy-Walker malformations are caused by dysgenesis (Dandy-Walker variant) or agenesis of the cerebellar vermis and are associated with midline central nervous system abnormalities, including lateral and third ventricle hydrocephalus, encephalocele, and agenesis of the corpus callosum. Additional abnormalities of the body, including cardiac and renal abnormalities, may be found (Fig. 71-11).

23. What is the significance of the nuchal skin?

Directly posterior to the occiput is a thin rim of soft tissue that normally measures 6 mm or less in the second trimester. An increased nuchal skin thickness greater than 6 mm is concerning for Down syndrome. The sensitivity of this finding is 50%, and the false-positive rate is less than 1%.

24. Which open neural tube defect contains elements of spinal cord?

A myelomeningocele contains spinal cord elements; *myelo* is the Latin prefix referring to the spine. The herniation of meninges alone through an open neural tube defect is known simply as a *meningocele.* On US, these defects usually appear as a cystic structure projecting through splayed posterior elements, most commonly in the lumbosacral region. If the cyst is completely anechoic, a meningocele is likely present. Hyperechoic strands representing neural elements within the cystic projection indicate that the likely diagnosis is myelomeningocele (Fig. 71-12).

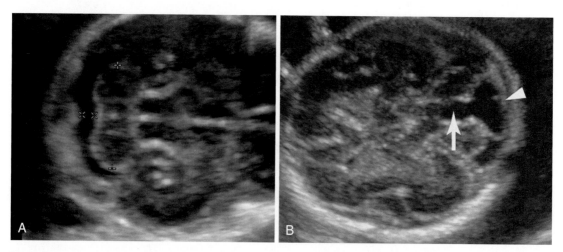

Figure 71-11. A, Transabdominal US image shows normal posterior fossa. Cross hairs measure the cerebellum (*plus sign*) and cisterna magna (*x*). **B,** Dandy-Walker malformation with absent vermis (*arrow*) and enlarged cisterna magna (*arrowhead*).

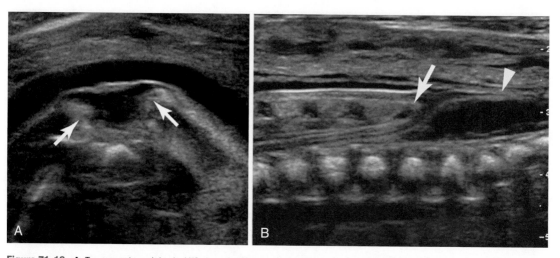

Figure 71-12. A, Transverse transabdominal US view of myelomeningocele. The posterior elements are splayed (*arrows*). **B,** Sagittal view of spine shows a low-lying, tethered spinal cord (*arrow*) and cystic mass arising from the spine (*arrowhead*).

25. When an open neural tube defect is discovered, what else should be evaluated?

The fetal head should be thoroughly evaluated whenever an open neural tube defect is discovered. These defects are almost always associated with Arnold-Chiari type II malformations, in which the cerebellar hemispheres herniate downward through the foramen magnum. Two US signs are associated with this malformation: the "banana" sign and the "lemon" sign. With the "banana" sign, the cerebellum is shaped like a downward-curved C, and with the "lemon" sign, the bilateral frontoparietal bones are flattened. Both signs are sensitive and specific for open neural tube defects; the "banana" sign is seen in more than 90% of cases, and the "lemon" sign is present in approximately 98% of cases.

BIBLIOGRAPHY

[1] W.E. Brant, Ultrasound: The Core Curriculum, Lippincott Williams & Wilkins, Philadelphia, 2001.
[2] P.W. Callen, Ultrasonography in Obstetrics and Gynecology, third ed., Saunders, Philadelphia, 1994.
[3] A.B. Kurtz, W.D. Middleton, Ultrasound: The Requisites, Mosby, St. Louis, 1996.

VASCULAR ULTRASOUND

Denise Fog, DO, and
Beverly G. Coleman, MD

1. What is the incidence of deep venous thrombosis (DVT)?

The exact incidence of DVT is unknown because of the inherent difficulty in establishing the clinical diagnosis related to the nonspecific nature or lack of patient symptoms. More recent data estimate the incidence of DVT to be about 80 cases per 100,000 individuals annually, resulting in 600,000 hospitalizations for this diagnosis every year in the United States. Additionally, each year, approximately 200,000 deaths in the United States are attributed to pulmonary embolism resulting from DVT.

2. How do patients with lower extremity DVT present clinically?

No single physical finding or combination of signs and symptoms is sufficiently accurate to establish the diagnosis. The most common physical signs are:

- Edema, which is primarily unilateral
- Leg pain, which is extremely nonspecific—present in about 50%
- Leg tenderness—seen in about 75%
- Homans sign, which is calf pain with dorsiflexion of the foot—present in less than one third
- Increase in skin temperature with fever

Many patients are asymptomatic, however, making the diagnosis even more difficult.

3. List the risk factors associated with the development of DVT.

- Malignancy
- Recent surgery
- Pregnancy
- Hypercoagulable states
- Stroke
- Trauma
- Cardiac failure
- Respiratory failure
- Immobilization
- Patient age younger than 40
- Obesity
- Oral contraceptive use

4. Describe how to perform an ultrasound (US) examination of the lower extremity when looking for DVT.

Evaluation of the lower extremity for DVT may be performed in the US suite or portably at the patient's bedside. The patient is scanned with a linear array 7-MHz to 10-MHz transducer in the supine position from the inguinal ligament to the proximal calf, with the leg mildly abducted and externally rotated and with slight knee flexion. The deep venous structures are evaluated with B-mode gray-scale images in the transverse plane, compressing every 2 cm. Pulsed Doppler images are also obtained with and without augmentation maneuvers by manually squeezing the more distal portion of the extremity to assess flow. Color images are obtained to evaluate patency of the lumen further.

5. How do the US findings of acute and chronic DVT differ?

See Table 72-1 and Figs. 72-1 and 72-2.

6. How accurate is US in establishing the diagnosis of DVT?

In symptomatic patients, studies that have directly compared US with venography have shown average sensitivities and specificities of 95% and 98%. The results are poorer, however, in asymptomatic, high-risk, or postoperative patients.

Table 72-1. Ultrasound Findings of Acute and Chronic Deep Venous Thrombosis (DVT)

ACUTE DVT	CHRONIC DVT
Loss of complete compressibility of vein	Decreased venous diameter, atretic segment (most sensitive and specific sign)
Isoechoic/hypoechoic intraluminal thrombus	Thickened irregular venous wall
Venous enlargement	Echogenic weblike filling defect
Absent Doppler signal	Venous collaterals
Loss of phasicity	Calcification
Loss of flow augmentation	

Collectively, results from six studies have shown a decrease in average sensitivity to 58%, whereas specificity was maintained at 98%. Reasons for the decrease in sensitivity in this group include small thrombus size, nonocclusive nature of certain thrombi, and higher prevalence of thrombus isolated to the calf.

7. **Discuss treatment options for patients with DVT.**
Proper treatment of patients with DVT is important to help prevent a potentially fatal pulmonary embolism, to decrease associated morbidity, and to reduce the patient's chance of developing postphlebitic syndrome. Several treatment options are available for acute DVT. Anticoagulation, the mainstay of initial therapy, begins with heparin (regular unfractionated heparin or low-molecular-weight heparin), with subsequent conversion to warfarin for 3 to 6 months. Catheter-directed thrombolysis can also be done, resulting in prompt resolution and restoration of normal venous flow. Surgical thrombectomy is also an option and is usually reserved for patients in whom limb salvage is at risk.

8. **List the US findings of a pseudoaneurysm.**
   - Hypoechoic fluid collection immediately adjacent to the injured artery
   - Variable amount of peripheral thrombus
   - Swirling color flow ("yin-yang") as blood flows in and out of the pseudoaneurysm
   - "To-and-fro" pattern of flow at the pseudoaneurysm neck on pulsed Doppler with a normal systolic upstroke as blood enters the pseudoaneurysm
   - Pandiastolic flow reversal because of the compliant nature of the pseudoaneurysm walls, as blood in the pseudoaneurysm cavity is ejected back into the artery during diastole (Fig. 72-3)

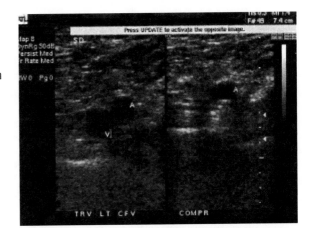
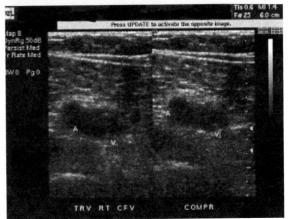

Figure 72-1. Normal vein versus acute DVT. *Left upper frame* shows normal anechoic vein (*V*) without compression, which is equal in size to the adjacent artery (*A*). *Right upper frame* with applied pressure shows that the normal vein is completely compressible. *Left and right lower frames,* performed with and without pressure, show echogenic thrombus distending the lumen of the vein (*V*) and loss of venous compressibility, which is consistent with acute DVT.

9. How may a pseudoaneurysm be treated nonsurgically?

There are two nonsurgical methods for treatment of a pseudoaneurysm.

- Transcutaneous US-guided compression can be performed by applying pressure over the pseudoaneurysm neck. This is a time-consuming process and can be painful for the patient and fatiguing for the physician performing the compression. Success rates are variable and are better when the pseudoaneurysm is acute or subacute and when the neck is narrow.
- A second option is direct thrombin injection into the pseudoaneurysm under US guidance. Compared with transcutaneous US-guided compression, this technique is faster, less painful for the patient, and more successful (success rate is approximately 90%), and it does not require termination of anticoagulation therapy.

10. Summarize the differential diagnoses for a perivascular mass seen on gray-scale imaging.

- *Pseudoaneurysm*: Pseudoaneurysm is a complication of arterial puncture/penetrating trauma, recognized by internal flow with features previously described.
- *Hematoma*: The gray-scale appearance may be identical to pseudoaneurysm, but hematoma is avascular; transmitted pulsation from adjacent artery should not be mistaken for true flow.
- *Hyperplastic lymph node*: A hyperplastic lymph node can be mistaken for a pseudoaneurysm because of the vascularity at its hilum, but it lacks a communicating neck, "yin-yang" flow, and "to-and-fro" pattern
- *Arterial aneurysm*: When fusiform, arterial aneurysm is easily recognized by its appearance or position within the arterial wall; when saccular, it can be difficult to differentiate from a pseudoaneurysm because they may share color Doppler flow patterns.

11. What are the characteristic findings of an arteriovenous fistula (AVF) on US?

Color and pulsed Doppler imaging techniques are extremely important to make this diagnosis because no gray-scale abnormality is seen. With color imaging, a perivascular tissue vibration at the fistula site can be seen, resulting in a color bruit (Doppler artifact with random assignment of red and blue pixels in the perivascular soft tissue). Pulsed Doppler findings include localized low-resistance arterial flow, shown by increased diastolic flow velocity and continuous forward flow throughout the cardiac cycle. This is in contrast to the normally absent or reversed diastolic flow seen in most peripheral arteries. On the venous end, localized turbulent or arterialized flow is seen because of direct arterial inflow (Fig. 72-4).

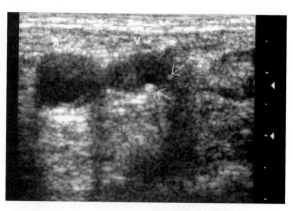

Figure 72-2. Chronic DVT. An echogenic thrombus is identified within the lumen of the vein (*V*), as with acute DVT. There is, however, calcification (*arrows*) within this long-standing clot, a feature of chronic thrombus.

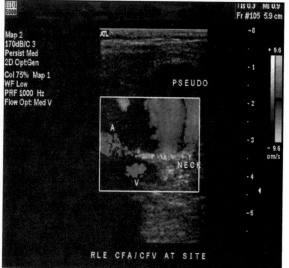

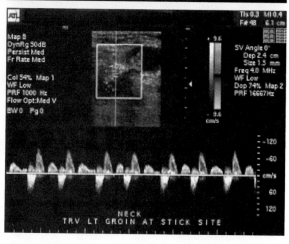

Figure 72-3. Pseudoaneurysm. *Top,* Color Doppler image reveals characteristic "yin-yang" appearance as blood swirls within this post-traumatic groin pseudoaneurysm, which is labeled "pseudo." Note the thin linear attachment of the pseudoaneurysm to the adjacent artery (*A*), labeled "neck." *Bottom,* Pulsed Doppler image at the neck of the pseudoaneurysm shows normal antegrade systolic flow and diastolic flow reversal, the "to-and-fro" pattern.

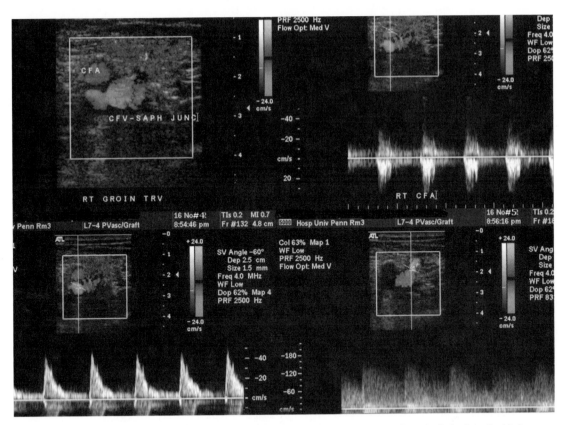

Figure 72-4. AVF. *Upper left panel* shows an example of a color bruit artifact (random assignment of extraluminal color pattern) in the region of an AVF, located above and to the right of the common femoral artery (CFA) in this image. *Upper right panel* shows abnormally low-resistance flow when Doppler sampled the affected artery. *Lower right panel* shows there is abnormal pulsatility and arterialization of the venous waveform. *Lower left panel* shows that a sample taken at the site of the AVF resulted in a mixed low-resistance waveform.

12. Where in the femoral vasculature do AVFs most commonly occur?

AVFs have increased in frequency because of the more common use of larger catheters and anticoagulation in various vascular interventional procedures. Most AVFs are asymptomatic. When large, however, they can result in high-output cardiac failure or lower extremity ischemia. AVFs are almost always located distal to the femoral bifurcation. Above the bifurcation, the femoral artery and vein are positioned side by side. Below the femoral bifurcation, the femoral vein is posterior to the artery, making it more likely that AVF will develop, especially as complication of a procedure.

13. Identify common indications for performing a carotid US examination.

- Evaluation of patients with transient ischemic attack or cerebrovascular accident
- Evaluation of a neck bruit or pulsat ile neck mass
- Postoperative follow-up after carotid endarterectomy
- Preoperative screening before major cardiovascular surgical procedures

14. Name the three components of a carotid US examination.

- *B-mode* is two-dimensional gray-scale imaging in the transverse and longitudinal planes. It is used to identify wall thickening and the presence of plaque, to characterize plaque, and to estimate the degree of luminal narrowing.
- *Spectral analysis* is a quantitative graphic display of the velocity and direction of flowing blood within a selected Doppler sample volume.
- *Color Doppler* provides simultaneous hemodynamic and anatomic information by showing flow direction, providing velocity information, and clarifying pulsed wave Doppler image mismatch.

15. What spectral analysis findings are indicative of stenosis?

Depending on where the Doppler sample is obtained, the waveform findings are variable. There is an increase in resistance of flow proximal to the level of stenosis, which is manifested as decreased diastolic flow. At and distal to the level of stenosis, turbulence causes broadening of the spectral waveform. After the luminal diameter narrows approximately 40% to 50%, the velocity increases with increasing severity of stenosis except in some cases of critical stenosis (>95%), in which case the velocity may decrease or become normal again because of reduced flow volume.

16. What parameters are used to grade the degree of carotid artery stenosis?

Several parameters can be used in isolation or in combination:

- Peak systolic velocity
- End-diastolic velocity
- Ratio of internal carotid artery (ICA) to common carotid artery (CCA) peak systolic velocity
- Ratio of ICA to CCA end-diastolic velocity

17. What degree of carotid stenosis is considered clinically significant in symptomatic and asymptomatic patients?

Two large multicenter trials, North American Symptomatic Carotid Endarterectomy Trial (NASCET) and European Carotid Surgery Trial (ECST), have shown that carotid endarterectomy is more beneficial than medical management in symptomatic patients when the degree of ICA stenosis is between 70% and 99%. The Asymptomatic Carotid Atherosclerosis Study (ACAS) has shown that asymptomatic patients with a stenosis greater than 60% can benefit from carotid surgery. Patients with lesser degrees of stenosis with demonstrated carotid artery ulceration may also benefit from surgical management.

18. In an area of critical stenosis, what is the significance of showing a "string" sign?

When dealing with a critical stenosis (>95%), care must be taken to optimize flow sensitivity and gain settings to help facilitate the identification of a remaining trickle, or "string," of residual flow. This is important from a management standpoint because patients with a critical stenosis may be treated surgically, whereas patients with complete occlusion are not operative candidates. With US, color and power Doppler techniques are best at differentiating critical stenosis with a remaining trickle of flow from complete carotid occlusion, which sometimes may be difficult to determine. When needed, angiography may be performed for confirmation.

19. Name several potential pitfalls of carotid US.

- Elevated or low baseline velocities can cause an overestimation or underestimation of the degree of stenosis (overestimation seen with hypertension/contralateral stenosis or occlusion and underestimation seen with decreased cardiac output/more proximal stenosis).
- Tandem lesions (additional areas of stenosis) may not be identified and may reduce anticipated velocity shifts.
- Paradoxic dampening of velocities may occur in a critical area of stenosis (>95%).
- Underlying cardiac abnormalities, such as cardiac dysrhythmias, aortic valvular lesions, and severe cardiomyopathies, can cause significant alterations in the shape of the underlying carotid waveforms, and can affect the systolic and diastolic velocities.

20. Can US be used to diagnose subclavian steal syndrome?

US is the preferred imaging modality for showing subclavian steal syndrome, caused by stenosis or occlusion of the subclavian artery proximal to the origin of the vertebral artery. To maintain adequate perfusion, the distal subclavian artery and upper extremity receive blood via retrograde flow through the ipsilateral vertebral artery, bypassing the stenosis. This situation can lead to significant neurologic symptoms as blood is "stolen" through the circle of Willis from the contralateral vertebral artery. A spectrum of pulsed Doppler abnormalities can be seen, ranging from a transient decrease in mid-systolic velocity (early) to complete flow reversal (late) in the ipsilateral vertebral artery.

21. What does a parvus tardus waveform indicate?

Normal arterial waveforms have a rapid early systolic upstroke related to fast acceleration of blood at the initiation of systole and a significantly higher peak in systole compared with diastole. Parvus tardus waveforms have a slow systolic upstroke and a systolic peak that is reduced in amplitude compared with the amount of diastolic flow. This parvus (reduced) tardus (delayed) morphology is indicative of a significant, more proximal arterial stenosis (Fig. 72-5).

22. What is the role of US in establishing the diagnosis of renovascular hypertension?

Hypertension affects approximately 50 million people in the United States. A renovascular cause is potentially curable, and although renovascular hypertension occurs in only 1% to 5% of cases of hypertension, development of a screening test to identify patients with renovascular hypertension is important. Duplex US is a suitable screening test for this diagnosis because it is a relatively inexpensive, noninvasive modality that avoids the use of nephrotoxic contrast material, which is important in patients with underlying renal disease. In contrast to other modalities, this examination is highly operator-dependent.

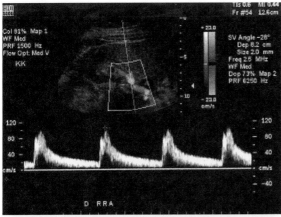

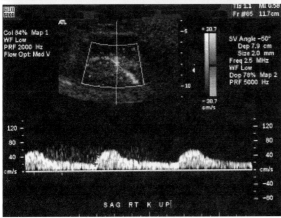

Figure 72-5. Parvus tardus waveform. *Top,* Normal pulsed Doppler waveform of a renal artery with a rapid, sharp systolic upstroke. *Bottom,* Abnormal parvus tardus waveform downstream from a stenosis, identified by a slower upstroke with reduced amplitude, resulting in a more rounded and flattened appearance.

23. What are the most common causes of renovascular hypertension?

In adults, most cases are due to atherosclerosis (65%). Fibromuscular dysplasia is the next most common cause (30% to 35%), followed by many, much less common etiologic factors, including aortic or renal artery dissection, aortic coarctation, vasculitides such as Takayasu arteritis and polyarteritis nodosa, prior radiation therapy, renal artery aneurysm, and post-transplant stenosis.

Key Points: Clinical Characteristics of Renovascular Hypertension
1. Abdominal bruit
2. Onset of hypertension before age 25 or after age 50
3. Refractory hypertension (diastolic pressure >100 mm Hg with patient taking three or more antihypertensive agents)
4. Worsening of hypertension after treatment with an angiotensin-converting enzyme inhibitor
5. Unexplained azotemia in an elderly hypertensive patient

24. What parameters are used to make the diagnosis of renovascular hypertension on US?

The renal arteries are first localized using color Doppler, and then spectral analysis is performed. Using this information, several criteria have been suggested to establish this diagnosis, including elevated velocity (peak systolic velocity in the main renal artery >100 cm/sec), ratio of the main renal artery to aortic peak systolic velocity (>3.5), systolic acceleration time (<370 to 470 cm/sec), time of acceleration (>0.05 to 0.08. sec), and spectral analysis pattern recognition (parvus tardus waveform).

25. How does US compare with other modalities in establishing the diagnosis of renovascular hypertension?

In establishing this diagnosis, US has the advantage of being less expensive, does not require the use of a nephrotoxic contrast agent, and is often more accessible than other modalities. Disadvantages are that it is extremely operator dependent, has a higher technical failure rate (10% to 20%) than other modalities, and is limited in the evaluation of accessory renal arteries. Studies have shown that when done properly, the ability of US to establish the diagnosis of renovascular hypertension accurately is comparable with that of nuclear medicine, computed tomography (CT) angiography, and magnetic resonance angiography (MRA) (Table 72-2).

Table 72-2. Diagnostic Accuracy of Noninvasive Detection of Renovascular Hypertension

	SENSITIVITY (%)	SPECIFICITY (%)
Duplex US	85-90	95
Captopril nuclear scan	90	95
MRA	95	90
CT angiography	92	83

WEBSITES

http://www.aium.org

http://www.jultrasoundmed.org

BIBLIOGRAPHY

[1] J.J. Cronan, Venous thromboembolic disease: the role of US, Radiology 186 (1993) 619–630.
[2] K.S. Freed, L.K. Brown, B.A. Carroll, The extracranial cerebral vessels, in: C.M. Rumack, S.R. Wilson, J.W. Charboneau (Eds.), Diagnostic Ultrasound, second ed., Mosby, St. Louis, 1998, pp. 885–919.
[3] A. Kawashima, C.M. Sandler, R.D. Ernst, et al., CT evaluation of renovascular disease, RadioGraphics 20 (2000) 1321–1340.
[4] B.D. Lewis, The peripheral veins, in: C.M. Rumack, S.R. Wilson, J.W. Charboneau (Eds.), Diagnostic Ultrasound, second ed., Mosby, St. Louis, 1998, pp. 943–958.
[5] W.D. Middleton, Duplex and color Doppler sonography of postcatheterization arteriovenous fistulas, Semin. Interv. Radiol. 7 (1990) 192–197.
[6] J.F. Polak, The peripheral arteries, in: C.M. Rumack, S.R. Wilson, J.W. Charboneau (Eds.), Diagnostic Ultrasound, second ed., Mosby, St. Louis, 1998, pp. 921–941.
[7] G. Soulez, V.L. Oliva, S. Turpin, et al., Imaging of renovascular hypertension: respective values of renal scintigraphy, renal Doppler US, and MR angiography, RadioGraphics 20 (2000) 1355–1368.
[8] E.E. Weinmann, E.W. Salzman, Deep vein thrombosis, N. Engl. J. Med. 331 (1994) 1630–1641.

ABDOMINAL ULTRASOUND

CHAPTER 73

Keith A. Ferguson, MD, and
Susan Hilton, MD

1. **What anatomic landmarks can be used to determine in which hepatic segment an abnormality is located?**

   The hepatic veins can be useful in placing an abnormality within a segment (Fig. 73-1).

   - The *right hepatic vein* separates the anterior and posterior segments of the right hepatic lobe.
   - The *middle hepatic vein* separates the anterior segment of the right hepatic lobe from the medial segment of the left hepatic lobe.
   - The *left hepatic vein* separates the medial and lateral segments of the left hepatic lobe.
   - Similar to the middle hepatic vein, the *gallbladder* separates the anterior segment of the right lobe and the medial segment of the left lobe.
   - The ligamentum teres separates the medial and lateral segments of the left hepatic lobe.

2. **What is the normal echogenicity of the liver?**

   The liver should normally be equal to or slightly more echogenic than the right kidney and less echogenic than the pancreas.

3. **Can one differentiate between hepatic and portal veins on ultrasound (US)?**

   Yes. Because the portal veins travel with hepatic arteries and biliary radicles and are surrounded by periportal fibrofatty tissue, there is a rim of increased echogenicity surrounding the portal veins. The hepatic veins have no such echogenic rim.

4. **Name the common benign and malignant focal hepatic lesions.**

   See Table 73-1.

5. **What is the significance of a target lesion?**

   Features that characterize a target lesion are an echogenic center with a hypoechoic peripheral rim. This appearance is important because it is relatively specific for malignancy, more commonly metastatic disease and less commonly hepatocellular carcinoma. Hepatic adenomas can also have this appearance, but are relatively rare.

6. **What are the possible growth patterns of hepatocellular carcinoma; when should one highly consider the diagnosis?**

   Hepatocellular carcinoma may be solitary, multifocal, or infiltrative. Although US features are generally nonspecific, invasion of the hepatic or portal veins is a feature commonly associated with hepatocellular carcinoma. True invasion can be differentiated from bland (non-neoplastic) thrombus by detecting arterial flow within the thrombus using Doppler imaging or by showing enhancement of the thrombus on computed tomography (CT) or magnetic resonance imaging (MRI). Additionally, hepatocellular carcinoma occurs almost exclusively in patients with cirrhosis, so the presence of a mass in a cirrhotic liver should be considered hepatocellular carcinoma until proven otherwise.

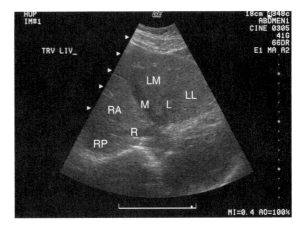

Figure 73-1. Transverse US image of the liver shows hepatic venous and segmental anatomy. The right hepatic vein (*R*) separates the right hepatic lobe into anterior (*RA*) and posterior (*RP*) segments. The middle hepatic vein (*M*) separates the anterior segment of the right hepatic lobe from the medial segment of the left hepatic lobe (*LM*), and the left hepatic vein (*L*) separates the left lobe into medial (*LM*) and lateral (*LL*) segments.

Table 73-1. Characteristics of Common Focal Hepatic Lesions

LESION	US APPEARANCE	ADDITIONAL INFORMATION
Cysts	Anechoic lumen, imperceptible wall, increased through-transmission, well-defined posterior wall; may contain septations	These characteristics apply to cysts in other organs as well (see Fig. 73-11 for an example of a renal cyst)
Fatty infiltration of the liver (Fig. 73-2)	Liver is more echogenic than the right kidney; common locations for focal fatty infiltration: adjacent to falciform ligament and anterior to the portal vein bifurcation	May be focal or diffuse
Hemangiomas (Fig. 73-3)	Homogeneously echogenic (typical hemangiomas) or echogenic periphery with hypoechoic center (atypical hemangiomas); increased through-transmission in a few lesions	More common in women; 10% are multiple
Focal nodular hyperplasia	Variable appearance; central scar characteristic but rarely seen on US	Benign lesion composed of normal hepatocytes, Kupffer cells, and bile ducts; more common in women
Adenomas	Variable appearance; when hemorrhagic, may have a complex or cystic appearance	Benign neoplasm composed of hepatocytes, but not Kupffer cells or bile ducts; association with oral contraceptive pills; usually resected due to propensity to hemorrhage
Metastases	Wide range of appearances, including echogenic, calcified, or complex cystic lesions; usually multiple	Most common cause of focal solid liver lesions
Hepatocellular carcinoma	May be solitary, multifocal, or infiltrating; portal or hepatic vein invasion	Usually occurs in cirrhotic livers
Abscess	Complex cystic or solid appearance, increased through-transmission, gas in lesion may cause shadowing	Often occur secondary to seeding from intestinal sources

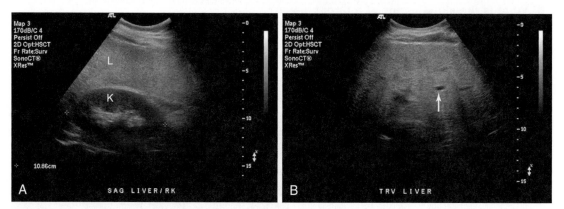

Figure 73-2. Diffuse fatty infiltration of the liver. **A,** Sagittal scan. The liver (*L*) is markedly more echogenic than the kidney (*K*). **B,** Transverse scan. There is decreased conspicuity of the portal vein (*arrow*), and the sound beam fails to penetrate through the liver.

7. What are the US findings of cirrhosis?

A nodular liver surface is highly suggestive of cirrhosis. Findings of portal hypertension—including ascites, splenomegaly, portal vein enlargement, and recanalization of the paraumbilical veins—are also indicative of cirrhosis.

8. In addition to location, what imaging features help to differentiate focal fatty infiltration from a mass lesion?

Focal fatty infiltration does not exert mass effect on the hepatic vessels and tends to have a more geographic distribution.

9. Describe the US appearance of gallstones.

A gallstone has a curvilinear, hyperechoic (bright) leading edge with posterior acoustic shadowing (Fig. 73-4). The posterior shadowing is caused by absorption of the sound beam by the gallstones and should be seen with stones bigger than 3 mm. Gallstones are also typically mobile, although they may occasionally adhere to the gallbladder wall.

10. What is meant by the "WES" sign?

The "wall-echo-shadow (WES)" sign may be seen when the gallbladder is completely filled with stones (Fig. 73-5). This sign consists of two curvilinear structures followed by a shadow. The first line is hypoechoic and represents the gallbladder wall. The second is echogenic, representing multiple gallstones, with their associated shadowing making up the third portion of the sign. The "WES" sign may be difficult to differentiate from a gas-filled bowel loop.

11. How does the US appearance of gallstones differ from that of other intraluminal abnormalities?

Similar to gallstones, tumefactive sludge (sludge balls) is typically mobile, but does not shadow. Gallbladder polyps are nonmobile and do not shadow.

12. What is the normal gallbladder wall thickness, and what diseases can produce gallbladder wall thickening?

The normal thickness of the gallbladder wall is 3 mm or less. Gallbladder wall thickening may be seen in numerous disease processes of biliary and nonbiliary origin. Biliary causes of gallbladder wall thickening include acute or chronic cholecystitis, adenomyomatosis, acquired immunodeficiency syndrome (AIDS) cholangiopathy, sclerosing cholangitis, and gallbladder carcinoma. Nonbiliary causes include hepatitis, cirrhosis, portal hypertension, hypoproteinemia, and heart failure.

13. Describe the US signs of early or uncomplicated acute cholecystitis.

Findings on US in early or uncomplicated acute cholecystitis may include gallstones (which may be impacted in the gallbladder neck or cystic duct), gallbladder wall thickening, and gallbladder distention. A sonographic Murphy sign (focal tenderness over the gallbladder when compressed by the US transducer) may also be elicited. The combination of gallstones and Murphy sign has a positive predictive value of 92% and a negative predictive value of 95% for acute cholecystitis.

14. What are additional findings in advanced or complicated cholecystitis?

Signs of advanced acute cholecystitis include pericholecystic fluid, a striated appearance of the thickened gallbladder wall, and intraluminal

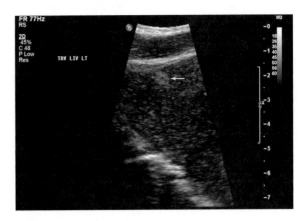

Figure 73-3. Hepatic hemangioma. Sagittal scan shows well-circumscribed echogenic lesion (*arrow*) seen in the left lobe of the liver, typical for hemangioma.

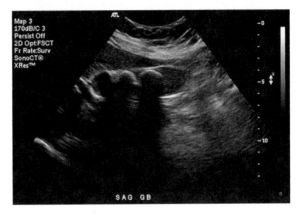

Figure 73-4. Gallstones on sagittal scan. Characteristics of gallstones include a curvilinear, echogenic leading edge and posterior acoustic shadowing.

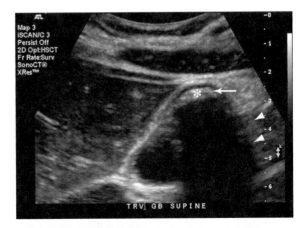

Figure 73-5. WES complex consists of a hypoechoic line (*arrow*), which represents the gallbladder wall, followed by an echogenic line (*asterisk*), which represents the leading edge of the gallstones, and posterior shadowing (*arrowheads*).

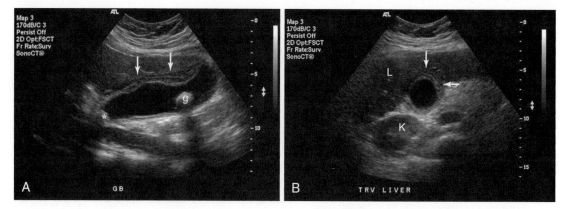

Figure 73-6. Cholecystitis. **A** and **B,** Sagittal (**A**) and transverse (**B**) scans. Gallbladder wall is thickened and striated (*arrows*). Two gallstones (*g*) are present, one of which (*asterisk*) is impacted in the gallbladder neck. The liver (*L*) and right kidney (*K*) are also seen.

membranes caused by sloughed gallbladder mucosa (Fig. 73-6). Emphysematous cholecystitis is most commonly seen in elderly patients with diabetes, in whom the gallbladder becomes infected by gas-producing organisms. The presence of gas in the gallbladder wall or lumen results in bright reflections along the nondependent portion of the gallbladder wall, with "dirty" posterior shadowing.

15. Describe the US appearances of gallbladder carcinoma, and tell which is the most common.
Most commonly, gallbladder carcinoma appears as a soft tissue mass centered in the gallbladder fossa, completely or partially replacing the gallbladder lumen. In a few cases, gallbladder carcinoma may also appear as asymmetric gallbladder wall thickening or as a polypoid intraluminal mass. In the latter case, the mass is usually larger than 1 cm, which helps to distinguish it from benign cholesterol polyps.

16. What malignancy has the highest propensity to metastasize to the gallbladder?
Melanoma has the highest propensity to metastasize to the gallbladder.

17. What is the normal measurement of the common duct?
The *normal common duct* (a term generally used to refer to the common hepatic duct and the common bile duct because these are difficult to distinguish on US) may vary in size based on the patient's age and cholecystectomy status, and where the measurement is taken. Generally, the normal common duct should measure less than 7 mm in patients younger than 60. In older patients and patients who have had previous cholecystectomy, the common duct should measure less than 10 mm.

18. Name three causes of extrahepatic biliary dilation.
- Choledocholithiasis
- Biliary stricture
- Tumor within or adjacent to the biliary tree

19. Does a normal-appearing pancreas exclude the diagnosis of pancreatitis?
No. Although the pancreas may be diffusely or focally enlarged and hypoechoic in patients with pancreatitis, it may also have a normal appearance.

20. Because the pancreas may appear normal in pancreatitis, what is the role of US in patients suspected to have pancreatitis?
One major role of US is to evaluate for the presence of stones in the biliary tree as the cause of pancreatitis, which may alter clinical management of a patient with pancreatitis. Additionally, US can evaluate for complications of pancreatitis, such as peripancreatic fluid collections and pseudocysts, thrombosis of the splenic or superior mesenteric vein, and pseudoaneurysm formation.

21. What is the differential diagnosis of a hypoechoic pancreatic mass lesion?
The top two considerations of a hypoechoic pancreatic mass lesion are *pancreatic adenocarcinoma* and *focal pancreatitis* (Fig. 73-7). A helpful finding in differentiating these entities is the presence of vascular encasement or metastases, which would support the diagnosis of adenocarcinoma. Pancreatic ductal dilation may be seen in either

process, although the obstructed pancreatic duct in adenocarcinoma is typically smoothly dilated, whereas the duct in chronic pancreatitis most often has an irregular appearance. Other differential diagnostic considerations include islet cell tumors, pancreatic lymphoma, metastases, and peripancreatic lymph nodes.

22. What are the two major types of cystic pancreatic neoplasm?

* *Serous pancreatic cystadenoma,* also known as *microcystic adenoma,* usually manifests as a large pancreatic mass composed of multiple small cysts. A calcified central scar may be present. This lesion is benign, most commonly located within the pancreatic tail and most commonly seen in elderly women.
* *Mucinous pancreatic tumors* (*macrocystic adenomas*) either have malignant potential or are frankly malignant. They are typically composed of fewer larger cysts, which may contain internal septations or mural nodules. These are most common in middle-aged women and most often occur in the pancreatic body or tail.

23. What genetic diseases are associated with pancreatic cysts?

von Hippel-Lindau disease is an autosomal dominant disease associated with pancreatic cysts and neoplasms; cerebellar, retinal, and spinal cord hemangioblastomas; renal cysts; renal cell carcinoma; and pheochromocytoma. Autosomal dominant polycystic kidney disease may be associated with pancreatic cysts in less than 5% of cases.

24. Describe the normal US appearance of a kidney.

Kidneys have a more complex US appearance than the other abdominal organs (Fig. 73-8). The central renal sinus is predominantly composed of fat and appears hyperechoic on US. Occasionally, renal blood vessels or the collecting system may be seen as anechoic tubular structures within the sinus. The renal pyramids are hypoechoic triangular or slightly rounded structures that abut the renal sinus. The renal cortex is slightly more echoic than the renal pyramids. The renal cortex should be equally or less echogenic than the liver and much less echogenic than the spleen. In normal adults, the kidneys should measure 9 to 13 cm in length.

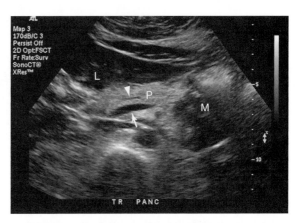

Figure 73-7. Hypoechoic mass (*M*) in the pancreatic tail on transverse scan. The remainder of the pancreas (*P*) is normal in appearance. Note the liver (*L*) anterior to the pancreas and the splenic vein (*arrow*) posterior to the pancreas. A small portion of the pancreatic duct is seen (*arrowhead*).

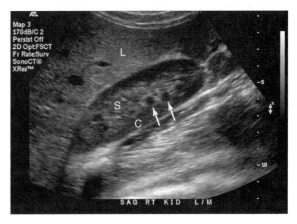

Figure 73-8. Normal sagittal image of kidney. Note normal renal architecture, which includes echogenic renal sinus (*S*), intermediately echogenic renal cortex (*C*), and hypoechoic medullary pyramids (*arrows*). The renal cortex is slightly less echogenic than the liver (*L*), which is normal.

25. What is the main function of US in the setting of acute renal failure?

US is very beneficial in determining whether urinary obstruction is present. Although urinary obstruction is an uncommon cause of acute renal failure (accounting for approximately 5% of cases), early detection and treatment are crucial to prevent permanent damage to the kidneys.

26. What are the US findings of obstruction?

The hallmark for the diagnosis of obstruction on US is the detection of hydronephrosis (Fig. 73-9). A dilated renal collecting system appears as multiple anechoic structures conforming to the expected location of the renal calyces, all connecting with a dilated renal pelvis centrally. Patients with other processes, such as prior obstruction, pregnancy, bladder distention, vesicoureteral reflux, and diuresis, can also present with a dilated collecting system. The lack of ureteral jets in the bladder and elevated resistive indices can be helpful in differentiating acute obstruction from these other processes.

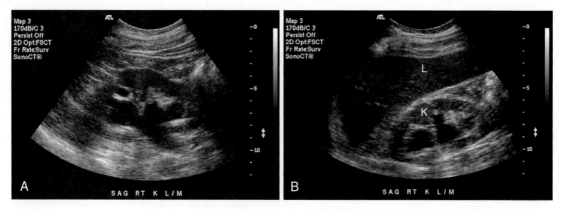

Figure 73-9. Hydronephrosis. **A** and **B,** Sagittal images of right kidney (*K*) show moderately dilated collecting structures. The liver (*L*) is also seen.

27. Describe the US appearance of renal calculi.

Renal stones appear as hyperechoic foci within the renal sinus. Stones of sufficient size show posterior acoustic shadowing, whereas smaller stones may not. Technical factors, such as transducer frequency, focal zone depth, and beam width, should be optimized to maximize the chance of detecting a shadow. Because the renal sinus is normally echogenic, renal stones are more difficult to detect on US than gallstones, which are surrounded by fluid. The composition of a renal calculus does not affect its US appearance.

28. What is the most common renal mass lesion?

US characteristics of simple cysts in the liver, kidney, or elsewhere are described in Table 73-1. Cysts may be present in 50% of people older than 50. Cysts that contain thin internal septations, small peripheral thin calcification, or hemorrhagic or proteinaceous debris are termed *minimally complex cysts,* and, similar to simple cysts, are benign. The presence of thick septations or more extensive calcification is more suggestive of a cystic renal neoplasm and should be evaluated further with dedicated renal CT or MRI or followed up closely with US to evaluate for growth.

29. Are any diseases associated with renal cysts?

Yes. See Table 73-2 and Fig. 73-10.

30. What is the most common solid renal mass?

Renal cell carcinoma is the most common solid renal mass.

Table 73-2. Diseases Associated with Renal Cysts

DISEASE	CYST CHARACTERISTICS	ASSOCIATED RENAL ABNORMALITIES	OTHER ORGAN SYSTEM INVOLVEMENT
Autosomal dominant polycystic disease	Multiple cysts of various sizes; hemorrhage into cysts common	Enlarged kidneys, renal failure, hypertension	Liver and pancreatic cysts, cerebral berry aneurysms
Acquired cystic disease	Multiple small cysts; hemorrhage common	Occurs in dialysis patients; kidneys are small and echogenic; increased risk of renal cell carcinoma	
von Hippel-Lindau disease	Multiple bilateral renal cysts; risk of neoplasm arising in cyst walls	Multiple bilateral renal cell carcinomas	Cerebellar and spinal cord hemangioblastomas, retinal angiomas, pancreatic cysts and neoplasms, pheochromocytomas
Tuberous sclerosis	Cysts develop most commonly in infancy and childhood	Multiple bilateral angiomyolipomas	Mental retardation, seizures, central nervous system tumors, cardiac rhabdomyomas, pulmonary lymphangiomyomatosis

31. Describe the imaging features of renal cell carcinoma.

Most renal cell carcinomas are slightly hyperechoic or isoechoic to the renal parenchyma. Approximately 10% are hypoechoic, and another 10% are much more echogenic than the normal kidney. They may contain areas of calcification, necrosis, or hemorrhage. Predominantly cystic renal cell carcinomas also occur, but are uncommon. Renal cell carcinoma has a propensity to invade the renal veins and inferior vena cava, and these should be evaluated in patients with a solid renal mass. Other benign and malignant neoplasms may involve the kidney and produce a solid mass.

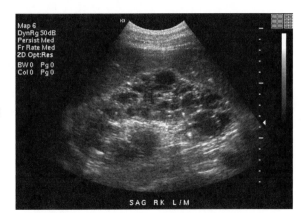

Figure 73-10. Autosomal dominant polycystic kidney disease. Sagittal scan of right kidney. Normal renal parenchyma is replaced by cysts of varying sizes.

32. Discuss the differential diagnosis for a markedly echogenic renal mass.

Angiomyolipomas are usually well-defined, markedly hyperechoic renal masses. These benign lesions consist of varying degrees of fat, vessels, and muscle; the presence of fat accounts for the hyperechoic appearance. As previously noted, a few renal cell carcinomas may also be much more echogenic, however, than the renal parenchyma. Malignancy must also be considered in the differential diagnosis for a hyperechoic renal mass. The presence of posterior acoustic shadowing without calcification is more suggestive of angiomyolipoma, whereas areas of calcification or cystic regions suggest renal cell carcinoma. Nevertheless, CT or MRI is usually indicated to characterize these lesions further.

Key Points: Diagnoses to Consider for a Solid Renal Mass

1. Renal carcinoma is the most common cause.
2. Angiomyolipoma is usually hyperechoic, but some carcinomas mimic angiomyolipoma on US.
3. Other neoplasms include oncocytoma, renal lymphoma, transitional cell carcinoma of the renal collecting system, and metastasis to the kidney.

---

33. Does pyelonephritis have a characteristic appearance on US?

Most patients with pyelonephritis have normal-appearing kidneys on US. In more severe cases, there may be focal areas of masslike enlargement or heterogeneous echotexture of the kidneys. The most important role of US in pyelonephritis is in excluding complications, however, such as renal or perinephric abscess or urinary obstruction.

34. What is meant by renal parenchymal disease?

Renal parenchymal disease, or medical renal disease, is a term used to describe kidneys of increased cortical echogenicity (Fig. 73-11). Kidneys that are more echogenic than the liver or equal to or greater in echogenicity than the spleen are too echogenic. Numerous disease processes result in this same US appearance, and biopsy may be necessary to differentiate among them when clinically appropriate. Renal size is helpful to differentiate acute from chronic renal disease.

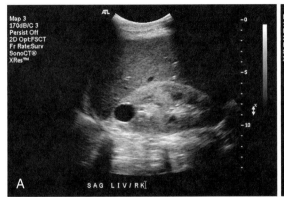
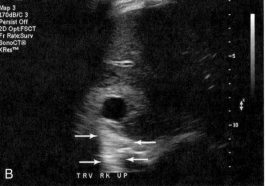

Figure 73-11. Renal parenchymal disease. **A** and **B,** Sagittal (**A**) and transverse (**B**) images show right kidney to be much more echogenic than the liver. Also note the upper pole renal cyst, with its typical features of an anechoic lumen, well-defined posterior wall, and increased through-transmission (*arrows*).

BIBLIOGRAPHY

[1] G.L. Bennett, E.J. Balthazar, Ultrasound and CT evaluation of emergent gallbladder pathology, Radiol. Clin. North. Am. 41 (2003) 1203–1216.
[2] A. Kurtz, W. Middleton, Ultrasound: The Requisites, Mosby, St. Louis, 1996.
[3] C.M. Rumack, C.R. Wilson, J.W. Charboneau (Eds.), Diagnostic Ultrasound, second ed., Mosby, St. Louis, 1998.

TRAINING PATHWAYS IN DIAGNOSTIC IMAGING

CHAPTER 74

E. Scott Pretorius, MD

1. What is the usual training pathway to become a radiologist in the United States?

After medical school, candidates complete an internship (PGY-1). After internship, radiology residency is 4 years (PGY 2-5). Most residents choose to pursue fellowship subspecialist training after residency. In most cases, this takes 1 year (PGY-6), but most neuroradiology fellowships and pediatric radiology fellowships take 2 years.

2. Do I have to match for a separate preliminary year?

In most cases, yes. A few radiology programs are affiliated with specific preliminary years, but most allow candidates to train in any accredited PGY-1 year (most commonly. transitional, medicine, or surgery; less commonly. obstetrics/gynecology, pediatrics, family medicine, emergency medicine, or neurology). The American Board of Radiology (ABR) requires at least 9 months of clinical training. Candidates seeking board certification in radiology must complete this clinical requirement and training requirements in diagnostic radiology. The requirement in clinical training may be met by internship in any of the aforementioned fields.

3. Is it difficult to get a residency position in diagnostic radiology?

Yes. Diagnostic radiology has become one of the most competitive fields in which to match. It is not unusual for top programs to receive 100 applications for every open spot.

4. What can I do to help my chances of matching in radiology?

For starters, do extremely well in medical school and score high on the United States Medical Licensing Examination (USMLE). Demonstrate commitment to the field by undertaking a research project in radiology. If you are interested in a particular program, try to make personal connections to people in that department. Some of the ways to do this include an audition elective rotation or a research project.

5. What information should my personal statement contain?

Ideally, the personal statement includes information about how you came to this point in life—applying for radiology residency—and also tells something about where you expect your medical training to lead you. Do you see yourself in academic practice or private practice? What are your reasons for choosing radiology? Explain to your reader—without succumbing to arrogance—what personal qualities or achievements might separate you from other applicants.

6. Does it matter who writes my letters of recommendation?

Many candidates aspire to have a letter from a particular well-known physician in their institution. That's fine, as long as he or she knows you well and is comfortable writing a very strong letter for you. In medicine, fame is often local or regional, however, and the surgeon who is "famous" in Los Angeles is likely to be unknown to radiologists in Philadelphia. In general, you are better off soliciting letters from physicians who know you very well and who are comfortable writing very positive things about you.

7. Do I need letters of recommendation from radiologists?

At least one of your letters should be from a radiologist. Without at least one such letter, it may seem that pursuing radiology is something that has only recently occurred to you and that you have not investigated the field. All of your letters do not need to come from radiologists, however. Again, you should choose people who know you very well. If you are an MD PhD, at least one of your letters should come from someone who has worked with you on a clinical service. As spectacular as your research may be, you will be spending most of your residency working with patients and interacting with clinicians. Applicants who have references only from their laboratory experiences place themselves at a disadvantage.

8. Are radiology positions offered outside of the National Resident Matching Program (NRMP) match?

Most positions in radiology are offered through the NRMP match (www.nrmp.org). Positions available outside of the match occasionally become available when residents choose to switch specialties or leave medicine altogether. Residency programs that are part of the NRMP match are not allowed to offer positions to U.S. senior medical students outside of the match. International medical graduates or U.S. medical graduates who are not seniors (e.g., candidates who previously went unmatched or who matched in some other field but now wish to switch to radiology) may accept such offers. Such positions are extremely rare, however.

9. To how many residency programs should I apply?

It depends on how competitive an applicant you are. If you are in the top 10% of your class in a good medical school with USMLE scores of 250 or more, you should feel comfortable applying to 12 to 15 top programs only. If you are a less competitive applicant, you should consider widening your application pool; 30 applications are not unreasonable for someone who is a good-but-not-spectacular applicant. If you are in the bottom half of your class, even at a top-ranked school with average USMLE scores, you need to consider seriously less competitive residencies at regional or community hospitals. If you have geographic restrictions because of spouse, family, or some other reason, you should apply to every program in that geographic area and be willing to go anywhere you match. Almost all programs use the Electronic Residency Application Service of the Association of American Medical Colleges (www.aamc.org/students/eras/start.htm).

10. To what kind of residency programs should I apply?

Radiology residency programs are designed to train physicians for either academic medicine or private practice. If you want to work in academic medicine, you should go someplace where you will get dedicated research time, training in research methods, and opportunities to develop teaching skills. Such programs often offer opportunities to develop subspecialty interests during residency training. Programs such as these are not optimal for training individuals for private practice. For that, you are better off going to programs that focus on clinical work only. You want places that have few or no fellows so that all procedures are available for residents because you will need those experiences to develop broad and versatile clinical skills.

11. How do I become board-certified in diagnostic radiology?

You must pass the written and oral examinations of the ABR (www.theabr.org). The written examination consists of a physics portion and a clinical portion. You may take the physics portion in your second, third, or fourth year of radiology training. The clinical written portion is taken in the fall of your fourth year, and the oral examination is taken in Louisville, Kentucky, in June of your fourth year of residency.

12. I am an international medical graduate. What must I do to apply for a diagnostic radiology residency position in the United States?

You must be a medical school graduate and be certified by the Educational Commission for Foreign Medical Graduates (www.ecfmg.org). You should take at least USMLE Step 1. If you have completed a clinical year in your home country, that training, in most cases, can be counted as your clinical year toward ABR certification. Most radiology programs are inundated with applicants, however, and generally prefer candidates who have done some part of their training in the United States or Canada. You may wish to complete a U.S. or Canadian internship, even if you have completed similar training in your home country.

Some international medical graduate candidates may have completed all training requirements in diagnostic radiology in their home country. Even so, if such an individual wishes to become certified by the ABR, he or she must complete a U.S. or Canadian residency or must serve as a resident or faculty member for 4 consecutive years in the same Accreditation Council for Graduate Medical Education/Royal College of Physicians and Surgeons of Canada (ACGME/RCPSC)–accredited institution to become eligible to take the ABR's examination (www.theabr.org/DRAppAndFeesinFrame.htm).

Key Points: Training Pathways in Diagnostic Imaging

1. Not every residency is right for every person.
2. Consider your ultimate career goals and the residency's curriculum before ranking or applying to a program.

---

13. What is a research track residency position?

Research track residency positions allow candidates to use 1 of their 4 years of radiology training to do research. Such positions are relatively new, but are increasing in number and are offered primarily by large, academic, research-driven departments. This is different from the Holman track, in which candidates complete 2 full years of research (www.theabr.org/ Holman.htm).

14. Do I have to complete a fellowship after residency?

Fellowship is not required, but approximately 70% of residency graduates pursue fellowship training. Failure to complete a fellowship may place one at a competitive disadvantage in the job market. Fellowship training is virtually required at most academic institutions to secure an academic appointment.

15. In what subspecialties is fellowship training offered?

Subspecialties in interventional radiology, neuroradiology, thoracic imaging, musculoskeletal radiology, nuclear medicine, magnetic resonance imaging (MRI), breast imaging, abdominal imaging (ultrasound [US], computed tomography [CT], and MRI), and women's imaging (mammography, US, and usually MRI) are offered.

16. What is the training pathway for nuclear medicine?

Nuclear imaging is studied as part of diagnostic radiology residency, and graduates of diagnostic radiology residencies may practice nuclear medicine. One may also pursue nuclear medicine alone. An internship (PGY-1) is required, and candidates then spend 2 more years (PGY-2 and PGY-3) pursuing residency training in nuclear medicine.

17. How do I become board-certified in nuclear medicine?

Candidates must pass the written examination of the American Board of Nuclear Medicine (ABNM). To be eligible, a candidate must have completed an intern year, followed by 2 years of training in a nuclear medicine residency. Candidates who have completed an internship and a diagnostic radiology residency may take the ABNM examination after completion of a 1-year fellowship in nuclear imaging. Such candidates are eligible to seek board certification from the ABR and ABNM.

18. What is a certificate of added qualification (CAQ)?

The ABR offers CAQs to appropriately trained individuals in certain subspecialties, including nuclear radiology, vascular and interventional radiology, neuroradiology, and pediatric radiology. Attainment of this distinction requires completion of fellowship training, clinical experience, and passage of an oral examination.

WEBSITES

http://www.theabr.org

http://www.theabr.org/DRAppAndFeesinFrame.htm

http://www.ecfmg.org

http://www.aamc.org/students/eras/start.htm

http://www.theabr.org/Holman.htm

http://www.nrmp.org

http://www.abnm.org

75 CHAPTER MEDICOLEGAL ISSUES IN DIAGNOSTIC IMAGING

Saurabh Jha, MBBS

"There but for the grace of God, go I."
—John Bradford, heretic, 1550 A.D.

1. Define medical negligence.

Negligence is the failure to possess and apply the knowledge that is possessed or applied by reasonable physicians practicing in similar circumstances.

2. What must be proven for a physician to be found liable for malpractice?

- Establishment of a duty of care (i.e., physician-patient relationship)
- Breach of the duty of care, or negligence
- Adverse outcome with injury or harm
- Direct causality between negligence and outcome

> **Key Points: Legal Requirements for a Finding of Malpractice**
>
> 1. Establishment of a duty of care (i.e., physician-patient relationship)
> 2. Breach of the duty of care, or negligence
> 3. Adverse outcome with injury or harm
> 4. Direct causality between negligence and outcome

3. Outline the history behind current malpractice law. What is unique about the legal determination of medical negligence in the United States?

The relevant legal framework in the United States originates from the work of Blackstone, a renowned English legal scholar whose *Commentaries on the Laws of England,* published in 1768, described the term *mala praxis* for injuries resulting from professional neglect or want of skill, specifically by physicians. *Malpractice* is derived from this term. Malpractice law is part of the tort, or personal injury, law. The plaintiff (injured party) files a suit against the defendant (physician) in a civil court in front of a jury composed of ordinary (not belonging to the medical profession) citizens. This adversarial system is different from the practice in countries such as the United Kingdom and Germany, where medical negligence is adjudicated by a panel of judges or medical experts.

4. List factors that have been responsible for the expansion of medical litigation in the United States.

- The ethos of marketplace professionalism (no special status to medical societies) and antiegalitarian sentiments of the early 19th century forced physicians to raise the level of their professionalism and medical organizations to stipulate standards of practice that, ironically, would be used against them.
- Medical innovations made physicians victims of their own advancement.
- Liability insurance ensured an available financial pool for compensation.
- Plaintiffs had nothing to lose by filing a lawsuit because of the contingent "no win–no fees" basis of legal representation and because of the fact that both adversarial parties had to bear their own legal costs regardless of the outcome.

5. There can be no malpractice without established practice. Who sets the established practice, and who determines whether the established practice has been breached?

The expected standard may be defined in textbooks, presented in other medical literature, or stated by professional organizations such as the American Medical Association and the American College of Radiology. The jury decides whether a physician's conduct is below that expected of a reasonable physician. The expert witness (an individual of the same or similar clinical discipline as the defendant) outlines the standard to which the physician should be held, however. The attorneys for the plaintiff and the defendant can retain an expert witness.

6. **Would a general radiologist who misses a lesion on a brain magnetic resonance imaging (MRI) study be held to the standard of a neuroradiologist?**
No. The legal requirement is that the radiologist must possess the knowledge and skill that is ordinarily possessed by a reasonable peer. He or she is not required to possess the highest skill level to which some aspire. A general radiologist would be held to the standard of a reasonable generalist, but not a specialist.

7. **The average plaintiff award in the United States is $3.5 million. What is the aim of the award, and what are the types of damage awarded by the jury?**
The ethos behind the jury award is restitution, not punishment. The award aims to compensate the patient and to deter further such episodes of negligence from occurring.

Three types of damages are considered:

* Economic losses, such as the injured plaintiff's health care costs and loss of wages
* Noneconomic losses, such as pain and suffering
* Punitive damages for cases in which the defendant exhibited wanton disregard for the plaintiff's well-being (this type of damage is awarded very rarely).

8. **Can an exculpatory waiver signed by a patient shield the physician of a certain degree of liability?**
It is common for instructional facilities for scuba diving, skydiving, and similar risky activities to ask participants to sign exculpatory waivers shielding them from lawsuits if injury or death results. Such a waiver implies a "contract" because the parties have theoretically agreed in advance on acceptable and unacceptable outcomes. The patient-physician relationship is not a contract, however, but rather a professional bond in which the physician assumes a position of responsibility as the possessor of knowledge and skill beyond the ordinary toward patients who may not know their own best interests. The signing of a waiver by a patient does not alter the legal course when medical negligence is alleged.

9. **A radiologist in an outpatient facility reads radiographs without ever meeting the patients. Does he or she still form a physician-patient relationship?**
Although a physician-patient relationship typically is a consensual one, a radiologist forms that relationship when he or she renders an interpretation on an imaging study for the patient. This is true even if the radiologist never meets or speaks with the patient or referring physician. This fact is important to appreciate because the basis of any malpractice claim is the establishment of a duty of care by formation of a physician-patient relationship.

10. **It is estimated that in any given year a lawsuit may be brought against 1 in 10 radiologists. What are the most common reasons radiologists get sued?**
* Failure of diagnosis (includes perceptual errors, insufficient knowledge, incorrect judgment, and failure to correct poor patient positioning and exposure)
* Failure to communicate findings in an appropriate and timely manner
* Failure to suggest the next appropriate procedure

Of these, failure to diagnose is the largest cause (70%), and two thirds of these cases are due to perceptual errors.

> **Key Points: Most Common Reasons Radiologists Are Sued**
>
> 1. Failure to diagnose
> 2. Failure to communicate findings in an appropriate and timely manner
> 3. Failure to suggest the next appropriate procedure

11. **What are the groundbreaking findings of the Institute of Medicine's report *To Err is Human: Building a Safer Health System*?**
The report, published in 2000, received much media interest and put medical errors in the spotlight. On reviewing the 1984 patient files of New York hospitals and the 1992 files of Colorado and Utah hospitals retrospectively for adverse events, the report concluded that medical error alone could account for 44,000 to 98,000 deaths annually in U.S. hospitals. This figure exceeds the number of deaths attributable annually to AIDS, motor vehicle accidents, or breast cancer.

12. Radiology has its unique set of errors. What is the most common radiologic error, and how often is this error estimated to occur?

Failure-to-diagnose errors, which are the most common, are of two major types: cognitive, in which an abnormality is seen, but its nature is misinterpreted (e.g., an infiltrate on a chest x-ray that represents cancer is interpreted as pneumonia), and perceptual, or the "miss," in which a radiologic abnormality is simply not seen by the radiologist on initial interpretation. Since Garland's seminal study in 1944, in which he found significant interobserver and intraobserver variation in the interpretation of chest x-rays by radiologists, several studies have confirmed that perceptual errors occur at an alarmingly high frequency. A University of Missouri study in 1976 reported an average error rate of 30% among experienced radiologists interpreting chest, bone, and gastrointestinal radiographs.

13. What is hindsight bias, and why is it important medicolegally?

Medicolegally, radiology is unique in that the evidence for examination (the image) remains for subsequent scrutiny, in contrast to physical examination findings or findings at endoscopy. It also lends itself to a phenomenon known as the *hindsight bias*—the tendency for people with knowledge of the actual event to believe falsely that they would have predicted the correct outcome. On 90% of chest films of patients with lung cancer that were reported as normal, the cancer was seen in hindsight. When a radiologist makes a perceptual error, and the finding is subsequently seen, it is difficult to determine whether the finding was seen only in retrospect and in lieu of all the clinical information. In other words, it is difficult to determine when a "miss" is negligent, and when it is simply an error of perception.

14. List ways to minimize the occurrence of perceptual errors.

- Adequate radiographic technique
- Appropriate clinical history: the knowledge of the site of pain reduces the "miss" of subtle fractures by 50%
- Comparison with old studies whenever possible
- Avoidance of "satisfaction of search," where the presence of an overt finding diminishes the chances of making a second, more subtle finding
- Double reading and spending more time examining the radiograph (controversial)
- Computer-aided detection (still experimental)

15. In 1997, the Wisconsin Court of Appeals issued a decision that has had a positive effect for radiologists sued for perceptual errors. Outline the decision.

Wisconsin's Medical Examining Board sought to revoke the medical license of a radiologist who had been sued for perceptual errors twice in a 10-year career. The case eventually reached the appeals court, which affirmed a decision in favor of the radiologist. The principles of the decision are as follows:

- Medicine is not an exact science.
- Error in and of itself is not negligence.
- A "miss" may not constitute negligence, even if the finding could be determined by a majority of radiologists as long as the radiologist "conformed to the accepted standards of practice."

16. What is the "Aunt Minnie" approach to film interpretation, and how may this approach lead to errors in judgment?

The attachment of an interpretation to a radiographic finding with a strong preconceived notion is akin to spotting a familiar face: "I know that's my Aunt Minnie because it looks like my Aunt Minnie!" Researchers believe that such an approach results in errors in interpretation because the self-imposed-limited mindset leads to a failure to include a differential diagnosis. If a diagnosis is not considered, it is not investigated, and if it is not investigated, it is not found.

17. How may errors in judgment be minimized?

- Analyze—not simply recognize—radiographic findings.
- Keep an open mind; always try to incorporate a differential diagnosis.
- Expand and maintain a comprehensive knowledge base.
- Avoid alliterative errors (i.e., the influence of another radiologist's opinion). Look at a prior radiograph with a fresh set of eyes.

18. Explain the following terms in the medicolegal context: proximate cause, law of intervening cause, and joint and several liabilities.

- *Proximate cause* is the connection between an alleged act of negligence and the injury sustained by a patient.
- *Law of intervening cause* is when an intervening act of negligence breaks the causal link between the initial act of negligence and injury.
- *Joint and several liabilities* is the fact that more than one person can be blamed for an injury (i.e., there can be multiple proximate causes).

The effect imaging has in clinical decision making makes radiologists vulnerable to erroneous medical decisions of their referring physicians if it can be shown that a radiographic report resulted in an error in subsequent clinical judgment. Radiologists may feel aggrieved at being named a co-defendant and ascribed a proximate cause for a plaintiff's injury, given that their report was followed by another's act of negligence, particularly because the referring physician has the bulk of clinical information. Courts are generally reluctant, however, to allow the law of intervening cause to apply. Their stance is well summarized in an appeals court decision: "Where an original act is negligent and in a natural and continuous sequence produces an injury that would not have taken place without the act, proximate cause is established, and the fact that some other intervening act contributes to the original act to cause injury does not relieve the initial offender from liability...."

19. Explain the following terms in the medicolegal context: vicarious liability and respondeat superior.

- *Vicarious liability* is the placing of the negligence of one person on another.
- Respondeat superior is a Latin term meaning "let the superior respond" and is a form of vicarious liability incurred by the employer (hospital or radiologist) because of the negligent acts of employees (nurses, physician assistants, or technologists), with the rationale that because an employer gains financial benefit through the actions of an employee, so should the employer be responsible for any harm as a result of an employee's actions.

20. Who is responsible for the negligent action of a technologist?

Negligence of the technologist is vicariously incurred by the employer (i.e., the medical facility [hospital or private medical imaging group]) through the respondeat superior principle. If the negligence occurs during a procedure when a radiologist is normally present (e.g., fluoroscopy or interventional radiology), the supervising radiologist is liable through a legal doctrine known as "borrowed servant" (the radiologist temporarily assumes authority over the actions of the technologist).

21. What is meant by the term *res ipsa loquitur*? Give some examples.

Res ipsa loquitur means that the "situation speaks for itself" and is a legal concept that asserts that certain acts cannot, by definition, occur without negligence. In such situations, the burden of proof does not rest with the plaintiff. Medicolegal examples include retention of surgical instruments in the body; transfusion complications resulting from administration of the wrong person's blood; and, in radiologic practice, rectal perforation during a barium enema.

22. A radiologist renders a report on an intensive care unit portable chest x-ray that reads, "Endotracheal tube in the right main bronchus should be withdrawn by 2 inches to lie within distal trachea; left lower lobe atelectasis; otherwise normal." What additional step should the radiologist take?

The radiologist should phone the physician or nurse treating the patient and include this in the final report. The American College of Radiology's Practice Guidelines advise that the radiologist should directly communicate a report to the physician (or other responsible personnel) or the patient (or responsible legal guardian) in the following situations:

- Discrepancy between the preliminary and final reads, which could affect management
- Conditions for which immediate treatment is required (e.g., pneumothorax or a misplaced support line)
- Significant unexpected findings (e.g., cancer)

23. A radiologist renders a report on a posteroanterior chest x-ray of a 60-year-old man with dyspnea that reads, "Infiltrate in the right lower lobe, likely pneumonia, clinical correlation is advised." Is this report adequate?

No. Although the infiltrate in the right lower lobe may represent pneumonia, malignancy should be considered either as a differential diagnosis or as an etiologic factor of the pneumonia, and the recommendation for follow-up films to ensure diagnostic resolution should be made clear. Failure to include a differential diagnosis may lead to an error in judgment. Failure to suggest the next appropriate step is a recognized area for malpractice.

24. A radiologist renders a report on a barium enema that reads, "Filling defect in the splenic flexure with abrupt shelflike margins, cannot rule out malignancy; colonoscopy may be of help if clinically indicated." What is wrong with this report?

When a radiologist suspects a malignancy (or any other significant finding), there is no merit in being ambiguous when reporting the findings. The report should use more assertive language (e.g., "Filling defect in the splenic flexure with abrupt shelflike margins, findings are highly suggestive of colonic cancer and should be confirmed with colonoscopy and biopsy. Findings were conveyed to..."). Ambiguous reporting can lead to a lawsuit.

25. A patient develops anaphylactic shock from iodinated contrast material for excretory urography performed to rule out renal calculi. This older examination (rather than the current standard—a noncontrast helical computed tomography [CT] scan) was performed at the insistence of the referring urologist. Who is to blame, the radiologist or urologist?

The blame lies with the radiologist. Certain risk management principles should be obvious. The radiologist must follow the principle of *primum non nocere*—"first, do no harm." A hazardous procedure should be avoided if a safer alternative is available. Although anaphylaxis is a recognized complication of iodinated contrast material, the physician is considered negligent for not using an examination that is safer than an excretory urogram and is at least as equally diagnostic. It is important for radiologists to keep referring physicians up-to-date with progress in radiology. In this example, the accepted method of diagnosing renal calculi is no longer with excretory urography, but with a noncontrast CT scan. The ultimate responsibility for the performance of a radiographic procedure is the radiologist's, not the referring physician's. It is radiologists who decide which patients should or should not receive iodinated contrast material.

26. A radiologist reports that a case of trauma to the lateral cervical spine is "normal except for straightening, which could be positional." Later the patient has weakness in the legs, and a CT scan shows "fracture-dislocation" at C7/T1—an area not covered by the lateral film. How was the original reading substandard?

The report did not mention specifically that the C7/T1 junction was not visualized. It is the radiologist's duty to comment on the adequacy (or inadequacy) of a radiographic examination and to suggest repeat or alternative radiographs. This must be done as a matter of routine, and it must not be assumed that other clinicians would realize the inadequacy of a study.

27. A radiologist reports an upper gastrointestinal study as follows: "Findings are highly suggestive of a scirrhous carcinoma of the stomach, endoscopy with biopsy is advised." Biopsy results are negative. What should the radiologist do next?

The radiologist must advise the physician to repeat the biopsy or assume the diagnosis without further pathologic findings. There are a few situations in imaging in which the findings of malignancy are so strong that negative biopsy results do not exclude the diagnosis. Radiologists should be aware of these situations. Conversely, there are situations in which the findings are so typically benign that it would be negligent to advise a biopsy.

28. Failure to diagnose breast cancer is the number one cause for litigation in radiology. Summarize how may one practice safe mammography.

- Communicate with the patients about their examination and the need for follow-up. Communicate with referring physicians.
- Correlate and follow up on pathologic findings.
- Compare findings with findings of old radiographs, not just the most recent ones, but even the more remote films.
- Participate in continuing medical education—breast imaging (and most of radiology) is expanding at an alarming pace.
- Comply with the Practice Guidelines of the American College of Radiology.
- Use computer-aided detection (still experimental).

29. Only 2% of medical negligence injuries result in claims, and only 17% of claims apparently involve negligent injuries. About 60 cents of every malpractice dollar is taken by administrative and legal costs. The current tort system is inefficient. What are some reforms that have been suggested?

- Creating a "no-fault" system, such as worker's compensation; in this case, patients would be compensated for all adverse events that are avoidable, even if the event may not be negligent.
- Capping of noneconomic damages (e.g., for pain and suffering).
- Eliminating the collateral rule, which prohibits jurors from knowing about payments the plaintiffs have already received from other sources.
- Eliminating joint and several liability.
- Eliminating the doctrine of *res ipsa loquitur*.
- Relocating responsibility from a personal to an institutional level (enterprise liability).

30. A 45-year-old man with uncontrollable hypertension is referred for "magnetic resonance angiography with contrast" to exclude renal artery stenosis by his cardiologist. His glomerular filtration rate is 25 mL/min/1.73 m². He is not on dialysis. What should be your course of action?

The administration of gadolinium-based MRI contrast agents has been linked to a rare and debilitating multisystem condition, nephrogenic systemic fibrosis. This progressive, nonremitting, and generally untreatable condition is characterized by skin thickening and contractures. Although nephrogenic systemic fibrosis is almost invariably associated with gadodiamide and related compounds in patients with advanced renal failure and on dialysis, the exact pathophysiology is unknown. Nonetheless, the U.S. Food and Drug Administration (FDA) cautions against using gadolinium-based agents in renal impairment, and this means that the radiologist needs to counsel the referring physician and patient regarding the risks involved and the alternatives. The risk of nephrogenic systemic fibrosis may be difficult to extrapolate to this group because of the absence of long-term studies, but a figure of 3% to 6% would be prudent to quote.

The radiologist should ascertain the history and pretest probability of renal artery stenosis. Alternative strategies include magnetic resonance angiography (MRA) without gadolinium (e.g., time of flight, phase contrast, and balanced steady-state free precession) or duplex ultrasound (US). These modalities may be less accurate than contrast-enhanced MRI, but safety supersedes accuracy initially. CT with contrast agent is a possibility. The patient is not on dialysis, however, and the nephrotoxicity of iodinated contrast material should be borne in mind. If the suggested alternatives have not affected clinical decision making, the examination is still deemed necessary, and the referring clinician and the patient are aware of the risks and wish to go ahead, after careful documentation the examination may be performed with reduction of the contrast agent dose (which may be aided by increasing the field strength) and use of an agent other than gadodiamide. Emphasis that the added safety of the maneuvers remains unproven is recommended.

31. A report states "History—suspected pulmonary embolus.... Technique—CT scan of the chest was performed...." If all reports in this radiology practice were of similar disposition, why would this practice expect to hemorrhage money?

The report is inadequate for billing purposes. First, the history does not state the history, but the suspected diagnosis. Patients do not complain of "suspected pulmonary embolus," but of symptoms pertaining to the diagnosis, such as dyspnea, chest pain, or syncope. Payers are very particular that the right study be done for the right reason, and the onus is on the imagers to ensure that the content of the report reflects appropriateness of the imaging examination in the clinical context. Second, if the patient received iodinated contrast agent (which is likely for the exclusion of pulmonary embolus) that has not been mentioned in the technique section of the report, the practice cannot bill for the use of contrast agent. The report must contain a sufficient description in the technique section that reflects the reason for imaging and type and complexity of the examination, so that the reimbursement is appropriate and unambiguous. Insufficient description risks nonpayment for the procedure and accusation of fraud.

BIBLIOGRAPHY

[1] American College of Radiology: ACR Standard for Communication: Diagnostic Radiology, in: Standards 2000–01, American College of Radiology, Reston, VA, 2001.
[2] L. Berlin, Malpractice Issues in Radiology, second ed., American Roentgen Ray Society, Leesburg, VA, 2003.
[3] H. Forster, J. Schwartz, E. DeRenzo, Reducing legal risk by practicing patient centered medicine, Arch. Intern. Med. 162 (2002) 1217–1219.
[4] R.M. Friedenberg, Malpractice reform, Radiology 231 (2004) 3–6.
[5] K. Juluru, J. Vogel-Claussen, K.J. Macura, et al., MR imaging in patients at risk for developing nephrogenic systemic fibrosis: protocols, practices, and imaging techniques to maximize patient safety, RadioGraphics 29 (2009) 9–22.
[6] J.C. Mohr, American medical malpractice litigation in historical perspective, JAMA 283 (2000) 1731–1737.
[7] J.R. Muhm, W.E. Miller, R.S. Fontana, et al., Lung cancer detected during a screening program using four-month chest radiographs, Radiology 148 (1983) 609–615.
[8] P.J. Robinson, Radiology's Achilles' heel: error and variation in the interpretation of the roentgen image, Br. J. Radiol. 70 (1997) 1085–1098.
[9] S. Studdert, Medical malpractice, N. Engl. J. Med. 350 (2004) 283–292.
[10] W.T. Thorwarth, Get paid for what you do: dictation patterns and impact on billing accuracy, J. Am. Coll. Radiol. 2 (2005) 665–669.

76 CHAPTER

RADIOLOGY ORGANIZATIONS

E. Scott Pretorius, MD

1. What is the Radiological Society of North America (RSNA)?

The mission of the RSNA, founded 1915, is "to promote and develop the highest standards of radiology and related sciences through education and research." The RSNA is the world's largest organization of its kind. The RSNA publishes the "gray journal," *Radiology*. The annual meeting of the RSNA is in Chicago during the last week of November or first week of December.

2. What is the American Roentgen Ray Society (ARRS)?

The ARRS was founded in 1900, shortly after Roentgen's discovery of the x-ray, with the stated goal of "advancement of medicine through the science of radiology and its allied sciences." The ARRS publishes the "yellow journal," the *American Journal of Roentgenology,* which has officially shortened its name to *AJR*. The ARRS meets annually in April or May at varying sites throughout the United States and Canada.

3. What is the Association of University Radiologists (AUR)?

The AUR is the organization of academic radiologists. Subgroups of the AUR include the Society of Chairmen of Academic Radiology Departments, the Association of Program Directors in Radiology, and the American Association of Academic Chief Residents in Radiology. The AUR and its constituent organizations meet annually at varying sites throughout the United States and Canada. It publishes the journal *Academic Radiology*.

4. What is the American Board of Radiology?

The American Board of Radiology, based in Tucson, Arizona, is the organization that administers the written and oral examinations in radiology. The diagnostic radiology written examination is given each September at sites throughout the United States and Canada. The diagnostic radiology oral examination is given annually in early June in Louisville, Kentucky.

5. What is the American College of Radiology (ACR)?

The ACR performs several important functions. It accredits sites that perform mammography, ultrasound (US), nuclear medicine, and magnetic resonance imaging (MRI) to maintain appropriate quality standards. Through its American College of Radiology Imaging Network (ACRIN), the ACR conducts multicenter studies in diagnostic radiology. Educational CD-ROMs in all subspecialties of radiology are produced by the ACR. Finally, the ACR has an important role in advocacy for the interests of radiologists, medical physicists, and their patients through work with Congress, the U.S. Food and Drug Administration (FDA), and state and local governments.

6. What is the American Council of Graduate Medical Education (ACGME)?

The ACGME is the body that accredits American residency training programs in radiology and all other fields of graduate medical education. The ACGME develops requirements and guidelines for residency training programs in all fields. Among its most noted recent actions are the limiting of the resident work week to 80 hours and the requirement that diagnostic radiology residencies include 3 months of training in breast imaging.

7. What are the major subspecialty societies in radiology?

There are many subspecialty societies, and most of them have discounted memberships available for medical students or residents (Table 76-1).

8. What are the leading academic journals within diagnostic radiology?

Radiology, the journal of the RSNA, and the *American Journal of Roentgenology,* the journal of the American Roentgen Ray Society, are the two leading general-purpose radiology journals. There are numerous important subspecialty journals, including the *Journal of Interventional Radiology, American Journal of Neuroradiology* (*AJNR*), *Pediatric Radiology, Magnetic Resonance in Medicine, Journal of Magnetic Resonance Imaging, Abdominal Imaging,* and *Journal of Nuclear Medicine* (see Table 76-1).

Table 76-1. Radiology Organizations and National Societies

SOCIETY	ABBREVIATION	JOURNAL	WEBSITE
Radiological Society of North America	RSNA	*Radiology* and *RadioGraphics*	www.rsna.org
American Board of Radiology	ABR	None	www.theabr.org
American College of Radiology	ACR	*Journal of the American College of Radiology (JACR)*	www.acr.org
American Institute of Ultrasound in Medicine	AIUM	*Journal of Ultrasound in Medicine (JUM)*	www.aium.org
American Roentgen Ray Society	ARRS	*American Journal of Roentgenology (AJR)*	www.arrs.org
American Society of Neuroradiology	ASNR	*American Journal of Neuroradiology (AJNR)*	www.asnr.org
Association of University Radiologists	AUR	*Academic Radiology*	www.aur.org
British Institute of Radiology	BIR	*British Journal of Radiology*	www.bir.org.uk
Canadian Association of Radiologists	CAR	*Canadian Association of Radiologists Journal*	www.car.ca
European Association of Radiology	EAR	*European Radiology*	www.eurorad.org
International Society of Magnetic Resonance in Medicine	ISMRM	*Journal of Magnetic Resonance Imaging (JMRI); Magnetic Resonance in Medicine (MRM)*	www.ismrm.org
International Society of Radiology	ISR	None	www.isradiology.org/isr/
Radiological Society of South Africa	RSSA	*South African Journal of Radiology*	www.rssa.co.za
Royal Australian and New Zealand College of Radiologists	RANZCR	*Australasian Radiology*	www.ranzcr.edu.au
Society of Breast Imaging	SBI	None	www.sbi-online.org
Society for Imaging Informatics in Medicine	SIIM	*Journal of Digital Imaging*	www.scarnet.org
Society of Interventional Radiology	SIR	*Journal of Vascular and Interventional Radiology (JVIR)*	www.sirweb.org
Society of Nuclear Medicine	SNM	*Journal of Nuclear Medicine (JNM)*	www.snm.org
Society for Pediatric Radiology	SPR	*Pediatric Radiology*	www.pedrad.org
Society of Skeletal Radiology	SSR	*Skeletal Radiology*	www.skeletalrad.org
Society of Thoracic Radiology	STR	*Thoracic Radiology*	www.thoracicrad.org

9. What is the NIBIB?

The National Institute of Biomedical Imaging and Bioengineering is the newest research institute within the National Institutes of Health. Its stated mission is to "improve health by promoting fundamental discoveries, design and development, and translation and assessment of technological capabilities." It has become an important source of funding for hypothesis-driven research in the imaging sciences (http://www.nibib.nih.org).

Key Points: Radiology Organizations

1. In the United States, the RSNA and ARRS are the two most important general-interest organizations for radiologists and have broad missions in terms of radiology education and research.
2. The American Board of Radiology administers the written and oral examinations that allow candidates to become board-certified in radiology.
3. The ACR accredits sites that perform diagnostic imaging studies and maintains quality standards.

INDEX